General
Ophthalmology

. . . *Now do you not see that the eye embraces the beauty of the whole world? It is the lord of astronomy and the maker of cosmography; it counsels and corrects all the arts of mankind; it leads men to the different parts of the world; it is the prince of mathematics, and the sciences founded on it are absolutely certain. It has measured the distances and sizes of the stars; it has found the elements and their locations; it . . . has given birth to architecture, and to perspective, and to the divine art of painting. Oh excellent thing, superior to all others created by God! . . . What peoples, what tongues will fully describe your true function? The eye is the window of the human body through which it feels its way and enjoys the beauty of the world. Owing to the eye the soul is content to stay in its bodily prison, for without it such bodily prison is torture.*

—*Leonardo da Vinci (1452–1519)*

a LANGE medical book

1989

General Ophthalmology

Twelfth Edition

Daniel Vaughan, MD
Clinical Professor of Ophthalmology
University of California, San Francisco
Member, Francis I. Proctor Foundation
for Research in Ophthalmology

Taylor Asbury, MD
Clinical Professor of Ophthalmology
College of Medicine
University of Cincinnati

Khalid F. Tabbara, MD
Professor and Chairman
Department of Ophthalmology
College of Medicine
King Saud University
Riyadh, Saudi Arabia

Illustrated by
Laurel V. Schaubert

APPLETON & LANGE
Norwalk, Connecticut/San Mateo, California

0-8385-3107-5

Notice: Our knowledge in clinical sciences is constantly changing. As new
information becomes available, changes in treatment and in the use of drugs
become necessary. The authors and the publisher of this volume have taken
care to make certain that the doses of drugs and schedules of treatment are
correct and compatible with the standards generally accepted at the time of
publication. The reader is advised to consult carefully the instruction
and information material included in the package insert of each drug or
therapeutic agent before administration. This advice is especially
important when using new or infrequently used drugs.

Prentice Hall International (UK) Limited, *London*
Prentice Hall of Australia Pty. Limited, *Sydney*
Prentice Hall Canada, Inc., *Toronto*
Prentice Hall of Hispanoamericana, S.A., *Mexico*
Prentice Hall of India Private Limited, *New Delhi*
Prentice Hall of Japan, Inc., *Tokyo*
Simon & Schuster Asia Pte. Ltd., *Singapore*
Editora Prentice Hall do Brasil Ltda., *Rio de Janeiro*
Prentice Hall, *Englewood Cliffs, New Jersey*

ISBN: 0-8385-3107-5
ISSN: 0891-2084

Production Editor: Laura K. Giesman
Designer: Steven M. Byrum

PRINTED IN THE UNITED STATES OF AMERICA

This edition of
General Ophthalmology
is dedicated to
Dr. Eslie Asbury

6. Cornea

7. Sclera

The Authors

Taylor Asbury, MD
Clinical Professor of Ophthalmology, University of Cincinnati School of Medicine, Cincinnati.

Roderick Biswell, MD
Assistant Clinical Professor of Ophthalmology, University of California School of Medicine, San Francisco.

David F. Chang, MD
Assistant Clinical Professor of Ophthalmology, University of California School of Medicine, San Francisco.

Pamela S. Chavis, MD
Chief of Neuro-ophthalmology, King Khaled Eye Specialist Hospital, Riyadh, Saudi Arabia.

J. Brooks Crawford, MD
Clinical Professor of Ophthalmology, University of California School of Medicine, San Francisco.

Howard M. Eggers, MD
Assistant Professor of Clinical Ophthalmology, Columbia University School of Medicine, New York.

Philip P. Ellis, MD
Professor of Ophthalmology and Chairman of Department of Ophthalmology, University of Colorado School of Medicine, Denver.

Eleanor E. Faye, MD
Ophthalmologic Director, Lighthouse Low Vision Service, New York; Attending Ophthalmologist, Manhattan Eye and Ear Hospital, New York.

F. T. Fraunfelder, MD
Professor of Ophthalmology and Chairman of Department of Ophthalmology, The Oregon Health Sciences University, Portland, Oregon.

Elizabeth M. Graham, MRCP, DO
Consultant Medical Ophthalmologist, St. Thomas' Hospital and National Hospital for Nervous Diseases, London.

David L. Guyton, MD
Professor of Ophthalmology, The Johns Hopkins University School of Medicine, Baltimore.

William F. Hoyt, MD
Professor of Ophthalmology, Neuro-ophthalmology, and Neurosurgery, University of California School of Medicine, San Francisco.

S. Martha Meyer, BS
Research Associate, Department of Ophthalmology, The Oregon Health Sciences University, Portland, Oregon.

G. Richard O'Connor, MD
Professor of Ophthalmology Emeritus, University of California School of Medicine, San Francisco; Director Emeritus, Francis I. Proctor Foundation for Research in Ophthalmology, San Francisco.

Conor O'Malley, MD
San Jose, California.

Patrick O'Malley, MD
South Bend, Indiana.

Paul Riordan-Eva, FRCS, MA, MB, BChir
Registrar in Ophthalmology, St. Thomas' and Greenwich District Hospitals, London.

Michael D. Sanders, FRCP, FRCS
Consultant Ophthalmologist, St. Thomas' Hospital and National Hospital for Nervous Diseases, London.

John P. Shock, MD
Professor of Ophthalmology and Chairman of Department of Ophthalmology, University of Arkansas School of Medicine, Little Rock, Arkansas.

John H. Sullivan, MD
Clinical Professor of Ophthalmology, University of California School of Medicine, San Francisco.

Khalid F. Tabbara, MD
Professor of Ophthalmology and Chairman of Department of Ophthalmology, College of Medicine, King Saud University, Riyadh, Saudi Arabia.

Daniel Vaughan, MD
Clinical Professor of Ophthalmology, University of California School of Medicine, San Francisco; Member, Francis I. Proctor Foundation for Research in Ophthalmology, San Francisco.

Orson W. White, MD
Associate Clinical Professor of Ophthalmology, University of Utah School of Medicine, Salt Lake City.

James B. Wise, MD
Clinical Professor of Ophthalmology, University of Oklahoma Health Sciences Center, Oklahoma City; Chairman of Ophthalmology, Baptist Medical Center of Oklahoma, Oklahoma City.

Preface

For three decades, *General Ophthalmology* has served as the most concise, current, and authoritative review of the subject for medical students, ophthalmology residents, practicing ophthalmologists, nurses, optometrists, and colleagues in other fields of medicine and surgery as well as allied health personnel. In keeping with that goal, the twelfth edition has been meticulously revised and updated throughout. It contains the following changes from the eleventh edition:

■ A thoroughly revised chapter on NEURO-OPHTHALMOLOGY
■ A new chapter on OPTICS and REFRACTION
■ A new chapter on LOW VISION
■ A new chapter on LASERS IN OPHTHALMOLOGY
■ Major revisions of the chapters on ANATOMY AND EMBRYOLOGY and on the UVEAL TRACT
■ A major revision of the chapter on EXAMINATION OF THE EYE, with many new illustrations

References have been brought up to date, and the following further improvements have been incorporated into the text:

■ J. Brooks Crawford's excellent chapter on TUMORS has been updated and integrated into the chapters on the lids and lacrimal apparatus, conjunctiva, retina, and orbit.
■ A new section on CHILDHOOD CATARACT has been added to the lens chapter.
■ New illustrations have been added to the chapter on the ORBIT.
■ The chapter on PREVENTIVE OPHTHALMOLOGY has been revised throughout.
■ The chapter on OCULAR DISORDERS ASSOCIATED WITH SYSTEMIC DISEASES incorporates the latest information on AIDS.

To achieve this major revision, we have relied on the assistance of many authorities in special fields who have given us the benefit of their advice. Camille Matta, John Cavender, and Richard Forster made substantial contributions to this effort. We wish in particular to express our gratitude to Robert N. Shaffer for his review of the chapter on glaucoma.

Daniel Vaughan
Taylor Asbury
Khalid F. Tabbara

August 1989

Acknowledgments

Arthur K. Asbury
Crowell Beard
Laurie Vaughan Campbell
John Cavender
Patricia Cunnane
Chandler Dawson
Richard Forster
Hans Beat Gassmann
Margaret Henry
Harry Hind
Geraldine Hruby
Marianne Thalman Huslid
Vicente Jocson

Philip Knapp
Heinrich König
Camille Matta
G. Richard O'Connor
Bruce Ostler
Patricia Pascoe
Margot Riordan-Eva
Kenneth D. Rogers
Joel G. Sacks
Lionel W. Sorenson
Rosalind Stevens
Ralph T. Sutton
Phillips Thygeson

Anatomy & Embryology of the Eye

1

Khalid F. Tabbara, MD

I. NORMAL ANATOMY

OCULAR ADNEXA

EYEBROWS

The eyebrows are folds of thickened skin covered with hair. The skin fold is supported by underlying muscle fibers. The glabella is the hairless prominence between the eyebrows.

EYELIDS

The upper and lower eyelids (palpebrae) are modified folds of skin that can close to protect the anterior eyeball (Fig 1–1). Blinking helps spread the tear film, which protects the cornea and conjunctiva from dehydration. The upper lid ends at the eyebrows; the lower lid merges into the cheek.

The skin of the eyelids differs from skin on most other areas of the body in that it is thin, loose, and elastic and possesses few hair follicles and no subcutaneous fat.

The eyelids consist of 5 principal planes of tissues. From superficial to deep, they are the skin layer, a layer of striated muscle (orbicularis oculi), areolar tissue, fibrous tissue (tarsal plates), and a layer of mucous membrane (palpebral conjunctiva).

Palpebral Fissure

The palpebral fissure is the elliptic space between the 2 open lids. The fissure terminates at the medial and lateral optic canthi (optic angles). The lateral canthus is about 0.5 cm from the lateral orbital rim and forms an acute angle. The medial canthus is more elliptic than the lateral canthus and surrounds the lacrimal lake (lacus lacrimalis).

Two structures are identified in the lacrimal lake: (1) the **lacrimal caruncle,** a yellowish elevation of modified skin containing large modified sweat glands and sebaceous glands that open into follicles which contain fine hair (Fig 1–2); and (2) the **plica semilunaris,** a vestigial remnant of the third eyelid of lower animal species.

In Orientals, a skin fold known as **epicanthus** passes from the medial termination of the upper lid to the medial termination of the lower lid, hiding the caruncle. Epicanthus may be present normally in young infants of all races and disappears with development of the nose bridge but persists throughout life in Orientals.

Lid Margins

The free lid margin is 25–30 mm long and about 2 mm wide. It is divided by the gray line (mucocutaneous junction) into anterior and posterior margins.

A. Anterior Margin:

1. Eyelashes–The eyelashes project from the margins of the eyelids and are arranged irregularly. The upper lashes are longer and more numerous than the lower lashes and turn upward; the lower lashes turn downward.

2. Glands of Zeis–These are small modified sebaceous glands that open into the hair follicles at the base of the eyelashes.

3. Glands of Moll–These are modified sweat glands that open in a row near the base of the eyelashes.

B. Posterior Margin: The posterior lid margin is in close contact with the globe, and along this margin are the small orifices of modified sebaceous glands (meibomian, or tarsal, glands). A surgical incision through the gray line splits the lid into anterior and posterior segments.

C. Punctum Lacrimale: At the medial end of the posterior margin of the lid, a small elevation with a central small opening (punctum lacrimale) can be seen on the upper and lower lids. The puncta serve to carry the tears down through the corresponding canaliculus to the lacrimal sac.

Structure of the Lids

A. Tarsal Plate: The main supporting structure of

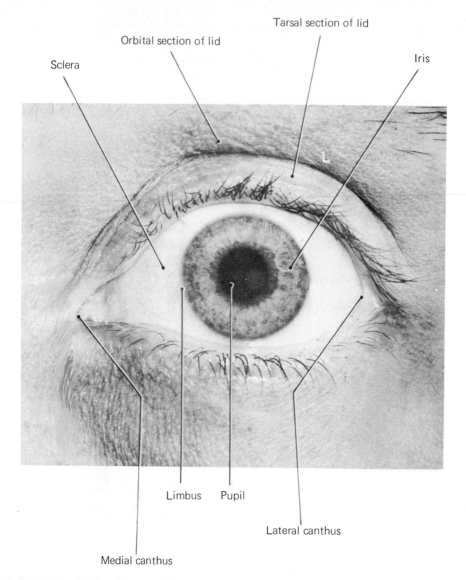

Tarsal section of lid

Orbital section of lid

Iris

Sclera

L

Limbus   Pupil

Lateral canthus

Medial canthus

Figure 1–1. External landmarks of the eye. The sclera is covered by transparent conjunctiva. (Photo by HL Gibson, from: *Medical Radiography and Photography.* Labeling modified slightly.)

the eyelids is a dense fibrous tissue layer that—along with a small amount of elastic tissue—is called the tarsal plate. The lateral and medial angles and extensions of the tarsal plates are attached to the orbital margin by the lateral and medial palpebral ligaments. The upper and lower tarsal plates are also attached by a condensed, thin fascia to the upper and lower orbital margins. This thin fascia forms the orbital septum (Fig 1–3).

B. Levator Palpebrae Superioris Muscle: The levator muscle arises from the apex of the orbit and passes forward to insert into the anterior surface of the superior tarsus and into the overlying skin.

C. Conjunctiva: The lids are lined posteriorly by a layer of mucous membrane, the **palpebral conjunctiva,** which adheres firmly to the tarsus.

Orbital Septum

The orbital septum is the fascia behind that portion of the orbicularis muscle that lies between the orbital rim and the tarsus and serves as a barrier between the lid and the orbit.

The orbital septum is pierced by the lacrimal vessels and nerves, the supratrochlear artery and nerve, the supraorbital vessels and nerves, the trochlear nerve, the anastomosis between the angular and ophthalmic veins, and the levator palpebrae superioris muscle.

The **superior orbital septum** blends with the tendon of the levator palpebrae superioris and the superior tarsus; the **inferior orbital septum** blends with the inferior tarsus.

Unstriated muscle fibers, known as **Müller's muscle,** lie deep to the orbital septum. They originate

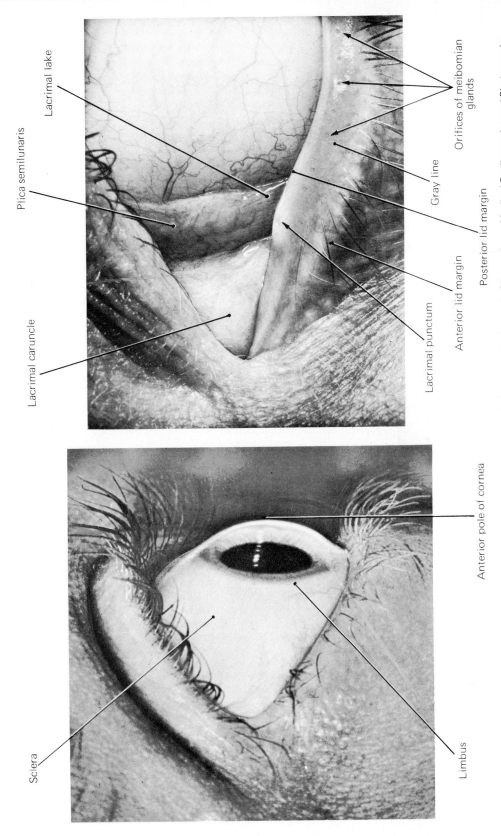

Figure 1–2. External landmarks of the eye. The sclera is covered by transparent conjunctiva. (Photo by HL Gibson, from: *Medical Radiography and Photography.* Labeling modified slightly.)

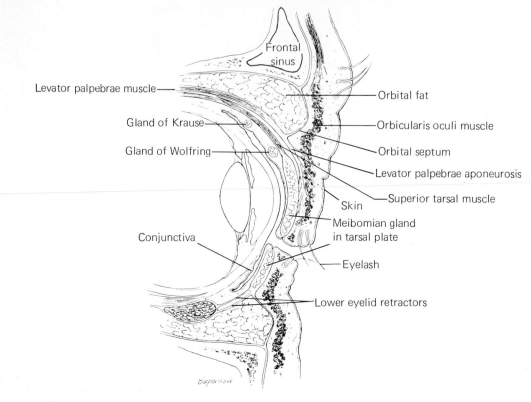

Figure 1–3. Cross section of the upper lid. (Courtesy of C Beard.)

from the levator aponeurosis and insert into the attached margins of the tarsus. Müller's muscle is innervated by sympathetic nerve fibers; its function is to widen the palpebral fissure.

Orbicularis Oculi Muscle

The orbicularis oculi muscle is supplied by the facial nerve; its function is to close the lids. Its muscle fibers surround the palpebral fissure in concentric fashion and spread for a short distance around the orbital margin. Some fibers run onto the cheek and the forehead. The portion of the muscle that is in the lids is known as its palpebral portion; the portion over the orbital septum is the preseptal portion. The segment outside the lid is called the orbital portion.

The submuscular areolar tissue that lies deep to the orbicularis oculi muscle communicates with the subaponeurotic layer of the scalp.

Nerve Supply

The sensory nerve supply to the eyelids is derived from the first and second divisions of the trigeminal nerve (V). The small lacrimal, supraorbital, supratrochlear, infratrochlear, and external nasal nerves are branches of the ophthalmic division of the fifth nerve. The infraorbital, zygomaticofacial, and zygomaticotemporal nerves are branches of the maxillary (second) division of the trigeminal nerve.

Blood Supply & Lymphatics

The blood supply to the lids is derived from the lacrimal and ophthalmic arteries by their lateral and medial palpebral branches. Anastomoses between the lateral and medial palpebral arteries form the tarsal arcades that lie in the submuscular areolar tissue.

Venous drainage from the lids empties into the ophthalmic vein and the veins that drain the forehead and temple. The veins are arranged in pre- and posttarsal plexuses (Fig 1–4).

Lymphatics from the lateral segment of the lids run into the preauricular and parotid nodes. Lymphatics draining the medial side of the lids empty into the submandibular lymph nodes.

LACRIMAL APPARATUS

The lacrimal complex consists of the lacrimal gland, the accessory lacrimal glands, the canaliculi, the lacrimal sac, and the nasolacrimal duct (Fig 1–5).

The lacrimal gland consists of the following structures:

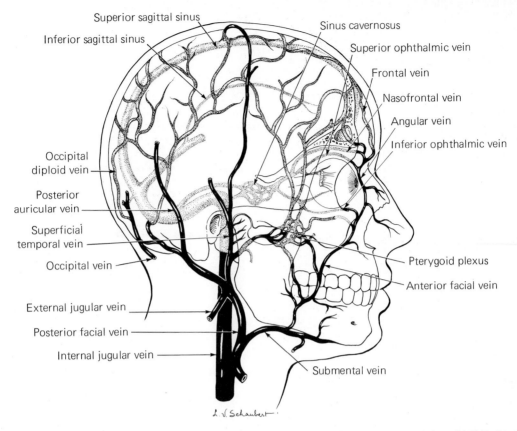

Figure 1–4. Venous drainage system of the eye. (Redrawn and reproduced, with permission, from Wolff E: *Anatomy of the Eye and Orbit,* 4th ed. Blakiston-McGraw, 1954.)

(1) The almond-shaped **orbital portion,** located in the lacrimal fossa in the anterior upper temporal segment of the orbit, is separated from the palpebral portion by the lateral horn of the levator palpebrae muscle. To reach this portion of the gland surgically, one must incise the skin, the orbicularis oculi muscle, and the orbital septum.

(2) The smaller **palpebral portion** is located just above the temporal segment of the superior conjunctival fornix. Lacrimal secretory ducts, which open by approximately 10 fine orifices, connect the orbital and palpebral portions of the lacrimal gland to the superior conjunctival fornix. Removal of the palpebral portion of the gland cuts off all of the connecting ducts and thus prevents secretion by the entire gland.

The **lacrimal sac** lies in the lacrimal fossa. The nasolacrimal duct continues downward from the fossa and opens into the inferior meatus of the nasal cavity lateral to the inferior turbinate. Tears are directed into the puncta by capillary attraction and gravity and by the blinking action of the eyelids. The combined forces of capillary attraction in the canaliculi, gravity, and the pumping action of Horner's muscle, which is an extension of the orbicularis oculi muscle to a point behind the lacrimal sac, all tend to continue the flow of tears down the nasolacrimal duct into the nose.

Blood Supply & Lymphatics

The blood supply of the lacrimal gland is derived from the lacrimal artery. The vein that drains the gland joins the ophthalmic vein. The lymphatic drainage joins with the conjunctival lymphatics to drain into the preauricular lymph nodes.

Nerve Supply

The nerve supply to the lacrimal gland is by (1) the lacrimal nerve (sensory), a branch of the trigeminal first division; (2) the great superficial petrosal nerve (secretory), which comes from the superior salivary nucleus; and (3) sympathetic nerves accompanying the lacrimal artery and the lacrimal nerve.

Related Structures

The **medial palpebral ligament** connects the upper and lower tarsal plates to the frontal process at the inner canthus anterior to the lacrimal sac. The portion of the lacrimal sac below the ligament is covered by a few fibers of the orbicularis oculi muscle. These fibers offer little resistance to swelling and distention of the lacrimal sac. The area below the medial palpebral ligament becomes swollen in acute dacryocystitis, and fistulas commonly open in the area.

The angular vein and artery lie just deep to the skin,

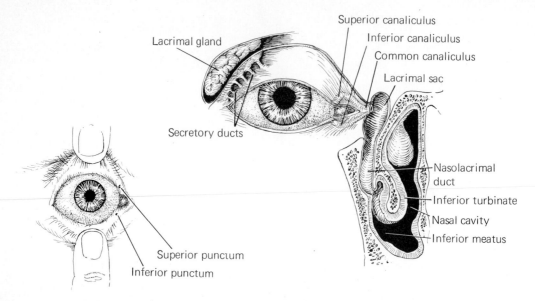

Figure 1–5. The lacrimal drainage system. (Redrawn with modifications and reproduced, with permission, from Thompson J, Elstrom ER: Radiography of the nasolacrimal passageways. *Med Radiogr Photogr* 1949;**25[3]**:66.)

8 mm to the nasal side of the inner canthus. Skin incisions made in surgical procedures on the lacrimal sac should always be placed 2–3 mm to the nasal side of the inner canthus to avoid these vessels.

THE EYEBALL

The Conjunctiva

The conjunctiva is a thin, transparent layer of mucous membrane that covers the posterior surface of the lids (the palpebral conjunctiva) and the anterior surface of the sclera (bulbar conjunctiva). It is continuous with the skin at the lid margin (mucocutaneous junction) and with corneal epithelium at the limbus.

The **palpebral conjunctiva** lines the posterior surface of the lids and adheres firmly to the tarsus. At the upper and lower margins of the tarsus, the conjunctiva is reflected backward and attaches to and covers the sclera as the bulbar conjunctiva.

The **bulbar conjunctiva** is loosely attached to the orbital septum in the region of the fornices and is folded many times. This allows the eye to move quite freely and enlarges the conjunctival secretory surface. The ductules of the lacrimal glands open into the upper temporal aspect of the superior fornix. Except at the limbus, where Tenon's capsule and the conjunctiva are fused for a distance of about 3 mm, the bulbar conjunctiva is loosely attached to Tenon's capsule and to the underlying sclera.

The **semilunar fold**—a soft, moveable, thickened fold of bulbar conjunctiva—is located at the inner canthus and corresponds to the nictitating membrane of some of the lower animals. A small, fleshy epidermoid structure, the **caruncle,** is attached superficially to the inner portion of the semilunar fold and is a transition zone containing both cutaneous and mucous membrane elements.

Blood Supply, Lymphatics, & Nerve Supply

The conjunctival arteries are derived from the anterior ciliary and palpebral arteries. The 2 arteries anastomose freely and—along with the numerous conjunctival veins that generally follow the arterial pattern—form a considerable conjunctival vascular network. The conjunctival lymphatics are arranged in superficial and deep layers and join with the lymphatics of the eyelids to form a rich lymphatic plexus. The conjunctiva receives its nerve supply from the first (ophthalmic) division of the fifth nerve. It possesses a relatively small number of pain fibers.

THE CORNEA

The cornea is an avascular, transparent tissue comparable in size and structure to the crystal of a small wristwatch (Fig 1–2). The cornea is inserted into the sclera at the limbus, seen as a circumferential depression called the scleral sulcus. The cornea is the refracting and protective membranous window through which light rays pass to the retina. Its refractive power is equivalent to a 43-diopter lens. The adult cornea is about 1 mm thick at the periphery, about 0.8 mm at the center, and about 11.5 mm in diameter. It is composed of 5 layers: epithelium, Bowman's layer or membrane, stroma, Descemet's membrane, and endothelium.

The cornea receives nourishment from the aqueous and the tears and from blood vessels at the limbus. The superficial cornea derives its oxygen from the atmosphere. The sensory nerves of the cornea are derived from the ophthalmic division of cranial nerve V. A rich network of nerve fibers in the corneal epithelium produces a sensation of pain whenever the fibers are exposed. The pain is felt even with minor abrasions of the corneal epithelium.

THE SCLERA

The sclera is the fibrous protective coating of the eye (Fig 1–6). It is white, dense, and continuous with the cornea anteriorly and the dural sheath of the optic nerve posteriorly. It is generally about 1 mm thick. A few strands of modified scleral tissue pass over the optic disk (lamina cribrosa). The outer layer of the sclera is composed of a thin, fine elastic tissue—the episclera—that contains the sclera's nourishing blood vessels. The lamina fusca, the brownish inner scleral

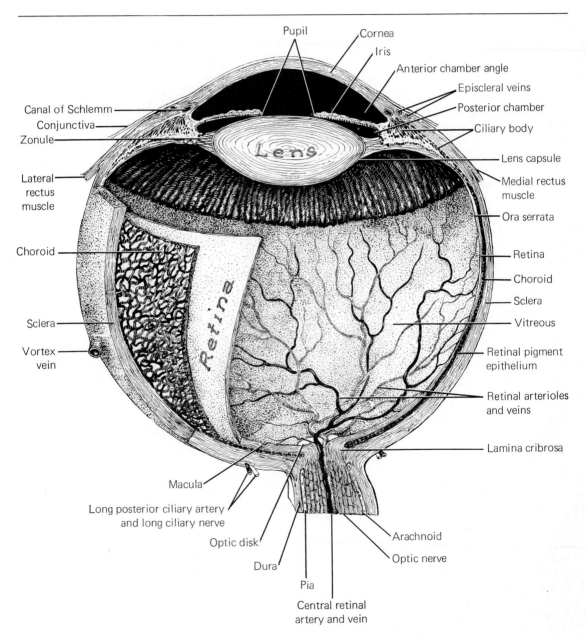

Figure 1–6. Internal structures of the human eye. (Redrawn from an original drawing by Paul Peck and reproduced, with permission, from: *The Anatomy of the Eye.* Courtesy of Lederle Laboratories.)

layer, is continuous along the sclera; at the choroid, it is related to the optic nerve. The sclera is penetrated by the long and short posterior ciliary arteries and the long and short ciliary nerves. About 4 mm behind the limbus, the 4 anterior ciliary arteries and veins penetrate the sclera. Just behind the equator of the globe, the 4 vortex veins exit the sclera—usually one in each quadrant.

THE UVEAL TRACT

The uveal tract is composed of the iris, the ciliary body, and the choroid (Fig 1–6). The tract is the middle vascular layer of the eye and is protected by cornea and sclera. It contributes blood supply to the retina.

The Iris

The **iris** is the anterior extension of the ciliary body. It presents as a flat surface with a medially placed round aperture, the pupil. It forms the posterior wall of the anterior chamber and the anterior wall of the posterior chamber. The iris is in front of the lens and aqueous posteriorly and behind the aqueous anteriorly. Within the stroma of the iris are the sphincter and dilator muscles of the pupil. There are 2 heavily pigmented layers on the posterior surface of the iris. These layers represent the anterior extension of the pigment epithelium of the retina.

The Ciliary Body

The **ciliary body** extends forward from the anterior end of the choroid to the root of the iris (about 6 mm). It consists of a corrugated anterior zone, the corona ciliaris, and a flattened posterior zone, and the pars plana.

The **ciliary muscle** is composed of a combination of longitudinal, circular, and radial fibers that contract and relax the zonular fibers. This alters the tension on the capsule of the lens, giving the lens a variable focus for both near and distant objects in the visual field. The blood vessels supplying the ciliary body are derived from the major circle of the iris. The sensory nerve supply of the iris is through the ciliary nerves.

The Choroid

The choroid is the posterior segment of the uveal tract between the retina and the sclera. It is composed of 3 layers of choroidal blood vessels: large, medium, and small. The deeper the vessels are placed in the choroid, the wider their lumens. The choroid is firmly attached posteriorly to the margins of the optic nerve. Anteriorly, the choroid joins with the ciliary body.

The iris controls the amount of light that enters the eye. Control is governed by a reflex that constricts the pupil under the influence of light and dilates the pupil in darkness. The ciliary body forms the root of the iris and through its muscular fibers governs the size of the lens in accommodation. Aqueous humor

is secreted by the ciliary processes into the posterior chamber. The aggregate of choroidal blood vessels serves to nourish the outer portion of the underlying retina (Fig 1–7).

THE LENS

The lens is a biconvex, avascular, colorless, and almost completely transparent structure about 4 mm thick and 9 mm in diameter. It is suspended behind the iris by the zonule, which connects it with the ciliary body. Anterior to the lens is the aqueous; and posterior to it, the vitreous. The lens capsule is a semipermeable membrane that will admit water and electrolytes. The zonule, or suspensory ligament of the lens, is composed of numerous fibrils that arise from the surface of the ciliary body and insert into the equator of the lens.

The sole purpose of the lens is to focus light on the retina. The physiologic interplay of ciliary body, zonule, and lens that focuses a nearby object on the retina is called accommodation. As the lens ages, its accommodative power is gradually reduced. There are no pain fibers, blood vessels, or nerves in the lens.

THE VITREOUS

The vitreous is a clear, avascular gelatinous body that comprises two-thirds of the volume and weight of the eye. It fills the space bounded by the lens, retina, and optic disk. It helps maintain the shape and transparency of the eye. The outer surface of the vitreous, the hyaloid membrane, is in contact with the posterior lens capsule, the zonular fibers, the epithelium of the pars plana, the retina, and the optic nerve head. The attachment of the vitreous to the lens capsule and optic nerve head is firm in early life but soon loosens. For this reason, intracapsular cataract extraction without prolapse of the vitreous is possible in adults but not in children.

THE AQUEOUS

The aqueous fills the anterior and posterior chambers of the eye. It is an alkaline liquid, composed mainly of water, that is secreted by the ciliary process. It is present only in small quantity (125 /mu/L). From the posterior chamber the fluid passes through the pupil into the anterior chamber. In the anterior chamber, the aqueous flows toward the filtering trabecular meshwork at the periphery and into the canal of Schlemm. About 30 collector channels and about 12 aqueous veins conduct the fluid into the venous system. There is a constant exchange of nonelectrolytes and a major exchange of water in the iris stroma. A small amount of aqueous leaves the eye through the uveal vessels and the sclera. Close to the sclerocorneal junction, the inner surface of the sclera projects as a

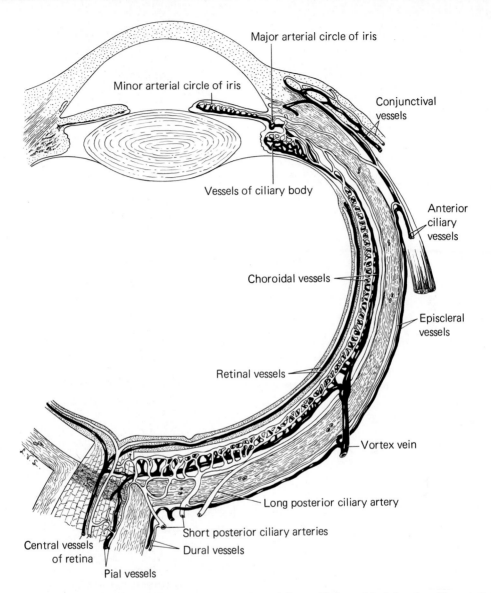

Figure 1–7. Vascular supply to the eye. All arterial branches originate with the ophthalmic artery. Venous drainage is through the cavernous sinus and the pterygoid plexus.

ridge, the scleral spur, to which the iris and the ciliary muscle are attached (Fig 1–8).

Anterior to this spur is a circular trough, the scleral sulcus, which is crossed by trabecular tissue that separates the angle of the anterior chamber from the canal of Schlemm (Fig 1–9). In the trabeculae, the spaces of Fontana connect on one side with the anterior chamber and on the other side with the pectinate villi through which the aqueous humor passes on its way to the venous sinus of the sclera and into the anterior ciliary veins (Fig 1–10). Drainage of the aqueous is similar to drainage of subarachnoid fluid through the dural granulations into the dural sinuses.

THE RETINA

The retina is the thin, semitransparent layer of nerve tissue that forms the innermost coat of the eye. It consists of 10 histologically distinct layers of highly organized, delicate tissue. Its outer surface is related to the choroid; its inner surface touches the vitreous. Posteriorly, the retina is continuous with the optic nerve. It extends almost as far anteriorly as the ciliary body, ending at that point in a ragged edge (ora serrata). At the ora serrata, the nerve tissue of the retina terminates, but a thin rim of the pigment layer of the retina moves farther anteriorly to relate to the

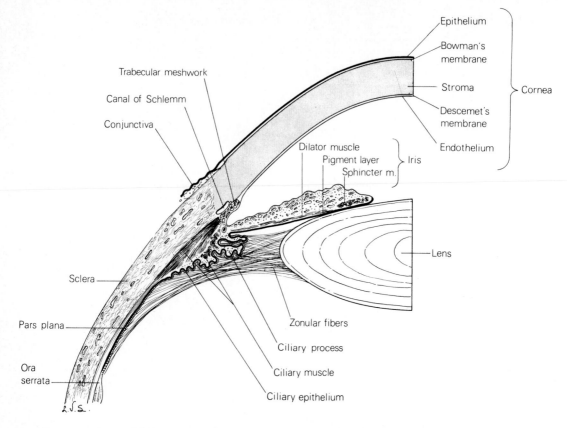

Figure 1–8. Anterior chamber angle and surrounding structures.

posterior surfaces of the ciliary processes and the iris. In the center of the posterior segment of the retina is the macula lutea, an oval, yellowish spot whose center is depressed (fovea centralis). At this point, the retina is very thin, and one can see the darkness of the choroid coat through it. About 3 mm to the medial side of the macula is the optic disk, marking the position of the optic nerve. A small niche in the center of the disk is the point of entrance of the central artery of the retina. Since the disk is insensitive to light, it is called the physiologic blind spot.

The layers of the retina are as follows: (1) internal limiting membrane, (2) a layer of nerve fibers, (3) a ganglion cell layer, (4) inner plexiform layer, (5) inner nuclear layer, (6) outer plexiform layer, (7) outer nuclear layer, (8) external limiting membrane, (9) layer of rods and cones, and (10) pigment epithelium (Fig 1–11).

The outer third of the retina receives its blood supply from the choriocapillaris. The inner two-thirds are supplied by branches from the central retinal artery, a branch of the ophthalmic artery. The central macular area is avascular.

Arteriovenous crossings are frequent in the temporal quadrants of the retina. Veins are located deep to the arteries at these crossings.

THE FASCIA BULBI (Tenon's Capsule)

The fascia bulbi is a fibrous membrane that envelops the globe from the limbus to the optic nerve, touching the sclera. Its lower segment is thick and fuses with the fascia of the inferior rectus and the inferior oblique muscles to form the suspensory ligament of Lockwood. The fusion forms a sling on which the globe rests. At the point where the fascia bulbi is pierced by the tendons of the extraocular muscles, it sends a tubular reflection around each of these muscles. These fascial reflections become continuous with the fascia of the muscles, the fused fasciae sending expansions to the surrounding structures and to the orbital bones. The fascial extensions are quite tough and limit the action of the extraocular muscles and are therefore known as **check ligaments.**

EXTRAOCULAR MUSCLES

There are 6 extraocular muscles: 4 recti and 2 obliques.

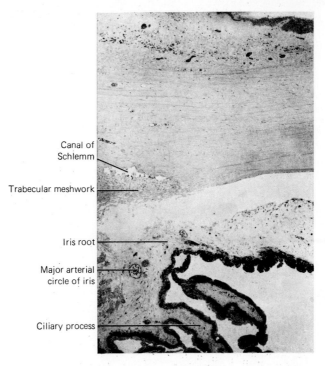

Figure 1–9. Photomicrograph of anterior chamber angle and related structures. (Courtesy of I Wood and L Garron.)

Nerve Supply

The oculomotor nerve (III) divides and innervates the medial, inferior, and superior rectus muscles and the inferior oblique muscle. The abducens nerve (VI) innervates the lateral rectus muscle; the trochlear nerve (IV) innervates the superior oblique muscle.

Blood Supply

The blood supply to the extraocular muscles is derived from the muscular branches of the ophthalmic artery. The lateral rectus and inferior oblique muscles are also supplied by branches from the lacrimal artery and the infraorbital artery, respectively.

RECTUS MUSCLES

The 4 rectus muscles originate in the tendinous ring—annulus of Zinn—surrounding the optic nerve at the posterior apex of the orbit (Fig 1–12). The rectus muscles insert into the sclera on the medial, lateral, inferior, and superior surfaces of the eyeball anterior to its equator. They are named by site of insertion, ie, medial rectus, lateral rectus, inferior rectus, and superior rectus muscles. The fibers of all 4 rectus muscles are loosely united and easily separated by blunt dissection. The muscles are about 40 mm long and become tendinous at their insertions.

The medial and lateral rectus muscles have only a single action. The inferior and superior rectus muscles have primary and secondary actions. The lateral rectus abducts and the medial rectus adducts the eye. The superior rectus elevates and adducts the eye and is concerned with intorsion. The inferior rectus depresses the eye, adducts it, and is concerned with extorsion.

OBLIQUE MUSCLES

The **superior oblique** is the longest and thinnest of the ocular muscles. It originates above and medial to the optic foramen and partially overlaps the origin of the levator palpebrae superioris muscle. The superior oblique has a thin, fusiform belly (40 mm long) and passes anteriorly in the form of a tendon to its trochlea, or pulley. It is then reflected backward and downward to attach in a fan shape to the sclera beneath the superior rectus. The trochlea is a cartilaginous structure attached to the frontal bone 3 mm behind the orbital rim. The superior oblique tendon is enclosed in a synovial sheath as it passes through the trochlea. The superior oblique directs the eye laterally and inferiorly.

The **inferior oblique** muscle originates from the nasal side of the orbital wall just behind the inferior orbital rim and lateral to the nasolacrimal duct. It passes beneath the inferior rectus and then under the lateral rectus muscle to insert onto the sclera with a short tendon. The insertion is into the posterotemporal segment of the globe and just over the macular area.

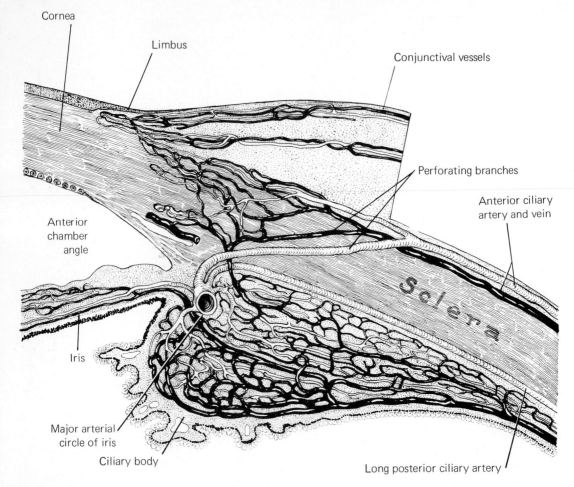

Cornea

Limbus

Conjunctival vessels

Perforating branches

Anterior ciliary
artery and vein

Anterior
chamber
angle

Sclera

Iris

Major arterial
circle of iris

Ciliary body

Long posterior ciliary artery

Figure 1–10. Vascular supply of the anterior segment. (Modified, redrawn, and reproduced, with permission, from Wolff E: *Anatomy of the Eye and Orbit,* 4th ed. Blakiston-McGraw, 1954.)

The muscle is 37 mm long. Its action directs the eye superiorly and laterally.

LEVATOR PALPEBRAE SUPERIORIS MUSCLE

The levator palpebrae muscle arises with a short tendon from the undersurface of the lesser wing of the sphenoid above and ahead of the optic foramen. The tendon blends with the underlying origin of the superior rectus muscle. The levator belly passes forward, forms an aponeurosis, and spreads like a fan. The muscle passes through the fibers of the orbicularis oculi and inserts into the skin of the eyelid at an area below the superior palpebral furrow (sulcus). It also inserts into the anterior or inferior surface of the upper tarsus (Müller's muscle) and into the superior fornix of the conjunctiva. The 2 extremities of the levator aponeurosis are called its medial and lateral horns. The medial horn is thin and is attached below the frontolacrimal suture and into the medial palpebral ligament. The lateral horn passes between the orbital and palpebral portions of the lacrimal gland and inserts into the orbital tubercle and the lateral palpebral ligament.

The sheath of the levator palpebrae superioris is attached to the superior rectus muscle inferiorly. The superior surface, at the junction of the muscle belly and the aponeurosis, forms a thickened band that is attached medially to the trochlea and laterally to the lateral orbital wall, the band forming the check ligaments of the muscle. The band is also known as Whitnall's ligament.

The levator is supplied by the superior branch of the oculomotor nerve (III); Müller's muscle is supplied by sympathetics.

Blood supply to the levator palpebrae superioris is derived from the lateral muscular branch of the ophthalmic artery. The action of the levator palpebrae superioris is to raise the upper eyelid. The palpebral segment of the orbicularis oculi muscle acts as the antagonist of the levator palpebrae.

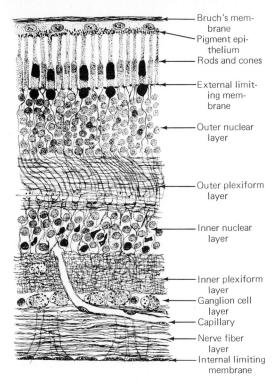

Bruch's membrane
Pigment epithelium
Rods and cones
External limiting membrane
Outer nuclear layer
Outer plexiform layer
Inner nuclear layer
Inner plexiform layer
Ganglion cell layer
Capillary
Nerve fiber layer
Internal limiting membrane

Figure 1–11. Layers of the retina. (Redrawn and reproduced, with permission, from Wolff E: *Anatomy of the Eye and Orbit,* 4th ed. Blakiston-McGraw, 1954.)

THE OPTIC NERVE

The trunk of the optic nerve consists of about 1 million axons that arise from the ganglion cells of the retina (nerve fiber layer). The optic nerve emerges from the posterior surface of the globe through a short, circular opening in the sclera about 1 mm below and 3 mm nasal to the posterior pole of the eye (Fig 1–13). The orbital segment of the nerve is 25–30 mm long; it travels within the optic muscle cone, enters the bony optic foramen, and gains access to the cranial cavity. After a 10-mm intracranial course, the nerve joins the opposite optic nerve, forms the optic chiasm, and continues posteriorly to the lateral geniculate bodies. Eighty percent of the nerve consists of visual fibers that synapse in the lateral geniculate body on neurons whose axons terminate in the primary visual cortex of the occipital lobes. The nerve fibers become myelinated on leaving the eye. Twenty percent of the fibers are pupillary and bypass the geniculate body en route to the pretectal area. Since the ganglion cells of the retina and their axons are part of the central nervous system, they will not regenerate if severed.

The fibrous wrappings of the optic nerve are continuous with the meninges. The pia mater is closely attached to the nerve in most of its intracranial and all of its intraorbital course, but it is only loosely attached in the optic chiasm. The pia divides the optic nerve fibers into bundles by sending multiple septa into the nerve substance and continues onto the sclera. The arachnoid sheaths the nerve from the intracranial end of the optic foramen to the globe, where it terminates in the sclera and the overlying dura mater. The dura mater lining the inner surface of the cranial vault meets the optic nerve as it leaves the optic foramen. As the nerve enters the orbit through the optic foramen, the dura splits, one layer lining the orbital cavity and the other forming the outer cover of the optic nerve. The tough, fibrous dura becomes continuous with the outer two-thirds of the sclera.

II. EMBRYOLOGY OF THE EYE

The eye is derived from 3 primitive embryonic layers: surface ectoderm, neural ectoderm, and mesoderm. Entoderm does not enter into the formation of the eye.

The **surface ectoderm** gives rise to the lens, the epithelium of the cornea, the conjunctiva, the lacrimal gland and its drainage system, and, in conjunction with the mesoderm, the vitreous.

The **neural ectoderm** gives rise to a portion of the vitreous, to the epithelium of the iris, the ciliary body, the retina, the sphincter and dilator components of the pupillary muscle, the optic nerve, and the cranial nerves that innervate the eye and the orbit.

The **mesoderm** gives rise to the sclera, the endothelium of the cornea, the substantia propria of the conjunctiva, the iris, the ciliary body, the choroid, the extraocular muscles, the lids (except their epithelium), the sheaths of the optic nerve, and the connective tissue and blood vessels of the eye, bony orbit, and vitreous.

Optic Vesicle Stage

The embryonic plate is the earliest stage in fetal development during which ocular structures can be differentiated. At the 2.5-mm (2-week) stage, the edges of the neural groove thicken to form the neural folds (Fig 1–14). The folds then fuse to form the neural tube, which sinks into the underlying mesoderm and detaches itself from the surface epithelium. The site of the optic groove or optic sulcus is in the cephalic neural folds on either side of and parallel to the neural groove. This occurs when neural folds begin to close at 3 weeks.

At the 9-mm (4-week) stage, just before the anterior portion of the neural tube closes completely, neural ectoderm grows outward and toward the surface ec-

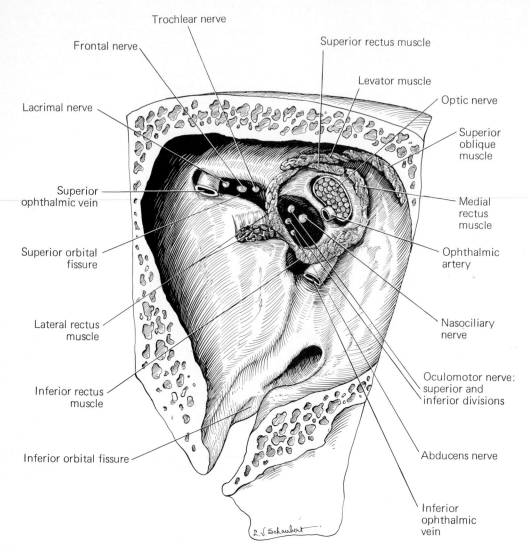

Figure 1–12. Anterior view of apex of right orbit.

toderm on either side to form the spherical optic vesicles. The optic vesicles are connected to the forebrain by the optic stalks. At this stage also, a thickening of the surface ectoderm (lens plate) begins to form opposite the ends of the optic vesicles.

Optic Cup Stage

As the optic vesicle invaginates to produce the optic cup, the original outer wall of the vesicle approaches its inner wall. The invagination of the ventral surface of the optic stalk and of the optic vesicle occurs simultaneously and creates a groove, the choroidal (fetal) fissure. The margins of the optic cup then grow around the choroidal fissure. At the same time, the lens plate invaginates to form first a cup and then a hollow sphere known as the lens vesicle. By the 9-mm (4-week) stage, the lens vesicle separates from

the surface ectoderm and lies free in the rim of the optic cup.

The choroidal fissure allows the vascular mesoderm to enter the optic stalk and eventually to form the hyaloid system of the vitreous cavity. As invagination is completed, the choroidal fissure narrows and closes during the 13-mm (6-week) stage, leaving one small permanent opening at the anterior end of the optic stalk through which the hyaloid artery passes. At the 100-mm (4-month) stage, the retinal artery and vein pass through this opening. At this stage also, the ultimate general structure of the eye has been determined.

Further development of the eye consists in differentiation of the individual optic structures. In general, differentiation of the optic structures occurs more rapidly in the posterior than in the anterior segment of

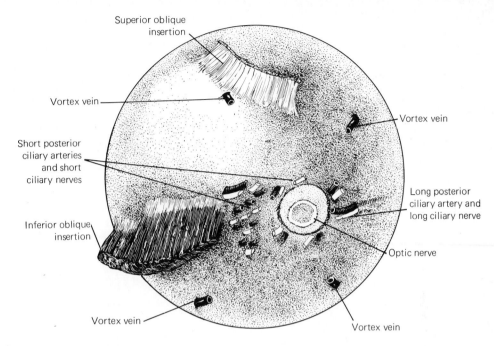

Superior oblique
insertion

Vortex vein

Vortex vein

Short posterior
ciliary arteries
and short
ciliary nerves

Long posterior
ciliary artery and
long ciliary nerve

Inferior oblique
insertion

Optic nerve

Vortex vein

Vortex vein

Figure 1–13. Posterior view of left eye. (Redrawn and reproduced, with permission, from Wolff E: *Anatomy of the Eye and Orbit,* 4th ed. Blakiston-McGraw, 1954.)

the eye during the early stages and more rapidly in the anterior segment during the later stages of gestation.

CONGENITAL OCULAR ABNORMALITIES

Congenital defects of the ocular structures fall into 2 main categories: (1) developmental anomalies, or dysplasia, of embryonal origin; and (2) tissue reactions to intrauterine insults (infections, drugs, etc). Examples of the first category are the colobomas, dermoid tumors, cyclopia, microphakia, anophthalmos, cryptophthalmos, and microphthalmos. Examples of the second category are chorioretinitis and some forms of cataract. Heredity plays a major role in the development of certain congenital deformities. Any failure of regression of primitive vascular tissue at the proper stage or of fusion of embryonic tissue can lead to a defect of development of iris or choroid.

Failure of Invagination of the Optic Vesicle

Failure of invagination of the optic vesicle leads to a congenital cystic eye. Colobomas of eyelid, iris, retina, or choroid result from failure of closure of the fetal fissure.

Anophthalmos & Microphthalmos

An eye may be missing (anophthalmos) or smaller than normal (microphthalmos). In microphthalmos, normal optic function usually is not present.

Congenital Lens Opacities

Congenital opacities of the lens may occur at any time during formation of the lens, and the stage during which the opacity started to develop is often measurable by the depth of the opacity. The innermost fetal nucleus of the lens forms early in embryonic life and is surrounded by the embryonic nucleus. During adult life, further growth in the lens is peripheral and subcapsular.

Extraocular Dermoids

Congenital rests of mesodermal and surface ectodermal tissues may lead to formation of dermoids that occur frequently in the extraocular structures.

EMBRYOLOGY OF SPECIFIC STRUCTURES

Lens

Soon after the lens vesicle lies free in the rim of the optic cap (13-mm or 6-week stage), the cells of its posterior wall elongate, encroach on the empty cavity, and finally fill it in (26-mm or 7-week stage). At about this stage (13-mm or 6-week), a hyaline capsule is secreted by the lens cells. Secondary lens fibers elongate from the equatorial region and grow forward under the subcapsular epithelium, which remains as a single layer of cuboid epithelial cells, and backward under the lens capsule. These fibers meet to form the lens sutures (upright "Y" anteriorly and inverted "Y" posteriorly), which are complete by the seventh month. (This growth and proliferation of sec-

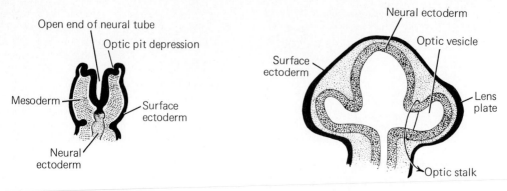

Open end of neural tube

Optic pit depression

Mesoderm

Surface ectoderm

Neural ectoderm

2.5-mm stage

Neural ectoderm

Surface ectoderm

Optic vesicle

Lens plate

Optic stalk

Forebrain of 4-mm embryo, optic vesicle stage

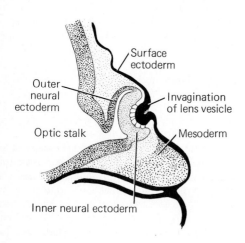

Surface ectoderm

Outer neural ectoderm

Invagination of lens vesicle

Optic stalk

Mesoderm

Inner neural ectoderm

5-mm stage. Beginning formation of optic cup by invagination.

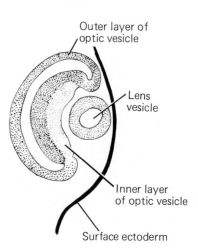

Outer layer of optic vesicle

Lens vesicle

Inner layer of optic vesicle

Surface ectoderm

9-mm stage. Lens vesicle has separated from surface ectoderm and lies free in rim of optic cup.

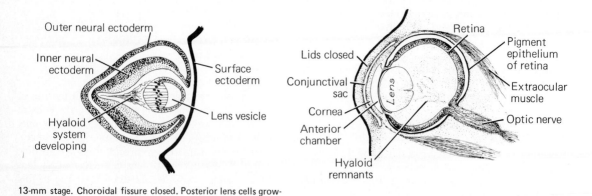

Outer neural ectoderm

Inner neural ectoderm

Surface ectoderm

Hyaloid system developing

Lens vesicle

13-mm stage. Choroidal fissure closed. Posterior lens cells growing forward.

Retina

Lids closed

Conjunctival sac

Cornea

Anterior chamber

Hyaloid remnants

Pigment epithelium of retina

Extraocular muscle

Optic nerve

Lens

65-mm stage (3 months)

Figure 2–1. Embryologic development of ocular structures. (Redrawn and reproduced, with permission, from Mann IC: *The Development of the Human Eye,* 2nd ed. British Medical Association, 1950.)

ondary lens fibers continues at a decreasing rate throughout life; the lens therefore continues to enlarge slowly, causing compression of the lens fibers.)

Retina

The outer layer of the optic cup remains as a single layer and becomes the pigment epithelium of the retina. Pigmentation begins at the 10-mm (5-week) stage. The inner layer undergoes a complicated differentiation into the other 9 layers of the retina. This occurs slowly throughout gestation. By the seventh month, the outermost cell layer (consisting of the nuclei of the rods and cones) is present as well as the bipolar, amacrine, and ganglion cells and nerve fibers. The macular region is thicker than the rest of the retina until the eighth month, when macular depression begins to develop. Macular development is not complete until 6 months after birth.

Optic Nerve

The axons of the ganglion cell layer of the retina form the inner nerve fiber layer. The fibers slowly form the optic stalk and then the optic nerve (26-mm stage). Mesodermal elements enter the surrounding tissue to form the vascular septa of the nerve. Medullation extends from the brain peripherally down the optic nerve, and at birth has reached the lamina cribrosa. Medullation is completed by age 3 months.

Iris & Ciliary Body

During the third month (50-mm stage), the rim of the optic cup grows forward in front of the lens as a double row of epithelium and lies posterior to mesoderm, which becomes the stroma of the iris. These 2 epithelial layers become pigmented in the iris, whereas only the outer layer is pigmented in the ciliary body. Folds appear in the epithelial layers of the ciliary body; mesoderm grows into this fold to form the ciliary processes. By the fifth month (150-mm stage), the sphincter muscle of the pupil is developing from a bud of nonpigmented epithelium derived from the anterior epithelial layer of the iris near the pupillary margin. Soon after the sixth month, the dilator muscle appears in the anterior epithelial layer near the ciliary body.

Choroid

At the 6-mm (3½-week) stage, a network of capillaries encircles the optic cup and develops into the choroid. By the 13-mm (6-week) stage, the outer neural epithelial layer has secreted Bruch's membrane. By the third month, the intermediate and large venous channels of the choroid are developed and drain into the vortex veins to exit from the eye.

Vitreous

A. First Stage: (Primary vitreous, 4.5- to 13-mm or 3- or 6-week stage.) At about the 4.5-mm stage, fibrils grow in from the inner layer of the optic vesicle to join elements from the lens vesicle that—along with some mesoderm fibrils associated with the hyaloid

artery—form the primary vitreous. This stage ends as the lens capsule appears, precluding any further lens participation in vitreous formation. The primary vitreous does not atrophy and ultimately lies just behind the posterior pole of the lens as the hyaloid canal.

B. Second Stage: (Secondary vitreous, 13- to 65-mm or 3- to 10-week stage.) Müller's fibers of the retina become continuous with vitreous fibrils, so that the secondary vitreous is mainly derived from retinal ectoderm. The hyaloid system develops a set of vitreous vessels as well as vessels on the lens capsule surface (tunica vasculosa lentis). The hyaloid system is at its height at 40 mm and then atrophies from posterior to anterior.

C. Third Stage: (Tertiary vitreous, 65 mm or 10 weeks on.) During the third month, the marginal bundle of Drualt is forming. This consists of vitreous fibrillar condensations extending from the future ciliary epithelium of the optic cup to the equator of the lens. Condensations then form the suspensory ligament of the lens, which is well developed by the 100-mm or 4-month stage. The hyaloid system atrophies completely during this stage.

Blood Vessels

Long ciliary arteries bud off from the hyaloid at the 16-mm (6-week) stage and anastomose around the optic cup margin with the major circle of the iris by the 30-mm (7-week) stage.

The hyaloid system (see Vitreous) atrophies completely by the eighth month. The hyaloid artery gives rise to the central retinal artery and its branches (100-mm or 4-month stage). Buds begin to grow into the retina and develop the retinal circulation, which reaches the ora serrata at 8 months. The branches of the central retinal vein develop simultaneously.

Cornea

The epithelium is derived from surface ectoderm, whereas the rest of the cornea comes from mesodermal structures. The earliest differentiation is seen at about the 12-mm (5-week) stage, when endothelial cells appear. Descemet's membrane is secreted by the flattened endothelial cells by the 75-mm (12-week) stage. The stroma slowly thickens, largely by an increase in the number of elastic fibers, and forms an anterior condensation just under the epithelium that is recognizable at 100 mm (4 months) as Bowman's layer. A definite corneoscleral junction is present at 4 months.

Anterior Chamber

The anterior chamber of the eye first appears at 20 mm (7 weeks) and remains very shallow until birth. At 65 mm (9–10 weeks), Schlemm's canal appears as a vascular channel at the level of the recess of the angle and gradually assumes a relatively more anterior location as the angle recess develops. The iris, which in the early stages of development is quite anterior, gradually lies relatively more posteriorly as the chamber angle recess develops, most likely because of the difference in rate of growth of the anterior segment structures. The trabecular meshwork develops from the loose vascular mesodermal tissue lying originally at the margin of the optic cup. The aqueous drainage system is ready to function before birth.

Sclera & Extraocular Muscles

The sclera and extraocular muscles are formed from condensations of mesoderm encircling the optic cup and are first identifiable at the 20-mm (7-week) stage. Development of these structures is well advanced by the fourth month. Tenon's capsule appears about the insertions of the rectus muscles at the 80-mm (12-week) stage and is complete at 5 months.

Lids & Lacrimal Apparatus

The lids develop from mesoderm except for the skin and conjunctiva. The lid buds are first seen at 16 mm (6 weeks) growing in front of the eye, where they meet and fuse at the 37-mm (8-week) stage. They separate during the fifth month, and lashes and meibomian and other lid glands develop. The lacrimal gland (including the accessory glands and the conjunctiva) and drainage system develop from ectoderm. The canaliculi, lacrimal sac, and nasolacrimal duct are developed by burying a solid epithelial cord between the maxillary and nasal processes. This cord canalizes just before birth.

III. GROWTH & DEVELOPMENT OF THE EYE

Eyeball

At birth, the eye is larger in relation to the rest of the body than is the case in children and adults. In relation to its ultimate size (reached at 7–8 years), it is comparatively short, averaging 17.3 mm in anteroposterior length (the only optically significant dimension). This would make the eye quite hyperopic if it were not for the refractive power of the nearly spherical lens.

Cornea

The newborn infant has a relatively large cornea that reaches adult size by the age of 2 years. It is flatter than the adult cornea, and its curvature is greater at the periphery than in the center. (The reverse is true in adults.)

Almost all astigmatic refractive errors are produced by differences in curvature in the various meridians of the cornea. In the infant, the vertical meridian usually has the greatest curvature. In adult life the cornea tends to flatten, and the flattening is more marked in the vertical than the horizontal, changing the axis of astigmatism. However, the degree of astigmatism changes very little throughout life.

Lens

At birth, the lens is more nearly spherical in shape than later in life, producing a greater refractive power that helps to compensate for the short anteroposterior diameter of the eye. The lens grows throughout life as new fibers are added to the periphery, making it flatter.

The consistency of the lens material changes throughout life. At birth, it may be compared with soft plastic; in old age, the lens is of a glasslike consistency. This accounts for the greater resistance to change of shape in accommodation as one grows older.

Refractive State

About 80% of children are born hyperopic, 5% myopic, and 15% emmetropic. Hyperopia often gradually decreases prior to puberty and may even become myopia. Myopia usually increases after age 7–8 years and develops in some children not previously affected. The increase in the myopic refractive error usually ceases or is much diminished by age 16 years. Refractive errors tend to stabilize during the 20s and 30s. The onset of presbyopia is at age 42–46 years in nearly everyone.

Iris

At birth, there is little or no pigment on the anterior surface of the iris; the posterior pigment layer showing through the translucent tissue gives the eyes of most infants a bluish color. As the pigment begins to appear on the anterior surface, the iris assumes its definitive color. If considerable pigment is deposited, the eyes become brown. Less iris stroma pigmentation results in blue, hazel, or green.

Position

During the first 3 months of age, eye movements may be so poorly coordinated (because of the normally slow development of reflexes) that doubt may exist about the straightness of the eyes. Most of the binocular reflexes should be well developed by 6 months of age. Deviation that persists beyond age 6 months should be investigated (see Chapter 13).

Nasolacrimal Apparatus

The cord of cells that hollows out to form the nasolacrimal duct between the tear sac and the nose usually becomes patent at about the time of birth. Failure to function may not be noticed for some time because of lack of tear secretion in the first few weeks of life. Failure of tear production by 3 months of age demands attention.

Optic Nerve

The completion of the medullation process around the optic nerve fibers usually occurs within a few weeks after birth.

Ophthalmologic Examination

2

David F. Chang, MD

Of all the organs of the body, the eye is most accessible to direct examination. Visual function can be measured by simple subjective testing. The external anatomy of the eye is visible to inspection with the unaided eye and with fairly simple instruments. Even the interior of the eye is visible through the clear cornea. The eye is the only part of the body where blood vessels and central nervous system tissue (retina and optic nerve) can be viewed without x-rays or incisions, which means that some of the important systemic effects of infectious, autoimmune, neoplastic, and vascular diseases may be visible from the internal eye examination.

The purpose of sections I and II of this chapter is to provide an overview of the ocular history and basic complete eye examination as performed by an ophthalmologist. In section III, more specialized examination techniques will be presented.

I. OCULAR HISTORY

The **chief complaint** is characterized according to its duration, frequency, intermittency, and rapidity of onset. The location, the severity, and the circumstances surrounding onset are important as well as any associated symptoms. Current eye medications being used and all other current and past ocular disorders are recorded, and a review of other pertinent ocular symptoms is performed.

The **past medical history** centers on the patient's general state of health and principal systemic illnesses if any. Vascular disorders commonly associated with ocular manifestations—such as diabetes and hypertension—should be asked about specifically. Just as a medical history should include ocular medications being used, the eye history should list the patient's systemic medications. This provides a general indication of health status and may include medications that affect ocular health, such as corticosteroids. Finally, any drug allergies should be recorded.

The **family history** is pertinent for ocular disorders such as strabismus, amblyopia, glaucoma, cataracts, and retinal problems, such as retinal detachment or macular degeneration. Medical diseases such as diabetes may be relevant as well.

COMMON OCULAR SYMPTOMS

A basic understanding of ocular symptomatology is necessary for performing a proper ophthalmic examination. Ocular symptoms can be divided into 3 basic categories: abnormalities of vision, abnormalities of ocular appearance, and abnormalities of ocular sensation—pain and discomfort.

Symptoms and complaints should always be fully characterized. Was the **onset** gradual, rapid, or asymptomatic? (Was blurred vision in one eye not discovered until the opposite eye was inadvertently covered?) Was the **duration** brief, or has the symptom continued until the present visit? If the symptom was intermittent, what was the frequency? Is the **location** focal or diffuse, and is involvement unilateral or bilateral? Finally, is the **degree** characterized by the patient as mild, moderate, or severe?

One should also determine what therapeutic measures have been tried and to what extent they have helped. Has the patient identified circumstances that trigger or worsen the symptom? Have similar instances occurred before, and are there any other associated symptoms?

The following is a brief overview of common ocular complaints. Representative examples of some causes are given here and discussed more fully elsewhere in this book.

ABNORMALITIES OF VISION

Visual Loss

Loss of visual acuity may be due to abnormalities anywhere along the optical and neurologic visual pathway. One must therefore consider refractive (focusing) error, lid ptosis, clouding or interference from the ocular media (eg, corneal edema, cataract, or hemorrhage in the vitreous or aqueous space), and malfunction of the retina (macula), optic nerve, or intracranial visual pathway.

A distinction should be made between decreased central acuity and peripheral vision. The latter may be focal, such as a scotoma, or more expansive as with hemianopia. With the exception of cortical blindness and amblyopia, abnormalities of the intracranial visual pathway usually disturb the visual field rather than central visual acuity.

Transient loss of central or peripheral vision is frequently due to circulatory changes anywhere along the neurologic visual pathway from the retina to the occipital cortex. Examples would be amaurosis fugax or migrainous scotoma.

The degree of visual impairment may vary under different circumstances. For example, uncorrected nearsighted refractive error may seem worse in dark environments. This is because pupillary dilatation allows more misfocused rays to reach the retina, increasing the blur. A central focal cataract may seem worse in sunlight. In this case, pupillary constriction prevents more rays from entering and passing around the lens opacity. Blurred vision from corneal edema may improve as the day progresses owing to corneal dehydration from surface evaporation.

Visual Aberrations

Glare or **haloes** may result from uncorrected refractive error, scratches on spectacle lenses, excessive pupillary dilatation, and hazy ocular media, such as corneal edema or cataract. **Visual distortion** (apart from blurring) may be manifested as an irregular pattern of dimness, wavy or jagged lines, and image magnification or minification. Causes may include the aura of migraine, optical distortion from strong corrective lenses, or lesions involving of the macula and optic nerve. **Flashing** or **flickering** lights may indicate retinal traction (if instantaneous) or migrainous scintillations that last for several seconds or minutes. **Floating spots** may represent normal vitreous strands due to vitreous "syneresis" or separation (see Chapter 10), or the pathologic presence of pigment, blood, or inflammatory cells. **Oscillopsia** is a shaking field of vision that may be due to harmless lid twitching ("myokymia") or to certain forms of nystagmus.

It must be determined whether **double vision** is monocular or binocular (ie, disappears if one eye is covered). **Monocular diplopia** is often a split shadow or ghost image. Causes include uncorrected refractive error, such as astigmatism, or focal media abnormalities such as cataracts or corneal irregularities (eg, scars, keratoconus). **Binocular diplopia** (see Chapters 13 and 15) can be vertical, horizontal, diagonal, or torsional. If the deviation occurs or increases in one gaze direction as opposed to others, it is called "incomitant." Neuromuscular dysfunction or mechanical restriction of globe rotation is suspected. "Comitant" deviation is one that remains constant regardless of the direction of gaze. It is usually due to inability to fuse 2 eyes with a strong, natural tendency to deviate, called a "phoria." An acquired phoria can be induced by certain types of spectacle correction.

ABNORMALITIES OF APPEARANCE

Complaints of "red eye" call for differentiation between redness of the lids and periocular area versus redness of the globe. The latter can be caused by subconjunctival hemorrhage or by vascular congestion of the conjunctiva, sclera, or episclera (connective tissue between the sclera and conjunctiva). Causes of such congestion may be either external surface inflammation, such as conjunctivitis and keratitis, or intraocular inflammation such as iritis and acute glaucoma. Color abnormalities other than redness may include jaundice (yellow) and hyperpigmented spots on the iris or outer ocular surface.

Other changes in appearance of the **globe** that may be noticeable to the patient include focal lesions of the ocular surface, such as a pterygium, and asymmetry of pupil size, called "anisocoria." The **lids** and **periocular tissues** may be the source of visible signs such as edema, redness, focal growths and lesions, and abnormal position or contour, such as ptosis. Finally, the patient may notice bulging or displacement of the globe, as with exophthalmos.

PAIN & DISCOMFORT

"Eye pain" may be periocular, ocular, retrobulbar (behind the globe), or poorly localized. Examples of **periocular** pain may be tenderness of the lid, tear sac, sinuses, or temporal artery. **Retrobulbar** pain can be due to orbital inflammation of any kind. Certain locations of inflammation, such as optic neuritis or orbital myositis, may produce pain on eye movement. Many **nonspecific** complaints such as "eyestrain," "pulling," "pressure," "fullness," and certain kinds of "headaches" are poorly localized. Causes may include fatigue from ocular accommodation or binocular fusion, or referred discomfort from nonocular muscle tension or fatigue.

Ocular pain itself may seem to emanate from the surface or from deeper within the globe. Corneal epithelial damage typically produces a superficial sharp pain or foreign body sensation exacerbated by blinking. Topical anesthesia will immediately relieve this pain. Examples of deeper internal aching pain would include acute glaucoma, iritis, endophthalmitis, and scleritis. The globe is often tender to palpation in these situations. Reflex spasm of the ciliary muscle and iris sphincter can occur with iritis or keratitis, producing brow ache and painful "photophobia" (light sensitivity). This discomfort is markedly improved by cycloplegic dilating drops (see Chapter 26).

Eye Irritation

Superficial ocular discomfort usually results from surface abnormalities. **Itching,** as a primary symptom, is often a sign of allergic sensitivity. Symptoms of **dryness,** burning, grittiness, and mild foreign body sensation can occur with dry eyes or other types of mild corneal irritation. **Tearing** may be of 2 general types. Sudden reflex tearing is usually due to irritation of the ocular surface. In contrast, chronic watering and "epiphora" (tears rolling down the cheek) may indicate abnormal lacrimal draining (see Chapter 3).

Ocular **secretions** are often diagnostically nonspecific. Severe amounts of discharge that cause the lids to be glued shut upon awakening usually indicate viral or bacterial conjunctivitis. More scant amounts of mucoid discharge can also be seen with allergic and noninfectious irritations. Dried matter and crusts on the lashes may occur acutely with conjunctivitis or chronically with blepharitis (lid margin inflammation).

II. BASIC OPHTHALMOLOGIC EXAMINATION

The opthalmologic physical examination can be organized conceptually into the evaluation of function and the evaluation of individual anatomic structures. The former can be subdivided into visual and nonvisual functions, such as eye movements and alignment. Eye problems can be anatomically separated into those involving the adnexa (lids and periocular tissue), the globe, and the orbit. A basic and complete examination would include all of these areas except for the orbit, which can be examined in detail only with the aid of specialized techniques discussed later in this chapter.

VISION

Just as assessment of vital signs is a part of every physical examination, any ocular examination must include assessment of vision, regardless of whether vision is mentioned as part of the chief complaint. Good vision results from a combination of an intact neurologic visual pathway, a structurally healthy eye, and proper focus of the eye. An analogy might be made to a video camera, requiring a functioning cable connection to the monitor, a mechanically intact camera body, and a proper focus setting. Measurement of visual acuity is subjective rather than objective, since it requires responses on the part of the patient.

Refraction

The unaided distant focal point of the eye varies among normal individuals depending on the shape of the globe and the cornea (Fig 2–1). An **emmetropic** eye is in optimal focus for distance vision naturally. An **ametropic** eye needs corrective lenses to be in proper focus for distance. This optical requirement is called **refractive error. Refraction** is the procedure by which this natural optical error is characterized and quantified (Fig 2–2).

Refraction is often necessary to distinguish between blurred vision caused by refractive (ie, optical) error or by medical abnormalities of the visual system. Thus, in addition to being the basis for prescription of corrective glasses or contact lenses, refraction serves a diagnostic function.

Testing Central Vision

Vision can be divided into central vision and peripheral vision. Central visual acuity is measured with

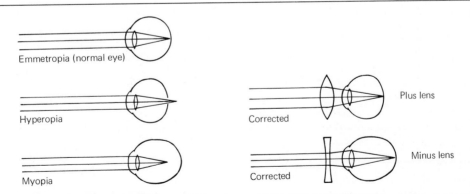

Figure 2–1. Common imperfections of the optical system of the eye **(refractive errors).** Ideally, light rays from a distant target should automatically arrive in focus on the retina if the retina is situated precisely at the eye's natural focal point. Such an eye is called **emmetropic.** In **hyperopia** ("farsightedness"), the light rays from a distant target instead come to a focus behind the retina, causing the retinal image to be blurred. A biconvex (+) lens corrects this by increasing the refractive power of the eye, and shifting the focal point forward. In **myopia** ("nearsightedness"), the light rays come to a focus in front of the retina, as though the eyeball is too long. Placing a biconcave (−) lens in front of the eye diverges the incoming light rays; this effectively weakens the optical power of the eye enough so that the focus is shifted backward and onto the retina. (Modified and reproduced, with permission, from Ganong WF: *Review of Medical Physiology,* 14th ed. Lange, 1989.)

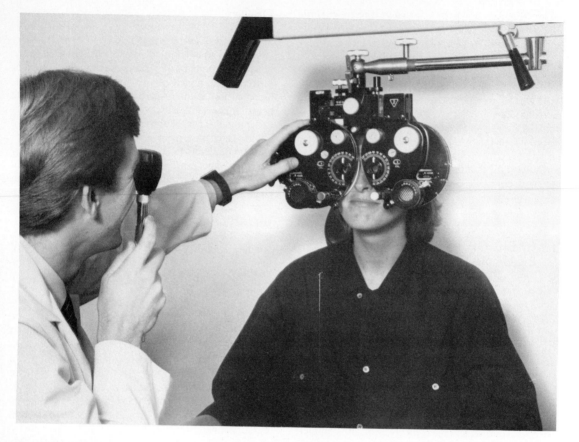

Figure 2–2. Refraction being performed using a "phoropter." This device contains the complete range of corrective lens powers which can quickly be changed back and forth, allowing the patient to subjectively compare various combinations while viewing the eye chart at a distance. (Photo by M Narahara.)

a display of different-sized targets shown at a standard distance from the eye. For example, the familiar "Snellen chart" is composed of a series of progressively smaller rows of random letters used to test distance vision. The letters within each row are of uniform and standardized size, and acuity is graded according to the smallest letter that can be read.

By convention, vision can be measured either at a distance at 20 feet (6 meters) or at near, 14 inches away. For diagnostic purposes, distance acuity is the standard for comparison and is always tested separately for each eye. Acuity is scored as a set of 2 numbers (eg, "20/20")—which, despite the form of notation, is not a true fraction. The first number ("numerator") represents the testing distance in feet between the chart and the patient. The "denominator" signifies the size of the smallest letter the patient can read from this testing distance.

A "size 20" letter is the basis for comparison and is the smallest letter a normal eye should be able to see 20 feet away. The normal eye seeing this letter has "20/20 vision." A "size 40" letter is twice as large and should be seen by the normal eye even when shown 40 feet away. A "200" letter is 10 times larger

than the standard and could normally still be recognized 200 feet away. Thus, the second number represents the actual distance at which a normal eye could still recognize a letter of that size. To say that an eye has "20/30 vision" means that at 20 feet from the chart it could at best only read a letter large enough for a normal eye to read 30 feet away. It should be obvious now that "20/60 vision" is even worse, signifying that letters large enough to be read by a normal eye at 60 feet were the largest this eye could read from a 20-foot distance.

Charts containing numerals can be used for patients not familiar with the English alphabet. The "illiterate E" chart is used to test small children or if there is a language barrier. "E" figures are randomly rotated in each of 4 different orientations throughout the chart. For each target, the patient is asked to point in the same direction as the 3 "bars" of the E (Fig 2–3). Most children can be tested in this manner beginning at about age 3½.

Uncorrected visual acuity is measured without glasses or contact lenses. **Corrected** acuity means that these aids were worn. Since poor uncorrected distance acuity may simply be due to refractive (ie, focusing)

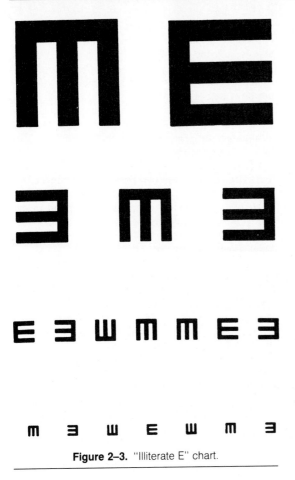

Figure 2–3. "Illiterate E" chart.

error, corrected visual acuity is a more relevant assessment of ocular health.

Testing Poor Vision

The patient unable to read the largest letter on the chart (eg, the "20/200" letter) should be moved closer to the chart until that letter can be read. The distance from the chart is then recorded as the numerator. Visual acuity of "5/200" means that the patient can just make out the largest letter from a distance of 5 feet. An eye unable to read any letters is tested by the ability to count fingers. A notation on the chart that reads "CF at 2 ft" indicates that the eye was able to count fingers held 2 feet away but not farther away.

If counting fingers is not possible, the eye may be able to detect a hand moving vertically or horizontally ("HM," or "hand motions" vision). The next lower level of vision would be the ability to perceive light ("LP," or "light perception"). An eye that cannot perceive light is considered totally blind ("NLP," or "no light perception").

Testing Peripheral Vision

Because it is much grosser than central acuity, side vision is harder to test quantitatively. Specialized tests described in the next section are used when peripheral vision measurements are needed, such as for the diagnosis of early glaucoma.

Gross screening of the peripheral field of vision can be quickly performed using **confrontation testing.** Since the visual fields of the 2 eyes overlap, each eye must be tested separately. The patient is seated facing the examiner several feet away and begins by covering the left eye while the right eye fixes on the examiner's left eye.

The examiner then briefly shows several fingers of one hand (usually one, 2, or 5 fingers) peripherally in one of the 4 quadrants. The patient must identify the number flashed while maintaining straight-ahead fixation. Since patient and examiner are staring eye to eye, any loss of fixation will be noticed. The upper and lower temporal and the upper and lower nasal quadrants are all tested in this fashion for each eye.

If the examiner closes the right eye while the patient covers the left eye—and if the targets (fingers) are presented at a distance halfway between the patient and the examiner—their respective peripheral fields should be the same. This allows comparison of the patient's field with the examiner's own. Consistent errors indicate gross deficiencies in the quadrant tested, as seen with retinal detachments, optic nerve abnormalities, and ischemic or mass injuries to the intracranial visual pathway. Since dense visual field abnormalities are often asymptomatic, confrontation testing should be included in complete ophthalmologic examinations.

A subtle form of right or left homonymous hemianopia may exist that can only be elicited by simultaneously presenting targets on both sides of the midline—not when targets are presented on one side at a time. To perform simultaneous confrontation testing, the examiner holds both hands out peripherally, one on each side. The patient must signify on which side (right, left, or both) the examiner is intermittently wiggling the fingers. Surprisingly, a patient with a mild left hemianopia may still be able to detect one hand wiggling fingers to the left side and may fail to see them (to the left) only when the examiner is simultaneously wiggling the fingers on both hands. This interesting finding indicates partial or relative inattention to the left side as both sides are being equally—and simultaneously—stimulated.

More sophisticated means of visual field testing are discussed later in this chapter.

PUPILS

Basic Examination

The pupils should appear symmetric, and each one should be examined for size, shape (circular or irregular), and reactivity to both light and accommodation. Pupillary abnormalities may be due to (1) neurologic disease, (2) acute intraocular inflammation causing either spasm or atony of the pupillary sphincter, (3) previous inflammation causing adhesions of the iris,

(4) prior surgical alteration, (5) the effect of systemic or eye medications, and (6) benign variations of normal.

To avoid accommodation, the patient is asked to stare in the distance as a penlight is directed toward each eye. Dim lighting conditions help to accentuate the pupillary response and may best demonstrate an abnormally small pupil. Likewise, an abnormally large pupil may be more apparent in brighter background illumination. The **direct response** to light refers to constriction of the illuminated pupil. The reaction may be graded as either brisk or sluggish. Normally, a **consensual** constriction will simultaneously occur in the opposite nonilluminated pupil. This is usually a slightly weaker response. The neuroanatomy of the pupillary pathway is discussed in Chapter 15.

Swinging Penlight Test for Marcus Gunn Pupil

As a light is swung back and forth in front of the 2 pupils, one can compare the direct and consensual reactions of each pupil. Since the direction reaction is usually stronger than the consensual, each pupil as the light falls directly on it should immediately constrict slightly more. Start by shining the light into the right eye, causing consensual constriction of the left pupil. As the light is then swung toward the left eye, the left pupil should constrict slightly more due to the direct light response. The right pupil should behave similarly as the light is swung back toward the right eye.

If the afferent conduction of light in the left optic nerve is impaired as a consequence of disease, the left pupil will have a weak direct response but its consensual efferent response will remain unchanged. As the light is swung from the right to the left eye, the left pupil will then paradoxically *widen* (since its abnormal direct response is weaker than the consensual response initiated by the healthy right optic nerve). This phenomenon is called a Marcus Gunn pupil, or afferent pupillary defect, since the paradoxic dilation in response to direct illumination occurs in the eye with the abnormal afferent pathway (ie, optic nerve or retina). Because the Marcus Gunn pupil reacts and is often of normal size, the swinging flashlight test may be the only means of demonstrating it.

Marcus Gunn pupil is further discussed and illustrated in Chapter 15.

OCULAR MOTILITY

The objective of ocular motility testing is to evaluate the alignment of the eyes and their movements, both individually ("ductions") and in tandem ("versions"). A more complete discussion of motility testing and abnormalities is presented in Chapter 13.

Testing Alignment

Normal patients have binocular vision. Since each eye generates a visual image separate from and independent of that of the other eye, the brain must be able to fuse the 2 images in order to avoid "double vision." This is achieved by having each eye positioned so that both foveas are simultaneously fixating on the object of regard.

A simple test of binocular alignment is performed by having the patient look toward a penlight held several feet away. A pinpoint light reflection, or "reflex," should appear on each cornea and should be centered over each pupil if the 2 eyes are straight in their alignment. If the eye positions are convergent, such that one eye points inward ("esotropia"), the light reflex will appear temporal to the pupil in that eye. If the eyes are divergent, such that one eye points outward ("exotropia"), the light reflex will be located more nasally in that eye.

The **cover test** (see Fig 13–6) is a more accurate method of verifying normal ocular alignment. The test requires good vision in both eyes. The patient is asked to gaze at a distant target with both eyes open. If both eyes are fixating together on the target, covering one eye should not affect the position or continued fixation of the other eye.

To perform the test, the examiner suddenly covers one eye and carefully watches to see that the second eye does not move (indicating that it was fixating on the same target already). If the second eye was not identically aligned but was instead turned abnormally inward or outward, it could not have been simultaneously fixating on the target. Thus, it will have to quickly move to find the target once the previously fixating eye is covered. Fixation of each eye is tested in turn.

An abnormal cover test is expected in patients with diplopia. However, diplopia is not present in many patients with abnormal ocular alignment. When the test is abnormal, prism lenses of different power can be used to neutralize the refixation movement of the misaligned eye. In this way, the amount of eye deviation can be quantified. A more complete discussion of this test and its variations is presented in Chapter 13.

Testing Extraocular Movements

The patient is asked to follow a target with both eyes as it is moved in each of the 4 cardinal directions of gaze. The examiner notes the speed, smoothness, range, and symmetry of movements and observes for unsteadiness of fixation (eg, nystagmus).

Impairment of eye movements can be due to neurologic problems (eg, cranial nerve palsy), primary extraocular muscular weakness (eg, myasthenia gravis), or mechanical constraints within the orbit limiting rotation of the globe (eg, orbital floor fracture with entrapment of the inferior rectus muscle). If the amount of deviation of ocular alignment is the same in all directions of gaze, is is called "comitant." It is "incomitant" if the amount of deviation varies with the direction of gaze.

EXTERNAL EXAMINATION

Before studying the eye under magnification, a general external examination of the ocular adnexa (eyelids and periocular area) is performed. Skin lesions, growths, and inflammatory signs such as swelling, erythema, warmth, and tenderness are evaluated by gross inspection and palpation.

The positions of the eyelids are checked for abnormalities such as ptosis or lid retraction. Asymmetry can be quantified by measuring the width (in millimeters) of the "palpebral fissure"—the space between the upper and lower lid margins. Abnormal motor function of the lids, such as impairment of upper lid elevation or forceful lid closure, may be due to either neurologic or primary muscular abnormalities.

Gross malposition of the globe, such as proptosis, may be seen with certain orbital diseases. Palpation of the bony orbital rim and periocular soft tissue should always be done in instances of suspected orbital trauma, infection, or neoplasm. The general facial examination may contribute other pertinent information as well. Depending on the circumstances, checking for enlarged preauricular lymph nodes, sinus tenderness, temporal artery prominence, or skin or mucous membrane abnormalities may be diagnostically relevant.

SLIT LAMP EXAMINATION

Basic Slit Lamp Biomicroscopy

The slit lamp (Fig 2–4) is a table-mounted binocular microscope with a special adjustable illumination source attached. A linear slit beam of incandescent light is projected onto the globe, illuminating an optical cross section of the eye (Fig 2–5). The angle of illumination can be varied along with the width, length, and intensity of the light beam. The magnification can be adjusted as well (normally $10\times$ to $16\times$ power). Since the slit lamp is a binocular microscope, the view is "stereoscopic," or 3-dimensional.

The patient is seated while being examined, and the head is stabilized by an adjustable chin rest and forehead strap. Using the slit lamp alone, the anterior half of the globe—the "anterior segment"—can be visualized. Details of the lid margins and lashes, the palpebral and bulbar conjunctival surfaces, the tear film and cornea, the iris, and the aqueous can be studied. Through a dilated pupil, the crystalline lens and the anterior vitreous can be examined as well.

Because the slit beam of light provides an optical cross section of the eye, the precise anteroposterior location of abnormalities can be determined within each of the clear ocular structures (eg, cornea, lens, vitreous body). The highest magnification setting is sufficient to show the abnormal presence of cells within the aqueous, such as red or white blood cells or pigment granules. Aqueous turbidity, called "flare," resulting from increased protein concentration can be detected with intraocular inflammation. Normal aqueous is optically clear, without cells or flare.

Adjunctive Slit Lamp Techniques

The eye examination with the slit lamp is supplemented by the use of various techniques. Tonometry is discussed separately in a subsequent section.

A. Lid Eversion: Lid eversion to examine the undersurface of the upper lid can be performed either at the slit lamp or without the aid of that instrument. It should always be done if the presence of a foreign body is suspected. A semirigid plate of cartilage called the tarsus gives each lid its contour and shape. In the upper lid, the superior edge of the tarsus lies centrally about 8–9 mm above the lashes. On the undersurface of the lid, it is covered by the tarsal palpebral conjunctiva.

Following topical anesthesia, the patient is positioned at the slit lamp and instructed to look down. The examiner gently grasps the upper lashes with the thumb and index finger of one hand while using the other hand to position an applicator handle just above the superior edge of the tarsus (Fig 2–6). The lid is everted by applying slight downward pressure with the applicator as the lash margin is simultaneously lifted. The patient continues to look down, and the lashes are held pinned to the skin overlying the superior orbital rim, as the applicator is withdrawn. The tarsal conjunctiva is then examined under magnification. To undo eversion the lid margin is gently stroked downward as the patient looks up.

B. Fluorescein Staining: Fluorescein is a specialized dye that stains the cornea and highlights any irregularities of its epithelial surface. Sterile paper strips containing fluorescein are wetted and touched against the inner surface of the lower lid, instilling the yellowish dye into the tear film (Fig 2–7). The illuminating light of the slit lamp is made blue with a filter, causing the dye to fluoresce.

A uniform film of dye should cover the normal cornea. If the corneal surface is abnormal, excessive amounts of dye will absorb into or collect within the affected area. Abnormalities can range from tiny punctate dots, such as those resulting from excessive dryness or ultraviolet light damage, to large geographic defects in the epithelium such as those seen in corneal abrasions or infectious ulcers (see Fig 6–6).

C. Special Lenses: Special examining lenses can expand and further magnify the slit lamp examination of the eye's interior. A goniolens (Fig 2–29) provides visualization of the anterior chamber "angle" formed by the iridocorneal junction. Other lenses placed on or in front of the dilated eye allow slit lamp evaluation of the posterior half of the globe's interior—the "posterior segment." Since the slit lamp is a binocular microscope, these lenses provide a magnified 3-dimensional view of the posterior vitreous, the fundus, and the disk. Examples are the Goldmann-style

A

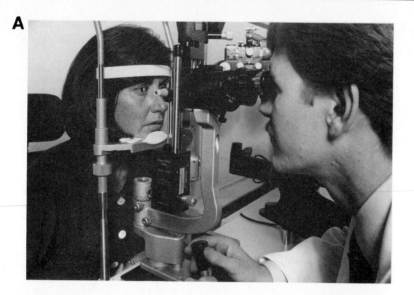

B

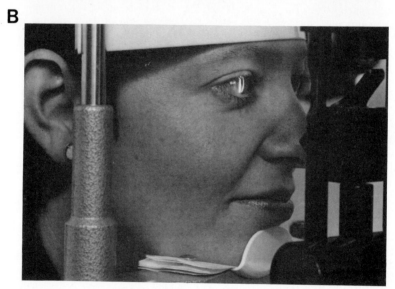

Figure 2–4. **A:** Slit lamp examination. **B:** Close-up view showing the slit beam of illuminating light. The anterior line of light is reflected from the cornea, while the posterior light is a reflection from the iris. (Photos by M Narahara.) (Courtesy of the American Academy of Ophthalmology.)

3-mirror lens (Fig 2–29), the Hruby lens, and the Volk-style 90-diopter biconvex lens.

D. Special Attachments: Special attachments to the slit lamp allow it to be used with a number of techniques requiring microscopic visualization. Special camera bodies can be attached for photographic documentation and for special applications such as corneal endothelial cell studies. Special instruments for study of visual potential (see p 82) require attachment to the slit lamp. Finally, laser sources are always attached to a slit lamp to allow microscopic control of eye treatment (Fig 2–30B).

TONOMETRY

The globe can be thought of as an enclosed compartment through which there is a constant circulation of aqueous humor. This fluid maintains the shape and a relatively uniform pressure within the globe. Tonometry is the method of measuring the intraocular fluid pressure using calibrated instruments that indent or flatten the corneal apex. As the eye becomes firmer, a greater force is required to cause the same amount of indentation. Pressures between 10 and 20 mm Hg are considered within the normal range.

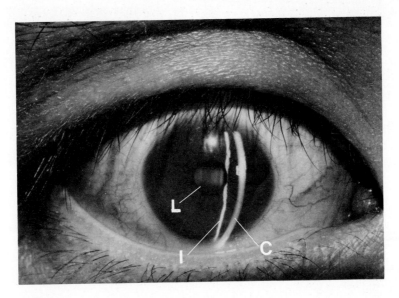

Figure 2–5. Slit lamp photograph of a normal right eye. The curved slit of light to the right is reflected off of the cornea (C), while the slit to the left is reflected off of the iris (I). As the latter slit passes through the pupil, the anterior lens (L) is faintly illuminated in cross section. (Photo by M Narahara.)

The 2 most common types of tonometry are the **Schiotz** and **applanation** methods. The Schiotz tonometer measures the amount of corneal indentation produced by a preset weight or force. The softer the eye, the more a given force will be able to indent the cornea. As the eye becomes firmer, less corneal indentation will result from the same amount of force.

In contrast to the Schiotz tonometer, the applanation tonometer can vary and measure the amount of force applied. The ocular pressure is determined by the force required to flatten the cornea by a predetermined standard amount. At lower intraocular pressures, less tonometer force is needed to achieve the standard degree of corneal flattening than at higher intraocular pressures. Since both methods employ devices that touch the patient's cornea, they require topical anesthetic and disinfection of the instrument tip prior to use. While retracting the lids with any method of tonometry, care must be taken to avoid pressing on the globe and artificially increasing its pressure. A new portable electronic tonometer, the Tono-Pen, has been developed, but clinical experience has been limited to date.

Schiotz Tonometry

The advantage of this method is that it is simple, requiring only a portable hand-held instrument—the Schiotz tonometer (Fig 2–8). It can be used in any clinic or emergency room setting, at the hospital bedside, or in the operating room. It is a practical device for the nonophthalmologist, who might use it to screen patients for glaucoma or to diagnose acute angle closure glaucoma in an emergency situation.

The 3 separate components of the tonometer should be cleaned, assembled, and then disassembled with each use. The tonometer **body** consists of a cylindric hollow plunger barrel fixed to a measuring scale with an indicator needle. The attached handle, which can slide along the outside of the cylindric barrel, supports the weight of the tonometer when it is not resting on the eye. The **plunger** is a slender blunt-tipped rod that is inserted into the barrel shaft, where it can slide back and forth. One end will touch the cornea, while the other end will deflect the needle of the measuring scale. The 5.5-g **weight** screwed onto the upper end of the plunger (farthest from the patient) keeps it from falling out of the shaft.

The patient is placed supine, and topical anesthetic is instilled into each eye. As the patient looks straight ahead, the lids are kept gently opened by lightly retracting the skin against the bony orbital rims. The tonometer is lowered with the other hand until the tip of the barrel balances on the cornea (Fig 2–9). Once the weight of the tonometer is fully supported by the globe, gravity—and not the examiner's hand—determines the force by which the instrument body rests on the eye.

The tip of the tonometer barrel has a concavity contoured to fit over the cornea, like a contact lens. The weight of the body is actually borne by the scleral wall and the limbus. With a force proportionate to its own separate weight, the blunt protruding plunger will press into and slightly indent the central cornea. The corneal resistance, which is proportionate to the intraocular pressure, will displace the plunger upward. As the plunger slides upward within the barrel, it will deflect the needle on the scale. The higher the intraocular pressure, the greater the corneal resistance to indentation, the more the plunger will be displaced

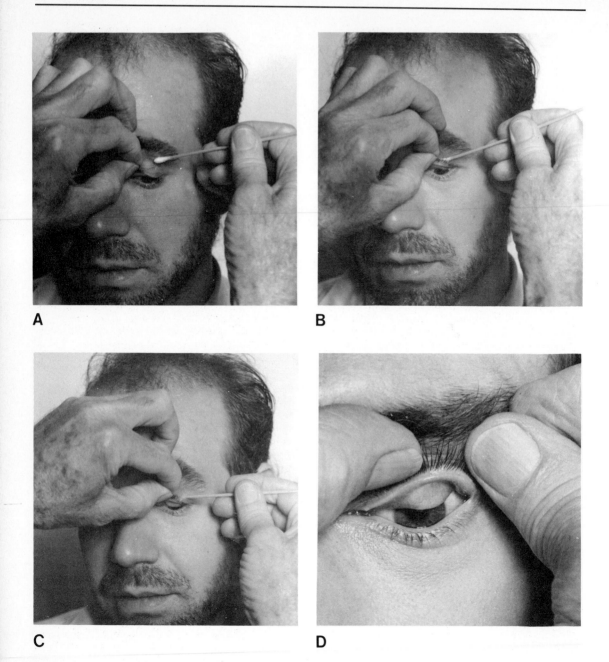

Figure 2–6. Technique of lid eversion. **A:** With the patient looking down, the upper lashes are grasped with one hand as an applicator stick is positioned at the superior edge of the upper tarsus (at the upper lid crease). **B and C:** As the lashes are lifted, slight downward pressure is simultaneously applied with the applicator stick. **D:** The thumb pins the lashes against the superior orbital rim, allowing examination of the undersurface of the tarsus. (Photos by M Narahara.)

upward, and the farther the needle will be deflected along the calibrated scale.

A conversion chart is used to translate the reading from the scale into millimeters of mercury. If the eye is firm, additional weights (7.5 g and 10 g) can be added to the plunger to increase the force brought to bear on the cornea. Calibration is checked by placing the tonometer on a ''cornea-shaped'' metal block that

should deflect the needle maximally so that it aligns with the ''0'' end of the scale.

Applanation Tonometry

The Goldmann applanation tonometer (Fig 2–10) is attached to the slit lamp and measures the amount of force required to flatten the corneal apex by a standard amount. The higher the intraocular pressure, the

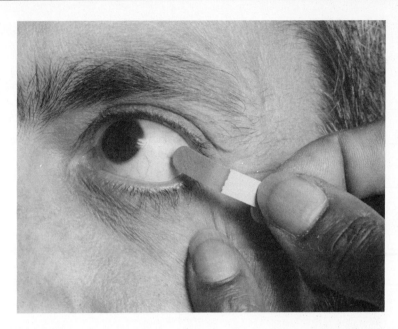

Figure 2–7. Instillation of fluorescein dye. (Photo by M Narahara.) Fluorescein staining of a dendritic epithelial defect due to herpes simplex keratitis is shown in Fig 6–6.

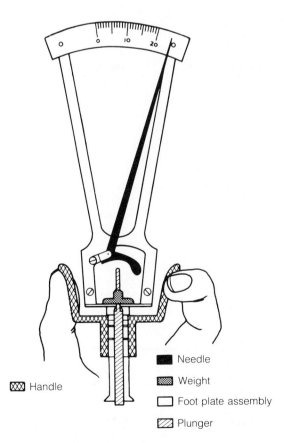

Figure 2–8. Diagram of Schiotz tonometer. The plunger is shown with the 5.5-g weight attached at one end.

greater the force required. Since Goldmann applanation tonometer is a more accurate method than Schiotz tonometry, it is preferred by ophthalmologists.

Following topical anesthesia and instillation of fluorescein, the patient is positioned at the slit lamp and the tonometer is swung into place. To visualize the fluorescein, the cobalt blue filter is used with the brightest illumination setting. After grossly aligning the tonometer in front of the cornea, the examiner looks through the slit lamp ocular just as the tip contacts the cornea. A manually controlled counterbalanced spring varies the force applied by the tonometer tip.

Upon contact, the tonometer tip flattens the central cornea and produces a thin circular outline of fluorescein. A prism in the tip visually splits this circle into 2 semicircles that appear green while viewed through the slit lamp oculars. The tonometer force is adjusted manually until the 2 semicircles just overlap, as shown in Fig 2–11. This visual end point indicates that the cornea has been flattened by the set standard amount. The amount of force required to do this is translated by the scale into a pressure reading in millimeters of mercury.

DIAGNOSTIC MEDICATIONS

Topical Anesthetics

Eyedrops such as proparacaine, tetracaine, and benoxinate provide rapid onset, short-acting topical anesthesia of the cornea, and conjunctiva. They are used

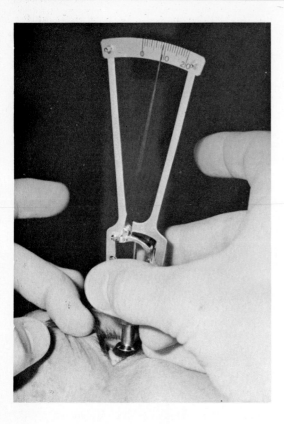

Figure 2–9. Schiotz tonometer placed on cornea. Handle is being held by thumb and third finger of right hand in this photo. (Photo by Diane Beeston.)

prior to ocular contact with diagnostic lenses and instruments such as the tonometer. Other diagnostic manipulations utilizing topical anesthetics will be discussed later. These include corneal and conjunctival scrapings, lacrimal canalicular and punctal probing, and scleral depression.

Mydriatic (Dilating) Drops

The pupil can be pharmacologically dilated by either stimulating the iris dilator muscle with a sympathomimetic agent (eg, 2.5% phenylephrine) or by inhibiting the sphincter muscle with an anticholinergic eye drop (eg, 0.5% or 1% tropicamide). Anticholinergic medications also inhibit accommodation, an effect called "cycloplegia." This may aid the process of refraction but causes further inconvenience for the patient. Therefore, drops with the shortest duration of action (usually several hours) are used for diagnostic applications. Combining drops from both pharmacologic classes produces the fastest onset (15–20 minutes) and widest dilation. Cholinergic "reversal" drops, such as pilocarpine, are not effective in speeding recovery from the effects of dilation.

Because dilatation can cause a small rise in intraocular pressure, tonometry should always be performed before these drops are instilled. There is also a risk of precipitating an attack of acute angle-closure glaucoma if the patient has preexisting narrow anterior chamber angles (between the iris and cornea). Such an eye can be identified using the technique illustrated in Fig 12–8. Finally, excessive instillation of these drops should be avoided because of the systemic absorption that can occur through the nasopharyngeal mucous membranes following lacrimal drainage.

A more complete discussion of diagnostic drops is found in Chapter 26.

DIRECT OPHTHALMOSCOPY

Instrumentation

The hand-held direct ophthalmoscope (Fig 2–12) provides a magnified (15×) monocular image of the ocular media and fundus. Because of its portability and the detailed view of the disk and retinal vasculature it provides, direct ophthalmoscopy is a standard part of the general medical examination as well as the ophthalmologic examination.

Darkening the room usually causes enough natural pupillary dilatation to allow evaluation of the central fundus, including the disk, the macula, and the proximal retinal vasculature. Pharmacologically dilating the pupil greatly enhances the view and permits a more extensive examination of the peripheral retina. The fundus examination is also optimized by holding the ophthalmoscope as close to the patient's pupil as possible (approximately 1–2 inches), just as one can see more through a keyhole by getting as close to it as possible. This requires using the examiner's right eye and hand to examine the patient's right eye and the left eye and hand to examine the patient's left eye (Fig 2–13). If the examiner wears spectacles, they can either be left on or off.

The intensity, color, and spot size of the illuminating light can be adjusted as well as the ophthalmoscope's point of focus. The latter is changed using a wheel of progressively higher power lenses that the examiner dials into place. These lenses are sequentially arranged and numbered according to their power in units called "diopters." The descending scale of black numbers designates the (+) converging lenses, whereas the ascending scale of red numbers designates the (−) divergent lenses.

As one dials this focusing wheel counterclockwise from high plus (+) lenses down to zero and on through increasingly minus (−) lenses, the focus is shifted progressively farther away from the ophthalmoscope toward the patient. By starting with a higher (+) lens and dialing in this direction, the examiner will eventually bring the cornea and iris into focus, followed several steps later by the retina. The refractive error (ie, "prescriptions") of the patient's and the examiner's eyes will determine the lens power needed to bring the fundus into optimal focus.

Fundus Examination

The primary value of the direct ophthalmoscope is

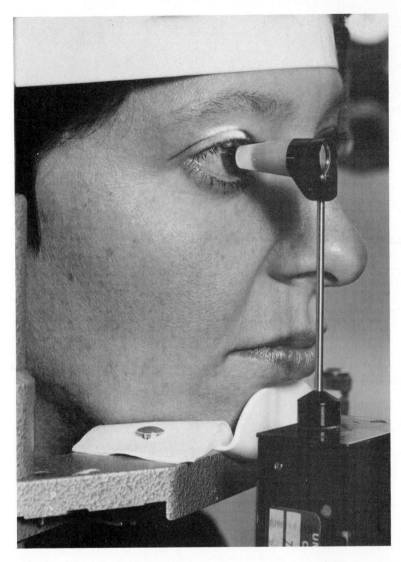

Figure 2–10. Applanation tonometry, using the Goldmann tonometer attached to the slit lamp. (Photo by M Narahara. Courtesy of the American Academy of Ophthalmology.)

Dial reading greater than pressure of globe

Dial reading less than pressure of globe

Dial reading equals pressure of globe

Figure 2–11. Appearance of fluorescein semicircles, or "mires," through the slit lamp ocular, showing the end point for applanation tonometry.

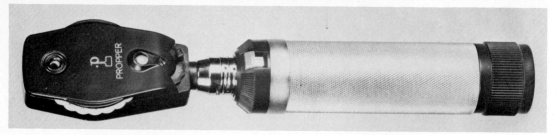

Figure 2–12. Direct ophthalmoscope. (Courtesy of Propper Manufacturing Co., Inc.)

in examination of the fundus (Fig 2–14). The view may be impaired by cloudy ocular media, such as a cataract, or by insufficient pupillary dilation. As the patient fixates on a distant target with the opposite eye, the examiner first brings retinal details into sharp focus. Since the retinal vessels all arise from the disk, the latter is located by following any major vascular branch back to this common origin. At this point, the ophthalmoscope beam will be aimed slightly nasal to the patient's line of vision, or "visual axis." One should study the shape, size, and color of the disk (Fig 2–15), the distinctness of its margins (Fig 2–16), and the size of the pale central "physiologic cup." The ratio of cup size to disk size is of diagnostic importance in glaucoma (Figs 2–17 and 2–18).

The macular area (Fig 2–14) is located approximately 2 "disk diameters" temporal to the edge of the disk. A small pinpoint white reflection or "reflex" marks the central fovea. This is surrounded by a more darkly pigmented and poorly circumscribed area called the macula. The retinal vascular branches approach from all sides but stop short of the fovea. Thus, its location can be confirmed by the focal absence of retinal vessels or by asking the patient to stare directly into the light.

The major retinal vessels are then examined and followed as far distally as possible in each of the 4 quadrants (superior, inferior, temporal, and nasal). The veins are darker and wider than their paired arteries. The vessels are examined for color, tortuosity,

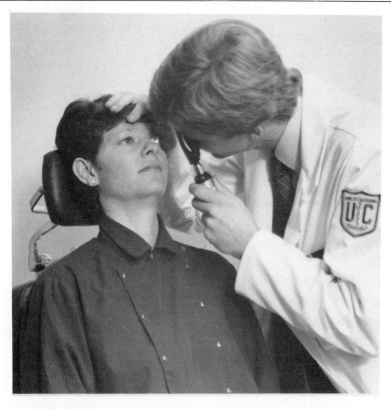

Figure 2–13. Direct ophthalmoscopy. The examiner uses the left eye to evaluate the patient's left eye. (Photo by M Narahara. Courtesy of the American Academy of Ophthalmology.)

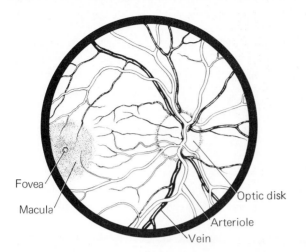
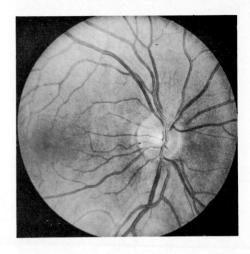

Fovea

Macula

Optic disk

Arteriole

Vein

Figure 2–14. Photo and corresponding diagram of a normal fundus. Note that the retinal vessels all stop short of and do not cross the fovea. (Photo by Diane Beeston.)

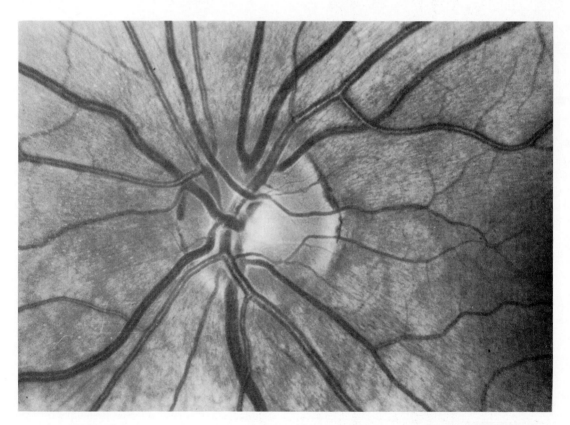

Figure 2–15. Ophthalmoscopic view of normal optic disk and peripapillary retina. (Courtesy of WF Hoyt.)

and caliber as well as for associated abnormalities such as aneurysms, hemorrhages, or exudates (see Fig 11–7). Sizes and distances within the fundus are often measured in "disk diameters (DD)." The typical optic disk is approximately 1.5 mm in diameter. Thus, one might describe a "1-DD area of hemorrhage located 2.5 DD inferotemporal to the fovea."

Dilating the pupil pharmacologically enables more

of the periphery to be visualized. The patient is asked to look in the direction of the quadrant one wishes to examine. Thus, the temporal retina of the right eye is seen when the patient looks temporally to the right, while the superior retina is seen when the patient looks up. This principle works because as the globe rotates about a point in the center of the eye, the retina and the cornea move in opposite directions. As the patient

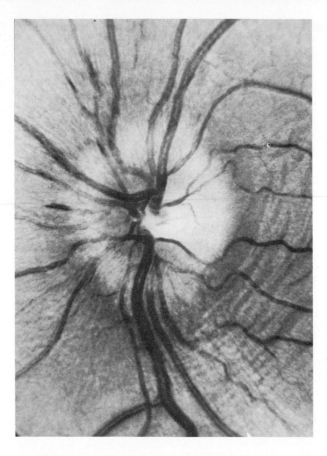

Figure 2–16. Early papilledema showing blurring of disk margins and peripapillary nerve fiber layer. The larger veins are engorged, while the smaller vessels crossing the edge of the disk are obscured by the surrounding edema. (See also Fig 15–8.) (Courtesy of WF Hoyt.)

looks up, the superior retina rotates downward into the examiner's line of vision.

The spot size and color of the illuminating light can be varied. If the pupil is well dilated, the large spot size of light affords the widest area of illumination. With a smaller pupil, however, much of this light would be reflected back toward the examiner's eye by the patient's iris, interfering with the view. For this reason, the smaller spot size of light is selected for undilated pupils. The green "red-free" filter can be used to highlight texture and small details within the retina. This filter eliminates the bright reddish-orange color of the fundus, providing more of a "black and white" rather than a "color" picture. This is helpful for studying the subtle striations of the nerve fiber layer as they course toward the disk (see Fig 15–7).

Anterior Segment Examination

As discussed earlier, the direct ophthalmoscope can be focused more anteriorly so as to provide a magnified view of the conjunctiva, cornea, and iris. The slit lamp allows a far superior and more magnified ex-amination of these areas, but it is not portable and may be unavailable.

Red Reflex Examination

If the illuminating light is aligned directly along the visual axis of a dilated pupil, the pupillary space will appear as a homogeneous bright reddish-orange color. This so-called red reflex is a reflection of the fundus color (actually the combined color of the choroidal vasculature and pigmentation) back through clear ocular media—the vitreous, lens, aqueous, and cornea. The red reflex is best observed by holding the ophthalmoscope at arm's length from the patient as he looks toward the illuminating light. By dialing the lens wheel, the bright red reflex will appear when the ophthalmoscope is focused on the plane of the pupil.

Any opacity located along this central optical pathway will block all or part of this bright reflex and appear as a dark spot or shadow. If a small opacity is seen, have the patient look momentarily away and then back toward the light. If the opacity is still moving or floating, it is located within the vitreous (eg, small hemorrhage). If it is stationary, it is probably in the

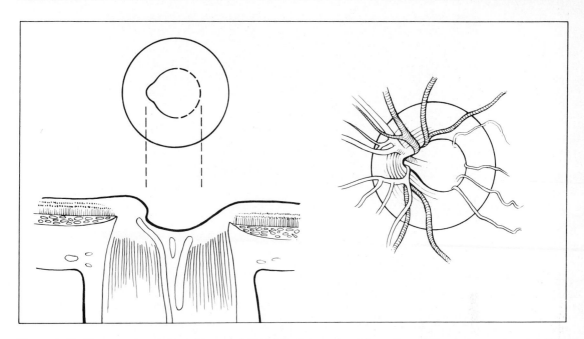

Figure 2–17. Diagram of a moderately cupped disk viewed on end and in profile, with an accompanying sketch for the patient's record. The width of the central cup divided by the width of the disk is the "cup-to-disk ratio." The cup-to-disk ratio of this disk is approximately 0.5.

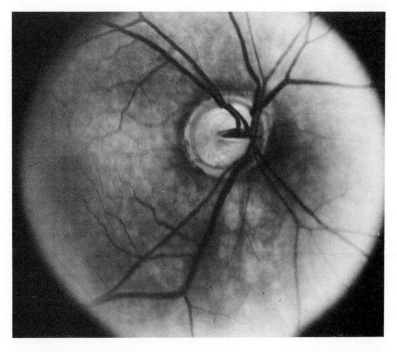

Figure 2–18. Cup-to-disk ratio of 0.9 in a patient with end-stage glaucoma. The normal disk tissue is compressed into a peripheral thin rim surrounding a huge pale cup.

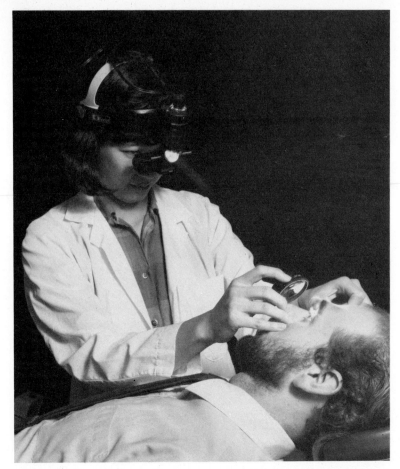

Figure 2–19. Examination with head-mounted binocular indirect ophthalmoscope. A 20-diopter hand-held condensing lens is used. (Photo by M Narahara.)

lens (eg, focal cataract) or on the cornea (eg, scar). Less red reflex is visible with a small pupil, limiting the usefulness of this test.

INDIRECT OPHTHALMOSCOPY

Instrumentation

The binocular indirect ophthalmoscope (Fig 2–19) complements and supplements the direct ophthalmoscopic examination. Since it requires wide pupillary dilatation and is difficult to learn, this technique is used primarily by ophthalmologists. The patient can be examined while seated, but the supine position is preferable.

The indirect ophthalmoscope is worn on the examiner's head and allows binocular viewing through a set of lenses of fixed power. A bright adjustable light source attached to the headband is directed toward the patient's eye. As with direct ophthalmoscopy, the patient is told to look in the direction of the quadrant being examined. A convex lens is hand-held several inches from the patient's eye in precise orientation so as to simultaneously focus light onto the retina and an image of the retina in midair between the patient and the examiner. Using the preset head-mounted ophthalmoscope lenses, the examiner can then "focus on" and visualize this midair image of the retina.

Comparison of Indirect & Direct Ophthalmoscopy

Indirect ophthalmoscopy is so called because one is viewing an "image" of the retina formed by a hand-held "condensing lens." In contrast, direct ophthalmoscopy allows one to focus on the retina itself. Compared with the direct ophthalmoscope ($15 \times$ magnification), indirect ophthalmoscopy provides a much wider field of view (Fig 2–20) with less overall magnification (approximately $3.5 \times$ using a standard 20-diopter hand-held condensing lens). Thus, it presents a wide panoramic fundus view from which specific areas can be selectively studied under higher magnification using either the direct ophthalmoscope or the slit lamp with special auxiliary lenses.

Indirect ophthalmoscopy has 3 distinct advantages

A

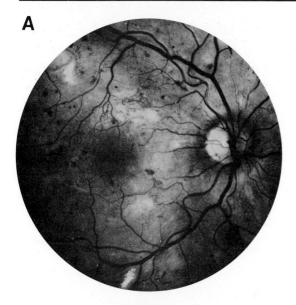

B

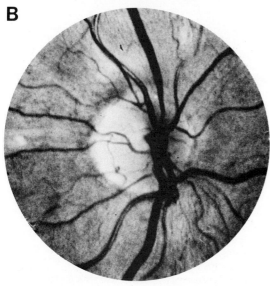

Figure 2–20. Comparison of view within the same fundus using the indirect ophthalmoscope **(A)** and the direct ophthalmoscope **(B).** The field of view with the latter is approximately 10 degrees, compared with approximately 37 degrees using the indirect ophthalmoscope. In this patient with diabetic retinopathy, an important overview is first seen with the indirect ophthalmoscope. The direct ophthalmoscope can then provide magnified details of a specific area. (Photos by M Narahara.)

over direct ophthalmoscopy. One is the brighter light source that permits much better visualization through cloudy media. A second advantage is that by using both eyes, the examiner enjoys a stereoscopic view, allowing visualization of elevated masses or retinal detachment in 3 dimensions. Finally, indirect ophthalmoscopy can be used to examine the entire retina even out to its extreme periphery, the ora serrata. This

is possible for 2 reasons. Optical distortions caused by looking through the peripheral lens and cornea interfere very little with the indirect ophthalmoscopic examination, compared with the direct ophthalmoscope. In addition, the adjunct technique of scleral depression can be used.

Scleral depression (Fig 2–21) is performed as the peripheral retina is being examined with the indirect ophthalmoscope. A smooth, thin metal probe is used to gently indent the globe externally through the lids at a point just behind the corneoscleral junction (limbus). As this is done, the ora serrata and peripheral retina are pushed internally into the examiner's line of view. By depressing around the entire circumference, the peripheral retina can be viewed in its entirety.

Because of all of these advantages, indirect ophthalmoscopy is used preoperatively and intraoperatively in the evaluation and surgical repair of retinal detachments. A minor disadvantage of indirect ophthalmoscopy is that it provides an inverted image of the fundus, which requires a mental adjustment on the examiner's part. Its brigher light source can also be more uncomfortable for the patient.

EYE EXAMINATION BY THE NONOPHTHALMOLOGIST

The preceding sequence of tests would comprise a complete routine or diagnostic ophthalmologic evaluation. A general medical examination would often include many of these same testing techniques.

Assessment of pupils, extraocular movements, and confrontation visual fields is part of any complete neurologic assessment. Direct ophthalmoscopy should always be performed to assess the appearance of the disk and retinal vessels. Separately testing the visual acuity of each eye (particularly with children) may uncover either a refractive or a medical cause of decreased vision. Finally, screening tonometry measurements using the Schiotz tonometer may detect the asymptomatic elevated intraocular pressure of glaucoma, a prevalent condition among the elderly.

The 3 most common preventable causes of permanent visual loss in developed nations are amblyopia, diabetic retinopathy, and glaucoma. All can remain asymptomatic while the opportunity for prevention is gradually lost. During this time, the pediatrician or general medical practitioner may be the only physician the patient visits.

By testing children for visual acuity in each eye, examining and referring diabetics for regular dilated fundus ophthalmoscopy, and referring patients with suspicious discs or tonometry readings to the ophthalmologist, the nonophthalmologist may indeed be the one who truly ''saves'' that patient's eyesight. This represents both an important opportunity and responsibility for every primary care physician.

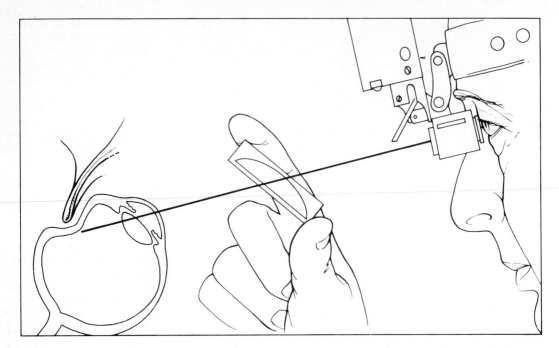

Figure 2–21. Diagrammatic representation of indirect ophthalmoscopy with scleral depression to examine the far peripheral retina. Indentation of the sclera through the lids brings the peripheral edge of the retina into visual alignment with the dilated pupil, the hand-held condensing lens, and the head-mounted ophthalmoscope.

III. SPECIALIZED OPHTHALMOLOGIC EXAMINATIONS

This section will discuss ophthalmologic examination techniques with more specific indications that would not be performed on a routine basis. They will be grouped according to the function or anatomic area of primary interest.

DIAGNOSIS OF VISUAL ABNORMALITIES

1. PERIMETRY

Perimetry is used to examine the central and peripheral visual fields. This technique, which is performed separately for each eye, measures the combined function of the retina, the optic nerve, and the intracranial visual pathway. It is used clinically to detect or monitor field loss due to disease at any of these locations. Damage to specific parts of the neurologic visual pathway may produce characteristic patterns of change on serial field examinations.

The visual field of the eye is measured and plotted in degrees of arc. Measurement of degrees of arc remains constant regardless of the distance from the

eye the field is checked. The sensitivity of vision is greatest in the center of the field (corresponding to the fovea) and least in the periphery. Perimetry relies on subjective patient responses, and the results will depend on the patient's psychomotor as well as visual status. Perimetry must always be performed and interpreted with this in mind.

The Principles of Testing

Although perimetry is subjective, the methods discussed below have been standardized to maximize reproducibility and permit subsequent comparison. Perimetry requires (1) steady fixation and attention by the patient; (2) a set distance from the eye to the screen or testing device; (3) a uniform, standard amount of background illumination and contrast; (4) test targets of standard size and brightness; and (5) a universal protocol for administration of the test by examiners.

As the patient's eye fixates on a central target, test objects are randomly presented at different locations throughout the field. If they are seen, the patient responds either verbally or with a hand-held signaling device. Varying the target's size or brightness permits quantification of visual sensitivity of different areas in the field. The smaller or dimmer the target seen, the better the sensitivity of that location.

There are 2 basic methods of target presentation—static and kinetic—that can be used alone or in combination during an examination. In **static perimetry,** different locations throughout the field are tested one at a time. A difficult test object, such as a dim light, is first presented at a particular location. If it is not seen, the size or intensity of the light is incrementally increased until it is just large enough or bright enough to be detected. This is called the "threshold" sensitivity level of that location. This sequence is repeated at a series of other locations, so that the light sensitivity of multiple points in the field can be evaluated and combined to form a profile of the visual field.

In **kinetic perimetry,** the sensitivity of the entire field to one single test object (of fixed size and brightness) is first tested. The object is slowly moved toward the center from a peripheral area until it is first spotted. By moving the same object inward from multiple different directions, a boundary called an **"isopter"** can be mapped out which is specific for that target. The isopter outlines the area within which the target can be seen and beyond which it cannot be seen. Thus, the larger the isopter, the better the visual field of that eye. The boundaries of the isopter are measured and plotted in degrees of arc. By repeating the test using objects of different size or brightness, multiple isopters can then be plotted for a given eye. The smaller or dimmer test objects will produce smaller isopters.

Methods of Perimetry

The **tangent screen** is the simplest apparatus for standardized perimetry. It utilizes different-sized white pins on a black wand presented against a black screen and is used primarily to test the central 30 degrees of visual field. The advantages of this method are its simplicity and rapidity, the possibility of changing the subject's distance from the screen, and the option of using any assortment of fixation and test objects, including different colors.

The more sophisticated **Goldmann perimeter** (Fig 2–22) is a hollow white spherical bowl positioned a set distance in front of the patient. A light of variable size and intensity can be presented by the examiner (seated behind the perimeter) in either static or kinetic fashion. This method can test the full limit of peripheral vision and was for years the primary method for plotting fields in glaucoma patients.

Computerized automated perimeters (Fig 2–23) now constitute the most sophisticated and sensitive equipment available for visual field testing. These instruments display test lights of varying brightness and size but use a quantitative static threshold testing format that is more precise and comprehensive than other methods. Numerical scores (Fig 2–24) corresponding to the threshold sensitivity of each test location can be stored in the computer memory and compared statistically with results from previous examinations or from other normal patients. The higher the numerical score, the better the visual sensitivity of that location in the field. Another important advantage is that the test presentation is programmed and automated, eliminating any variability on the part of the examiner.

2. AMSLER GRID

The Amsler grid is used to test the central 20 degrees of the visual field. The grid (Fig 2–25) is viewed by each eye separately at normal reading distance and with reading glasses on if the patient uses them. It is most commonly used to test macular function.

While fixating on the central dot, the patient checks to see that the lines are all straight, without distortion,

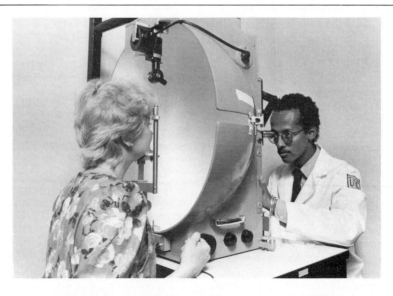

Figure 2–22. Goldmann perimeter. (Photo by M Narahara.)

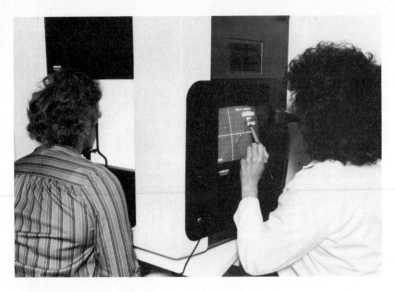

Figure 2–23. Computerized automated perimeter. (Photo by M Narahara.)

and that no spots or portions of the grid are missing. One eye is compared with the other. A scotoma or blank area—either central or paracentral—can indicate disease of the macula or optic nerve. Wavy distortion of the lines (metamorphopsia) can indicate macular edema or submacular fluid.

The grid can be used by patients at home to test their own central vision. For example, patients with age-related macular degeneration (see Chapter 11) can use the grid to monitor for sudden metamorphopsia. This often is the earliest symptom of acute fluid accumulation beneath the macula arising from leaking subretinal neovascularization. Since these abnormal vessels can be treatable with the laser, early detection is important.

3. BRIGHTNESS ACUITY TESTING

The visual abilities of patients with media opacities may vary depending on conditions of lighting. For example, when dim illumination makes the pupil larger, one may be able to "see around" a central focal cataract, whereas bright illumination causing pupillary constriction would have the contrary effect. Bright lights may also cause disabling glare in patients with corneal edema or diffuse clouding of the crystalline lens.

Because the darkened examining room may not accurately reflect the patient's functional difficulties in real life, instruments have been developed to test the effect of varying levels of brightness or glare on visual acuity. Distance acuity with the Snellen chart is usually tested under standard levels of incrementally increasing illumination, and the information may be helpful in making therapeutic or surgical decisions. Asking cataract patients specific questions about how their vision is affected by various lighting conditions is even more important.

4. COLOR VISION TESTING

Normal color vision requires healthy function of the macula and optic nerve. The most common abnormality is X-linked red-green "color blindness," which is present in approximately 8% of the male population. This is due to an X-linked congenital deficiency of one specific type of retinal photoreceptor. Depressed color vision may also be a sensitive indicator of certain kinds of acquired macular or optic nerve disease. For example, in optic neuritis or optic nerve compression (eg, by a mass), abnormal color vision is often an earlier indication of disease than visual acuity, which may still be 20/20.

The most common testing technique utilizes a series of polychromatic plates, such as those of Ishihara or Hardy-Rand-Rittler (Fig 2–26). The plates are made up of dots of the primary colors printed on a background mosaic of similar dots in a confusing variety of secondary colors. The primary dots are arranged in simple patterns (numbers or geometric shapes) that cannot be recognized by patients with deficient color perception.

5. CONTRAST SENSITIVITY TESTING

Contrast sensitivity is the ability of the eye to discern subtle degrees of contrast. Retinal and optic nerve

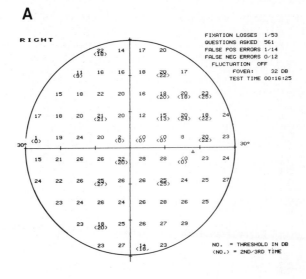

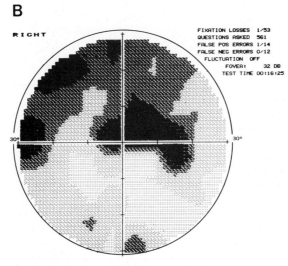

Figure 2–24. *A:* Numerical printout of threshold sensitivity scores derived by using the static method of computerized perimetry. This is the 30-degree field of a patient's right eye with glaucoma. The higher the numbers, the better the visual sensitivity. The computer retests many of the points (bracketed numbers) to assess consistency of the patient's responses. *B:* Diagrammatic "gray scale" display of these same numerical scores. The darker the area, the poorer the visual sensitivity at that location.

disease and clouding of the ocular media (eg, cataracts) can impair this ability. Like color vision, contrast sensitivity may become depressed before Snellen visual acuity is affected in many situations.

Contrast sensitivity is best tested by using standard preprinted charts with a series of test targets (Fig 2–27). Since illumination greatly affects contrast, it must be standardized and checked with a light meter. Each separate target consists of a series of dark parallel lines in one of 3 different orientations. They are displayed against a lighter, contrasting gray background. As the contrast between the lines and their background is progressively reduced from one target to the next, it becomes more difficult for the patient to judge the orientation of the lines. The patient can be scored

according to the lowest level of contrast at which the pattern of lines can still be discerned.

6. ASSESSING POTENTIAL VISION

When opacities of the cornea or lens coexist with disease of the macula or optic nerve, the visual potential of the eye is often in doubt. The benefit of corneal transplantation or cataract extraction will depend on the severity of coexisting retinal or optic nerve impairment. Several methods are available for assessing central visual potential under these circumstances.

Even with a totally opaque cataract that completely

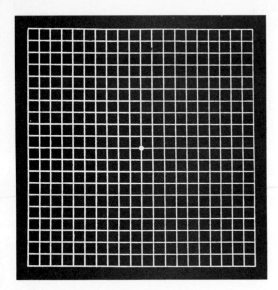

Figure 2–25. Amsler grid.

prevents a view of the fundus, the patient should still be able to identify the direction of a light directed into the eye from different quadrants. When a red lens is held in front of the light, the patient should be able to differentiate between white and red light. The presence of a Marcus Gunn afferent pupillary defect (see p 24) indicates significant disease of the retina or optic nerve and thus a poor visual prognosis.

A gross test of macular function involves the patient's ability to perceive so-called **entoptic phenomena.** For example, as the eyeball is massaged with a rapidly moving penlight through the closed lids, the patient should be able to visualize an image of the paramacular vascular branches if the macula is healthy. These may be described as looking like ''the veins of a leaf.'' Because this test is highly subjective and subject to interpretation, it is only helpful if the patient is able to recognize the vascular pattern in at least one eye. Absence of the pattern in the opposite eye then suggests macular impairment.

In addition to these gross methods, sophisticated quantitative instruments have been developed for more direct determination of visual potential in eyes with media opacities. These instruments project a narrow beam of light containing a pattern of images through any relatively clear portion of the media (eg, through a less dense region of a cataract) and onto the retina. The patient's vision is then graded according to the size of the smallest patterns that can be seen.

Two different types of patterns are used. **Laser interferometry** employs laser light to generate interference fringes or gratings, which the patient sees as a series of parallel lines. Progressively narrowing the width and spacing of the lines causes an end point to be reached where the patient can no longer discern the orientation of the lines. The narrowest image width the patient can resolve is then correlated with a Snellen acuity measurement to determine the visual potential of that eye. The **potential acuity meter** projects a standard Snellen acuity chart onto the retina (Fig 2–28). The patient is then graded in the usual fashion, according to the smallest line of letters read.

Although both instruments appear useful in measuring potential visual acuity, false-positive and false-negative results do occur, with a frequency dependent on the type of disease present. Thus, these methods are helpful but not completely reliable in determining the visual prognosis of eyes with cloudy media.

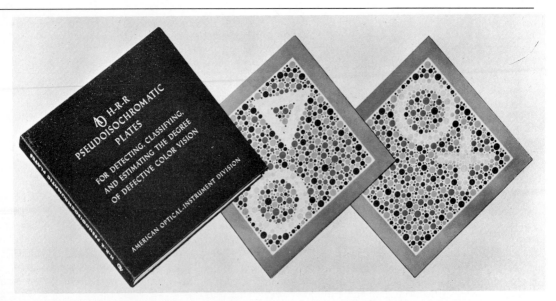

Figure 2–26. Hardy-Rand-Rittler (H-R-R) pseudoisochromatic plates for testing color vision.

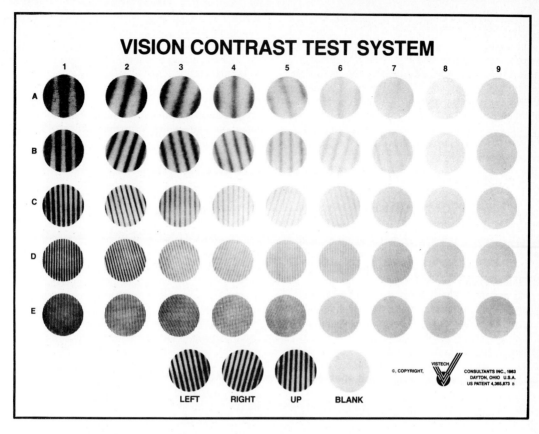

Figure 2–27. Contrast sensitivity test chart. (Courtesy of Vistech Consultants, Inc.)

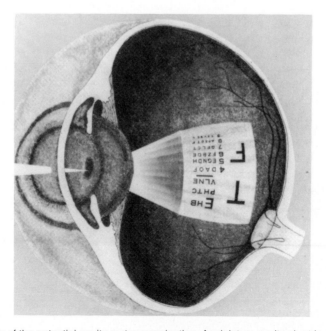

Figure 2–28. The principle of the potential acuity meter examination. A miniature acuity chart is projected directly onto the retina by selectively aiming it through the clearest portion of the cataract. This helps to estimate what the vision could be if the retina were unobstructed by media opacity. (Courtesy of Mentor O & O, Inc.)

7. TESTS FOR FUNCTIONAL VISUAL LOSS

The measurement of vision is subjective, requiring responses on the part of the patient. The validity of the test may therefore be limited by the alertness or cooperation of the patient. "Functional" visual loss is a subjective complaint of impaired vision without any demonstrated organic or objective basis. Examples include hysterical blindness and malingering.

Recognition of functional visual loss or malingering depends on the use of testing variations in order to elicit inconsistent or contradictory responses. An example would be eliciting "tunnel" visual fields using the tangent screen.

A patient claiming "poor vision" and tested at the standard distance of 1 meter may map out a narrow central zone of intact vision beyond which even large objects—such as a hand—allegedly cannot be seen. The borders ("isopter") of this apparently small area are then marked.

The patient is then moved back to a position 2 meters from the tangent screen. From this position, the field should be twice as large as the area plotted from 1 meter away. If the patient outlines an area of the same size from both testing distances, he will have produced a response that is not physically possible. This would raise a strong suspicion of malingering.

A variety of other different tests can be chosen to assess the validity of different degrees of visual loss that may be in question.

DIAGNOSIS OF OCULAR ABNORMALITIES

1. MICROBIOLOGY & CYTOLOGY

Like any mucous membrane, the conjunctiva can be cultured with swabs for the identification of bacterial infection. Specimens for cytologic examination are obtained by lightly scraping the palpebral conjunctiva (ie, lining the inner aspect of the lid) with a small platinum spatula following topical anesthesia. For the cytologic evaluation of conjunctivitis, Giemsa's stain is used to identify the types of inflammatory cells present, while Gram's stain may demonstrate the presence (and type) of bacteria. These applications are discussed at length in Chapter 5.

The cornea is normally sterile. The base of any suspected infectious corneal ulcer should be scraped with the platinum spatula for Gram staining and culture. This procedure is performed at the slit lamp following topical anesthesia. Because in many cases only trace quantities of bacteria are recoverable, the spatula should be used to plate the specimen directly onto the culture plate without the intervening use of transport media. Any amount of culture growth, no matter how scant, is considered significant, but many cases of infection may still be "culture-negative."

Culture of intraocular fluids is the only reliable method of diagnosing or ruling out infectious endophthalmitis. Aqueous can be tapped by inserting a short 25-gauge needle on a tuberculin syringe through the limbus parallel to the iris. Care must be taken not to traumatize the lens. The diagnostic yield is better if vitreous is cultured. Vitreous specimens can be obtained by a needle tap through the pars plana or by doing a surgical vitrectomy. In the evaluation of noninfectious intraocular inflammation, cytology specimens are occasionally obtained using similar techniques.

2. TECHNIQUES FOR CORNEAL EXAMINATION

Several additional techniques are available for more specialized evaluation of the cornea. The **keratometer** is a calibrated instrument that measures the radius of curvature of the cornea in 2 meridians 90 degrees apart. If the cornea is not perfectly spherical, the 2 radii will be different. This is called **astigmatism** and is quantified by measuring the difference between the 2 radii of curvature. Keratometer measurements are used in contact lens fitting and for intraocular lens power calculations prior to cataract surgery.

Many corneal diseases result in distortion of the otherwise smooth surface of the cornea, which impairs its optical quality. The **keratoscope** is an instrument that assesses the uniformity and evenness of the surface by reflecting a pattern of concentric circles onto it. This pattern, which can be visualized and photographed through the instrument, should normally appear perfectly regular and uniform. Focal corneal irregularities will instead distort the circular patterns reflected from that particular area.

The endothelium is an irreplaceable monolayer of cells lining the posterior corneal surface. These cells function as fluid pumps and are responsible for keeping the cornea thin and dehydrated, thereby maintaining its optical clarity. If these cells become impaired or depleted, corneal edema and thickening result, ultimately decreasing vision. Central corneal thickness can be accurately measured with a **pachymeter,** a device for quantifying and monitoring these changes. The endothelial cells themselves can be photographed with a special slit lamp camera, enabling one to study cell morphology and perform cell counts.

3. GONIOSCOPY

The anterior chamber—the space between the iris and the cornea—is filled with liquid aqueous humor. The aqueous, which is produced behind the iris by the ciliary body, exits the eye through a tiny sievelike drainage network called the trabecular meshwork. The meshwork is arranged as a thin circumferential band of tissue just anterior to the base of the iris and within the angle formed by the iridocorneal junction (Fig 12–1). This angle recess can vary in its anatomy, pig-

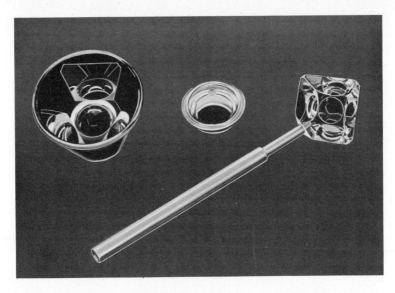

Figure 2–29. Three types of goniolenses. **Left:** Goldmann 3-mirror lens. Besides the goniomirror, there are also 2 peripheral retinal mirrors and a central fourth mirror for examining the central retina. **Center:** Koeppe lens. **Right:** Posner/Zeiss-type lens. (Photo by M Narahara.)

mentation, and width of opening—all of which may affect aqueous drainage and be of diagnostic relevance for glaucoma.

Gonioscopy is the method of examination of the anterior chamber angle anatomy using binocular magnification and a special **goniolens.** The Goldmann and Posner/Zeiss types of goniolenses (Fig 2–29) have special mirrors angled so as to provide a line of view parallel with the iris surface and directed peripherally toward the angle recess.

After topical anesthesia, the patient is seated at the slit lamp and the goniolens is placed on the eye (Fig 2–30A). Magnified details of the anterior chamber angle are viewed stereoscopically. By rotating the mirror, the entire 360-degree circumference of the angle can be examined. The same lens can be used to direct laser treatment toward the angle as therapy for glaucoma (Fig 2–30B).

A third type of goniolens, the Koeppe lens, requires a special illuminator and a separate handheld binocular microscope. It is used with the patient lying supine and can thus be used in the office or in the operating room (either diagnostically or for surgery).

4. GOLDMANN THREE-MIRROR LENS

The Goldmann lens is a versatile adjunct to the slit lamp examination (Fig 2–29). Three separate mirrors, all with different angles of orientation, allow the examiner's line of sight to be directed peripherally at 3 different angles while using the standard slit lamp. The most anterior and acute angle of view is achieved with the goniolens, discussed above.

Through a dilated pupil, the other 2 mirrored lenses

angle the examiner's view toward the retinal mid periphery and far periphery, respectively. As with gonioscopy, each lens can be rotated 360 degrees circumferentially and can be used to aim laser treatment. A fourth central lens (no mirror) is used to examine the posterior vitreous and the centralmost area of the retina. The stereoscopic magnification of this method provides the greatest 3-dimensional detail of the macula and disk.

The patient's side of the lens has a concavity designed to fit directly over the topically anesthetized cornea. A clear, viscous solution of methylcellulose is placed in the concavity of the lens prior to insertion onto the patient's eye. This eliminates interference from optical interfaces, such as bubbles, and provides mild adhesion of the lens to the eye for stabilization.

5. FUNDUS PHOTOGRAPHY

Special retinal cameras are used to document details of the fundus for study and future comparison. Standard film is used for 35 mm color slides which can be easily stored. As with any form of ophthalmoscopy, a dilated pupil and clear ocular media provide the most optimal view. All of the fundus photographs in this textbook were taken with such a camera.

One of the most common applications is disk photography, used in the evaluation for glaucoma. Since the slow progression of glaucomatous optic nerve damage may be evident only by subtle alteration of the disk's appearance over time (see Chapter 13), precise documentation of its morphology is needed. By slightly moving the camera angle on two consecutive shots, a "stereo" pair of slides can be produced

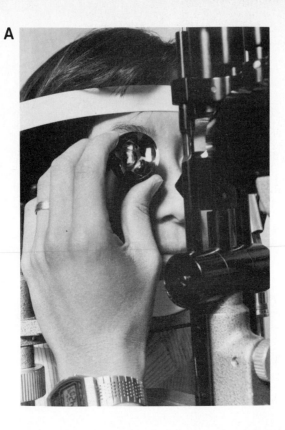

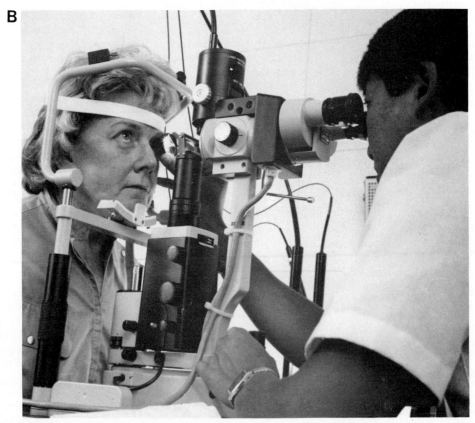

Figure 2–30. *A:* Gonioscopy with slit lamp and Goldmann type lens. (Photo by M Narahara.) *B:* Laser treatment for glaucoma can also be performed in this manner.

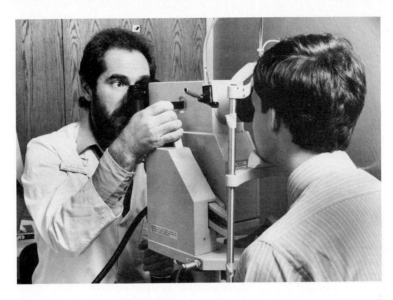

Figure 2–31. Fluorescein angiography with fundus camera. (Photo by M Narahara.)

which will provide a three-dimensional image when studied through a stereo slide viewer. Stereo disk photography thus provides the most sensitive means of detecting increases in glaucomatous cupping.

6. FLUORESCEIN ANGIOGRAPHY

The capabilities of fundus photographic imaging can be tremendously enhanced by fluorescein, a dye whose molecules emit green light when stimulated by blue light. When photographed, the dye highlights vascular and anatomic details of the fundus. Fluorescein angiography has become indispensable in the diagnosis and evaluation of many retinal conditions. Because it can so precisely delineate areas of abnormality, it is an essential guide for planning laser treatment of retinal vascular disease.

Technique
The patient is seated in front of the retinal camera following pupillary dilation (Fig 2–31). After a small amount of fluorescein is injected into a vein in the arm, it circulates throughout the body before eventually being excreted by the kidneys. As the dye passes through the retinal and choroidal circulation, it can be visualized and photographed because of its properties of fluorescence. Two special filters within the camera produce this effect. A blue **"excitatory"** filter bombards the fluorescein molecules with blue light from the camera flash, causing them to emit a green light. The **"barrier"** filter allows only this emitted green light to reach the photographic film, blocking out all other wavelengths of light. A black and white photograph results in which only the fluorescein image is seen.

Because the fluorescein molecules do not diffuse

out of normal retinal vessels, the latter are highlighted photographically by the dye, as seen in Fig 2–32. The diffuse, background "ground glass" appearance results from fluorescein filling of the separate underlying choroidal circulation. The choroidal and retinal circulations are anatomically separated by a thin, homogeneous monolayer of pigmented cells—the "retinal pigment epithelium." Denser pigmentation located in the macula obscures more of this background choroidal fluorescence (Fig 2–32) causing the

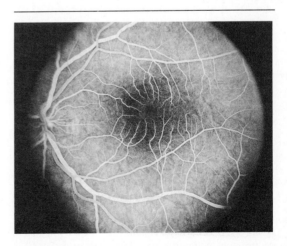

Figure 2–32. Normal angiogram of the central retina. The photo has been taken after the dye (appearing white) has already sequentially filled the choroidal circulation (seen as a diffuse, mottled whitish background), the arterioles and the veins. The macula appears dark due to heavier pigmentation which obscures the underlying choroidal fluorescence that is visible everywhere else. (Photo courtesy of R Griffith and T King.)

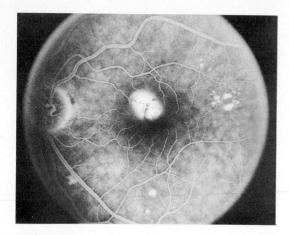

Figure 2–33. Abnormal angiogram in which dye-stained fluid originating from the choroid has pooled beneath the macula. This is one type of abnormality associated with age-related macular degeneration (see Chapter 11). Secondary atrophy of the overlying retinal pigment epithelium in this area causes heightened, unobscured visibility of this increased fluorescence. (Photo courtesy of R Griffith and T King.)

darker central zone on the photograph. In contrast, focal atrophy of the pigment epithelium causes an abnormal increase in visibility of the background fluorescence (Fig 2–33).

Applications

A high-speed motorized film advance allows for rapid sequence photography of the dye's transit through the retinal and choroidal circulations over time. A fluorescein study or "angiogram" therefore consists of multiple black and white photos of the fundi taken at different times following dye injection (Fig 2–34). Early phase photos document the dye's initial rapid, sequential perfusion of the choroid, the retinal arteries, and the retinal veins. Later phase photos may, for example, demonstrate the gradual, delayed leakage of dye from abnormal vessels. This extravascular dye-stained edema fluid will persist long after the intravascular fluorescein has exited the eye.

Fig 2–34 illustrates several of the retinal vascular abnormalities that are well demonstrated by fluorescein angiography. The dye delineates structural vascular alterations, such as aneurysms or neovascularization. Changes in blood flow such as ischemia and vascular occlusion are seen as an interruption of the normal perfusion pattern. Abnormal vascular permeability is seen as a leaking cloud of dye-stained edema fluid increasing over time. Hemorrhage does not stain with dye but rather appears as a dark, sharply demarcated void. This is due to blockage and obscuration of the underlying background fluorescence.

In addition to the fundus, vascular details of the iris can be evaluated with fluorescein angiography as well. The clinical usefulness of this technique is limited however.

7. ELECTRORETINOGRAPHY

Physiologically, "vision" is a series of neurologic synapses and events initiated in the retina and ending in the occipital cortex. Electroretinography and visual evoked response testing are 2 methods of evaluating the neurologic integrity of the visual pathway.

Technique

Since the retina is neurologic tissue, the normal retina exhibits certain electrical responses when stimulated by light. Electroretinography measures the normal change in electrical potential of the eye caused by a diffuse flash of light. A recording electrode is placed on the cornea by means of a special contact lens. Following a light stimulus, it detects the change in electrical potential and records it as a single, composite oscilloscope waveform composed of several components. This is called the electroretinogram, or ERG.

The retina is a complex tissue composed of several uniformly arranged layers of neurons (see Fig 11–2). The outermost layer contains the photoreceptor cells (rods and cones), which sense the light and are responsible for the initial electrical component of the ERG waveform. This photoreceptor-generated impulse is called the "a wave." The photoreceptors next synapse with a series of interneurons located within the middle layer of the retina, called bipolar cells. This electrical event produces the "b wave" deflection of the ERG waveform. The interneuron bipolar cells finally synapse with the ganglion cells of the innermost layer of the retina. The axons of the ganglion cells comprise the retinal nerve fiber layer and the optic nerve. Because their axons do not synapse until they reach the brain, the retinal ganglion cells do not contribute to the electrical potentials (ERG) measured by the corneal electrode.

Interpretation

The pattern, the amplitude, and the latency of the ERG waveform and its component parts are examined. A normal ERG waveform signifies functional integrity of the retina, exclusive of the ganglion cell layer. Thus, disease involving the ganglion cells and the optic nerve (ie, the ganglion cell axons) will not be detected by the ERG. Because it measures the composite electrical potential of the entire retina, ERG abnormalities indicate generalized retinal dysfunction. as is seen with congenital dystrophies or widespread inflammation and damage. Focal disease, such as of the macula alone, will not affect the mass response recorded by the ERG.

Since it will not detect disorders of the macula or optic nerve, the importance of electroretinography is in the evaluation of generalized retinal disease. Examples might include retinitis pigmentosa (progressive degeneration of photoreceptor cells), massive ischemia, disseminated infection, or toxic effects from drugs or chemicals (eg, iron intraocular foreign body). The ERG is invaluable for diagnosing congenital ret-

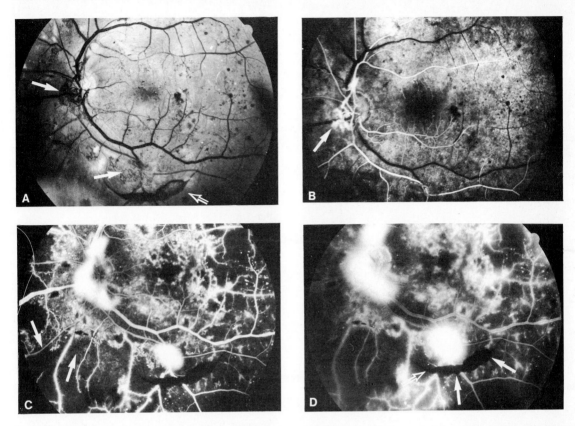

Figure 2–34. Fluorescein angiographic study of an eye with proliferative diabetic retinopathy demonstrating variations in the dye pattern over several minutes' time. **A:** Fundus photograph of left eye (before fluorescein) showing neovascularization (abnormal new vessels) on the disk and inferior to the macula (arrows). This latter area has bled, producing the arcuate preretinal hemorrhage at the bottom of the photo (open arrow). **B:** Early phase angiogram of the same eye, in which fluorescein has initially filled the arterioles and highlighted the area of the disk neovascularization. **C:** Midphase angiogram of the same eye in which dye has begun to leak out of the hyperpermeable areas of neovascularization. In addition to the irregular venous caliber and the microaneurysms (white dots), extensive areas of ischemia are apparent by virtue of the gross absence of vessels (and therefore dye) in many areas (see arrows). **D:** Late-phase photo demonstrating increasing amounts of dye leakage over time. Although the preretinal hemorrhage does not stain with dye, it is detectable as a solid black area since it obscures all underlying fluorescence (arrows). (Photos courtesy of University of California, San Francisco.)

inal dystrophies in which the retina may still appear normal by ophthalmoscopy. It is also particularly helpful if cloudy ocular media are present, since the latter may obscure visualization of the retina but not the bright light stimulus or electrical recording of the ERG.

8. VISUAL EVOKED RESPONSE

Like electroretinography, the visual evoked response (VER) measures the electrical potential resulting from a visual stimulus. However, because it is measured by scalp electrodes placed over the occipital cortex, the entire visual pathway from retina to cortex must be intact in order to produce a normal electrical waveform reading. Like the ERG wave, the VER pattern is plotted on a scale displaying both amplitude and latency (Fig 2–35).

Reduced speed of neuronal conduction, such as with demyelination, will result in an abnormally increased latency of the VER. Interruption of conduction will primarily be apparent from reduced amplitude of the VER. Unilateral **prechiasmal** (retinal or optic nerve) disease can be diagnosed by stimulating each eye separately and comparing the responses. **Postchiasmal** disease (eg, homonymous hemianopia) can be determined by comparing the electrode responses measured separately over each hemisphere.

Proportionately, the majority of the occipital lobe area is devoted to the macula. This large cortical area representing the macula is also closest in proximity to the scalp electrode, so that the clinically measured VER is primarily a response generated by the macula and optic nerve. An abnormal VER would thus indicate poor visual acuity, making it a valuable objective test in situations where subjective testing is un-

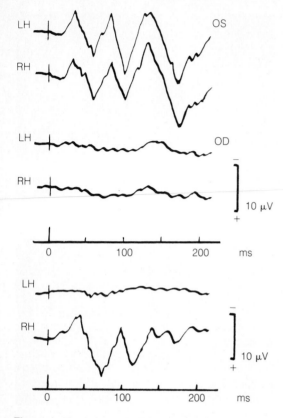

Figure 2–35. A: Normal VER generated by stimulating the left eye ("OS") is contrasted with the absent response form the right eye ("OD"), which has a severe optic nerve lesion. "LH" and "RH" signify recordings from electrodes over the left and right hemispheres of the occipital lobe. **B:** VER with right homonymous hemianopia. No response is recorded from over the left hemisphere. (Courtesy of M Feinsod.)

reliable. Such patients might include infants, unresponsive patients, and suspected malingerers.

Instead of a flash of light, an alternating patterned stimulus (such as a flashing "pattern reversal" checkerboard) can be used to specifically test the macula. By progressively reducing the pattern size, one eventually surpasses the limit of macular resolution, and the measured VER diminishes. This allows some quantitation of central vision and serves as a means of detecting and monitoring amblyopia in infants.

DIAGNOSIS OF EXTRAOCULAR ABNORMALITIES

1. LACRIMAL SYSTEM EVALUATION

Evaluation of Tear Production

Tears and their components are produced by the lacrimal gland and accessory glands in the lid and conjunctiva (see Chapter 4). The **Schirmer test** is a simple method for assessing gross tear production. Schirmer strips are disposable dry strips of filter paper in standard 5 × 35 mm sizes. The tip of one end is folded at the preexisting notch so that it can drape over the lower lid margin just lateral to the cornea.

Tears in the conjunctival sac will cause progressive wetting of the paper strip. The distance between the leading edge of wetness and the initial fold can be measured after 5 minutes, using a millimeter ruler. The ranges of normal measurements vary depending on whether or not topical anesthetic is used. Without anesthesia, irritation from the Schirmer strip itself will cause reflex tearing, thereby increasing the measurement. Without anesthesia, less than 5 mm of wetting after 5 minutes is considered abnormal.

Significant degrees of chronic dryness cause surface changes in the exposed areas of the cornea and conjunctiva. **Fluorescein** will stain punctate areas of epithelial loss on the cornea. In contrast, a second dye, **rose bengal,** will stain devitalized cells of the conjunctiva and cornea before they actually degenerate and drop off.

Evaluation of Lacrimal Drainage

The anatomy of the lacrimal drainage system is discussed in Chapter 3. The pumping action of the lids draws tears nasally into the upper and lower canalicular channels through the medially located "punctal" openings in each lid margin (Fig 3–10). After collecting in the lacrimal sac, the tears then drain into the nasopharynx via the nasolacrimal duct. Symptoms of watering are frequently due to increased tear production as a reflex response to some type of ocular irritation. However, the patency and function of the lacrimal drainage system must be checked in the evaluation of otherwise unexplained tearing.

The **Jones I** test evaluates whether the entire drainage system as a whole is functioning. Concentrated fluorescein dye is instilled into the conjunctival sac on the side of the suspected obstruction. After 5 minutes, a cotton Calgiswab is used to attempt to recover dye from beneath the inferior nasal turbinate. Alternatively, the patient blows his nose into a tissue which is checked for the presence of dye. Recovery of any dye indicates that the drainage system is functioning.

The **Jones II** test is performed if no dye is recovered, indicating some abnormality of the system. Following topical anesthesia, a smooth-tipped metal probe is used to gently dilate one of the punctae (usually lower). A 3-mL syringe with sterile water or saline is prepared and attached to a special lacrimal irrigating cannula (Fig 2–36). This blunt-tipped cannula is used to gently intubate the lower canaliculus, and fluid is injected as the patient leans forward. With a patent drainage system, fluid should easily flow into the patient's nasopharynx without resistance.

If fluorescein can now be recovered from the nose following irrigation, a partial obstruction might have been present. Recovery of clear fluid without fluorescein, however, may indicate inability of the lids to initially pump dye into the lacrimal sac with an

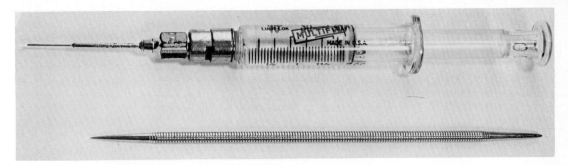

Figure 2–36. Punctum dilator (below) and blunt-tipped lacrimal cannula attached to a syringe (above), used for intubating and irrigating the lacrimal drainage system.

otherwise patent drainage apparatus. If no fluid can be irrigated through to the nasopharynx using the syringe, total occlusion is present. Finally, some drainage problems may be due to stenosis of the punctal lid opening, in which case the preparatory dilation may be therapeutic.

2. METHODS OF ORBITAL EVALUATION

Exophthalmometry

A method is needed to measure the anteroposterior location of the globe with respect to the bony orbital rim. The lateral orbital rim is a discrete, easily palpable landmark and is used as the reference point.

The exophthalmometer (Fig 2–37) is a hand-held instrument with 2 identical measuring devices (one for each eye), connected by a horizontal bar. The distance between the 2 devices can be varied by sliding one toward or away from the other, and each has a notch that fits over the edge of the corresponding

lateral orbital rim. When properly aligned, an attached set of mirrors reflects a side image of each eye profiled alongside a measuring scale, calibrated in millimeters. The tip of the corneal image aligns with a scale reading representing its distance from the orbital rim.

The patient is seated facing the examiner. The distance between the 2 measuring devices is adjusted so that each aligns with and abuts against its corresponding orbital rim. To allow reproducibility for repeat measurements in the future, the distance between the 2 devices is recorded from an additional scale on the horizontal bar. Using the first mirror scale, the patient's right eye position is measured as it fixates on the examiner's left eye. The patient's left eye is measured while fixating on the examiner's right eye.

The distance from the cornea to the orbital rim typically ranges from 12 to 20 mm, and the 2 eye measurements are normally within 2 mm of each other. A greater distance is seen in exophthalmos, which can be unilateral or bilateral. This abnormal forward protrusion of the eye can be produced by any

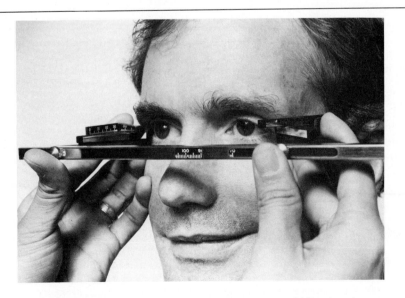

Figure 2–37. Hertel exophthalmometer. (Photo by M Narahara.)

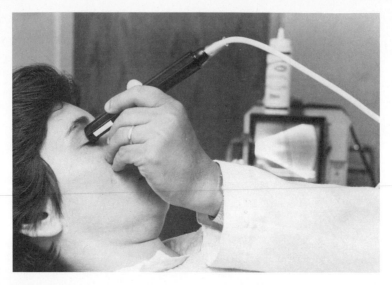

Figure 2–38. Ultrasonography using B-scan probe. The image will appear on the oscilloscope screen, visible in the background. (Photo by M Narahara.)

significant increase in orbital mass, because of the fixed size of the bony orbital cavity. Causes might include orbital hemorrhage, neoplasm, inflammation, or edema.

Ultrasonography

Ultrasonography utilizes the principle of sonar to study structures that may not be directly visible. It can be used to evaluate either the globe or the orbit. High-frequency sound waves are emitted from a special transmitter toward the target tissue. As the sound waves bounce back off the various tissue components, they are collected by a receiver that amplifies and displays them on an oscilloscope screen.

A single probe that contains both the transmitter

and receiver is placed against the eye and used to aim the beam of sound (Fig 2–38). Various structures in its path will reflect separate echoes (which arrive at different times) back toward the probe. Those derived from the most distal structures arrive last, having traveled the farthest.

There are 2 methods of clinical ultrasonography: A scan and B scan. In **A scan ultrasonography,** the sound beam is aimed in a straight line. Each returning echo is displayed as a spike whose amplitude is dependent on the density of the reflecting tissue and on how perpendicularly the tissue is oriented with respect to the probe (which optimizes the strength of reflection back toward the probe). The spikes are arranged in temporal sequence, with the latency of each signal's

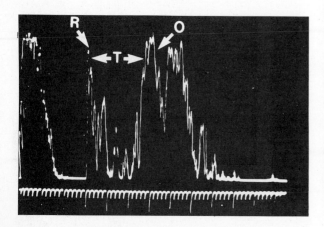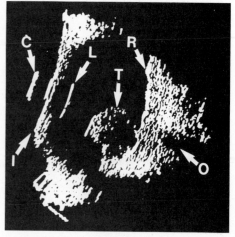

Figure 2–39. A scan *(left)* and B scan *(right)* of an intraocular tumor (melanoma). C = cornea; I = iris; L = posterior lens surface; O = optic nerve; R = retina; T = tumor. (Courtesy of RD Stone.)

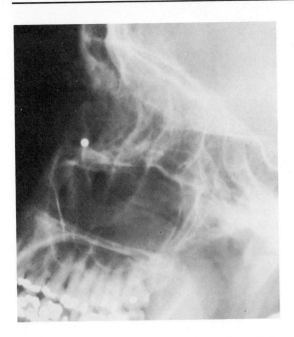

Figure 2–40. Lateral plain x-ray view of an ocular metallic foreign body. This view cannot differentiate an intraocular from an orbital foreign body, however.

arrival correlating with that structure's distance from the probe (Fig 2–39). If the same probe is now swept across the eye, a continuous series of individual A scans is obtained. From spatial summation of these multiple linear scans, a 2-dimensional image, or **B scan,** can be constructed.

Although therapeutic applications are being investigated, ophthalmic ultrasonography is currently used for diagnosis and measurement. Both A and B scans can be used to image and differentiate orbital disease or intraocular anatomy concealed by opaque media. In addition to defining the size and location of intraocular and orbital masses, A and B scans can provide clues to the tissue characteristics of a lesion (eg, solid, cystic, vascular, calcified).

For purposes of measurement, the A scan is the most accurate method. Sound echoes reflected from 2 separate locations will reach the probe at different times. This temporal separation can be used to calculate the distance between the points, based on the speed of sound in the tissue medium. The most commonly used ocular measurement is the axial length (cornea to retina). This is important in cataract surgery in order to calculate the power for an intraocular lens implant. A scans can also be used to quantify tumor size and monitor growth over time.

3. OPHTHALMIC RADIOLOGY (X-RAY, CT SCAN)

Plain x-ray, tomography, and CT scan (Figs 2–40 and 2–41) are useful in the evaluation of **orbital** and

intracranial conditions. CT scan in particular has become the most widely used method for localizing and characterizing structural disease in the extraocular visual pathway. Common orbital abnormalities demonstrated by CT scan include neoplasms, inflammatory masses, fractures, and extraocular muscle enlargement associated with Graves' disease.

The **intraocular** applications of radiology are primarily in the detection of foreign bodies following trauma and the demonstration of intraocular calcium in tumors such as retinoblastoma. CT scan is useful for foreign body localization because of its multidimensional reformatting capabilities and its ability to image the ocular walls.

4. MAGNETIC RESONANCE IMAGING

The evolving technique of magnetic resonance imaging (MRI) has many applications in orbital and intracranial diagnosis. Improvements such as surface

A

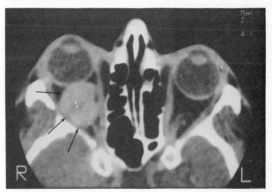

B

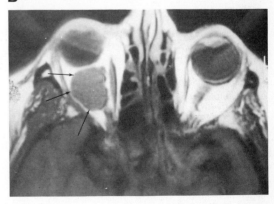

Figure 2–41. Cavernous hemangioma (arrows) of the right orbit as demonstrated by both CT scan **(A)** and MRI **(B).** The left side demonstrates the appearance of a normal orbit and globe. (Courtesy of D Char.)

receiver coils and thin section techniques have improved the anatomic resolution in the eye and orbit.

Unlike CT, the MRI technique does not expose the patient to ionizing radiation. Multidimensional views (axial, coronal, and sagittal) are possible without having to reposition the patient. However, the availability of MRI is more limited, and the examination takes longer than CT scanning, making it more difficult for the patient. Since MRI might cause movement of metal, it should not be used if a metallic foreign body is suspected.

Because it can better differentiate between tissues of different water content, MRI is superior to CT in its ability to image edema, areas of demyelination, and vascular lesions (Fig 2–41). Bone generates a weak MRI signal, allowing improved resolution of intraosseous disease and a clearer view of the intracranial posterior fossa. Additional examples of CT and MRI scans are presented in Chapters 14 and 15.

5. OPHTHALMODYNAMOMETRY

Ophthalmodynamometry gives an approximate measurement of the relative pressures in the central retinal arteries and is an indirect means of assessing carotid artery flow on either side. The test consists of exerting pressure on the sclera with a spring plunger while observing with an ophthalmoscope the vessels emerging from the optic disk. Ophthalmodynamometry is indicated in the neurologic evaluation of patients who complain of "blacking out" (amaurosis fugax) in one eye, spells of weakness on one side of the body, or other symptoms of transient cerebral ischemia. A difference of more than 20% in the diastolic pressures between the 2 eyes suggests insufficiency of the carotid arterial system on the side with the lower reading.

The test is often performed in conjunction with other noninvasive carotid artery flow studies.

REFERENCES

Anderson DR: *Perimetry: With and Without Automation,* 2nd ed. Mosby, 1987.

Beck RW et al: A clinical comparison of visual field testing with a new automated perimeter, the Humphrey Field Analyzer, and the Goldmann perimeter. *Ophthalmology* 1985;**92**:77.

Berkow JW et al: *Fluorescein Angiography: A Guide to the Interpretation of Fluorescein Angiograms,* 2nd ed. American Academy of Ophthalmology, 1984.

Boothe WA et al: The Tono-Pen: A monometric and clinical study. *Arch Ophthalmol* 1988;**106**:1214.

Drake M, Liegerman MF: *A Simplified Guide to Computerized Perimetry.* Slack, 1987.

Duane T (editor): *Clinical Ophthalmology.* 5 vols. Lippincott, 1987.

Ehrlich MI et al: Preschool vision screening for amblyopia and strabismus: Programs, methods, guidelines, 1983. *Surv Ophthalmol* 1983;**28**:145.

Faulkner W: Macular function testing through opacities. Vol 4, Module 2, in: *Focal Points 1986: Clinical Modules for Ophthalmologists.* American Academy of Ophthalmology, 1986.

Fish EF et al: A comparison of visual function tests in eyes with maculopathy. *Ophthalmology* 1986;**93**:1177.

Harrington DO: *The Visual Fields: A Textbook and Atlas of Clinical Perimetry,* 5th ed. Mosby, 1981.

Hirst LW: Clinical evaluation of the corneal endothelium. Vol 4, Module 8, in: *Focal Points 1986: Clinical Modules for Ophthalmologists.* American Academy of Ophthalmology, 1986.

Hoskins HD, Kass M: *Becker-Shaffer's Diagnosis and Therapy of the Glaucomas,* 6th ed. Mosby, 1988.

Hoyt CS et al: Ophthalmological examination of the infant. *Surv Ophthalmol* 1982;**26**:177.

Levi L, Schwartz B: Glaucoma screening in the health care setting. *Arch Ophthalmol* 1987;**105**:164.

Mannis MJ: Making sense of contrast sensitivity testing. *Arch Ophthalmol* 1987;**105**:627.

Miller BW: A review of practical tests for ocular malingering and hysteria. *Surv Ophthalmol* 1973;**17**:241.

Nelson ME, Orton HP: Counteracting the effects of mydriatics. *Arch Ophthalmol* 1987;**105**:486.

Owsley C, Sloane ME: Contrast sensitivity, acuity, and the perception of "real-world" targets. *Br J Ophthalmol* 1987;**71**:791.

Richard JM (editor): *A Manual for the Beginning Ophthalmology Resident,* 4th ed. American Academy of Ophthalmology, 1981.

Rosenthal ML, Fradin S: The technique of binocular indirect ophthalmoscopy. *Highlights Ophthalmol* 1966;**9**:179. (Reprinted as Appendix in: Hilton GF et al: *Retinal Detachment,* 4th ed. American Academy of Ophthalmology, 1981.)

Sassani JW, Osbakken MD: Anatomic features of the eye disclosed with nuclear magnetic resonance imaging. *Arch Ophthalmol* 1984;**102**:541.

Schatz H et al: *Interpretation of Fundus Fluorescein Angiography.* Mosby, 1978.

Shaffer RN et al: The use of diagrams to record changes in glaucomatous discs. *Am J Ophthalmol* 1975;**80**:460.

Shammas HJ: *Atlas of Ophthalmic Ultrasonography and Biometry.* Mosby, 1984.

Simons K: Visual acuity norms in young children. *Surv Ophthalmol* 1983;**28**:141.

Sokol S: Visually evoked potentials: Theory, techniques and clinical applications. *Surv Ophthalmol* 1976;**21**:18.

Stein HA et al: *The Ophthalmic Assistant: Fundamentals and Clinical Practice,* 5th ed. Mosby, 1988.

Thompson HS: Functional visual loss. *Am J Ophthalmol* 1985;**100**:209.

Thompson HS et al: How to measure the relative afferent pupillary defect. *Surv Ophthalmol* 1981;**26**:39.

Thompson HS et al: The relationship between visual acuity, pupillary defect, and visual field loss. *Am J Ophthalmol* 1982;**93**:681.

von Noorden GK: *Burian-von Noorden's Binocular Vision and Ocular Motility,* 3rd ed. Mosby, 1985.

Wirtschafter JD, Taylor S: *Computed Tomography: An Atlas for Ophthalmologists.* American Academy of Ophthalmology, 1982.

Zimmerman RA et al: Orbital magnetic resonance imaging. *Am J Ophthalmol* 1985;**100**:312.

Lids & Lacrimal Apparatus

3

John H. Sullivan, MD

I. LIDS

INFECTIONS & INFLAMMATIONS OF THE LID

HORDEOLUM

Hordeolum is infection of the glands of the eyelid. When the meibomian glands are involved, a large swelling occurs called internal hordeolum (Fig 3–1). The smaller and more superficial external hordeolum (sty) is an infection of Zeis's or Moll's glands.

Pain, redness, and swelling are the principal symptoms. The intensity of the pain is a function of the amount of lid swelling. An internal hordeolum may point to the skin or to the conjunctival surface. An external hordeolum always points to the skin.

Most hordeolums are caused by staphylococcal infections, usually *Staphylococcus aureus*. Culture is seldom indicated. Treatment consists of warm compresses 3 or 4 times a day for 10–15 minutes. If the process does not begin to resolve within 48 hours, incision and drainage of the purulent material is indicated. A vertical incision should be made on the conjunctival surface to avoid cutting across the meibomian glands. The incision should not be squeezed to express residual pus. If the hordeolum is pointing externally, a horizontal incision should be made on the skin to minimize scar formation.

Antibiotic ointment applied to the conjunctival sac every 3 hours is beneficial. Systemic antibiotics may be indicated if cellulitis develops.

CHALAZION

A chalazion (Fig 3–2) is an idiopathic sterile chronic granulomatous inflammation of a meibomian gland, usually characterized by painless localized swelling that develops over a period of weeks. It may begin with mild inflammation and tenderness resembling hordeolum—differentiated from hordeolum by the absence of acute inflammatory signs. Most chalazions point toward the conjunctival surface, which may be slightly reddened or elevated. If sufficiently large, a

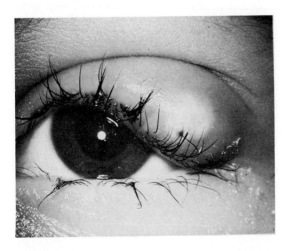

Figure 3–1. Internal hordeolum, left upper eyelid, pointing on skin side. This should be opened by a horizontal skin incision. (Courtesy of A Rosenberg.)

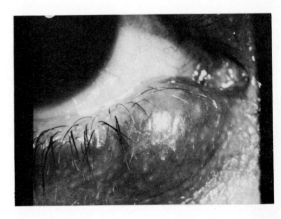

Figure 3–2. Chalazion, right lower eyelid. (Courtesy of K Tabbara.)

chalazion may press on the eyeball and cause astigmatism. If large enough to distort vision or to be a cosmetic blemish, excision is indicated.

Laboratory study is seldom indicated, but on pathologic examination there is proliferation of the endothelium of the acinus and a granulomatous inflammatory response that includes Langerhans-type gland cells. Biopsy is indicated for recurrent chalazion, since meibomian gland carcinoma may mimic the appearance of chalazion.

Surgical excision is performed via a vertical incision into the tarsal gland from the conjunctival surface followed by careful curettement of the gelatinous material and glandular epithelium. Intralesional steroid injections may also be useful alone for small lesions and in combination with surgery in difficult cases.

MARGINAL BLEPHARITIS
(Granulated Eyelids)

Blepharitis is a common chronic bilateral inflammation of the lid margins. There are 2 main types: staphylococcal and seborrheic. Staphylococcal blepharitis is usually ulcerative. Seborrheic blepharitis (nonulcerative) is usually associated with the presence of *Pityrosporum ovale,* although this organism has not been shown to be the etiologic factor. Often, both types are present (mixed infection). Seborrhea of the scalp, brows, and ears is frequently associated with seborrheic blepharitis.

The chief symptoms are irritation, burning, and itching of the lid margins. The eyes are "red-rimmed." Many scales or "granulations" can be seen clinging to the lashes of both the upper and lower lids. In the staphylococcal type, the scales are dry, the lids are red, tiny ulcerated areas are found along the lid margins, and the lashes tend to fall out. In the seborrheic type, the scales are greasy, ulceration does not occur, and the lid margins are less red. In the more common mixed type, both dry and greasy scales are present and the lid margins are red and may be ulcerated. *Staphylococcus aureus* and *P ovale* can be seen together or singly in stained material scraped from the lid margins.

Conjunctivitis, superficial keratitis of the lower third of the cornea, and chronic meibomianitis are the main complaints in the early morning hours. Seborrheic blepharitis is occasionally complicated by a mild keratitis. Persons with staphylococal blepharitis are prone to develop chalazions and hordeola.

The scalp, eyebrows, and lid margins must be kept clean, particularly in the seborrheic type of blepharitis, by means of soap and water shampoo. Scales must be removed from the lid margins daily with a damp cotton applicator and baby shampoo.

Staphylococcal blepharitis is treated with antistaphylococcal antibiotic or sulfonamide eye ointment applied on a cotton applicator once daily to the lid margins.

Meibomianitis is very resistant to treatment and requires repeated expression of the glands. It may be complicated by secondary infection with one of the prominent gram-negative organisms (eg, *Pseudomonas aeruginosa*).

The seborrheic and staphylococcal types usually become mixed and may run a chronic course over a period of months or years if not treated adequately; associated staphylococcal conjunctivitis or keratitis usually disappears promptly following local antistaphylococcal medication.

MEIBOMIANITIS

Bilateral, chronic inflammation of the meibomian glands is an uncommon disease of unknown cause that occurs during or after the middle years of life. It is generally preceded by or associated with blepharitis.

The patient complains of chronically red and irritated eyes and a slight but continuous discharge. The meibomian glands are prominent, the lid margins are red, and there is a frothy conjunctival discharge. A soft, cheesy, yellow material that contains no organisms can be expressed from the glands. An irritative conjunctivitis due to contact with meibomian secretion is a frequent complication, especially in the morning upon awakening.

The only treatment is repeated expression of the meibomian glands. However, because this treatment never produces dramatic results, the patient usually neglects to do it or have it done, and the disease process continues indefinitely with a slight tendency to become worse.

ANATOMIC LID DEFORMITIES

ENTROPION

Entropion—turning inward of the lid (Fig 3–3)—may be involutional (spastic, senile), cicatricial, or congenital. Involutional entropion is most common and by definition occurs as a result of aging. It always affects the lower lid and is the result of a combination of laxity of the lower lid retractors, upward migration of the preseptal orbicularis muscle, and buckling of the upper tarsal border.

Cicatricial entropion may involve the upper or lower lid and is the result of conjunctival and tarsal scar formation. It is most often found with chronic inflammatory diseases such as trachoma.

Congenital entropion is rare and should not be confused with congenital **epiblepharon,** which is most often found in Asians. In congenital entropion, the lid margin is rotated toward the cornea, whereas in epiblepharon the pretarsal skin and muscle cause the lashes to rotate around the tarsal border.

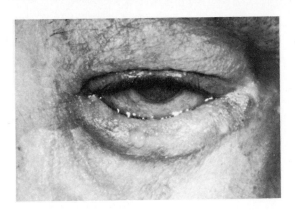

Figure 3–3. Entropion. (Courtesy of M Quickert.)

Trichiasis is impingement of eyelashes on the cornea and may be due to entropion, epiblepharon, or simply misdirected growth. It causes corneal irritation and encourages ulceration. Chronic inflammatory lid diseases such as blepharitis may cause scarring of the lash follicles and subsequent misdirected growth.

Distichiasis is accessory eyelashes, often growing from the orifices of the meibomian glands. It may be congenital or the result of metaplastic changes in the glands of the eyelid margin.

Surgery to evert the lid is effective in all kinds of entropion. A useful temporary measure in involutional entropion is to tape the lower lid to the cheek, with tension exerted temporally and inferiorly. Trichiasis without entropion can be temporarily relieved by plucking the offending eyelashes. Permanent relief may be achieved with electrolysis, surgery, or cryosurgery.

ECTROPION

Ectropion (sagging and eversion of the lower lid) (Fig 3–4), is usually bilateral and is a frequent finding in older persons. Ectropion may be caused by relax-ation of the orbicularis oculi muscle, either as part of the aging process or following seventh nerve palsy. The symptoms are tearing and irritation. Exposure keratitis may occur.

Marked ectropion is treated by surgical shortening of the lower lid in a horizontal direction. Cicatricial ectropion is caused by contracture of the anterior lamella of the lid. It requires surgical revision of the scar and often skin grafting for relief. Minor degrees of ectropion can be treated by several fairly deep electrocautery penetrations through the conjunctiva 4–5 mm from the lid margins at the inferior aspect of the tarsal plate. The fibrotic reaction that follows will often draw the lid up to its normal position.

DERMATOCHALASIS

Dermatochalasis (Fig 3–5) is skin redundancy and loss of elasticity such that the preseptal fold of the skin and orbicularis muscle cover the pretarsal portion of the lid. It is a function of aging and is very common. It results from loss of elasticity of skin and muscle and weakening of the orbital septum. In the upper lid, the preseptal skin and muscle, which normally forms a crease near the upper tarsal border in Caucasians, folds over the pretarsal muscle of the lid. Weakness of the orbicularis muscle and septum causes the preaponeurotic fat pad to bulge forward, accentuating the fullness of the lid. The medial fat pad also becomes visible. Marked dermatochalasis causes pseudoptosis and obstruction of the superior visual field.

Surgical correction may be indicated for visual or cosmetic reasons. A portion of eyelid tissue including skin, muscle, and fat is usually removed for best esthetic results. In the lower lid, redundant skin hangs loosely in the preseptal area, and the bulging fat pads contribute to the appearance of ''bags'' in the lower lids.

Surgery of the lower lids is performed for cosmetic

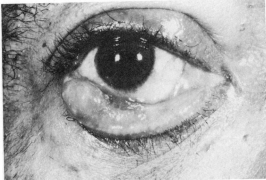

Figure 3–4. Ectropion. (Courtesy of M Quickert.)

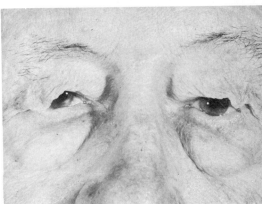

Figure 3–5. Dermatochalasis of upper lids and herniation of orbital fat of lower lids. (Courtesy of M Quickert.)

reasons unless extreme redundancy contributes to ectropion of the lid margin. A fairly large amount of fat and small amounts of skin and muscle are usually resected.

BLEPHAROCHALASIS

Blepharochalasis (Fig 3–6) is a rare condition caused by recurrent episodes of edema resulting in thin, wrinkled, and redundant eyelid skin, sometimes described as resembling cigarette paper. Atrophic changes of all eyelid tissue frequently produce ptosis and a sunken appearance at the location of the medial fat pad. Symptoms of edema begin around puberty and diminish with age. Surgery consists of removal of the redundant skin and repair of the levator aponeurosis. Medical management is directed at controlling the episodic angioneurotic edema.

EPICANTHUS

Epicanthus (Fig 3–7) is characterized by vertical folds of skin over the medial canthi. It is typical of Asians and is present to some degree in most children of all races. The skinfold is often large enough to cover part of the nasal sclera and cause "pseudoesotropia." The eye appears to be crossed when the medial aspect of the sclera is not visible. The most frequent type is **epicanthus tarsalis,** in which the superior lid fold is continuous medially with the epicanthal fold. In **epicanthus inversus,** the skinfold blends into the lower lid. Other types are less common. The cause of epicanthus is lack of vertical skin between the canthus and the nose. Surgical correction is directed at vertical lengthening and horizontal shortening. Epicanthal folds in normal children, however, diminish gradually as the child grows older and are seldom apparent by school age.

TELECANTHUS

The distance between the medial canthus of each eye—the intercanthal distance—is the same as the

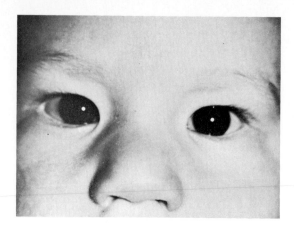

Figure 3–7. Epicanthus.

length of each palpebral fissure (approximately 30 mm in adults). A wide intercanthal distance may be the result of traumatic disinsertion or maldevelopment of the medial canthal tendon (eg, blepharophimosis syndrome). Reduction of the intercanthal distance in such instances can be accomplished by correcting the skin and underlying soft tissue. Major craniofacial reconstruction, however, is required when the orbits are widely separated, as in Crouzon's disease.

ANKYLOBLEPHARON

The horizontal length of the palpebral fissure may be shortened by scarring or congenital malformation. The usual means of correction is by lateral canthoplasty. The opposite condition, **euryblepharon,** is congenital enlargement of the lids without enlargement of the globe. It is associated with ectropion and sometimes ptosis and telecanthus.

COLOBOMA

Coloboma is a congenital segmental full-thickness defect of the eyelid. It is the result of incomplete fusion of fetal maxillary processes. Colobomas occur most frequently in the medial aspect of the upper lid. The lower lid is less likely to be involved.

Reconstruction can usually be delayed for years. Surgery should not be delayed if exposure keratitis is evident.

BLEPHAROSPASM

Benign essential blepharospasm is an uncommon type of involuntary muscle contraction characterized

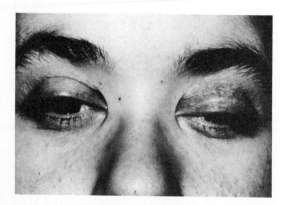

Figure 3–6. Blepharochalasis.

by persistent or repetitive spasm of the orbicularis oculi muscle. It is almost always bilateral and most common in the elderly. The spasms tend to progress in force and frequency, resulting in a grimacing expression and closure of the eyes. Patients may be incapacitated—able to catch only brief glimpses of vision between spasms. When the entire face and neck are involved, the condition is known as Meigs's syndrome.

The cause is not known. Emotional stress and fatigue sometimes make the condition worse, leading to speculation that this is a psychogenic affliction. Psychotherapy and psychoactive drugs, however, have had very limited success. A small percentage of patients have psychogenically induced spasms, but in most cases the dysfunction is thought to originate in the basal ganglia.

It is important to differentiate benign essential blepharospasm from hemifacial spasm. The latter condition tends to be unilateral and to involve the upper and lower face. Hemifacial spasm is thought to be related to compression of the facial nerve by an artery or posterior fossa tumor. Jenetta's neurosurgical decompression is the usual mode of treatment.

Other types of involuntary facial movements include **tardive dyskinesia,** which results from prolonged phenothiazine therapy and seldom affects the orbicularis muscle selectively; and **facial tics,** common in children, which are thought to be related to anxiety.

Treatment of blepharospasm begins with an attempt to identify the unusual instances of psychoneurotic behavior. Psychotherapy, neuroleptic drug treatment, biofeedback training, and hypnosis have occasionally been used with success. Most patients, however, require either repeated injections for neuromuscular blockade or surgery to ablate the action of the facial nerve.

Botulinum A toxin (Oculinum) has replaced alcohol as the preferred substance for intramuscular injection to produce temporary neuromuscular paralysis. When intolerance or unresponsiveness to the toxin occurs, the only recourse is selective surgical ablation of the facial nerve or extirpation of the orbicularis musculature.

BLEPHAROPTOSIS

Blepharoptosis is abnormally low position of one or both upper lids. The normal position of the upper lid is midway between the superior limbus and the upper pupillary margin. This may vary by 2 mm as long as the lids are symmetric. Blepharoptosis may be congenital or acquired and can be hereditary in either case.

Classification

It is important to be able to classify blepharoptosis in order to apply appropriate treatment. The following scheme, adapted from Beard, has been found to be useful.

A. True Congenital Ptosis: True congenital ptosis is caused by isolated dystrophy of the levator muscle affecting both contraction and relaxation of the fibers. The result is ptosis in the primary position of gaze, reduced movement of the lid in upgaze, and impaired closure on downgaze. This relative lagophthalmos is an important clue to diagnosis of true congenital ptosis. The different forms of congenital ptosis may be classified as follows:

1. Ptosis with normal superior rectus function–This type accounts for most cases of true congenital ptosis and is apparent shortly after birth.

2. Ptosis with weakness of the superior rectus–In 25% of cases of congenital ptosis, the superior rectus muscle shares the same dystrophic changes as the levator. Additional levator resection must be performed for a successful outcome.

3. Marcus Gunn syndrome (jaw winking)–In 5% of cases of true congenital ptosis, the eye opens when the mandible is opened or is deviated to the opposite side. The ptotic levator muscle is innervated by motor branches of the trigeminal nerve instead of the oculomotor nerve.

4. Blepharophimosis–Another unusual form of congenital ptosis is blepharophimosis, which accounts for 5% of cases. The patient usually has severe ptosis, with poor levator function, as well as telecanthus, epicanthal folds, and cicatricial ectropion of the lower lids.

B. Acquired Ptosis: Most cases of acquired ptosis are easily categorized on the basis of the history. However, acquired ptosis may be present at birth and can be confused with congenital ptosis.

1. Neurogenic ptosis–Partial or complete paralysis of the oculomotor nerve is most often a result of trauma. Aberrant regeneration is not uncommon and results in bizarre movements of the globe, eyelid, and pupil. Congenital third nerve paralysis is not associated with aberrant regeneration. When the lid is completely closed, deprivational amblyopia will develop unless the ptosis is treated. Strabismic amblyopia will also occur unless it too is treated early and vigorously.

Paralysis of Müller's muscle is almost always associated with Horner's syndrome, which may be congenital but is usually acquired. Rarely is there more than 2 mm of ptosis, and amblyopia is never a threat.

Ptosis and diplopia are often the initial manifestations of myasthenia gravis. The orbicularis oculi muscles are also frequently involved. Cogan's lid twitch is sometimes present—on rapid upgaze, the upper lid twitches as the eyes are looking up. Demonstration of lid fatigue, however, is more consistent. The diagnosis can be confirmed by intravenous administration of edrophonium, which temporarily reverses the weakness. Another useful test is the detection of circulating anti-acetylcholine receptor autoantibodies.

Medical management is usually effective initially, but ptosis surgery often becomes necessary. Thymectomy may be helpful in refractory cases. When lid closure and Bell's phenomenon have been impaired, ptosis surgery creates difficult problems with exposure keratitis.

Similar problems exist in the management of **chronic progressive external ophthalmoplegia.** This slowly progressive hereditary neuromuscular disease begins in mid life. In the form known as oculopharyngeal dystrophy, myopathy of the laryngeal muscles produces dysphagia. In Kearns-Sayer syndrome, ophthalmoplegia is associated with tapetoretinal degeneration and heart block.

2. Myogenic ptosis–Ptosis and facial weakness may also be found in **myotonic dystrophy.** Other findings include cataract, pupillary abnormalities, and frontal baldness.

Another very common form of myogenic ptosis occurs late in life and results from partial disinsertion or dehiscence of the levator aponeurosis from the tarsal plate. Typically there remain sufficient attachments to the tarsus to maintain excellent excursion of the lid with upgaze. The attachment of the retracted levator aponeurosis to the skin and orbicularis muscle creates an unusually high lid fold. Thinning of the lid may also occur, and on occasion the image of the iris may be seen through the skin of the upper lid. Trauma is often a precipitating cause of disinsertion of the levator. Ptosis following cataract surgery is thought to have this mechanism.

3. Traumatic ptosis–Trauma to the eyelid may induce ptosis on a neurogenic, myogenic, or mechanical basis. Traumatic ptosis often provides the most difficult reconstructive challenges.

4. Mechanical ptosis–The upper lid may be prevented from opening completely because of the mass effect of a neoplasm or the tethering effect of scar formation. Excessive horizontal shortening of the upper lid is a common cause of mechanical ptosis. Another form is that seen following enucleation, when absence of support to the levator by the globe permits the lid to drop.

C. Pseudoptosis: The appearance of ptosis may occur in the presence of hypotropia. When the eye looks down, the upper lid follows to a greater extent than the lower lid. The narrowed palpebral fissure and the ptotic upper lid are much more obvious than the hypotropic globe. Occlusion of the opposite eye, however, reveals the true condition. In severe dermatochalasis, a fold of pretarsal orbicularis and skin may conceal the lid margin and give the appearance of blepharoptosis.

Clinical Findings

The upper lid normally lies about 2 mm below the limbus and 2 mm above the pupillary margin. If the lid margin rests on the edge of the pupil, ptosis is considered mild; if the pupil is slightly covered, ptosis is moderate; and if the lid falls to the middle of the pupil or lower, ptosis is categorized as severe. The most important measurement, however, is the magnitude of lid excursion, which is an indication of levator function. In most instances, this measurement will determine the type and amount of surgery to be performed. With the eyebrow immobilized, a ruler is used to quantitate excursion of the lid margin from full downgaze to full upgaze. Eight millimeters or more of movement is good function; 4 mm or less is poor function. Absence of a lid crease suggests poor levator function.

Ocular motility disturbances are not uncommon in ptosis and may be important in surgical management. The presence of impaired superior rectus function is an indication for resection of additional levator to achieve adequate correction. Pupillary reactions may provide the first clue to Horner's syndrome or myotonic dystrophy. Facial features make the diagnosis of blepharophimosis and chronic progressive external ophthalmoplegia.

Treatment
(Fig 3–8)

With the exception of myasthenia gravis, all types of ptosis are treated surgically. In children, surgery can be performed when accurate evaluation can be obtained and the child is able to cooperate postoperatively. There may be an association of astigmatism and myopia with childhood ptosis. Early surgery might be helpful in preventing anisometropic amblyopia, but this has not been proved. Deprivational amblyopia probably occurs only with complete ptosis, as in third nerve palsy.

Symmetry is the goal of surgery, and symmetry in all positions of gaze is possible only if levator function is unimpaired. In most cases the best result that can be achieved is to balance the lids in the primary position. With unilateral ptosis, the degree of symmetry in other positions of gaze is inversely proportionate to levator function.

Most ptosis operations involve resection of the levator aponeurosis or superior tarsal muscle (or both). The superior portion of the tarsus is often resected for additional elevation. Many approaches, from both skin and conjunctiva, are currently in use. In recent years, emphasis has been placed on the advantages of confining the operation to advancement and resection of the levator aponeurosis, especially in acquired ptosis.

Patients with little or no levator function require an alternative elevating source. Suspension of the lids to the brow allows the patient to elevate the lids with the natural movement of the frontalis muscle. Autogenous fascia lata is usually considered the best means of suspension.

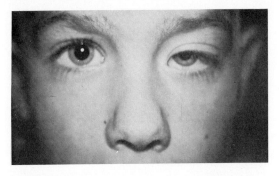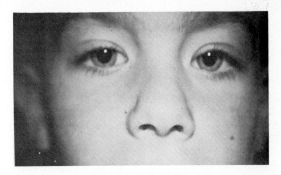

Figure 3–8. Surgical correction of ptosis. *Left:* Before operation, ptosis of the upper lid was present. *Right:* After the operation (levator resection), the ptosis was well corrected and a natural-appearing upper lid fold produced. (Courtesy of C Beard.)

COSMETIC MICROPIGMENTATION OF THE LIDS

Tattooing the lids of women is a controversial procedure whose purpose is to reduce the necessity for applying eyeliner. The procedure is also occasionally used to simulate eyelashes following reconstruction of the lid margin. It is performed under local anesthesia using a power-driven handpiece to implant various pigments adjacent to the eyelashes. It is known that subcutaneous impregnation of certain mercury-based dyes can cause a local inflammatory reaction, and these dyes have been abandoned. Carbon particle tattooing appears to be harmless, but the long-term consequences of dye impregnation at the lid margin are unknown.

As is true also of tattoos elsewhere on the body, the intensity and crispness of the image tends to fade with time. Complete removal of the pigmentation because of misplacement or change in fashion is difficult.

TUMORS OF THE EYELIDS
J. Brooks Crawford, MD

BENIGN LID TUMORS

Benign tumors of the lids are very common and increase in frequency with age. Most are readily distinguished clinically, and excision is done for cosmetic reasons. However, it is often impossible to recognize malignant lesions clinically, and biopsy should always be performed if there is any doubt about the diagnosis.

Nevus

Melanocytic nevi of the eyelids are common benign tumors with the same pathologic structure as nevi found elsewhere. They are usually congenital but may be relatively unpigmented at birth, enlarging and darkening during adolescence. Many never acquire visible pigment, and many resemble benign papillomas. Nevi rarely become malignant.

Nevi may be removed by shave excision if desired for cosmetic reasons.

Verrucae (Warts)

Warts commonly appear along the margins of the lids as fleshy, multilobulated, flat-based to pedunculated lesions. They are thought to be caused by viruses.

If treatment is indicated for cosmetic reasons, verrucae may be removed by excision with cauterization at the base of the lesion. Care must be exercised to avoid producing a marginal notch in the eyelid.

Molluscum Contagiosum (Fig 3–9)

The typical lesion of this unusual disorder is a small, flat, symmetric, centrally umbilicated growth along the lid margin. It is caused by a large virus and may produce conjunctivitis and even keratitis if the lesion sheds into the conjunctival space.

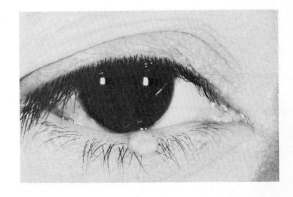

Figure 3–9. Molluscum contagiosum. Note central umbilication.

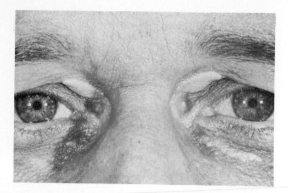

Figure 3–10. Xanthelasma. (Courtesy of M Quickert.)

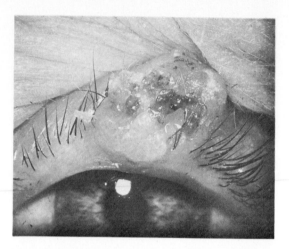

Figure 3–12. Squamous cell carcinoma of upper lid. (Courtesy of A Rosenberg.)

Cure can usually be obtained by incision, cautery, or excision.

Xanthelasma
(Fig 3–10)

Xanthelasma is a common disorder that occurs on the anterior surface of the eyelid, usually bilaterally near the inner angle of the eye. The lesions appear as yellow, wrinkled patches on the skin and occur more often in elderly people. Xanthelasma represents lipid deposits in histiocytes in the dermis of the lid. Clinical evaluation of serum cholesterol levels is indicated, but only rarely is a direct relationship found.

Treatment is indicated for cosmetic reasons. Surgical removal is simple. Cauterization of the smaller lesions is sometimes effective. Recurrence following removal is not unusual.

Hemangioma
(Fig 3–11)

Two main types of congenital vascular tumors occur in the lids: cavernous hemangiomas and capillary hemangiomas. **Cavernous hemangiomas** are composed of large venous channels lying in the subcutaneous tissue; they are bluish in color and change in size according to their distention with blood. **Capillary hemangiomas,** when superficial, are bright red (strawberry) spots. These and the more invasive type are composed of proliferating capillaries and endothelial cells. They may grow rapidly in the first few months of life. Both types frequently undergo spontaneous involution, usually by age 5.

Treatment is usually not indicated in infancy or childhood unless the defect is extensive enough to cause occlusion amblyopia. Refractive amblyopia can also occur owing to astigmatism or anisometropia produced by the tumor. It is important to detect this and treat it as it develops. If the hemangioma blocks the pupil or does not spontaneously involute, surgical excision may be necessary. Some of these hemangiomas respond to the injection of steroids.

PRIMARY MALIGNANT TUMORS OF THE LIDS

Carcinoma
(Figs 3–12 and 3–13)

Basal cell and squamous cell carcinomas of the lids are the most common malignant ocular tumors. These tumors occur most frequently in fair-complexioned individuals who have had chronic exposure to the sun. Ninety-five percent of lid carcinomas are of the basal cell type. The remaining 5% consist of squamous cell

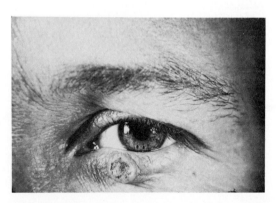

Figure 3–13. Basal cell carcinoma of left lower lid. (Courtesy of S Mettier, Jr.)

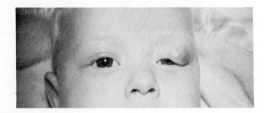

Figure 3–11. Cavernous hemangioma of left upper lid.

carcinomas and meibomian gland carcinomas. Keratoacanthomas and inverted follicular keratoses are benign lesions that resemble squamous cell carcinomas. In the past this was not recognized, and the incidence of squamous cell carcinomas was thought to be higher than it actually is. Diagnosis is based upon clinical appearance and biopsy.

Squamous cell carcinoma may spread via the lymphatic system to the preauricular and submaxillary lymph nodes. Most do not spread if they are recognized and treated. Basal cell tumors grow very slowly, are locally invasive, and do not spread to the regional lymph nodes.

Squamous cell carcinoma grows slowly and painlessly, and it may be present for many months before it is noted. It usually begins as a small warty growth with a keratotic covering, gradually eroding and fissuring until an ulcer develops. The base of the ulcer is indurated and hyperemic and the edges hard. Unless the tumor is excised early it grows through the skin, connective tissue, cartilage, and bone until large areas are destroyed in a fungating crater that may eventually reach the cranial cavity. Pain then becomes severe and constant. When sensory nerves are involved, the pain may be excruciating. The patient may die of hemorrhage, meningitis, or general debility.

Basal cell carcinoma begins in a similar manner, eventually forming the typical rodent ulcer with a raised nodular border and indurated base. It eventually erodes the surrounding tissue in somewhat the same way as squamous cell carcinoma but much more slowly. Biopsy of the tumor itself is a simple office procedure and is the only sure method of diagnosis.

Basal cell tumors of the lower lid near the inner canthus tend to invade the structures of the inner canthus and the orbit. Complete eradication of these tumors is important.

The sclerosing or morphealike basal cell carcinoma, an unusually aggressive variety of basal cell carcinoma, may lie beneath the skin surface and manifest its presence by subtle signs such as alopecia, lid notching, ectropion, or entropion.

Sebaceous gland carcinomas of the eyelid, most of which arise from the meibomian glands and the glands of Zeis, are potentially fatal neoplasms; about half of them may resemble benign inflammatory diseases such as chalazions and chronic blepharitis.

Any suspicious growths on the lids should be submitted for pathologic examination.

The objective of treatment is complete destruction of the tumor. Surgery is an effective method, particularly if frozen sections are used to ensure complete excision. Radiotherapy can also be effective for basal cell carcinomas and squamous cell carcinomas; cryotherapy has been successful in the treatment of some basal cell carcinomas.

Carcinoma Associated With Xeroderma Pigmentosum

This rare disease is characterized by the appearance of a large number of freckles in the areas of the skin exposed to the sun. These are followed by telangiectases, atrophic patches, and eventually a warty growth that may undergo carcinomatous degeneration. The eyelids are frequently affected and may be the first area to show degenerative changes, causing atrophy and ectropion with secondary inflammatory changes of the conjunctiva, symblepharon, corneal ulceration, and carcinoma of the lids. Malignant tumors include basal cell carcinomas, squamous cell carcinomas, and malignant melanomas. This condition is inherited as an autosomal recessive trait. Carriers can often be identified by excessive freckling.

The disease appears early in life and in most cases is fatal by adolescence as a result of metastasis. Life may be prolonged by carefully protecting the skin from actinic rays and treating carcinomatous tumors as rapidly as they appear.

Sarcoma

Sarcoma of the lids is rare and usually represents an anterior extension of an orbital sarcoma. Rhabdomyosarcomas involving the orbit and lids represent the most common malignant tumor in these tissues in the first decade of life. Other sarcomas (usually named after the predominant type of cell) also occur. Most are radiosensitive, but a combination of surgery and radiation is often required. They may be associated with similar lesions elsewhere in the body.

Malignant Melanoma

Malignant melanomas of the eyelids are similar to those elsewhere in the skin and include 3 distinct varieties: superficial spreading melanoma, lentigo maligna melanoma, and nodular melanoma. Not all malignant melanomas are pigmented. Most pigmented lesions on the eyelid skin are not melanomas. Therefore, biopsy should be used to establish the diagnosis. The prognosis for melanomas of the skin depends upon the depth of invasion or the thickness of the lesion.

II. LACRIMAL EXCRETORY APPARATUS

The lacrimal secretory apparatus consists of the lacrimal gland and the accessory lacrimal glands (see Fig 1–5). The excretory system is composed of the punctae, canaliculi, lacrimal sac, and nasolacrimal duct.

The main lacrimal gland is divided by the levator aponeurosis into orbital and palpebral lobes. The ductules from the orbital lobe pass through and join with the ductules of the palpebral lobe to empty into the superior temporal conjunctival fornix.

With each blink, the eyelids close like a zipper— beginning laterally, distributing moisture evenly across the cornea, and delivering it to the excretory system on the medial aspect of the lids. Passage of tears through the excretory system begins with their entrance into the punctum by capillary attraction.

The deep heads of the pretarsal and preseptal orbicularis muscles close the ampulla to prevent retrograde flow and simultaneously draw the tears into the lacrimal sac by traction on the fascia overlying the lacrimal sac. This dynamic pumping action is very important, and its absence in facial nerve palsy is the cause of epiphora. Once the tears are in the sac, gravity assists in carrying the fluid through the nasolacrimal duct into the inferior meatus of the nose. Valves are present in the sac that resist retrograde flow. The most important of these valves is at the junction of the common canaliculus and lacrimal sac, the sinus of Maier.

Tear production tends to diminish with age, and dryness of the eyes is a common complaint of the elderly. Drying of the corneal epithelium (keratitis sicca) is painful and can lead to loss of vision. Secretions from the glands of the conjunctiva provide the basic lubrication for the cornea and are more important than those of the lacrimal gland. Most patients who have had the lacrimal gland removed are asymptomatic under normal conditions.

The Schirmer test can be used to measure the function of both the lacrimal gland and the accessory glands (see Chapter 4 for detailed discussion). Inflammation of the lacrimal gland (dacryoadenitis) or tumor involving the gland may reduce tear production (alacrima). Absence of tears may also occur after disruption of the lacrimal secretory nerve by acoustic neuroma or following surgery involving the cerebellopontine angle. Congenital alacrima is a feature of Riley-Day syndrome.

INFECTIONS OF THE LACRIMAL APPARATUS

DACRYOCYSTITIS
(Fig 3–4)

Infection of the lacrimal sac is a common acute or chronic disease that usually occurs in infants or in persons over 40 years of age. Most adult cases occur in postmenopausal women. Dacryocystitis is uncommon in the intermediate age groups unless it follows trauma or is caused by a fungal dacryolith. In infants, chronic infection accompanies nasolacrimal duct obstruction, but acute dacryocystitis is uncommon.

Dacryocystitis is most often unilateral and always secondary to obstruction of the nasolacrimal duct. In many adult cases, the cause of obstruction remains unknown.

In acute dacryocystitis, the usual infectious agent is *Staphylococcus aureus* or occasionally β-hemolytic

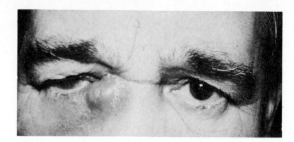

Figure 3–14. Acute dacryocystitis.

streptococci. In chronic dacryocystitis, *Streptococcus pneumoniae* or, rarely, *Candida albicans* is the predominant organism—mixed infections do not occur. The infectious agent can be identified microscopically by staining a conjunctival smear taken after expression of the tear sac.

Obstruction of the nasolacrimal duct sometimes occurs as a result of a fungal dacryolith. Spontaneous improvement follows passage of the stone, but recurrence is the rule.

Clinical Findings

The chief symptoms of dacryocystitis are tearing and discharge. In the acute form, inflammation, pain, swelling and tenderness are present in the tear sac area. Purulent material can be expressed from the sac. In the chronic form, tearing is usually the only sign. Mucoid material can usually be expressed from the sac.

It is curious that dacryocystitis is seldom complicated by conjunctivitis even though the conjunctival sac is constantly being bathed with pus exuding through the lacrimal puncta.

Corneal ulcer occasionally occurs following minor corneal trauma in the presence of pneumococcal dacryocystitis. Perforation of the skin and systemic treatment are indicated, and dacryocystectomy or dacryocystorhinostomy should be done without delay.

Treatment

In both adults and children, dacryocystitis responds well to systemic antibiotic therapy. Recurrences are common if the nasolacrimal duct obstruction is not removed.

The chronic form can be kept latent by using antibiotic drops, but relief of the obstruction is the only cure. The presence of a mucocele is evidence that the site of obstruction is in the nasolacrimal duct, and dacryocystorhinostomy is indicated. The patency of the canalicular system is assured if mucus or pus is regurgitated through the puncta on compression of the sac. Examination of the nose is important to ensure adequate space for drainage. Surgery consists of forming a permanent anastomosis between the lacrimal sac and the nose. Exposure is gained by an incision over the anterior lacrimal crest. A bony opening is made in the lateral wall of the nose, and the nasal mucosa is sutured to that of the lacrimal sac.

A. Adult Dacryocystitis:

1. Acute–Specific treatment for acute staphylococcal or pneumococcal dacryocystitis consists of penicillin or other antibiotic until the inflammation subsides.

2. Chronic–Since obstruction of the nasolacrimal duct is the basic cause of dacryocystitis, the disease is usually persistent until the obstruction is relieved. Probing is notably unsuccessful in adults, and dacryocystorhinostomy is usually necessary if symptoms are severe. If chronic tearing is the only symptom, some patients prefer the tearing to surgery.

B. Infantile Dacryocystitis: Normally, the lacrimal ducts open spontaneously before birth or during the first month of life. Failure of canalization is a common occurrence (5–7% of newborns), resulting in dacryostenosis. Forceful compression of the lacrimal sac will sometimes rupture the membrane and establish patency. If stenosis persists after 6 months or if dacryocystitis develops, probing of the duct is indicated. One probing is effective in 75% of cases. In the remainder, cure can almost always be achieved by repeated probing, by inward fracture of the inferior turbinate, or by a temporary silicone lacrimal splint. Probing should not be attempted in the presence of acute infection.

Acute dacryocystitis in children is often a result of *Haemophilus influenzae* infection. Prompt and aggressive treatment should be instituted in such cases because of the risk of orbital cellulitis.

CANALICULAR DISORDERS

Congenital anomalies of the canalicular system include imperforate punctae, accessory punctae, canalicular fistulas, and, rarely, agenesis of the canalicular system. Most cases of canalicular stenosis are acquired, usually the result of viral infections—notably varicella, herpes simplex, and adenovirus infection. Obstruction—even obliteration—may occur with Stevens-Johnson syndrome, pemphigoid, and other conjunctival shrinkage diseases. Systemic chemotherapy with fluorouracil and topical idoxuridine may also cause obstruction.

Canaliculitis is an uncommon chronic unilateral infection caused by *Actinomyces israelii* (Fig 3–15), *Candida albicans,* or *Aspergillus* species. It affects the lower canaliculus more often than the upper, occurs exclusively in adults, and causes a secondary purulent conjunctivitis that frequently escapes etiologic diagnosis. Untreated, it will result in canalicular stenosis.

The patient complains of a mildly red and irritated eye with a slight discharge. The punctum usually pouts, and material can be expressed from the canaliculus. The organism can be seen microscopically

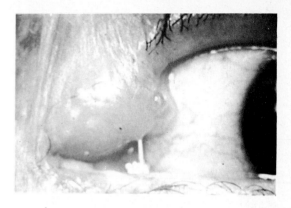

Figure 3–15. *Actinomyces israelii* canaliculitis, left eye. (Courtesy of P Thygeson.)

on a direct smear taken from the canaliculus. Curettage of the necrotic material in the involved canaliculus, followed by forceful irrigation, is usually effective. Canaliculotomy is sometimes necessary. Tincture of iodine should be applied to the lining of the canaliculus after canaliculotomy. Recurrence is not uncommon.

Total canalicular obstruction necessitates use of an artificial tear duct for relief of epiphora (conjunctivodacryocystorhinostomy). A Pyrex glass tube is placed between the conjunctival sac and the nasal cavity.

Closure of the punctum is sometimes performed in patients with keratitis sicca to allow tears to remain in the conjunctival sac. Temporary closure may be done with collagen plugs in the canaliculi or by sealing the punctum with a hot cautery. The obstruction will last several days, providing an opportunity to evaluate the effect. Permanent closure may be done by extensive cautery of the ampulla or by dividing the canaliculus surgically.

DACRYOADENITIS

Acute inflammation of the lacrimal gland is a rare condition most often seen in children as a complication of mumps, measles, or influenza and in adults in association with gonorrhea.

Chronic dacryoadenitis may be the result of benign lymphocytic infiltration, lymphoma, leukemia, or tuberculosis (see Chapter 16). It is occasionally seen bilaterally as a manifestation of sarcoidosis. When combined with parotid gland swelling, it is called Mikulicz's syndrome.

Considerable pain, swelling, and injection occur over the temporal aspect of the upper eyelid, which often imparts to it an S-shaped curve. If bacterial infection is present, systemic antibiotics are given. It is rarely necessary to surgically drain the infection.

REFERENCES

Anderson RL: Age of aponeurotic awareness. *Ophthalmic Plast Reconstr Surg* 1985;**1**:77.

Beard C: Malignancy of the eyelids. *Am J Ophthalmol* 1981;**92**:1.

Beard C: Observations on the treatment of basal cell carcinoma of eyelids. *Trans Am Acad Ophthalmol Otolaryngol* 1975;**79**:664.

Beard C: *Ptosis,* 3rd ed. Mosby, 1981.

Bedford MA: *Color Atlas of Ocular Tumors.* Year Book, 1979.

Boniuk M, Zimmerman LE: Sebaceous carcinoma of the eyelid, eyebrow, caruncle, and orbit. *Trans Am Acad Ophthalmol Otolaryngol* 1968;**72**:619.

Bullock JD, Beard C, Sullivan JH: Cryotherapy of basal cell carcinoma in oculoplastic surgery. *Am J Ophthalmol* 1976;**82**:841.

Callahan MA: Surgically mismanaged ptosis associated with double elevator palsy. *Arch Ophthalmol* 1981;**99**:108.

Char D: Therapeutic review: The management of lid and conjunctival malignancies. *Surv Ophthalmol* 1980;**24**:679.

Collin JRO: Basal cell carcinoma in the eyelid region. *Br J Ophthalmol* 1976;**60**:806.

Collin JRO, Rathbun JE: Involutional entropion. *Arch Ophthalmol* 1978;**96**:1058.

Custer PL, Tenzel RR, Kowalczyk AP: Blepharochalasis syndrome. *Am J Ophthalmol* 1985;**99**:424.

Frueh BR, Schoengarth LD: Evaluation and treatment of the patient with ectropion. *Ophthalmology* 1982;**89**:1049.

Garland PE, Patrinely JR, Anderson RL: Hemifacial spasm: Results of unilateral myectomy. *Ophthalmology* 1987;**94**:288.

Johnson CC: Developmental abnormalities of the eyelids. *Ophthalmic Plast Reconstr Surg* 1986;**2**:2.

Jones LT: The lacrimal secretory system and its treatment. *Am J Ophthalmol* 1966;**62**:47.

Jones LT, Wobig JL: *Surgery of the Eyelids and Lacrimal Apparatus.* Aesculapius, 1976.

Kushner BJ: Congenital nasolacrimal system obstruction. *Arch Ophthalmol* 1982;**100**:597.

Quickert MH: The eyelids. Pages 937–954 in: *Modern Ophthalmology.* Vols 3 and 4. Sorsby A (editor). Butterworth, 1972.

Sevel D: Ptosis and underaction of the superior rectus muscle. *Ophthalmology* 1984;**91**:1080.

Stewart WB (editor): *Ophthalmic Plastic and Reconstructive Surgery.* American Academy of Ophthalmology, Manuals Program, 1984.

Sullivan JH, Beard C, Bullock JD: Cryosurgery for treatment of trichiasis. *Am J Ophthalmol* 1976;**82**:117.

Thygeson P: Complications of staphylococcic blepharitis. *Am J Ophthalmol* 1969;**68**:446.

Tears

4

Khalid F. Tabbara, MD

SOURCE & FUNCTION OF THE TEARS

The tears are a mixture of secretions from the major and minor (accessory) lacrimal glands, the goblet cells, and the meibomian glands. Under normal circumstances, the tear fluid forms a thin layer approximately 7–10 μm thick that covers the corneal and conjunctival epithelium. The functions of this ultrathin layer are (1) to make the cornea a smooth optical surface by abolishing minute surface irregularities of its epithelium; (2) to wet the surface of the corneal and conjunctival epithelium, preventing damage to the epithelial cells; (3) to inhibit the growth of microorganisms on the conjunctiva and cornea by mechanical flushing and the antimicrobial action of the tear fluid; and (4) to provide the cornea with necessary nutrient substances.

The total mass of the accessory lacrimal glands has been estimated to be approximately one-tenth that of the lacrimal gland mass.

COMPOSITION OF THE TEARS

The normal tear volume is estimated to be 7 ± 2 μL in each eye, with 1.1 μL in the precorneal tear film, 2.9 μL in the marginal tear meniscus, and 4.5 μL in the cul-de-sac. When collected with minimal trauma, tear fluid contains a high concentration of proteins. Three fractions are demonstrable by paper electrophoresis: albumin, globulins, and lysozyme. Albumin accounts for 60% of the total proteins of tears, and the remainder is divided equally between globulin and lysozymes.

The gamma globulins found in the normal tear fluid are IgA, IgG, and IgE. The IgA predominates and is similar to the IgA found in other body secretions bathing mucous membrane surfaces such as saliva and the bronchial, nasal, and gastrointestinal secretions. The IgA found in tears differs from serum IgA, however, and is more concentrated, since it is not transudated from serum only but is produced by plasma cells. In certain allergic conditions such as vernal conjunctivitis, the IgE concentration of tear fluid increases.

Tear lysozymes form 21–25% of the total tear proteins and, acting synergistically with gamma globulins and other nonlysozyme antibacterial factors, represent an important defense mechanism against infection.

Although lysozyme is known to have a lytic effect on certain bacteria, its absence does not necessarily increase the risk of infection. Reduction in tear lysozyme concentration usually occurs early in the course of Sjögren's syndrome and is considered helpful in the diagnosis of that disorder. Lysozyme in tears can be measured by turbidimetric assays utilizing the microorganism *Micrococcus lysodeikticus* (heat-killed) as the substrate. This can be performed on tear samples collected on regular Schirmer strips. More recently, an antibacterial factor that is closely related to betalysin was identified and measured in human tears. It appears that betalysin is a normal constituent of human tears and complements the antibacterial action of lysozyme. Tear enzymes may also play a role in diagnosis of certain clinical entities, eg, hexoseaminidase assay for diagnosis of Tay-Sachs disease.

The average glucose concentration of the tears is 5 mg/dL. Unstable glucose levels have been demonstrated in tears of normal adults. Glucose levels were found to be less in tears in closed eyes than in open eyes.

The tears also contain a small amount of urea, with an average level of 0.04 mg/dL.

Changes in the blood concentrations of both glucose and urea parallel changes in the tear glucose and tear urea levels.

K^+, Na^+, and Cl^- occur in higher concentrations in tears than in plasma. The average pH of tears is 7.35, although a wide variation in normal individuals exists (5.2–8.35). pH is usually lowest on awakening and then gradually increases owing to loss of CO_2 as the eyes remain open. Under normal conditions, tear fluid is isotonic. Tear film osmolarity ranges from 295 to 309 mosm/L. In keratoconjunctivitis sicca, there is hyperosmolarity of the tear film.

If collection of the tear fluid is traumatic, the normal constituents of the tears may be altered and there may be transudation of substances from the conjunctival blood vessels. In certain inflammatory conditions of the conjunctiva, there is marked transudation of immunoglobulins directly from the blood to the tear fluid.

LAYERS OF THE PREOCULAR TEAR FILM

The tear film covering the corneal and conjunctival epithelium (preocular tear film) is composed of 3 layers (Fig 4–1): (1) The superficial lipid layer is a monomolecular layer derived from the secretions of the meibomian glands and thought to retard evaporation of the aqueous layer. (2) The middle aqueous layer is elaborated by the major and minor lacrimal glands and contains water-soluble substances (salts and proteins). The distinction between "basal" and "reflex" tears—from the accessory and main lacrimal gland, respectively—has been questioned recently. It is generally thought that all aqueous secretion is in response to stimuli from outside that decrease during sleep and under general anesthesia. (3) The deep mucinous layer is composed of glycoprotein mucin and overlies the corneal and conjunctival epithelial cells. The epithelial cell membranes are composed of lipoproteins and are therefore relatively hydrophobic. Such a surface cannot be wetted with an aqueous solution alone. Mucin (glycoprotein) plays an important role in wetting this surface. It is partly adsorbed onto the corneal epithelial cell membranes and is anchored by the microvilli of the surface epithelial cells. This provides a new hydrophilic surface for the aqueous tears to spread on,

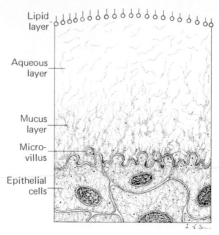

Figure 4–1. The 3 layers of the tear film covering the superficial epithelial layer of the cornea.

and the surface is wetted by a lowering of the tears' surface tension. Mucin is elaborated by the goblet cells of the conjunctiva, and recent studies have shown that the lacrimal gland contributes to its production.

Periodic resurfacing of the tear film is important to prevent dry spots and is accomplished by blinking.

Table 4–1. Etiology and diagnosis of dry eye syndrome.

I. Etology:
  A. Conditions Characterized by Hypofunction of the Lacrimal Gland:
   1. Congenital–
      a. Familial dysautonomia (Riley-Day syndrome).
      b. Aplasia of the lacrimal gland (congenital alacrima).
      c. Trigeminal nerve aplasia.
      d. Ectodermal dysplasia.
   2. Acquired–
      a. Systemic diseases–
         (1) Sjögren's syndrome.
         (2) Progressive systemic sclerosis.
         (3) Sarcoidosis.
         (4) Leukemia, lymphoma.
         (5) Amyloidosis.
         (6) Hemochromatosis.
      b. Infection–
         (1) Trachoma.
         (2) Mumps.
      c. Injury–
         (1) Surgical removal of lacrimal gland.
         (2) Irradiation.
         (3) Chemical burn.
      d. Medications–
         (1) Antihistamines.
         (2) Antimuscarinics: atropine, scopamine.
         (3) General anesthetics: halothane, nitrous oxide.
         (4) Beta-adrenergic blockers: timolol, practolol.
      e. Neurogenic–Neuroparalytic (facial nerve palsy).
  B. Conditions Characterized by Mucin Deficiency:
   1. Avitaminosis A.
   2. Stevens-Johnson syndrome.
   3. Ocular pemphigoid.
   4. Chronic conjunctivitis, eg, trachoma.
   5. Chemical burns.
      6. Medications–Antihistamines, antimuscarinic agents, beta-adrenergic blocking agents (eg, practolol).
      7. Folk remedies, eg, kermes.
  C. Conditions Characterized by Lipid Deficiency:
   1. Lid margin scarring.
   2. Blephatitis.
  D. Defective Spreading of Tear Film Caused by the Following:
   1. Eyelid abnormalities–
      a. Defects, coloboma.
      b. Ectropion or entropion.
      c. Keratinization of lid margin.
      d. Decreased or absent blinking.
         (1) Neurologic disorders.
         (2) Hyperthyroidism.
         (3) Contact lens.
         (4) Drugs.
         (5) Herpes simplex keratitis.
         (6) Leprosy.
      e. Lagophthalmos–
         (1) Nocturnal lagophthalmos.
         (2) Hyperthyroidism.
         (3) Leprosy.
   2. Conjunctival abnormalities–
      a. Pterygium.
      b. Symblepharon.
   3. Proptosis.
II. Diagnostic Tests:
  A. Biomicroscopy.
  B. Rose bengal staining.
  C. Fluorescein staining.
  D. Tear break-up time.
  E. Tear film osmolarity.
  F. Tear lysozyme.
  G. Schirmer test without anesthesia.
  H. Impression cytology.
  I. Ocular ferning test.

In the normal eye, blinking maintains a continuous tear film over the ocular surface.

DRY EYE SYNDROME
(Keratoconjunctivitis Sicca)

Inadequacy or instability of any of the tear film components or insufficient interaction between the tear film mucin layer and the cell surface membrane glycoproteins results in structural and functional alterations in the ocular surface, including the appearance of dry spots on the corneal and conjunctival epithelium, formation of filaments, loss of conjunctival goblet cells, abnormal enlargement of nongoblet epithelial cells, increased cellular stratification, and increased keratinization. Dryness of the eye may therefore result from any disease associated with deficiency of the tear film components (aqueous, mucin, or lipid; lid surface abnormalities, or epithelial abnormalities). Although there are many forms of keratoconjunctivitis sicca, those connected with rheumatoid arthritis and other autoimmune diseases are commonly referred to as Sjögren's syndrome.

Etiology

Many of the causes of dry eye syndrome affect more than one component of the tear film or lead to ocular surface alterations that secondarily cause tear film instability. Despite the diversity of underlying causes, however, the ocular surface changes show common histopathologic features, as mentioned above. The etiology and diagnosis of keratoconjunctivitis sicca are summarized in Table 4–1.

Clinical Findings

Patients with dry eyes complain most frequently of a scratchy or sandy (foreign body) sensation. Other common symptoms are itching, excessive mucus secretion, inability to produce tears, a burning sensation, photosensitivity, redness, pain, and difficulty in moving the lids. In most patients, the most remarkable feature of the eye examination is the grossly normal appearance of the eye.

The most characteristic feature on slit lamp examination is the interrupted or absent tear meniscus at the lower lid margin. Tenacious yellowish mucous strands are sometimes seen in the lower conjunctival fornix. The bulbar conjunctiva loses its normal luster and may be thickened, edematous, and hyperemic.

The damaged corneal and conjunctival epithelial cells stain with 1% rose bengal (Fig 4–2), and defects in the corneal epithelium stain with fluorescein. The corneal epithelium shows varying degrees of fine punctate stippling in the interpalpebral fissure.

In the late stages of keratoconjunctivitis sicca, filaments may be seen—one end of each filament attached to the corneal epithelium and the other end moving freely (Figs 4–3 and 4–4). Three types of corneal filaments have been recognized: (1) filaments

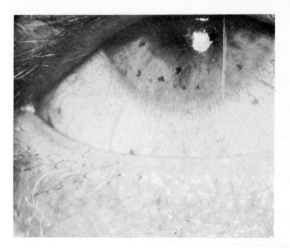

Figure 4–2. Rose bengal staining of corneal and conjunctival cells in a 54-year-old woman with keratoconjunctivitis sicca.

consisting entirely of mucus, (2) filaments consisting entirely of epithelial cells, and (3) filaments consisting of epithelial cells and mucus.

In patients with Sjögren's syndrome, conjunctival scrapings may show increased numbers of goblet cells (Fig 4–5). Lacrimal gland enlargement occurs uncommonly in patients with Sjögren's syndrome. Diagnosis and grading of the dry eye condition can be achieved with good accuracy using the following diagnostic methods:

A. Schirmer Test: The use of wettable filter paper strips as a device for measuring tear secretion was first described by Köster in 1900 in connection with a study of facial nerve paralysis. Köster placed one end of a filter paper strip 1 cm wide and 20 cm long

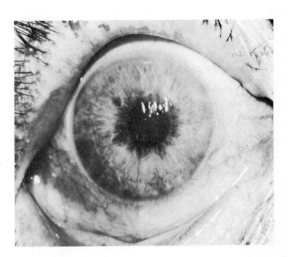

Figure 4–3. Corneal filaments in a 56-year-old patient with keratoconjunctivitis sicca.

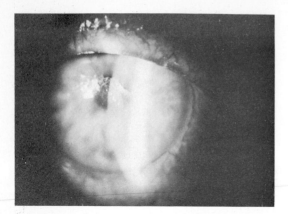

Figure 4–4. Slit lamp picture of a 48-year-old patient with keratoconjunctivitis sicca and corneal filaments.

in the conjunctival sac in each eye and noted the extent of wetting by the tear fluid. In 1903, Otto Schirmer modified Köster's method by reducing the width of the strips to 0.5 cm and their length to 3.5 cm utilizing Whatman filter paper No. 41. The test is done by inserting the Schirmer strips into the lower conjunctival cul-de-sac at the junction of the middle and temporal thirds of the lower lid, then measuring the moistened exposed portion 5 minutes after insertion. The normal range of the Schirmer test (without anesthesia) is 10–25 minutes.

Schirmer tests performed without topical anesthesia measure the function of the lacrimal gland, whose secretory activity is stimulated by the irritating nature of the filter paper. Schirmer tests performed after topical anesthesia (instillation of 0.5% tetracaine) measure the function of the accessory lacrimal glands (the basic secretors).

The Schirmer test is a good screening test—and definitely the simplest test—for the assessment of tear production. However, false-positive and false-negative results occur in 15% of eyes tested; a positive result (decreased wetting of the filter paper strip) should be confirmed and a negative result should by no means rule out dryness of the eyes, particularly if it is secondary to mucin deficiency.

A Schirmer test showing less than 10 mm of wetting in 5 minutes is considered abnormal. Many modifications of the Schirmer test have been introduced, but none have been shown to be superior.

B. Tear Film Break-Up Time: At present there is no practical method of measuring the mucin content of the tear fluid, but measurement of the tear film break-up time may sometimes be very useful. Deficiency in mucin may not affect the Schirmer test but may lead to instability of the tear film. This causes the film's rapid break-up. "Dry spots" (Fig 4–6) are formed in the tear film, and a baring of the corneal or conjunctival epithelium follows. This process ultimately damages the epithelial cells, which can then be stained with rose bengal. Damaged epithelial cells may be shed from the cornea, leaving areas susceptible to punctate staining when the corneal surface is flooded with fluorescein.

The tear film break-up time can be measured by applying a slightly moistened fluorescein strip to the bulbar conjunctiva and asking the patient to blink. The tear film is then scanned with the aid of a slit lamp while the patient refrains from blinking. A cobalt blue filter and a broad light beam are used for this purpose. The time that elapses before the first dry spot appears in the corneal fluorescein layer is the tear film break-up time. Normally, the break-up time is over 15 seconds, but it can be reduced appreciably by the

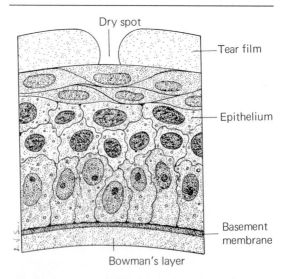

Figure 4–6. Baring of the corneal epithelium following formation of a dry spot in the tear film. (Modified and redrawn from Dohlman CH: The function of the corneal epithelium in health and disease. *Invest Ophthalmol* 1971;**10**:383.)

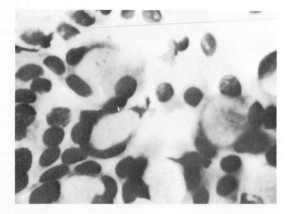

Figure 4–5. Goblet cells in conjunctival scrapings from a patient with Sjögren's syndrome. (Stained with Giemsa's stain.)

use of local anesthetics, by manipulating the eye, or by holding the lids open. The break-up time is shorter in eyes with aqueous tear deficiency and is always shorter than normal in eyes with mucin deficiency.

C. Rose Bengal Staining: Rose bengal is a sensitive dye capable of staining all desiccated nonvital epithelial cells. Three patterns of staining have been shown to be proportionate to the severity of conduction: **C-pattern (mild)** staining is scattered punctate staining of the exposed conjunctiva and minimal staining of the inferior cornea; **B-pattern (moderate)** staining consists of blotchy uptake of rose bengal in the entire interpalpebral area; and in **A-pattern (severe)** staining, filaments are present, with confluent staining as a wedge-shaped pattern on the interpalpebral part of the bulbar conjunctiva and the corneal surface.

Rose bengal staining is highly specific (about 100%), though sensitivity is only about 60%.

D. Ocular Ferning Test: A simple and inexpensive qualitative test for the study of conjunctival mucus has been described. The test is performed by spreading conjunctival scrapings on a clean glass slide and letting them dry. Microscopic arborization (ferning) is observed in normal eyes. In patients with cicatrizing conjunctivitis (ocular pemphigoid, Stevens-Johnson syndrome, diffuse conjunctival cicatrization), ferning of the mucus is either reduced or absent.

E. Fluorescein Staining: Touching the conjunctiva with a dry strip of fluorescein is a good indicator of its wetness, and the tear meniscus can be seen easily. Fluorescein will stain the eroded and denuded areas as well as microscopic defects of the corneal epithelium.

F. Tear Osmolarity: Hyperosmolarity of tears has been documented in many cases of keratoconjunctivitis sicca and in contact lens wearers. It can occur even with normal Schirmer test and rose bengal staining. The method's sensitivity and specificity depend on the reference value used.

G. Tear Lysozyme Assay: Patients with dry eye syndromes have low to absent levels of tear lysozymes. All methods used to determine lysozyme assay are difficult to standardize. The most common is spectrophotometric assay.

H. Impression Cytology: Impression cytology is a method by which goblet cell densities on the conjunctival surface can be counted. In normal individuals, the goblet cell population reaches its maximum in the inferonasal quadrant ($1500/mm^2$) and decreases to $400/mm^2$ on the interpalpebral bulbar conjunctiva. Loss of goblet cells has been documented in cases of keratoconjunctivitis sicca, trachoma, cicatricial ocular pemphigoid, Stevens-Johnson syndrome, and avitaminosis A.

Complications

Early in the course of keratoconjunctivitis sicca, vision is slightly impaired and a few patients develop corneal ulceration, corneal thinning, and perforation. Secondary bacterial infection occasionally occurs, and corneal scarring and vascularization may result in marked reduction in vision. Early treatment may prevent these complications.

Treatment

The patient should understand that dry eyes is a chronic condition and that definitive cure is unlikely except in early cases, when the corneal and conjunctival epithelial changes are usually reversible.

Aqueous deficiency can be treated by replacement of aqueous with artificial tears. Relief of symptoms can be achieved by control of environmental conditions and work habits and by using humidifiers, wraparound glasses, or moist chamber spectacles (Table 4–2). A slow-release artificial tear insert (Lacrisert) is now available. The insert is a solid 5-mg rod made of hydroxypropylcellulose. When inserted into the inferior cul-de-sac, the rod swells up to 10 times its original size by imbibition of fluid from the capillary bed, and the hydroxypropylcellulose is slowly released over a period of 12 hours. About half of patients with keratoconjunctivitis sicca achieve good relief with one insert in each eye in the morning. Some patients complain of irritation or burning sensations. Topical artificial tears may be used simultaneously with these preservative-free inserts.

Mucin deficiency can be partially compensated for by use of ophthalmic vehicles of high molecular weight—eg, water-soluble polymers—or by the use of diluted sodium hyaluronate (Amvisc, Healon) solutions or the patient's own serum as local eye drops. Serum used for this purpose must be kept refrigerated. It acts by lowering the surface tension of the tears, assisting in the spreading of the tears and wetting the epithelium. If the mucus is tenacious, as in Sjögren's syndrome, mucolytic agents (eg, acetylcysteine, 10%) will be of help.

Patients who have excessive tear lipids require specific instructions and demonstration of techniques for removal of lipid from the eyelid margin. Antibiotics either topically or as systemic tetracycline may be necessary in some cases.

Table 4–2. Local therapy of dry eye syndrome.

Mild syndrome
  (1) Artificial tears 4–5 times daily.
  (2) Lubricating ointment at bedtime.
Moderate syndrome
  (1) Artificial tears every 2 hours.
  (2) Lubricating ointment at bedtime.
  (3) Consider sustained-release tear insert (Lacrisert), one insert in each eye once daily.
  (4) Mucolytic agent (acetylcysteine, 10%, 4 times daily).
Severe syndrome
  (1) Artificial tears (or gum cellulose, 0.625%) every hour. Avoid benzalkonium chloride.
  (2) Tight goggles.
  (3) Punctal occlusion.
  (4) Lubricating ointment at bedtime.
  (5) Change environment; use humidifier.
  (6) Tretinoin (Retin–A), 0.1%, in patients with squamous metaplasia.

Treatment with tretinoin (Retin-A), 0.1%, relieved symptoms and improved visual acuity in patients with Sjögren's syndrome, Stevens-Johnson syndrome, ocular pemphigoid, and postoperative or postradiation dry eye syndrome. Fewer abnormalities were also seen with rose bengal staining or the Schirmer test in these patients. Topical vitamin A treatment causes reversal of squamous metaplasia.

OTHER DISORDERS OF THE LACRIMAL SYSTEM

Lacrimal Hypersecretion

The causes of excessive tearing are varied but are due to stimulation of the lacrimal gland.

Psychic lacrimation is normally associated with pain or emotional upsets. The fact that this type of lacrimation appears after the first few months of life explains why newborns do not produce tears when they cry.

Neurogenic lacrimation is brought about by reflex stimulation. Eyestrain, corneal injury, a blast of hot air, dry wind, or foreign body in the cornea or conjunctiva may cause reflex trigeminal irritation that excites lacrimation. Strong light causes reflex visual irritation and copious lacrimation. Irritation of the facial nerve, yawning, vomiting, and laughing are also associated with reflex lacrimation.

Epiphora may follow obstruction of the lacrimal drainage system. This can be caused by punctal eversion or occlusion or by canalicular or nasolacrimal duct obstruction. Most cases of nasolacrimal duct obstruction can be corrected surgically.

Paradoxic Lacrimation ("Crocodile Tears")

This is an acquired unilateral (very rarely bilateral) condition characterized by excessive tearing while eating. It occurs as a sequel to Bell's palsy (facial nerve palsy) and is the result of aberrant regeneration of the facial nerve fibers.

Bloody Tears

This is a rare clinical entity attributed to a variety of causes. It has been associated with menstruation ("vicarious menses"). Blood-tinged tears may be secondary to conjunctival hemorrhage due to any cause (trauma, blood dyscrasia, etc) or to tumors of the lacrimal sac. They have also recently been reported in a hypertensive patient suffering from epistaxis with extension through the nasolacrimal duct.

REFERENCES

Allansmith MR et al: Plasma cell content of main and accessory lacrimal glands and conjunctiva. *Am J Ophthalmol* 1976;**82**:819.

Allen M, Wright P, Reid L: The human lacrimal gland: A histochemical and organ culture study of the secretory cells. *Arch Ophthalmol* 1972;**88**:493.

Beitch I: The induction of keratinization in the corneal epithelium: A comparison of the "dry" and vitamin A-deficient eyes. *Invest Ophthalmol* 1970;**9**:827.

Brauninger GE, Centifanto YM: Immunoglobulin E in human tears. *Am J Ophthalmol* 1971;**72**:558.

Cotlier E: Tears for diagnosis of Tay-Sachs and other genetic diseases. Page 16 in: *The Fourth National Science Writer Seminar in Ophthalmology.* Research to Prevent Blindness Inc., 1973.

Crandall DC, Leopold IH: The influence of systemic drugs on tear constituents. *Ophthalmology* 1979;**86**:115.

Daum KM, Hill RM: Human tears: Glucose instabilities. *Acta Ophthalmol* 1984;**62**:472.

DeLuise VP, Tabbara KF: Quantitation of tear lysozyme levels in dry-eye disorders. *Arch Ophthalmol* 1983;**101**:634.

Dohlman CH: Punctal occlusion in keratoconjunctivitis sicca. *Ophthalmology* 1978;**85**:1277.

Farris RL: The dry eye: Its mechanisms and therapy, with evidence that contact lens wear is a cause. *CLAO J* 1986;**12**:234.

Ford LC, DeLange RJ, Petty RW: Identification of a non-lysozymal bactericidal factor (beta lysin) in human tears and aqueous humor. *Am J Ophthalmol* 1976;**81**:30.

Frayha RA, Tabbara KF, Geha RS: Familial CRST syndrome with sicca complex. *J Rheumatol* 1977;**4**:53.

Friedland BR, Anderson DR, Forster RK: Non-lysozyme antibacterial factor in human tears. *Am J Ophthalmol* 1972;**74**:52.

Gilbard JP, Farris RL, Santamaria J II: Osmolarity of tear microvolumes in keratoconjunctivitis sicca. *Arch Ophthalmol* 1978;**96**:677.

Gilbard JP et al: Morphologic effect of hyperosmolarity on rabbit corneal epithelium. *Ophthalmology* 1984;**91**:1205.

Gillette TE, Greiner JV, Allansmith MR: Immunohistochemical localization of human tear lysozyme. *Arch Ophthalmol* 1981;**99**:298.

Holly FJ, Lemp MA: Tear physiology and dry eyes. *Surv Ophthalmol* 1977;**22**:69.

Huth SW, Miller MJ, Leopold IH: Calcium and protein in tears: Diurnal variation. *Arch Ophthalmol* 1981;**99**:1628.

Hypher TJ: Uptake and loss of tears from filter paper discs employed in lysozyme tests. *Br J Ophthalmol* 1979; **63**:251.

Jones DB: Prospects in the management of tear-deficiency states. *Trans Am Acad Ophthalmol Otolaryngol* 1977; **83**:693.

Kassan SS, Gardy M: Sjögren's syndrome: An update and overview. *Am J Med* 1978;**64**:1037.

Katz IM, Blackman WM: A soluble sustained-release ophthalmic delivery unit. *Am J Ophthalmol* 1977;**83**:728.

Kurihashi K: A new thread tear test using silicone tubing. *Ophthalmologica* 1987;**195**:192.

Lamberts DW, Langston DP, Chu W: A clinical study of slow-releasing artificial tears. *Ophthalmology* 1978;**85**:794.

Lemp MA et al: Dry eye secondary to mucus deficiency. *Trans Am Acad Ophthalmol Otolaryngol* 1971;**75**:1223.

Mackie IA, Seal DV: Beta-blockers, eye complaints, and tear secretion. (Letter.) *Lancet* 1977;**2**:1027.

Mackie IA, Seal DV: The questionably dry eye. *Br J Ophthalmol* 1981;**65**:2.

Mackie IA, Seal DV, Pescod JM: Beta-adrenergic receptor blocking drugs: Tear lysozyme and immunological screening for adverse reaction. *Br J Ophthalmol* 1977; **61**:354.

Minton LR: Paralimbal ring keratitis and absence of lysozyme in lupus erythematosus. *Am J Ophthalmol* 1965; **60**:532.

Moses R: *Adler's Physiology of the Eye: Clinical Application,* 7th ed. Mosby, 1981.

Nielsen NV, Eriksen JS: Timolol transitory manifestations of dry eyes in long-term treatment. *Acta Ophthalmol* 1979;**57**:418.

Norn MS: The conjunctival fluid, its height, volume, density of cells, and flow. *Acta Ophthalmol* 1966;**44**:212.

Ohashi Y et al: The presence of cytotoxic autoantibody to lacrimal gland cells in NZB/W mice. *Invest Ophthalmol Vis Sci* 1985;**26**:214.

Spiers AS: Syndrome of "crocodile tears": Pharmacologic study of a bilateral case. *Br J Ophthalmol* 1970;**54**:330.

Tabbara KF: Sjögren's syndrome. Pages 309–314 in: *The Cornea: Scientific Foundation and Clinical Practice.* Smolin G, Thoft RA (editors). Little, Brown, 1983.

Tabbara KF, Okumoto M: Ocular ferning test: A qualitative test for mucus deficiency. *Ophthalmology* 1982;**89**:712.

Tabbara KF et al: Sjögren's syndrome: A correlation between ocular findings and labial salivary gland histology. *Trans Am Acad Ophthalmol Otolaryngol* 1974;**78**:467.

Tseng SC et al: Topical retinoid treatment for various dry-eye disorders. *Ophthalmology* 1985;**92**:717.

Van Bijsterveld OP: Diagnostic tests in the sicca syndrome. *Arch Ophthalmol* 1969;**82**:10.

Warwick R: *Eugene Wolff's Anatomy of the Eye and Orbit,* 7th ed. Saunders, 1977.

Werblin TP, Rheinstrom SD, Kaufman HE: The use of slow-release artificial tears in the long-term management of keratitis sicca. *Ophthalmology* 1981;**88**:78.

5

Conjunctiva

Daniel Vaughan, MD

ANATOMY & PHYSIOLOGY

The conjunctiva is the thin, transparent mucous membrane that covers the posterior surface of the lids (the palpebral conjunctiva) and the anterior surface of the sclera (the bulbar conjunctiva). It is continuous with the skin at the lid margin (a mucocutaneous junction) and with the corneal epithelium at the limbus.

The **palpebral conjunctiva** lines the posterior surface of the lids and is firmly adherent to the tarsus. At the superior and inferior margins of the tarsus, the conjunctiva is reflected posteriorly (at the superior and inferior fornices) and covers the episcleral tissue to become the bulbar conjunctiva.

The **bulbar conjunctiva** is loosely attached to the orbital septum in the fornices and is folded many times. This allows the eye to move and enlarges the secretory conjunctival surface. (The ducts of the lacrimal gland open into the superior temporal fornix.) Except at the limbus (where Tenon's capsule and the conjunctiva are fused for about 3 mm), the bulbar conjunctiva is loosely attached to Tenon's capsule and the underlying sclera.

A soft, movable, thickened fold of bulbar conjunctiva (the **semilunar fold**) is located at the inner canthus and corresponds to the nictitating membrane of some lower animals. A small, fleshy, epidermoid structure (the **caruncle**) is attached superficially to the inner portion of the semilunar fold and is a transition zone containing both cutaneous and mucous membrane elements.

Histology

The **conjunctival epithelium** consists of 2–5 layers of stratified columnar epithelial cells, superficial and basal. Conjunctival epithelium near the limbus, over the caruncle, and near the mucocutaneous junctions at the lid margins consists of stratified squamous epithelial cells. The **superficial epithelial cells** contain round or oval mucus-secreting goblet cells. The mucus, as it forms, pushes aside the goblet cell nucleus and is necessary for proper dispersion of the precorneal tear film. The **basal epithelial cells** stain more deeply than the superficial cells and near the limbus may contain pigment.

The **conjunctival stroma** is divided into an adenoid (superficial) layer and a fibrous (deep) layer. The ad-enoid layer contains lymphoid tissue and in some areas may contain "folliclelike" structures without germinal centers. The adenoid layer does not develop until after the first 2 or 3 months of life. This explains why inclusion conjunctivitis of the newborn is papillary in nature rather than follicular and why it later becomes follicular. The **fibrous layer** is composed of connective tissue that attaches to the tarsal plate. This explains the appearance of the papillary reaction in inflammations of the conjunctiva. The fibrous layer is loosely arranged over the globe.

The **accessory lacrimal glands** (glands of Krause and Wolfring), which resemble the lacrimal gland in structure and function, are located in the stroma. Most of the glands of Krause are in the upper fornix, the remaining few in the lower fornix. The glands of Wolfring lie at the superior margin of the upper tarsus.

The conjunctival blood vessels are derived from the anterior ciliary and palpebral arteries. The nerves arise from the ophthalmic division of the fifth cranial nerve. There are only a few pain fibers. The conjunctiva is rich in lymphatics.

CONJUNCTIVITIS

Inflammation of the conjunctiva (conjunctivitis) is the most common eye disease in the western hemisphere. It varies in severity from a mild hyperemia with tearing to a severe conjunctivitis with purulent discharge. The source is usually exogenous, sometimes endogenous.

The types of conjunctivitis and their commonest causes are set forth in Tables 5–1 and 5–2.

GENERAL CONSIDERATIONS

Because of its location, the conjunctiva is exposed to many microorganisms and other noxious substances. Resisting this bombardment are the tears. By diluting the infectious material and sluicing the conjunctival debris and organisms into the nasal passages for excretion, they greatly reduce the conjunctiva's

Table 5–1. Causes of conjunctivitis.

Bacterial
  Purulent
    Neisseria gonorrhoeae
    Neisseria meningitidis
  Acute catarrhal (pinkeye)
    Pneumococcus (*Streptococcus pneumoniae*)
      (temperate climates)
    Haemophilus aegyptius (Koch-Weeks bacillus)
      (tropical climates)
  Subacute catarrhal
    Haemophilus influenzae (temperate climates)
  Chronic, including blepharoconjunctivitis
    Staphylococcus aureus
    Moraxella lacunata (diplobacillus of
      Morax-Axenfeld)
  Rare types (acute, subacute, chronic)
    Streptococci
    Branhamella (*Neisseria*) *catarrhalis*
    Coliforms
    Proteus
    Corynebacterium diphtheriae
    Mycobacterium tuberculosis
    Treponema pallidum
Chlamydial
  Trachoma (*Chlamydia trachomatis*)
  Inclusion conjunctivitis (*Chlamydia oculogenitalis*)
  Lymphogranuloma venereum (LGV) (*Chlamydia
    lymphogranulomatis*)
  Psittacosis (*Chlamydia psittaci*)
  Rare types: Agents of feline pneumonitis and ovine
    abortion
Viral
  Acute viral follicular conjunctivitis
    Pharyngoconjunctival fever due to adenoviruses
      types 3 and 7
    Epidemic keratoconjunctivitis due to adenovirus
      types 8 and 19
    Herpes simplex virus
  Newcastle disease
    Acute hemorrhagic conjunctivitis due to enterovirus
      type 70; rarely, coxsackievirus type A28
  Chronic viral follicular conjunctivitis
    Molluscum contagiosum virus
  Viral blepharoconjunctivitis
    Vaccinia due to vaccinia-variola viruses
    Varicella, zoster due to varicella-zoster virus
    Measles virus
Rickettsial
  Nonpurulent conjunctivitis with hyperemia and
    minimal infiltration, often a feature of rickettsial
    diseases
    Typhus
    Murine typhus
    Scrub typhus
    Rocky Mountain spotted fever
    Mediterranean fever
    Q fever
Fungal (Rare.)
  Catarrhal, complicating blepharitis
    Candida
  Granulomatous
    Rhinosporidium seeberi
    Coccidioides immitis (San Joaquin Valley fever)
    Sporothrix schenckii
Parasitic (Rare but important.)
  Chronic conjunctivitis and blepharoconjunctivitis
    Onchocerca volvulus (Central America, Africa)
    Thelazia californiensis

Parasitic (Rare but important.) (cont'd)
  Chronic conjunctivitis and blepharoconjunctivitis
    (cont'd)
    Loa loa
    Ascaris lumbricoides
    Trichinella spiralis
    Schistosoma haematobium (bladder fluke)
    Taenia solium (cysticercus)
    Pthirus pubis (*Pediculus pubis,* pubic louse)
    Fly larvae (*Oestrus ovis,* etc) (ocular myiasis)
Immunologic (Allergic)
  Immediate (humoral) hypersensitivity reactions
    Hay fever conjunctivitis (pollens, grasses, animal
      dander, etc)
    Vernal keratoconjunctivitis
    Atopic keratoconjunctivitis
    Giant papillary conjunctivitis
  Delayed (cellular) hypersensitivity reactions
    Phlyctenulosis
    Mild conjunctivitis secondary to contact blepharitis
  Autoimmune disease
    Keratoconjunctivitis sicca associated with Sjögren's
      syndrome
    Cicatricial pemphigoid
    Midline lethal granuloma and Wegener's
      granulomatosis
Chemical or Irritative
  Iatrogenic
    Miotics
    Idoxuridine
    Other topically applied drugs
    Contact lens solutions
  Occupational
    Acids
    Alkalies
    Smoke
    Wind
    Ultraviolet light
    Caterpillar hair
Etiology Unknown
  Folliculosis
  Chronic follicular conjunctivitis (orphan's
    conjunctivitis, Axenfeld's conjunctivitis)
  Ocular rosacea
  Psoriasis
  Erythema multiforme major (Stevens-Johnson
    syndrome) and minor
  Dermatitis herpetiformis
  Epidermolysis bullosa
  Superior limbic keratoconjunctivitis
  Ligneous conjunctivitis
  Reiter's syndrome
  Mucocutaneous lymph node syndrome (Kawasaki
    disease)
Associated With Systemic Disease
  Conjunctivitis in thyroid disease
  Gouty conjunctivitis
  Carcinoid conjunctivitis
  Sarcoidosis
  Tuberculosis
  Syphilis
Secondary to Dacryocystitis or Canaliculitis
  Conjunctivitis secondary to dacryocystitis
    Pneumococci or beta-hemolytic streptococci
  Conjunctivitis secondary to canaliculitis
    Actinomyces israelii, Candida sp, *Aspergillus* sp
    (rarely)
  Conjunctivitis secondary to tumors of conjunctiva
    or lid margins

Table 5–2. Differentiation of the common types of conjunctivitis.

Clinical Findings and Cytology	Viral	Bacterial	Chlamydial	Allergic
Itching	Minimal	Minimal	Minimal	Severe
Hyperemia	Generalized	Generalized	Generalized	Generalized
Tearing	Profuse	Moderate	Moderate	Moderate
Exudation	Minimal	Profuse	Profuse	Minimal
Preauricular adenopathy	Common	Uncommon	Common only in inclusion conjunctivitis	None
In stained scrapings and exudates	Monocytes	Bacteria, PMNs[1]	PMSs,[1] plasma cells, inclusion bodies	Eosinophils
Associated sore throat and fever	Occasionally	Occasionally	Never	Never

[1] Polymorphonuclear cells.

vulnerability. They also contain lysozyme, betalysin, IgA, and IgG, all of which can inhibit bacterial growth.

The following factors make established conjunctivitis a self-limiting disease: tears, abundant lymphoid elements, constant epithelial exfoliation, a cool conjunctival sac due to tear evaporation, the pumping action of the tear drainage system (unimpeded when the lids are open), and the fact that bacteria are caught in the conjunctival mucus and then excreted.

Although organisms pathogenic for the genitourinary tract are also pathogenic for the conjunctiva, those that grow abundantly on the nasal mucosa tend to grow less well in the conjunctival sac, and vice versa. For example, whereas the conjunctiva is usually resistant to the viruses of the common cold, it is highly susceptible to the gonococcus and inclusion conjunctivitis agents, both of which are infectious for the genitourinary tract. Moreover, when these organisms are established on the conjunctiva, they are constantly washed down the nasolacrimal duct into the nose by the tears, yet they grow in the nose only rarely and with difficulty.

Cytology of Conjunctivitis

Damage to the conjunctival epithelium by a noxious agent may be followed by epithelial edema, cellular death and exfoliation, epithelial hypertrophy, or granulomas. There may also be edema of the conjunctival stroma (chemosis) and hypertrophy of the adenoid layer of the stroma (follicle formation). Inflammatory cells, including neutrophils, eosinophils, basophils, lymphocytes, and plasma cells, may be seen and often indicate the nature of the damaging agent. The inflammatory cells migrate from the conjunctival stroma through the epithelium to the surface. They then combine with fibrin and with the mucus produced by the conjunctival goblet cells to form the conjunctival exudate, which accounts for the gumming of the eyelids noted on waking.

The inflammatory cells appear in the exudate or in scrapings taken with a sterile platinum spatula from the anesthetized conjunctival surface. The material is stained with Gram's stain (to identify the bacterial organisms) and with Giemsa's stain (to identify the cell types). A predominance of polymorphonuclear leukocytes is characteristic of both bacterial and chlamydial conjunctivitis. As a rule, a predominance of mononuclear cells, especially lymphocytes, is characteristic of viral conjunctivitis except when a pseudomembrane forms, as it may in epidemic keratoconjunctivitis or herpes simplex virus conjunctivitis. Polymorphonuclear cells then predominate because of necrosis.

Eosinophils and basophils are found in allergic conjunctivitis, and scattered eosinophil granules and eosinophils are found in vernal keratoconjunctivitis. In all types of conjunctivitis there are plasma cells in the conjunctival stroma. They do not migrate through the epithelium, however, and are therefore not seen in smears of exudate or of scrapings from the conjunctival surface unless the epithelium has become necrosed, as it may in trachoma; in this event, the rupturing of a follicle allows the plasma cells to reach the epithelial surface. Since the mature follicles of trachoma rupture easily, the finding of large, palely staining, lymphoblastic (germinal center) cells in scrapings strongly suggests trachoma.

Symptoms of Conjunctivitis

The important symptoms of conjunctivitis are a foreign body sensation, a scratching or burning sensation, a sensation of fullness around the eyes, itching, and (when the cornea is also affected) photophobia.

Foreign body sensation and a scratching or burning sensation are often associated with the swelling and papillary hypertrophy that normally accompany conjunctival hyperemia. If there is pain, the cornea is probably also affected. Pain is suggestive of corneal or iridic involvement.

Signs of Conjunctivitis
(Table 5–2)

The important signs of conjunctivitis are hyperemia, tearing, exudation, pseudoptosis, papillary hypertrophy, chemosis, follicles, pseudomembranes and membranes, granulomas, and preauricular adenopathy.

Hyperemia is the most conspicuous clinical sign of acute conjunctivitis. The redness is most marked in the fornix and diminishes toward the limbus by virtue of the dilatation of the posterior conjunctival vessels. (A perilimbal dilatation suggests inflammation of the cornea or deeper structures.) A brilliant red suggests bacterial conjunctivitis, and a milky appearance suggests allergic conjunctivitis. Hyperemia without cellular infiltration suggests irritation from physical causes such as wind, sun, smoke, etc, and also occurs occasionally as part of a general vascular dilatation, eg, acne rosacea or carcinoid.

Tearing is often prominent in conjunctivitis, the tears resulting from the foreign body sensation, the burning or scratching sensation, or the itching. Mild transudation also arises from the hyperemic vessels and adds to the tearing. An abnormally scant secretion of tears suggests granulomatous conjunctivitis or keratoconjunctivitis sicca.

Exudation is a feature of all types of acute conjunctivitis. The exudate is flaky and amorphous in bacterial conjunctivitis and stringy in allergic conjunctivitis. A mild gumming of the lids on waking occurs in almost all types of conjunctivitis, and if the exudate is copious and the lids are firmly stuck together the conjunctivitis is probably bacterial or chlamydial.

Pseudoptosis is a drooping of the upper lid. This suggests edema or infiltration of Müller's muscle. The condition is seen in several types of severe conjunctivitis, eg, trachoma and epidemic keratoconjunctivitis.

Papillary hypertrophy is a nonspecific conjunctival reaction that occurs because the conjunctiva is bound down to the underlying tarsus or limbus by fine fibrils. When the tuft of vessels that forms the substance of the papilla (along with cellular elements and exudates) reaches the basement membrane of the epithelium, it branches over the papilla like the spokes in the frame of an umbrella. An inflammatory exudate accumulates between the fibrils, heaping the conjunctiva into mounds. In necrotizing disease (eg, trachoma), the exudate may be replaced by granulation tissue or connective tissue.

When the papillae are small, the conjunctiva usually has a smooth, velvety appearance. A red papillary conjunctiva suggests bacterial or chlamydial disease (eg, a velvety red tarsal conjunctiva is characteristic of stage IIb trachoma). When the papillae are large they are flat-topped, polygonal, and milky in color. On the upper tarsus they suggest vernal keratoconjunctivitis, and on the lower tarsus they suggest atopic keratoconjunctivitis. Giant papillae may also occur at the limbus, especially in the area that is normally exposed when the eyes are open (between 2 and 4 o'clock and between 8 and 10 o'clock). Here they appear as gelatinous infiltrates that may encroach on the cornea. Limbal papillae are characteristic of vernal keratoconjunctivitis, rare in atopic keratoconjunctivitis.

Chemosis of the conjunctiva strongly suggests acute hay fever conjunctivitis but may also occur in acute gonococcal or meningococcal conjunctivitis and especially in adenoviral conjunctivitis. Chemosis of the bulbar conjunctiva is seen in patients with trichinosis. Occasionally, chemosis may appear before there is any gross cellular infiltration or exudation.

Follicles are seen in most cases of viral conjunctivitis, in all cases of chlamydial conjunctivitis except neonatal inclusion conjunctivitis, and in some cases of toxic conjunctivitis induced by topical medications such as idoxuridine and miotics. Follicles in the fornix and at the tarsal margins have limited diagnostic value, but when they are located on the tarsi (especially the upper tarsus), a chlamydial, viral, or toxic conjunctivitis following topical medication should be suspected.

The follicle is a focal lymphoid hyperplasia within the adenoid layer of the conjunctiva and usually contains a germinal center. Clinically, it can be recognized as an avascular white or gray, round structure. On slit lamp examination, small vessels can be seen arising at the border of the follicle and encircling it.

Pseudomembranes and **membranes**—the result of a coagulating process and differing only in degree—are produced by infectious or toxic agents. A pseudomembrane is a coagulum on the *surface* of the epithelium, and when it is removed the epithelium remains intact. A membrane is a coagulum involving the *entire* epithelium, and when it is removed a raw, bleeding surface remains. Pseudomembranes or membranes may accompany epidemic keratoconjunctivitis, primary herpes simplex virus conjunctivitis, streptococcal conjunctivitis, diphtheria, and erythema multiforme major. They may also be an aftermath of chemical burns, especially alkali burns.

In a peculiar form of chronic conjunctivitis (ligneous), bilateral membranes or pseudomembranes form repeatedly on the upper and lower tarsal conjunctivas and often spread out from a granulomatous area. Sometimes simulating pseudomembranes are conjunctival mucous patches—minimally elevated, whitish, and surrounded by a narrow border of erythema—seen in secondary syphilis.

Granulomas of the conjunctiva always affect the stroma. Although they usually arise endogenously (eg, from tuberculosis, syphilis, coccidioidomycosis), there are also many exogenous causes (eg, cat-scratch disease, lymphogranuloma venereum conjunctivitis, tularemia). Both chalazions (lipogranulomas) and the lesions of Parinaud's oculoglandular syndrome are granulomas, and biopsies are often necessary to determine their causes.

Phlyctenules represent a delayed hypersensitivity reaction to microbial antigen, eg, staphylococcal or mycobacterial antigens.

Preauricular lymphadenopathy is an important sign. A grossly visible preauricular node is seen in Parinaud's oculoglandular syndrome and, rarely, in epidemic keratoconjunctivitis. A large or small preauricular node, sometimes slightly tender, occurs in primary herpes simplex conjunctivitis, epidemic keratoconjunctivitis, inclusion conjunctivitis, and trachoma. Small but nontender preauricular lymph nodes occur in pharyngoconjunctival fever, Newcastle disease conjunctivitis, and acute hemorrhagic conjunctivitis. Occasionally, preauricular lymphadenopathy may be observed in children with infections of the meibomian glands.

BACTERIAL CONJUNCTIVITIS

Two forms of bacterial conjunctivitis are recognized: acute (and subacute) and chronic. Acute bacterial conjunctivitis may be self-limited when caused by certain microorganisms such as *Haemophilus influenzae*. The course may take up to 2 weeks if proper treatment is not given.

Acute bacterial conjunctivitis may become chronic. Treatment with one of the many available antibacterial agents usually cures the condition in a few days. Purulent conjunctivitis caused by *Neisseria* spp (*Neisseria gonorrhoeae* or *Neisseria meningitidis*) may lead to serious ocular complications if not treated early.

Clinical Findings

A. Symptoms and Signs: The organisms listed in Table 5–1 account for most cases of bacterial conjunctivitis. They produce bilateral irritation and injection, a purulent exudate with sticky lids on waking, and occasionally lid edema. The infection usually starts in one eye and is spread to the other by the hands. It may spread from one person to another by fomites.

1. Acute (and subacute) bacterial conjunctivitis–Purulent conjunctivitis (caused by *N gonorrhoeae* and *N meningitidis*) is marked by a profuse

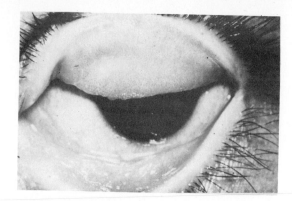

Figure 5–2. Acute catarrhal conjunctivitis caused by Koch-Weeks bacillus *(Haemophilus aegyptius)*. (Courtesy of HB Ostler.)

purulent exudate (Fig 5–1). Meningococcal conjunctivitis may be seen in children. The disease should be promptly diagnosed and treated to prevent the possibility of hematogenous spread and meningitis. Any severe, profusely exudative conjunctivitis demands immediate laboratory investigation and immediate treatment. If there is any delay, there may be severe corneal damage and the conjunctiva may become the portal of entry of the meningococcus to the bloodstream and meninges.

Acute mucopurulent (catarrhal) conjunctivitis often occurs in epidemic form and is called "pinkeye" by most laymen (Fig 5–2). It is characterized by an acute onset of conjunctival hyperemia and a moderate amount of mucopurulent discharge. The commonest causes are the pneumococcus in temperate climates and *H aegyptius* in warm climates. Rare causes are staphylococci and streptococci. The types caused by the pneumococcus (Fig 5–3) and *H aegyptius* may be accompanied by subconjunctival hemorrhages.

Subacute conjunctivitis is caused most often by *H influenzae* and occasionally by *Escherichia coli* and *Proteus* sp. *H influenzae* infection is characterized by a thin, watery, or flocculent exudate.

2. Chronic bacterial conjunctivitis–*Chronic bacterial conjunctivitis* occurs in patients with nasolacrimal duct obstruction and chronic dacryocystitis, which are usually unilateral. It may also be associated with chronic bacterial blepharitis or meibomianitis. Patients with floppy lid syndrome and ectropion may develop secondary bacterial conjunctivitis.

Rare bacterial conjunctivitides may be caused by *C diphtheriae* and *Streptococcus pyogenes*. Pseudomembranes or membranes caused by these organisms may form on the palpebral conjunctiva. The rare cases of chronic conjunctivitis produced by *B catarrhalis*, the coliform bacilli, *Proteus* spp, etc, are as a rule indistinguishable clinically. Both *Mycobacterium tuberculosis* and *Treponema pallidum* produce granulomatous conjunctival disease associated with large, grossly visible preauricular nodes.

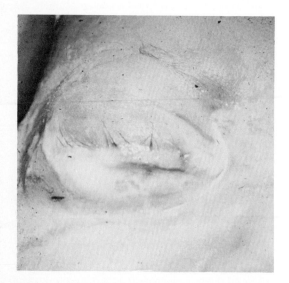

Figure 5–1. Gonorrheal conjunctivitis. Profuse purulent exudate. (Courtesy of P Thygeson.)

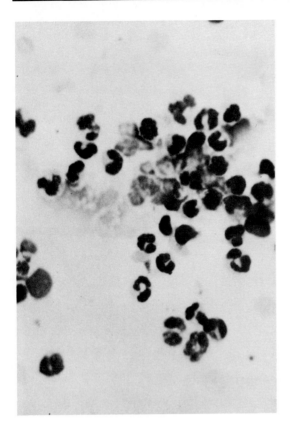

Figure 5-3. Polymorphonuclear reaction in Giemsa-stained scrapings from a patient with bacterial conjunctivitis. (Courtesy of M Okumoto.)

B. Laboratory Findings: In most cases of bacterial conjunctivitis, the organisms can be identified by the microscopic examination of conjunctival scrapings stained with Gram's stain or Giemsa's stain; this reveals numerous polymorphonuclear neutrophils (Fig 5-3). Direct examination and culture study are recommended for all cases and are mandatory if the disease is purulent, membranous, or pseudomembranous. Antibiotic sensitivity studies are also highly desirable, but empirical antibiotic therapy should be started. When the results of antibiotic sensitivity tests become available, specific antibiotic therapy can then be started.

Complications & Sequelae

A chronic marginal blepharitis may complicate an untreated staphylococcal conjunctivitis except in very young patients who are not subject to blepharitis. Conjunctival scarring may follow both pseudomembranous and membranous conjunctivitis, and in some cases corneal ulceration and perforation supervene.

Marginal corneal ulceration may follow infection with *N gonorrhoeae, H aegyptius, S aureus, Moraxella,* and *N meningitidis;* if the toxic products of *N gonorrhoeae* diffuse through the cornea into the anterior chamber, they may cause toxic iritis.

Treatment

Specific therapy of bacterial conjunctivitis depends on the identification of the etiologic agent. While waiting for the laboratory results, the physician can start topical therapy with a sulfonamide or an antibiotic. In any purulent conjunctivitis, an antibiotic suitable for treating *N gonorrhoeae* and *N meningitidis* infection should be selected, and both systemic and topical therapy should be started immediately after material for laboratory study has been collected.

In acute purulent and mucopurulent conjunctivitis, the conjunctival sac should be irrigated with saline solution as necessary to remove the conjunctival secretions. To prevent spread of the disease, the patient and family should be instructed to give special attention to their personal hygiene.

Course & Prognosis

Acute bacterial conjunctivitis is almost always self-limited. Untreated, it usually lasts 10–14 days; if properly treated, 1–3 days. The exceptions are staphylococcal conjunctivitis (which may progress to blepharoconjunctivitis and enter a chronic phase) and gonococcal conjunctivitis (which when untreated can lead to corneal perforation and endophthalmitis). Since the conjunctiva may be the portal of entry for the meningococcus to the bloodstream and meninges, septicemia and meningitis may be the end results of meningococcal conjunctivitis.

Chronic bacterial conjunctivitis may not be self-limited and may become a troublesome therapeutic problem.

CHLAMYDIAL CONJUNCTIVITIS

1. TRACHOMA

Trachoma is one of the most ancient of known diseases. It was recognized as a cause of trichiasis as early as the 27th century BC and affects all races. With over 400 million of the world's population afflicted, it is one of the most common of all chronic human diseases. Its regional variations in prevalence and severity can be explained on the basis of variations in the personal hygiene and standards of living of the world's peoples, the climatic conditions under which they live, the prevailing age at onset, and the frequency and type of the prevailing concomitant bacterial eye infections. Although sporadic cases occur in the white population of the USA, trachoma is rare here except among the American Indians of the southwestern states, where it is now mild and relatively uncomplicated.

Trachoma has a special affinity for the eye and is usually bilateral. Spread is by direct contact or fomites, usually from mother to child or grandmother to grandchild. Family members in contact with a child with trachoma should always be investigated and should be treated when found to harbor the disease.

Insect vectors, especially flies and gnats, may play a role in transmission. The acute forms of the disease are more infectious than the cicatricial forms, and the larger the inoculum the more severe the onset. Spread is often associated with epidemics of bacterial conjunctivitis and with the dry seasons in tropical and semitropical countries.

Clinical Findings

A. Symptoms and Signs: The incubation period of trachoma averages 7 days but varies from 5 to 14 days. In an infant or child the onset is usually insidious, and the disease may resolve with minimal or no complications. In the adult the onset is often subacute or acute, and complications may develop early. At onset, trachoma often resembles bacterial conjunctivitis, the signs and symptoms usually consisting of tearing, photophobia, pain, exudation, edema of the eyelids, chemosis of the bulbar conjunctiva, hyperemia, papillary hypertrophy, tarsal and limbal follicles (Fig 5–4), superior keratitis, pannus formation, and a small, tender preauricular node.

In established trachoma there may also be superior epithelial keratitis, subepithelial keratitis, pannus, superior limbal follicles, and ultimately the cicatricial remains of these follicles, known as **Herbert's pits.** Both the limbal follicles and Herbert's pits are pathognomonic of trachoma; the follicles are gelatinous, semiopaque, dome-shaped elevations surrounded by the pannus, and the pits are small depressions in the connective tissue of the limbocorneal junction. They are filled with epithelium and look like small, lucid circles or semicircles in a fibrovascular membrane arising at the limbus, from which vascular loops encroach on the cornea from above (Fig 5–5). All of the signs of trachoma are more severe in the upper than in the lower conjunctiva and cornea.

For prognostic purposes, a classification of the intensity of the inflammatory response has been developed, based on the scoring of papillae and follicles in the upper tarsal conjunctiva. The slightly simplified

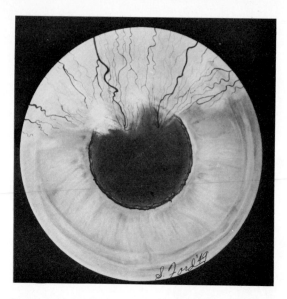

Figure 5–5. Trachomatous pannus. (Courtesy of P Thygeson.)

system presented here consists of 4 categories: severe, moderate, mild, and trivial or inactive (Table 5–3).

Other systems of classification have been devised for distortion of the eyelids due to conjunctival scarring, for trichiasis and entropion, and for corneal scarring, all of which represent potentially blinding lesions of trachoma. These grading systems may be helpful in epidemiologic studies.

B. Laboratory Findings: Giemsa-stained conjunctival scrapings show a predominantly polymorphonuclear reaction, but plasma cells, Leber cells (large macrophages containing phagocytosed debris), and follicle cells (lymphoblasts) may also be seen. Plasma cells and Leber cells suggest trachoma, but follicle cells are diagnostic. Unfortunately, they are not always present. When inclusion bodies, which cannot always be found in chronic active trachoma, appear in the Giemsa-stained preparations, they are dark purple, purplish-blue, or blue inclusions that cap the nucleus of the epithelial cell (Fig 5–6). Fluorescent antibody stains increase the likelihood of detecting inclusion bodies, but the technique is expensive and difficult.

The agent of trachoma resembles the agent of inclusion conjunctivitis morphologically, but the 2 can be differentiated serologically by microimmunofluoresence and by their pathogenicity patterns in monkeys and apes. Trachoma is caused by serotypes A, B, Ba, or C. Both agents can be isolated in tissue cultures, commonly using McCoy cells treated with cycloheximide, idoxuridine, or irradiation to favor the growth of chlamydiae or using the yolk sac of embryonated hen eggs. Identification of the organisms in tissue cultures is achieved by staining for inclusions with iodine, Giemsa's stain, or fluorescent antibody.

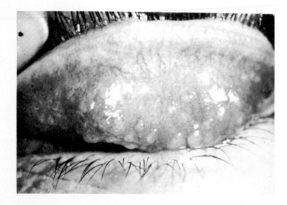

Figure 5–4. Trachoma. Papillae and follicles in upper tarsal conjunctiva. (Courtesy of P Thygeson.)

Table 5–3. Prognostic classification of trachoma according to intensity of inflammatory response.

Intensity	Papillae (P)	Follicles (F)
Severe	P3	F3 or F2 or F1
Moderate	P2	F3
Mild	P1 or P2	F1 or F2
Trivial or inactive	P1	F4

[1]Papillae and diffuse infiltration in the upper tarsal conjunctiva are scored as follows:

P0 Absent: normal appearance.

P1 Mild: individual papillae prominent but deep subconjunctival vessels not obscured.

P2 Moderate: more prominent papillae, and normal vessels appear hazy, even to the naked eye.

P3 Severe: pronounced papillae, conjunctiva thickened and opaque, normal tarsal vessels hidden over more than half the surface.

[2] For the purpose of scoring follicles, the upper tarsal conjunctival surface is divided into 3 approximately equal zones by 2 imaginary lines. The lines run approximately parallel with the upper tarsal border. Zone 1, nearest to the upper tarsal border, includes the entire upper tarsal border and adjacent tarsal surface. Zone 3 includes the tarsal conjunctiva adjacent to the central half of the lid margin. Upper tarsal follicles are scored as follows:

F0 Absent: no follicles.

F1 Mild: follicles present but not more than 5 altogether in zones 2 and 3.

F2 Moderate: more follicles in zones 1 and 2 but not more than 5 in zone 3.

F3 Severe: follicles present in all 3 zones but more than 5 in zone 3.

F4 Old follicles: yellowish, angular, and depressed follicles.

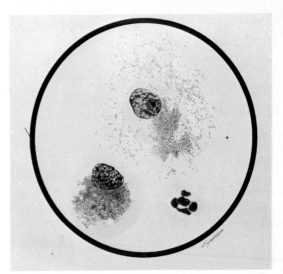

Figure 5–6. Cytoplasmic inclusion body in conjunctival epithelial cells in trachoma. Ruptured inclusion at right. Polymorphonuclear neutrophil (typical in conjunctival scrapings of trachoma) below. (Courtesy of P Thygeson and C Dawson.)

Recently, specific DNA probes have also become available.

Measurement of antibody levels in the patient's serum plays no significant role in the diagnosis of ocular chlamydial infections. The prevalence of positive serology among unaffected members of most populations is much too high. Serologic testing is, however, a useful epidemiologic tool.

Differential Diagnosis

In the differentiation of trachoma from viral infections, 2 differences are important: (1) With one exception (the follicular conjunctivitis associated with a molluscum contagiosum nodule on the lid margin), all viral conjunctivitides are of less than 3 weeks' duration; and (2) unless there is a pseudomembrane, all viral infections are associated with a predominantly mononuclear inflammatory reaction. Follicular conjunctivitis following treatment with idoxuridine, vidarabine, trifluridine, or miotics may simulate trachoma, but the drug-induced follicular reaction subsides when the drug is withdrawn, and a conjunctival scraping contains a limited and approximately equal number of polymorphonuclear and mononuclear cells. In children, folliculosis secondary to focal lymphoid hyperplasia may simulate trachoma grossly, but there are no associated corneal changes and no papillary hypertrophy, and the conjunctiva between follicles is normal.

The agents of inclusion conjunctivitis, feline pneumonitis, and psittacosis (all chlamydial infections) may produce follicular conjunctivitis, but except for the flat scars associated with the pseudomembranes that occasionally form in neonatal inclusion conjunctivitis, there is no scarring.

Parinaud's oculoglandular syndrome in children may have an associated follicular conjunctivitis, but a prominent feature of Parinaud's syndrome, not seen in trachoma, is a grossly visible preauricular node.

Vernal keratoconjunctivitis is occasionally mistaken for trachoma because of its upper tarsal lesions, but the conjunctiva in vernal keratoconjunctivitis has a milky appearance, polygonal, flat-topped giant papillae, and numerous eosinophils and eosinophil granules in conjunctival scrapings.

Complications & Sequelae

Conjunctival scarring is a frequent complication of trachoma and can shut off the ductules of the accessory lacrimal glands and obliterate the orifices of the lacrimal gland. These effects may drastically reduce the aqueous component of the precorneal tear film, and the film's mucous components may be reduced by loss of goblet cells. The scars may also cause entropion of the upper lid, and if there is an associated trichiasis the aberrant lashes may abrade the cornea. This often leads to corneal ulceration, bacterial corneal infections, and corneal scarring (Fig 5–7).

Ptosis (Fig 5–8), nasolacrimal duct obstruction, and dacryocystitis are other common complications of trachoma.

Treatment

Tetracycline, 1–1.5 g/d orally in 4 divided doses for 3–4 weeks; doxycycline, 100 mg orally twice daily for 3 weeks; or erythromycin, 1 g/d orally in 4 divided

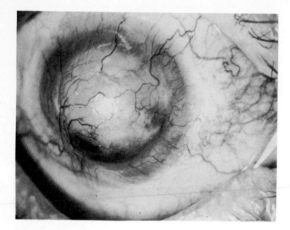

Figure 5–7. Advanced trachoma following corneal ulceration and scarring. (Courtesy of P Thygeson.)

doses for 3–4 weeks, will usually result in striking clinical improvement. Several courses are sometimes necessary for actual cure. Systemic tetracyclines should not be given to a child under 7 years of age or to a pregnant woman, since tetracycline binds to calcium in the permanent teeth and in the growing bone and may lead to congenital yellowish discoloration of the permanent teeth and skeletal abnormalities, eg, clavicular abnormalities.

Topical ointments or drops, including preparations of sulfonamides, tetracyclines, erythromycin, and rifampin, used 4 times daily for 6 weeks, have had some success.

From the time therapy is begun, its maximum effect is usually not achieved for 10–12 weeks. The persistence of follicles on the upper tarsus for some weeks after a course of therapy should therefore not be construed as evidence of therapeutic failure.

Course & Prognosis

Characteristically, trachoma is a chronic disease of long duration. In an ideal environment, however, about 20% of cases detected in any one year heal

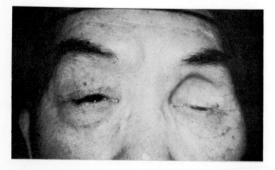

Figure 5–8. Ptosis with an "S"-shaped curve of lids associated with chronic trachoma. (Courtesy of P Thygeson.)

spontaneously; and when treatment is given early the prognosis is excellent. Unfortunately, however, because of unfavorable conditions and lack of treatment, about 20 million people in the world today have major visual loss from trachoma.

2. INCLUSION CONJUNCTIVITIS (Inclusion Blennorrhea)

Inclusion conjunctivitis, often bilateral, is a common disease, especially in sexually active young people. Characteristically, the chlamydial agent infects the urethra of the male and the cervix of the female. Transmission to the eyes of adults is usually from the genitourinary tract to the eye. Indirect transmission in inadequately chlorinated swimming pools can also occur, and in the newborn the agent is transmitted during birth by direct contamination of the conjunctiva with cervical secretions. The Credé prophylaxis does not protect against inclusion conjunctivitis.

Clinical Findings

A. Symptoms and Signs: Inclusion conjunctivitis may have an acute or a subacute onset. The patient frequently complains of redness of the eyes, pseudoptosis, and discharge, especially in the mornings. The newborn has a papillary conjunctivitis and a moderate amount of exudate, and in hyperacute cases pseudomembranes occasionally form and can lead to scarring. Since the newborn has no adenoid tissue in the stroma of the conjunctiva (see p 167), there is no follicle formation; but if the conjunctivitis persists for 2–3 months, follicles appear and the conjunctival picture is like that in older children and adults. In the newborn, chlamydial infection may cause pharyngitis, otitis media, and, occasionally, interstitial pneumonia.

In adults the conjunctivas of both tarsi, and especially of the lower tarsus, are loaded with both papillae and follicles (Fig 5–9). Since pseudomembranes do not usually form in the adult, scarring does not occur. A superficial keratitis may be noted superiorly and, less often, a small superior micropannus (< 1–2 mm). Rarely, subepithelial opacities, usually marginal, may develop. Otitis media may occur as a result of infection of the auditory tube.

B. Laboratory Findings: The examination of conjunctival scrapings shows (1) a predominantly polymorphonuclear neutrophil reaction; (2) no bacteria; (3) basophilic cytoplasmic inclusion bodies in epithelial cells, identical to those seen in trachoma; and (4) free elementary bodies, the extracellular form of chlamydial organisms. Bacterial cultures are negative.

In neonatal inclusion conjunctivitis, epithelial inclusions and free elementary bodies are plentiful. Giemsa staining is usually sufficient to establish the diagnosis and is useful in excluding other causes of acute conjunctivitis. In adult inclusion conjunctivitis, epithelial inclusions and free elementary bodies are less frequently seen; fluorescent antibody techniques

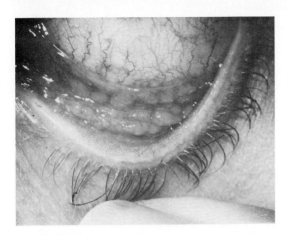

Figure 5–9. Acute follicular conjunctivitis caused by inclusion conjunctivitis in a 22-year-old male with urethritis. (Courtesy of K Tabbara.)

may be used to aid in their identification. The best method of diagnosis in these cases is isolation of the organism in tissue culture.

Inclusion conjunctivitis may be caused by serotypes D–K. Serologic determinations are not useful in the diagnosis of ocular infections, but measurement of IgM antibody levels is extremely valuable in the diagnosis of chlamydial pneumonia in infants.

Differential Diagnosis

Inclusion conjunctivitis can be clinically differentiated from trachoma on the following grounds: (1) Inclusion conjunctivitis is transmitted sexually; trachoma from eye to eye. (2) Conjunctival scarring, which is common in trachoma, occurs in inclusion conjunctivitis only in the newborn and only after the formation of a pseudomembrane. If scars develop under these circumstances, they are flat and diffuse rather than linear or stellate, as in trachoma. (3) Inclusion conjunctivitis sometimes causes a micropannus but never the gross pannus seen regularly in trachoma. (4) The corneal scarring and Herbert's pits (limbal scars) that occur in trachoma are not seen in inclusion conjunctivitis.

Treatment

In infants, 1% tetracycline ointment, erythromycin ophthalmic ointment (5 mg/g), or a sulfonamide drop (instilled 5–6 times daily for 14 days) is very effective. In adults, a 3-week course of oral tetracycline, 1–1.5 g/d; doxycycline, 100 mg orally twice daily; or erythromycin, 1 g/d, is curative. (Systemic tetracyclines should not be given to a pregnant woman or a child under 7 years of age since they cause epiphyseal problems in the fetus or staining of the young child's incisors.) The patient's sexual partners should be examined and treated.

When one of the standard therapeutic regimens is

followed, recurrences are rare. If untreated, inclusion conjunctivitis runs a course of 3–9 months or longer. The average duration is 5 months.

3. LYMPHOGRANULOMA VENEREUM CONJUNCTIVITIS

Lymphogranuloma venereum infections of the conjunctiva, which can result from accidental laboratory accidents or sexual transmission, are rare. The conjunctival reaction is nonfollicular and largely granulomatous, and there is a grossly visible preauricular node (bubo). Elephantiasis of the eyelids may occur because of lymph blockage and has been compared to the esthiomene of the female genitalia. The conjunctiva and cornea become diffusely scarred. In endogenous disease secondary to a genitourinary focus, optic neuritis, uveitis, episcleritis, and phlyctenulosis have all been reported.

The causal organism, *C lymphogranulomatis*, may be recovered by inoculating mouse brains or tissue cultures with scrapings from an infected conjunctiva. Examination of the scrapings may show typical inclusions within monocytes and macrophages but not in epithelial cells. In more than 50% of patients, the Frei test is positive, and a high titer of complement-fixing antibodies is the rule. Lymphogranuloma venereum conjunctivitis is caused by chlamydia of serotypes L1, L2, and L3.

A sulfonamide or broad-spectrum antibiotic, given systemically for 3–4 weeks, is curative.

4. PSITTACOSIS

One reported case of conjunctivitis due to an accidental laboratory infection with *C psittaci* of parakeet origin was characterized by chronic conjunctival infiltration and papillary hypertrophy of the upper tarsus and by epithelial keratitis. No inclusions were seen in epithelial cells, but cultures were positive for chlamydia. The conjunctivitis and keratitis responded only after long-term systemic tetracycline.

5. FELINE PNEUMONITIS

Two cases have been reported of follicular conjunctivitis associated with intimate exposure to domestic cats with feline pneumonitis (a chlamydial infection caused by *C psittaci*). In both cases the conjunctivitis was associated with central epithelial keratitis and cleared after 4 weeks of therapy with systemic tetracycline. There were no sequelae. Cytoplasmic epithelial cell inclusions were seen in Giemsa-stained scrapings from the conjunctiva. This was in sharp contrast to the absence of inclusions in the parakeet-derived disease.

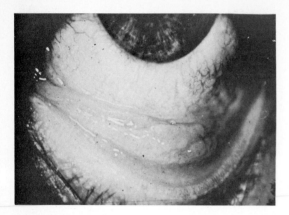

Figure 5–10. Acute follicular conjunctivitis due to adenovirus type 3. (Courtesy of P Thygeson.)

VIRAL CONJUNCTIVITIS

Viral conjunctivitis, a common affliction, can be caused by a wide variety of viruses. Some of these produce severe, disabling disease; others only mild, rapidly self-limited disease.

I. ACUTE VIRAL FOLLICULAR CONJUNCTIVITIS

1. PHARYNGOCONJUNCTIVAL FEVER

Pharyngoconjunctival fever is characterized by fever of 38.3–40 °C (101–104 °F), sore throat, and a follicular conjunctivitis in one or both eyes. The follicles are often very pominent on both the conjunctiva (Fig 5–10) and the pharyngeal mucosa. Bilateral and, less commonly, unilateral injection and tearing occur, and there may be transient superficial epithelial keratitis and occasionally some subepithelial opacities. Preauricular lymphadenopathy (nontender) is characteristic. The syndrome may be incomplete, consisting of only one or 2 of the cardinal signs (fever, pharyngitis, and conjunctivitis).

Pharyngoconjunctival fever is caused regularly by adenovirus type 3 and occasionally by types 4 and 7. The virus can be grown on HeLa cells and identified by neutralization tests. As the disease progresses, it can also be diagnosed serologically by a rising titer of neutralizing antibody to the virus. Clinical diagnosis is a simple matter, however, and clearly more practical.

Conjunctival scrapings contain predominantly mononuclear cells, and no bacteria grow in cultures. The condition is more common in children than in adults and can be transmitted in chlorinated swimming pools. There is no specific treatment, but the conjunctivitis is self-limited, usually lasting about 10 days.

2. EPIDEMIC KERATOCONJUNCTIVITIS

Epidemic keratoconjunctivitis is usually bilateral. The onset is often in one eye only, however, and as a rule the first eye is more severely affected. At onset the patient notes injection, moderate pain, and tearing, followed in 5–14 days by photophobia, epithelial keratitis, and round subepithelial opacities. Corneal sensation is normal. A large, tender preauricular node, rarely grossly visible, is characteristic. Edema of the eyelids, chemosis, and conjunctival hyperemia mark the acute phase, with follicles and subconjunctival hemorrhages often appearing within 48 hours. Pseudomembranes (and occasionally true membranes) may occur and may be followed by flat scars or symblepharons (Fig 5–11).

The conjunctivitis lasts for 3–4 weeks at most. The subepithelial opacities are concentrated in the central cornea, sparing the periphery, and may persist for months but heal without scars.

Epidemic keratoconjunctivitis is caused by adenovirus types 8 and 19, which can be cultivated on HeLa cells and identified by neutralization tests. Rising neutralizing antibody titers during the course of the disease are diagnostic. Scrapings from the conjunctiva show a primarily mononuclear inflammatory reaction (Fig 5–12); when pseudomembranes occur, neutrophils may also be prominent.

Epidemic keratoconjunctivitis in adults is confined to the external eye, but in children there may be such systemic symptoms of viral infection as fever, sore throat, and diarrhea. Spread takes place all too often by way of the physician's fingers or use of improperly sterilized ophthalmic instruments or contaminated solutions. Eye solutions, particularly topical anesthetics, can be contaminated when a dropper tip rubs the conjunctiva or cilia. There the virus may persist, and the solution becomes a source of spread.

The danger of contaminated solution bottles can be averted by the use of individual sterile droppers for each patient. Hand washing between examinations and

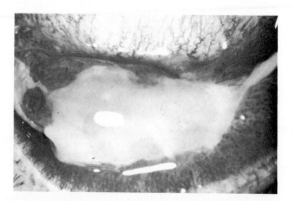

Figure 5–11. Epidemic keratoconjunctivitis. Thick white membrane in lower palpebral conjunctiva. (Courtesy of P Thygeson.)

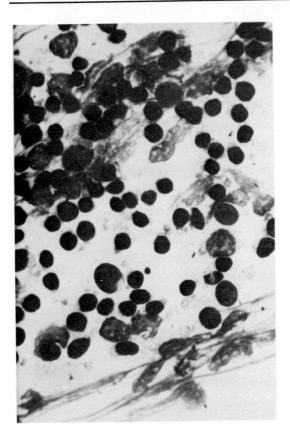

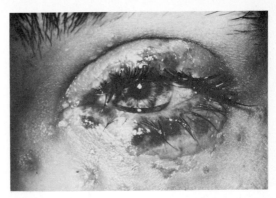

Figure 5–13. Primary ocular herpes. (Courtesy of HB Ostler.)

Figure 5–12. Mononuclear cell reaction in conjunctival scrapings of a patient with viral conjunctivitis caused by adenovirus type 8. (Courtesy of M Okumoto.)

meticulous sterilization, especially of tonometers, are also mandatory. The tonometer footplate should be cleansed carefully with a sterile stolution after each use, and the instrument should be sterilized by flame or in a hot air tonometer sterilizer after use on an inflamed eye. Applanation tonometers should be cleaned by rinsing with a sterile nonirritating solution and careful wiping several times with a facial tissue. (Epidemic keratoconjunctivitis is the only serious eye disease known to be transmissible by tonometry.)

3. HERPES SIMPLEX VIRUS CONJUNCTIVITIS

Herpes simplex virus conjunctivitis, a disease of young children, is an uncommon entity characterized by unilateral injection, irritation, mucoid discharge, pain, and mild photophobia. It occurs only in first attacks of herpes simplex virus infection, ie, in primary infections (Fig 5–13), and is often associated with herpes simplex virus keratitis, in which the cornea shows discrete epithelial lesions that usually coalesce to form single or multiple dendrites. The conjunctivitis is follicular or, less often, pseudo-membranous. (Patients receiving idoxuridine may develop follicular conjunctivitis that is not to be confused with primary herpes simplex virus conjunctivitis.) Herpetic vesicles often appear on the eyelids and lid margins, usually associated with severe edema of the eyelids. Typically, there is a large or small tender preauricular node.

No bacteria are found in scrapings or recovered in cultures. If the conjunctivitis is follicular, the predominant inflammatory reaction is mononuclear, but if it is pseudomembranous the predominant reaction is polymorphonuclear due to the chemotaxis of necrosis. Intranuclear inclusions cannot be seen in Giemsa-stained preparations (because of the margination of the chromatin), but they appear if Bouin fixation and the Papanicolaou stain are used. The finding of multinucleated giant epithelial cells has diagnostic value.

The virus can be isolated readily by gently rubbing a dry cotton-tipped applicator over an infected conjunctiva and then transferring the infected cells on the applicator directly to either an abraded rabbit cornea or a susceptible tissue culture.

Herpes simplex virus conjunctivitis may persist for 2–3 weeks, and if it is pseudomembranous it may leave fine linear or flat scars. Complications include corneal dendrites and vesicles on the skin. Although type 1 herpesvirus causes the overwhelming majority of cases, type 2 can be a rare cause in both the newborn and adult. In the newborn there may be generalized disease with encephalitis, chorioretinitis, hepatitis, etc.

Since the conjunctivitis is self-limited, therapy is usually not necessary. Corneal debridement may be performed, or idoxuridine vidarabine, or trifluridine may be applied 4 times daily for 7–10 days. Herpetic keratitis may be treated with 3% acyclovir ointment 5 times daily for 10 days. The use of steroids is contraindicated, since they aggravate herpes simplex infections and convert the disease from a short, self-limited process to a severe, greatly prolonged process.

4. NEWCASTLE DISEASE CONJUNCTIVITIS

Newcastle disease conjunctivitis is a rare disorder characterized by burning, itching, pain, redness, tearing, and (rarely) blurring of vision. It often occurs in small epidemics among poultry workers handling infected birds, or among veterinarians or laboratory helpers working with live vaccines or virus.

The disease often presents as chemosis and mild lid edema, and, although usually unilateral, it may sometimes affect both eyes at onset or within the first few days. There is a small nontender preauricular node, minimal discharge, and follicles that are more prominent on the lower tarsus than elsewhere. Rarely, there is corneal involvement in the form of fine epithelial keratitis or round, central subepithelial opacities. An influenzalike syndrome with mild fever, headaches, and mild arthralgia may develop. The disease subsides in less than a week, and there is no specific treatment.

No bacteria appear in scrapings or grow in cultures, and the inflammatory reaction is predominantly mononuclear. The virus can be isolated readily in embryonated hen eggs or tissue cultures, and complement-fixing, neutralizing, and hemagglutination-inhibiting antibodies can be found in the patient's serum.

5. ACUTE HEMORRHAGIC CONJUNCTIVITIS

All of the continents and most of the islands of the world have had major epidemics of acute hemorrhagic conjunctivitis. Because it was first recognized in Ghana in 1969 at the time of the Apollo XI moon trip, the disease has often been called Apollo XI conjunctivitis. It is caused by enterovirus type 70. Coxsackievirus type A24 has been found in some cases.

Characteristically, the disease has a short incubation period (8–48 hours) and course (5–7 days). The usual signs and symptoms are pain, photophobia, foreign body sensation, copious tearing, redness, lid edema, and subconjunctival hemorrhages (Fig 5–14). Che-

mosis sometimes also occurs. The subconjunctival hemorrhages are usually diffuse but may be punctate at onset, beginning in the upper bulbar conjunctiva and spreading to the lower. Most patients have preauricular lymphadenopathy, conjunctival follicles, and epithelial keratitis. Anterior uveitis has been reported; fever, malaise, and generalized myalgia have been observed in 25% of cases; and motor paralysis of the lower extremities has occurred in rare cases in India and Japan.

The virus is transmitted by close person-to-person contact and by such fomites as common linens, contaminated optical instruments, and water. Recovery occurs within 5–7 days, and there is no known treatment.

6. COXSACKIEVIRUS CONJUNCTIVITIS

Various coxsackieviruses have caused acute conjunctivitis accidentally in laboratory workers and in children with hand-foot-and-mouth disease.

II. CHRONIC VIRAL CONJUNCTIVITIS

1. MOLLUSCUM CONTAGIOSUM BLEPHAROCONJUNCTIVITIS

A molluscum nodule on the lid margin, especially if it is on the upper lid, may produce unilateral chronic conjunctivitis, superior keratitis, and superior pannus, all of which are also typical of trachoma. The inflammatory reaction is predominantly mononuclear (unlike the reaction in trachoma), and the round, waxy, pearl-white, noninflammatory lesion with an umbilicated center is typical of molluscum contagiosum (Fig

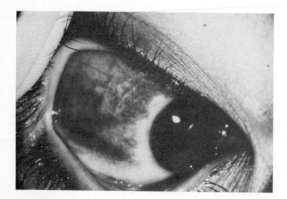

Figure 5–14. Acute hemorrhagic conjunctivitis. (Courtesy of K Tabbara.)

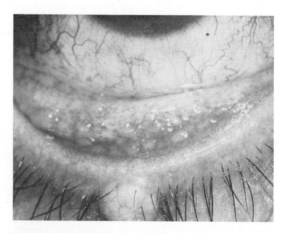

Figure 5–15. Molluscum contagiosum of lid margin with follicular conjunctivitis. (Courtesy of HB Ostler.)

5–15). Prolonged (24-hour) Giemsa staining of scrapings from the lid nodule shows small red elementary bodies, and biopsy shows eosinophilic cytoplasmic inclusions that fill the entire cytoplasm of the enlarged cell, pushing its nucleus to one side.

Excision or simple incision of the nodule to allow peripheral blood to permeate it cures the conjunctivitis. On very rare occasions (reports of only 2 cases have appeared in the literature), molluscum nodules have occurred on the conjunctiva. In these cases, excision of the nodule has also relieved the conjunctivitis.

2. VACCINIAL BLEPHAROCONJUNCTIVITIS

This was an important complication of smallpox vaccination at one time but is now of historical interest only.

3. VARICELLA-ZOSTER BLEPHAROCONJUNCTIVITIS

Hyperemia and an infiltrative conjunctivitis, associated with the typical vesicular eruption along the dermatomal distribution of the ophthalmic branch of the trigeminal nerve, are characteristic of herpes zoster (preferably called simply zoster). The conjunctivitis is usually papillary, but follicles, pseudomembranes, and transitory vesicles that later ulcerate have all been noted. A tender preauricular lymph node occurs early in the disease. Scarring of the lid, entropion, and the misdirection of individual lashes are rare sequelae.

The lid lesions of varicella, which are like the skin lesions (pox) elsewhere, may appear on both the lid margins and the lids and may leave scars on the lid margins. A mild catarrhal type of conjunctivitis often occurs, but discrete conjunctival lesions (except at the limbus) are very rare. Limbal lesions resemble phlyctenules and may go through all the stages of vesicle, papule, and ulcer. The adjacent cornea becomes infiltrated and may vascularize.

In both zoster and varicella, scrapings from lid vesicles contain giant cells and a predominance of polymorphonuclear neutrophil cells; scrapings from the conjunctiva in varicella and from conjunctival vesicles in zoster contain giant cells and monocytes. The virus can be recovered in tissue cultures of human embryo cells.

There is no satisfactory treatment, but studies with interferon and acyclovir are promising.

4. MEASLES KERATOCONJUNCTIVITIS

The characteristic enanthem of measles frequently precedes the skin eruption. At this early stage the conjunctiva may have a peculiar glassy appearance, followed within a few days by swelling of the semilunar fold (Meyer's sign). Several days before the skin eruption, a catarrhal conjunctivitis with a mucopurulent discharge develops, and at the time of the skin eruption Koplik's spots appear on the conjunctiva and occasionally on the caruncle. At some time (early in children, late in adults), epithelial keratitis supervenes.

In the immunocompetent patient, measles keratoconjunctivitis has few or no sequelae, but in malnourished or otherwise immunoincompetent patients the ocular disease is frequently associated with a secondary bacterial infection due to the pneumococcus, H influenzae, and other organisms. In this event there is often a severe purulent or even pseudomembranous conjunctivitis with associated corneal ulceration and perforation. In many developing countries, measles and the folk remedies used to treat measles-associated eye disease are major causes of blindness.

Conjunctival scrapings show a mononuclear cell reaction unless there are pseudomembranes or secondary infection. Giemsa-stained preparations contain giant cells. Since there is no specific therapy, only supportive measures are indicated unless there is secondary infection.

RICKETTSIAL CONJUNCTIVITIS

All rickettsiae recognized as pathogenic for humans are likely to attack the conjunctiva. The conjunctiva is in fact often their portal of entry, eg, in Q fever, Marseilles fever (boutonneuse fever), endemic (murine) typhus, scrub typhus, Rocky Mountain spotted fever, and epidemic typhus.

1. Q FEVER

In Q fever there is usually severe conjunctival hyperemia. Rarely there may also be severe inflammation followed by gangrene of the lids.

Conjunctival scrapings, in which neither bacteria nor inclusions are seen, show a predominantly polymorphonuclear cell response. Diagnosis can be verified serologically by complement fixation and the Weil-Felix reaction.

Treatment with systemic tetracyclines or chloramphenicol is curative.

2. MARSEILLES FEVER (Boutonneuse Fever)

The conjunctivitis associated with Marseilles fever is ulcerative or granulomatous and associated with a grossly visible preauricular lymph node (Parinaud's oculoglandular syndrome). The conjunctivitis usually precedes the systemic signs and symptoms by 5 or 6 days.

3. ENDEMIC (MURINE) TYPHUS, SCRUB TYPHUS, ROCKY MOUNTAIN SPOTTED FEVER

The conjunctivitis associated with these rickettsial diseases is usually mild, varying from a conjunctival hyperemia with photophobia to a mild catarrhal conjunctivitis.

4. EPIDEMIC TYPHUS

The signs of conjunctivitis in epidemic typhus vary from hyperemia alone to subconjunctival hemorrhages and a low-grade conjunctival inflammation. Small, purplish oval spots appear on the conjunctiva concurrently with the cutaneous manifestations of the disease.

FUNGAL CONJUNCTIVITIS

1. CANDIDAL CONJUNCTIVITIS

Candidal conjunctivitis, a rare phenomenon, appears as a white conjunctival plaque that can be mistaken for a pseudomembrane. There is often some exudate. In adults, candidal blepharitis may occur in diabetic patients accompanied by ulcerative or granulomatous conjunctivitis, which in rare cases may be followed by conjunctival scarring. The disease may occur in the newborn infant secondary to passage through an infected birth canal.

Scrapings show a polymorphonuclear cell inflammatory reaction. The organism grows readily on blood agar on Sabouraud's medium and can be readily identified as a budding yeast or, rarely, as pseudohyphae.

The fungus responds to amphotericin B (3–8 mg/mL) in aqueous (not saline) solution, or to applications of nystatin dermatologic cream (100,000 units/g) 4–6 times daily. The ointment must be applied carefully to be sure that it reaches the conjunctival sac and does not just build up on the lid margins.

2. SPOROTHRIX SCHENCKII CONJUNCTIVITIS

Occasionally, *S schenckii* invades the conjunctiva alone or in conjunction with granulomatous lesions on the lids. The conjunctival lesion is typically a small, yellow granuloma that may ulcerate. It is associated with a grossly visible preauricular node (Parinaud's oculoglandular syndrome). The lid lesions proceed along the lymphatic chain and gradually ulcerate. The infection usually follows injury or an abrasion with thorns, often barberry bush thorns.

Microscopic examination of a biopsy of the granuloma reveals gram-positive, cigar-shaped conidia

(spores). The lesions respond readily to systemic iodides, although in vitro the organism is not iodide-sensitive.

3. RHINOSPORIDIUM SEEBERI CONJUNCTIVITIS

R seeberi has many of the characteristics of a fungus but never has been cultivated. The ocular disease it causes may affect the conjunctiva, lacrimal sac, lids, canaliculi, and sclera.

The typica lesion is a polypoid granuloma arising from the upper or lower palpebral or bulbar conjunctiva. It is a painless, soft, pink lesion that sometimes has white spots on its surface. The patient often complains of a small mass that bleeds after minimal trauma. The rest of the conjunctiva appears to be normal, and there is no regional lymphadenopathy.

Histologic examination discloses a granuloma in which there are large spherules that contain myriads of endospores. Treatment is by simple excision of the lesion with cauterization of its base.

4. COCCIDIOIDOMYCOSIS (San Joaquin Valley Fever)

C immitis may on rare occasions cause a granulomatous conjunctivitis associated with a grossly visible preauricular node (Parinaud's oculoglandular syndrome). There is often a mucopurulent discharge and occasionally a thin, transparent pseudomembrane. The granulomas are raised, indolent, discrete or diffuse, reddish lesions showing tiny areas of focal necrosis. Primary ocular disease has not been recognized; the conjunctivitis is usually only a metastasis from the primary pulmonary infection. In disseminated coccidioidomycosis, the skin (including the skin of the lids) is more frequently affected than the conjunctiva.

The primary disease is an influenzalike illness with fever, malaise, cough, aches and pains, and night sweats. It is more common among dark-skinned than among light-skinned races, with Filipinos especially susceptible. Dissemination follows the rare failure of the body to limit the organism to its primary site.

Low titers of complement-fixing antibodies (< 1:16) indicate the usually limited spread of the disease; titers over 1:16 suggest widespread dissemination and a poor prognosis.

Histologic examination shows granulomatous lesions with spherules that are thick, doubly refractile, and filled with endospores. A fluffy, cotton-white colony grows on Sabouraud's medium.

Treatment with systemically administered amphotericin B yields the best results in disseminated cases, but transfer factor is now offering promise. In mild cases, only supportive therapy is needed.

PARASITIC CONJUNCTIVITIS*

1. *THELAZIA CALIFORNIENSIS* INFECTION

The natural habitat of this roundworm is the eye of the dog, but it can also infest the eyes of cats, sheep, black bears, horses, and deer. Accidental infection of the human conjunctival sac has occurred.

In the dog, the worms usually remain on the surface of the conjunctiva, causing irritation or tearing, but occasionally the corneal epithelium may be abraded. The eggs are laid in the lacrimal duct, conjunctival sac, or nictitating membrane, and the full life cycle may take place in the conjunctival sac and lacrimal apparatus. Transmission to other animals probably requires an intermediate arthropod host such as a fly (eg, *Fannia canicularis* or *Fannia benjamini*).

The disease can be treated effectively by removing the worms from the conjunctival sac with forceps or a cotton-tipped applicator.

2. *LOA LOA* INFECTION

L loa is the eye worm of Africa. It lives in the connective tissue of humans and monkeys, and the monkey may be its reservoir. The adult worm measures up to 55 mm in length. The female deposits the sheathed embryo (microfilaria) in its host's connective tissue, whence it migrates to the bloodstream and is taken up by the horse fly or mango fly as the fly bites its host. After 10 days the filariform larvae have developed, are infective, and are transferred to humans by the bite of the fly. (The fly feeds during the daylight hours only and especially in the middle of the day.)

The worm wanders in the connective tissue of humans for a year while it matures. During this time it may wander into the orbit or under the conjunctiva, sometimes giving pain or a feeling of vermiculation. Subcutaneous migration to the lid has also been seen, and the worm has been found in the anterior chamber, the vitreous, and (rarely) the retina.

Infestation with *L loa* is accompanied by a 60–80% eosinophilia, but diagnosis is made by identifying the worm on removal or by finding microfilariae in blood examined at midday.

Systemic diethylcarbamazine citrate (Hetrazan)† is the treatment of choice.

3. *ASCARIS LUMBRICOIDES* INFECTION (Butcher's Conjunctivitis)

Ascaris may cause a rare type of violent conjunctivitis. When butchers or persons performing postmortem examinations cut tissue containing *Ascaris*,

the tissue juice of some of the organisms may hit them in the eye. This can be followed by a violent, toxic, painful conjunctivitis marked by extreme chemosis and lid edema. Treatment consists of rapid and thorough irrigation of the conjunctival sac.

4. *TRICHINELLA SPIRALIS* INFECTION

This parasite does not cause a true conjunctivitis, but in the course of its general dissemination there is often a doughy edema of the upper and lower eyelids, and over 50% of patients have chemosis—a pale, lemon-yellow swelling most marked over the lateral and medial rectus muscles and fading toward the limbus. The chemosis may last a week or more, and there is often pain on movement of the eyes.

The diagnosis is verified by a positive serologic test, a positive skin test, or a positive muscle biopsy. There is always eosinophilia of 10–50%.

The conjunctival aspect of the infection does not require therapy, but thiabendazole may be of value in allaying symptoms and reducing the eosinophilia. Whether or not systemic corticosteroids should be used is controversial.

5. *SCHISTOSOMA HAEMATOBIUM* INFECTION

This parasitic disease (schistosomiasis, bilharziasis) is endemic in Egypt, especially in the region irrigated by the Nile. Granulomatous conjunctival lesions appearing as small, soft, smooth, pinkish-yellow tumors occur, especially in males. The symptoms are minimal. Diagnosis depends on the microscopic examination of biopsy material, which shows a granuloma containing lymphocytes, plasma cells, giant cells, and eosinophils surrounding the bilharzial ova in various stages of disintegration.

Treatment consists of excision of the conjunctival granuloma and systemic therapy with antimonials such as niridazole.

6. *TAENIA SOLIUM* INFECTION

This parasite occasionally causes conjunctivitis but more often invades the retina, choroid, or vitreous to produce ocular cysticercosis. As a rule, the affected conjunctiva shows a subconjunctival cyst in the form of a localized hemispherical swelling, usually at the inner angle of the lower fornix, which is adherent to the underlying sclera and painful on pressure. The conjunctiva and lid may be inflamed and edematous.

Diagnosis is based on a positive complement fixation or precipitin test or on the demonstration of the organism in the gastrointestinal tract. Eosinophilia is a constant feature.

The best treatment is to excise the lesion. The intestinal condition can be treated by niclosamide.

---

*Onchocerciasis is discussed in Chapter 8.
†Available in the USA only from Lederle Laboratories.

7. PTHIRUS PUBIS INFECTION (Pubic Louse Infection)

P pubis may infest the cilia and margins of the eyelids. Because of its size, the pubic louse seems to require widely spaced hair. For this reason it has a predilection for the widely spaced cilia as well as for pubic hair. The parasites apparently release an irritating substance (probably feces) that produces a toxic follicular conjunctivitis in children and an irritating papillary conjunctivitis in adults. The lid margin is usually red, and the patient may complain of intense itching.

Finding the adult organism or the ova-shaped nits cemented to the eyelashes is diagnostic.

Lindane (hexachlorocyclohexane [Kwell]) 1%, or RID (pyrethrins), applied to the pubic area and lash margins after removal of the nits, is usually curative. Application of lindane or RID to the lid margins must be undertaken with great care to avoid contact with the eye. Any ointment applied to the lid margin tends to smother the adult organisms. The patient's family and close contacts should be examined and treated. All clothes and fomites should be washed.

8. OPHTHALMOMYIASIS

Myiasis is an infestation with larvae of flies. In humans, myiasis is common in rural areas. Many different species of flies may produce myiasis. The ocular tissues may be injured by mechanical transmission of disease-producing organisms and by the parasitic activities of the larvae in the ocular tissues. The larvae are able to invade either necrotic or healthy tissue. Many become infected by accidental ingestion of the eggs or larvae or by contamination of external wounds or skin. Infants and young children, alcoholics, and debilitated unattended patients are common targets for infestation with myiasis-producing flies.

Clinical Findings

There are 3 types of ocular myiasis: (1) ocular surface myiasis, (2) intraocular myiasis, and (3) orbital myiasis.

A. Ocular Surface Myiasis: This is a common ocular condition caused by several species of flies. *Musca domestica,* the housefly, and *Fannia* latrine flies deposit their eggs at the lower lid margin or inner canthus. The larvae may remain on the surface of the eye without penetration into the tissues and receive their nutrients from the tear film. This type of myiasis causes irritation, pain, and conjunctival hyperemia.

B. Intraocular Myiasis: In this rare type of ophthalmomyiasis, maggots of certain species of flies penetrate the surface of the eye and gain access to the intraocular tissues. The maggot may stay under the retina or in the vitreous and may cause severe inflammatory reactions within the eye that may damage the ocular structures and lead to loss of vision.

C. Orbital Myiasis: The larvae of certain flies may penetrate and gain access to the orbital tissue, leading to orbital myiasis.

Diagnosis

A definitive diagnosis of myiasis can be made by identification of the larvae. When live maggots are obtained, they should be placed on a dish of raw meat in a glass jar containing moist sand and the jar plugged with cotton and allowed to stay at room temperature. The maggot develops in the meat and later leaves the meat and enters the sand in order to pupate. The emergent flies can then be examined and identified. Maggots may also be placed on blood agar and species identification made by studying the adult fly. In rare instances, however, genetic determination can be made on the basis of larval morphology.

Prevention

Prevention of myiasis requires control of infestation using larvicides and other hygienic measures. Adequate disposal of animal carcasses can reduce the breeding grounds for many species of flies. Window screens and fly traps may also be helpful in certain rural areas. Children and infants should not be allowed to sleep in the open.

Treatment

Treatment of ocular myiasis is by mechanical removal of the larvae after topical local anesthesia. Orbital myiasis may require operative debridement. Intraocular myiasis may be treated by photocoagulation of the larvae with simultaneous use of systemic steroids.

IMMUNOLOGIC (ALLERGIC) CONJUNCTIVITIS

I. IMMEDIATE (HUMORAL) HYPERSENSITIVITY REACTIONS

1. HAY FEVER CONJUNCTIVITIS

A mild, nonspecific conjunctival inflammation is commonly associated with hay fever (allergic rhinitis). There is usually a history of allergy to pollens, grasses, animal dander, etc. The patient complains of itching, tearing, and redness of the eyes and often states that his or her eyes seem to be sinking into the surrounding tissue. There is mild injection of the palpebral and bulbar conjunctiva, and during acute attacks there is often severe chemosis (which no doubt explains the concept that the eyes are "sinking into the surrounding tissue"). There may be a small amount of ropy discharge, especially if the patient has been rubbing the eyes. A few eosinophils are found in conjunctival scrapings. There are no conjunctival papillae or follicles.

Treatment consists of the instillation of local vasoconstrictors during the acute phase (epinephrine, 1:1000 solution applied topically, will relieve the chemosis and symptoms within 30 minutes). Cold compresses are helpful to relieve itching, and antihistamines by mouth are of some value. The immediate response to treatment is satisfactory, but recurrences are common unless the antigen is eliminated. Fortunately, the frequency of the attacks and the severity of the symptoms tend to moderate as the patient ages.

2. VERNAL KERATOCONJUNCTIVITIS

This disease, also known as seasonal or warm weather conjunctivitis, is an uncommon bilateral allergic disease that usually begins in the prepubertal years and lasts for 5–10 years. It occurs much oftener in boys than in girls. The identity of the specific allergen or allergens is still a mystery, but patients with vernal keratoconjunctivitis sometimes show other manifestations of allergy known to be related to grass pollen sensitivity. The disease is less common in temperate than in warm climates and is almost nonexistent in cold climates. It is almost always more severe during the spring, summer, and fall than in the winter.

The patient usually complains of extreme itching and a ropy discharge. There is often a family history of allergy (hay fever, eczema, etc) and sometimes in the young patient as well. The conjunctiva has a milky appearance, and there are many fine papillae in the lower tarsal conjunctiva. The upper palpebral conjunctiva often has giant papillae that give the conjunctiva a cobblestone appearance (Fig 5–16). Each giant papilla is polygonal, has a flat top, and contains tufts of capillaries.

A stringy conjunctival discharge and a fine, fibrinous pseudomembrane (Maxwell-Lyons sign) may be noted. In some cases, especially in the black race, the most prominent lesions are located at the limbus, where gelatinous swellings (papillae) are noted. A pseudogerontoxon (arcus) is often noted in the cornea adjacent to the limbal papillae. Tranta's dots are whitish dots seen at the limbus in some patients with vernal keratoconjunctivitis during the active phase of the disease. Many eosinophils and free eosinophil granules are found in Giemsa-stained smears of the conjunctival exudate.

Micropannus is often seen in both palpebral and limbal vernal keratoconjunctivitis, but total pannus is extremely rare. Conjunctival scarring usually does not occur unless the patient has been treated with cryotherapy, surgical removal of the papillae, irradiation, or other damaging procedure. Superficial corneal ulcers (oval and located superiorly) may form and may be followed by mild corneal scarring. A characteristic diffuse epithelial keratitis frequently occurs. None of the corneal lesions responds well to standard treatment.

The disease may be associated with keratoconus.

Treatment

Since vernal keratoconjunctivitis is a self-limited disease, it must be recognized that the medication used to treat the symptoms may provide short-term benefit but do long-term harm. Topical and systemic steroids, which relieve the itching, affect the corneal disease only minimally, and their side effects (glaucoma, cataract, and other complications) can be severely damaging. Topical disodium cromoglycate (cromolyn) is a useful prophylactic agent in moderate to severe cases. Vasoconstrictors, cold compresses, and ice packs are helpful, and sleeping (if possible, also working) in cool, air-conditioned rooms can keep the patient reasonably comfortable. Probably the best remedy of all is to move to a cool, moist climate. Patients able to do so are benefited if not completely cured.

The severe symptoms of an extremely photophobic patient who is unable to function can often be relieved by a short course of topical or systemic steroids followed by vasoconstrictors and cold packs. As has already been indicated, the prolonged use of steroids must be avoided since it is all too often followed by herpes simplex keratitis, cataract, glaucoma, and fungal and other opportunistic corneal ulcers. Recent clinical studies have shown that topical 1% cyclosporine

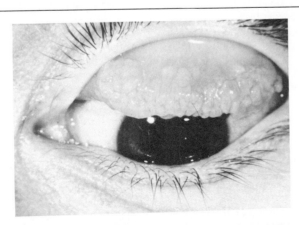

Figure 5–16. Vernal conjunctivitis. "Cobblestone" papillae in superior tarsal conjunctiva. (Courtesy of P Thygeson.)

eye drops are effective in severe unresponsive cases.

Desensitization to grass pollens and other antigens has not been rewarding. Staphylococcal blepharitis and conjunctivitis are frequent complications and should be treated. Recurrences are the rule, particularly in the spring and summer; but after a number of recurrences the papillae disappear completely, leaving no scars.

3. ATOPIC KERATOCONJUNCTIVITIS

Patients with atopic dermatitis (eczema) often also have atopic keratoconjunctivitis. The symptoms and signs are a burning sensation, mucoid discharge, redness, and photophobia. The lid margins are erythematous, and the conjunctiva has a milky appearance. There are fine papillae, but giant papillae are rare; when they occur they are on the lower tarsus (unlike the giant papillae of vernal keratoconjunctivitis, which are on the upper tarsus). Severe corneal signs appear late in the disease after repeated exacerbations of the conjunctivitis. Superficial peripheral keratitis develops and is followed by vascularization. In severe cases, the entire cornea becomes hazy and vascularized, and visual acuity is reduced. The disease is associated with keratoconus.

There is usually a history of allergy (hay fever, asthma, or eczema) in the patient or the patient's family. Most patients have had atopic dermatitis since 1 or 2 years of age. Scarring of the flexure creases of the antecubital folds and of the wrists and knees is common. Like the dermatitis with which it is associated, atopic keratoconjunctivitis has a protracted course and is subject to exacerbations and remissions. Like vernal keratoconjunctivitis, it tends to become inactive when the patient reaches the fifth decade.

Scrapings of the conjunctiva show eosinophils, although not nearly so many as are seen in vernal keratoconjunctivitis. Scarring of both the conjunctiva and cornea is often seen, and an atopic cataract, a posterior subcapsular plaque, or an anterior shieldlike cataract may develop. Keratoconus, retinal detachment, and herpes simplex keratitis are all more than usually frequent in patients with atopic keratoconjunctivitis, and there are many cases of secondary bacterial blepharitis and conjunctivitis, usually staphylococcal.

The management of atopic keratoconjunctivitis is often discouraging. Any secondary infection must of course be treated. A short course of topical steroids may relieve symptoms. In advanced cases with severe corneal complications, corneal transplantation may be needed to improve the visual acuity.

4. GIANT PAPILLARY CONJUNCTIVITIS (Pseudovernal Conjunctivitis)

A type of giant papillary conjunctivitis with signs and symptoms closely resembling those of vernal conjunctivitis may develop in patients wearing plastic artificial eyes or contact lenses. It is a sensitivity reaction, possibly to components of the plastic leached out by the action of the tears. Use of glass instead of plastic for prostheses and spectacle lenses instead of contact lenses is curative.

II. DELAYED HYPERSENSITIVITY REACTIONS

1. PHLYCTENULOSIS

Phlyctenular keratoconjunctivitis is a delayed hypersensitivity response to microbial proteins, including the proteins of the tubercle bacillus, *Staphylococcus*, *Candida albicans*, *Coccidioides immitis*, and *Chlamydia lymphogranulomatis*. Until recently, by far the most frequent cause of phlyctenulosis in the USA was delayed hypersensitivity to the protein of the human tubercle bacillus. This is still the commonest cause in developing countries where tuberculosis is still prevalent. In the USA, however, most cases are now associated with delayed hypersensitivity to *S aureus*.

The conjunctival phlyctenule begins as a small lesion (usually 1–3 mm in diameter) that is hard, red, elevated, and surrounded by a zone of hyperemia. At the limbus it is often triangular in shape, with its apex toward the cornea. In this location it develops a grayish-white center that soon ulcerates and then subsides within 10–12 days. The patient's first phlyctenule and most of the recurrences develop at the limbus, but there may also be bulbar and very rarely even tarsal phlyctenules.

Unlike the conjunctival phlyctenule, which leaves no scar, the corneal phlyctenule develops as an amorphous gray infiltrate and always leaves a scar. Consistent with this difference is the fact that scars form on the corneal side of the limbal lesion and not on the conjunctival side. The result is a triangular scar with its base at the limbus—a valuable sign of old phlyctenulosis when the limbus has been involved.

Conjunctival phlyctenules usually produce only irritation and tearing; it is the typical corneal phlyctenule that is accompanied also by photophobia—severe when the disease is tuberculoprotein-induced and mild when staphylococcus protein–induced. Phlyctenulosis is often triggered by active blepharitis, acute bacterial conjunctivitis, and dietary deficiencies. Acute bacterial conjunctivitis causes hyperemia, which facilitates transfer of the tuberculoprotein to the limbus in large amounts. Phlyctenular scarring (Fig 5–17), which may be minimal or extensive, is often followed by Salzmann's nodular degeneration.

Histologically, the phlyctenule is a focal subepithelial infiltration of small round cells, followed by a preponderance of polymorphonuclear cells when the overlying epithelium necrotizes and sloughs—a sequence of events characteristic of the delayed tuberculin type hypersensitivity reaction.

Phlyctenulosis induced by tuberculoprotein and the

proteins of other systemic infections responds dramatically to topical corticosteroids. There is a major reduction of symptoms within 24 hours and disappearance of the lesion in another 24 hours. In contrast, phlyctenulosis induced by the proteins of staphylococcus (from staphylococcal blepharitis) is relatively unresponsive to the corticosteroids. Treatment should be aimed at the underlying disease, and the steroids, when effective, should be used only to control acute symptoms. A well-balanced diet is most important, and any bacterial conjunctivitis must be controlled. Severe corneal scarring may call for corneal transplantation.

2. MILD CONJUNCTIVITIS SECONDARY TO CONTACT BLEPHARITIS

Contact blepharitis caused by atropine, neomycin, broad-spectrum antibiotics, and other topically applied medications is often followed by a mild infiltrative conjunctivitis that produces hyperemia, mild papillary hypertrophy, a mild mucoid discharge, and some irritation. The examination of Giemsa-stained scrapings often shows only a few degenerated epithelial cells, a few polymorphonuclear and mononuclear cells, and no eosinophils.

Treatment should be directed toward finding the offending agent and eliminating it. The contact blepharitis may clear rapidly with topical corticosteroids, but their use should be limited. Long-term use of steroids on the lids may lead to steroid glaucoma and to skin atrophy with disfiguring telangiectasis.

III. AUTOIMMUNE DISEASE CONJUNCTIVITIS

1. KERATOCONJUNCTIVITIS SICCA (Associated With Sjögren's Syndrome)

Sjögren's syndrome is a systemic disease characterized by a triad of disorders: keratoconjunctivitis sicca, xerostomia, and connective tissue dysfunction (arthritis). To establish the diagnosis of Sjögren's syndrome, at least 2 of the 3 disorders must be present. The disease is overwhelmingly more common in women at or beyond the menopause than in others, although men and younger women can also be affected. The lacrimal gland is infiltrated with lymphocytes and occasionally with plasma cells, and this leads to atrophy and destruction of the glandular structures.

Keratoconjunctivitis sicca is characterized by bulbar conjunctival hyperemia and symptoms of irritation that are out of proportion to the mild inflammatory signs. It often begins as a catarrhal conjunctivitis. Blotchy epithelial lesions appear on the cornea, more prominently in its lower half, and filaments may be seen. Pain builds up in the afternoon and evening but

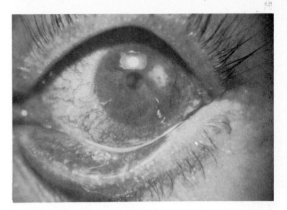

Figure 5–17. Postphlyctenulosis. Vascularized scar in temporal portion of left cornea.

is absent or only slight in the morning. The tear film is diminished and often contains shreds of mucus (Fig 5–18). Results of the Schirmer test are abnormal (see Chapter 4). Rose bengal staining is a helpful diagnostic test.

The diagnosis is confirmed by demonstrating lymphocytic and plasma cell infiltration of the accessory salivary glands in a labial biopsy obtained by means of a simple surgical procedure (Fig 5–19).

Treatment should be directed toward preserving and replacing the tear film with artificial tears, with obliteration of the puncta, and with moisture chambers and Buller shields. As a rule, the simpler things should be tried first. Clinical trials have suggested that topical vitamin A in conjunction with artificial tears may be helpful in certain cases.

2. CICATRICIAL PEMPHIGOID

This disease usually begins as a nonspecific chronic conjunctivitis that is resistant to therapy. The conjunctiva may be affected alone or in combination with the mouth, nose, esophagus, vulva, and skin. The

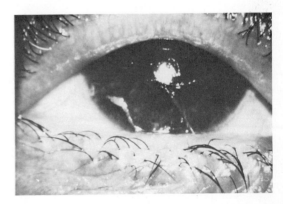

Figure 5–18. Keratoconjunctivitis sicca. (Courtesy of HB Ostler.)

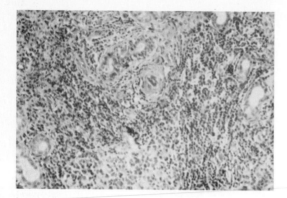

Figure 5–19. Mononuclear infiltration of the accessory salivary glands of a patient with Sjögren's syndrome. (Courtesy of K Tabbara.)

conjunctivitis leads to progressive scarring and obliteration of the fornices, especially the lower fornix (Fig 5–20). The patient complains of pain, irritation, and blurring of vision. The cornea is affected only secondarily as a result of obliteration of the fornix and lack of the precorneal tear film. The disease is more severe in women than in men. It is typically a disease of middle life, occurring only very rarely before age 45. In women it may progress to blindness in a year or less; in men, progress is slower and spontaneous remission sometimes takes place.

Conjunctival scrapings usually contain a few eosinophils. Oral dapsone and immunosuppressive therapy have been effective in some cases. Treatment must always be instituted at an early stage, prior to the onset of significant scarring. Generally, the course is long and the prognosis poor, with blindness due to

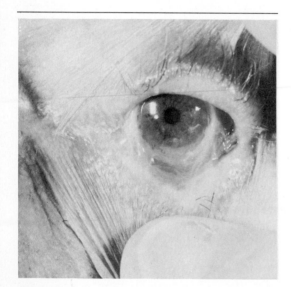

Figure 5–20. Cicatricial pemphigoid. (Courtesy of M Quickert.)

complete symblepharon and corneal desiccation the usual outcome.

3. MIDLINE LETHAL GRANULOMA & WEGENER'S GRANULOMATOSIS

Wegener's granulomatosis is a syndrome (assumed to be autoimmune in origin) that is characterized by necrotizing granulomatous lesions, generalized arteritis, and glomerulitis. The glomerulitis differentiates it from midline lethal granuloma. In both diseases there is progressive destruction of the soft tissues and bony structures of the ethmoid region. In Wegener's granulomatosis, the lower part of the respiratory tract may also be affected, and terminally there may be uremia.

In both of these diseases there may be one or more of the following ocular manifestations: exophthalmos, chemosis, exposure keratitis, papillitis by extension of the process into the orbit, episcleritis, scleritis, marginal corneal infiltration and ulceration, uveitis, and retinitis with hemorrhages and cytoid bodies. The typical conjunctival lesions are multiple small granulomas at the limbus.

Steroids and other immunosuppressives appear to reduce the severity of the lesions.

CHEMICAL OR IRRITATIVE CONJUNCTIVITIS

1. IATROGENIC CONJUNCTIVITIS FROM TOPICALLY APPLIED DRUGS

A toxic follicular conjunctivitis or an infiltrative, nonspecific conjunctivitis, followed by scarring, is often produced by the prolonged administration of miotics, idoxuridine, neomycin, and other drugs prepared in toxic or irritating preservatives or vehicles. Silver nitrate instilled into the conjunctival sac at birth (Credé prophylaxis) is a frequent cause of mild chemical conjunctivitis. If tear production is reduced by continual irritation, the conjunctiva can be further damaged by the lack of dilution of the noxious agent as it is instilled into the conjunctival sac.

Conjunctival scrapings often contain keratinized epithelial cells, a few polymorphonuclear neutrophils, and an occasional oddly shaped cell. The treatment is to stop the offending agent and to use bland drops or none at all. Often the conjunctival reaction persists for weeks or months after its source has been eliminated.

2. OCCUPATIONAL CONJUNCTIVITIS FROM CHEMICALS & IRRITANTS

Acids, alkalies, smoke, wind, and almost any irritating substance that enters the conjunctival sac may cause conjunctivitis. Some common irritants are fertilizers, soap, deodorants, hair sprays, tobacco, makeup preparations (mascara, etc), and various acids and alkalies. In certain areas, smog has become the commonest cause of mild chemical conjunctivitis. The specific irritant in smog has not been positively identified, and treatment is nonspecific. There are no permanent ocular effects, but affected eyes are frequently chronically red and irritated.

In acid burns, the acids denature the tissue proteins and the effect is immediate. Alkalies do not denature the proteins but tend to penetrate the tissues deeply and rapidly and to linger in the conjunctival tissue. Here they continue to inflict damage for hours or days, depending on the molar concentration of the alkali and the amount of it introduced. Adhesion between the bulbar and palpebral conjunctivas (symblepharon) and corneal leukoma are more likely to occur if the offending agent is an alkali. In either event, pain, injection, photophobia, and blepharospasm are the principal symptoms of caustic burns. A history of the precipitating event can usually be elicited.

Immediate and profuse irrigation of the conjunctival sac with water or saline solution is of first importance, and any solid material should be removed mechanically. Do not use chemical antidotes. General symptomatic measures include cold compresses for 20 minutes every hour, atropine 1% drops twice daily, and systemic analgesics as necessary. Corneal scarring may require corneal transplantation, and symblepharon may require a plastic operation on the conjunctiva. Severe conjunctival and corneal burns have a poor prognosis even with surgery, but if proper treatment is started immediately, scarring may be minimized and the prognosis improved.

3. CATERPILLAR HAIR CONJUNCTIVITIS (Ophthalmia Nodosum)

On rare occasions, caterpillar hairs are introduced into the conjunctival sac, where they produce one or many granulomas (ophthalmia nodosum). Under magnification, each granuloma is seen to contain a small foreign body.

Treatment by removal of each hair individually is effective. If a hair is retained, invasion of the sclera and uveal tract usually occurs.

CONJUNCTIVITIS OF UNKNOWN CAUSE

1. FOLLICULOSIS

Folliculosis is a widespread benign, bilateral noninflammatory conjunctival disorder characterzied by follicular hypertrophy. It is more common in children than in adults, and the symptoms are minimal. The follicles are more numerous in the lower than in the upper cul-de-sac and tarsal conjunctiva. There is no

associated inflammation or papillary hypertrophy, and complications do not occur.

There is no treatment for folliculosis, which disappears spontaneously after a course of 2–3 years. The cause is unknown, but folliculosis may be only a manifestation of a generalized adenoidal hypertrophy.

2. CHRONIC FOLLICULAR CONJUNCTIVITIS (Orphan's Conjunctivitis, Axenfeld's Conjunctivitis)

This is a bilateral transmissible disease of children characterized by numerous follicles in the upper and lower tarsal conjunctivas. There are minimal conjunctival exudates and minimal inflammation but no complications. Treatment is ineffective, but the disease is self-limited within 2 years.

3. OCULAR ROSACEA

Ocular rosacea is an uncommon complication of acne rosacea and occurs more often in light-skinned people, especially of Irish descent, than in dark-skinned people. It is usually a blepharoconjunctivitis, but the cornea is sometimes also affected. The patient complains of mild injection and irritation. There is frequently an accompanying staphylococcal blepharitis. The blood vessels of the lid margins are dilated and the conjunctiva is hyperemic, especially in the exposed interpalpebral region. Less often, there may be a nodular conjunctivitis with small gray nodules on the bulbar conjunctiva, especially near the limbus, which may ulcerate superficially. The lesions can be differentiated from phlyctenules by the fact that even after they subside, the large dilated vessels persist.

Microscopic examination of the nodules shows lymphocytes and epithelial cells. The peripheral cornea may ulcerate and vascularize, and the keratitis may have a narrow base at the limbus and a wider infiltrate centrally. The corneal pannus is often segmented or wedge-shaped inferiorly (Figs 5–21 and 5–22).

Treatment of ocular rosacea consists of the elimination of alcohol and hot, spicy food and drink that cause dilatation of the facial vessels. Any secondary staphylococcal infection should be treated. A course of oral tetracycline is often helpful and a small maintenance dose may be indicated.

The disease is chronic, recurrences are common, and the response to treatment is usually poor. If the cornea is not affected, the visual prognosis is good; but corneal lesions tend to recur and progress, and the vision grows steadily worse over a period of years.

4. PSORIASIS

Psoriasis vulgaris usually affects the areas of the skin not exposed to the sun, but in about 10% of cases

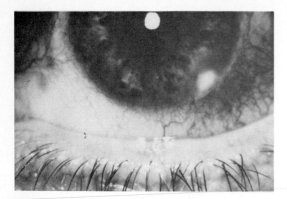

Figure 5–21. Conjunctivitis and corneal infiltrate in a patient with acne rosacea. (Courtesy of HB Ostler.)

lesions appear on the skin of the eyelids, and the plaques may extend to the conjunctiva, where they cause irritation, a foreign body sensation, and tearing. Psoriasis can also cause nonspecific chronic conjunctivitis with considerable mucoid discharge. Rarely, the cornea may show marginal ulceration or a deep, vascularized opacity.

The conjunctival and corneal lesions wax and wane with the skin lesions and are not affected by specific treatment. In rare cases, conjunctival scarring (symblepharon, trichiasis), corneal scarring, and occlusion of the nasolacrimal duct have occurred.

5. ERYTHEMA MULTIFORME (Major & Minor)

Erythema multiforme major (Stevens-Johnson syndrome) is a disease of the mucous membranes and skin. The skin lesion is an erythematous, urticarial bullous eruption that appears suddenly and is often distributed symmetrically. Bilateral conjunctivitis, often pseudomembranous, is a common manifestation. The patient complains of pain, irritation, discharge, and photophobia. The cornea is affected secondarily, and vascularization and scarring may seriously reduce vision. Stevens-Johnson syndrome is typically a disease of young people, occurring only rarely after age 35.

Cultures are negative for bacteria; conjunctival scrapings show a preponderance of polymorphonuclear cells. Systemic steroids are thought to shorten the systemic disease but have little or no effect on the eye lesions. Careful cleansing of the conjunctiva to remove the accumulated secretion is helpful, however, and tear replacement may be indicated. If trichiasis and entropion supervene, they should be corrected. Topical steroids probably have no beneficial effect, and their protracted use can cause corneal melting and perforation.

The acute episode of Stevens-Johnson syndrome usually lasts about 6 weeks, but the conjunctival scarring, loss of tears, and complications from entropion and trichiasis may result in prolonged morbidity and progressive corneal cicatrization (Fig 5–23). Recurrences are rare.

Erythema multiforme minor sometimes complicates a catarrhal conjunctivitis associated with tearing and mucoid discharge. The patient complains of irritation, redness, and discharge. The conjunctivitis is self-limited but may recur when the skin eruption recurs (usually in the spring and fall). Conjunctival scrapings show a polymorphonuclear cell reaction. Bacterial cultures are negative.

The cause is not definitely known, but there is growing evidence that the disease is a hypersensitivity disorder mediated by the deposition of circulating immune complexes in the superficial microvasculature of the skin and mucous membranes. The disease can be triggered by herpes simplex, by antibiotics, and especially by sulfonamides.

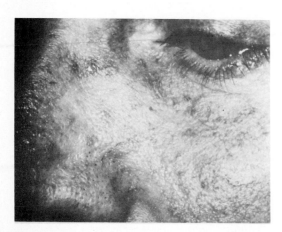

Figure 5–22. Skin lesions in acne rosacea. (Courtesy of HB Ostler.)

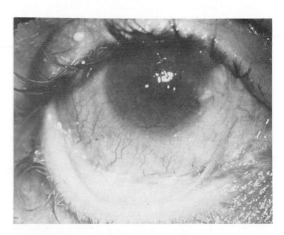

Figure 5–23. Late sequelae of Stevens-Johnson syndrome: conjunctival and corneal cicatrization and epidermalization. (Courtesy of P Thygeson.)

Erythema multiforme minor is self-limited, the conjunctiva clearing as the skin lesions clear. Steroids are often used systemically for the skin eruption. In contrast to ocular erythema multiforme major, this minor conjunctivitis does not leave scars and the cornea remains clear.

6. DERMATITIS HERPETIFORMIS

This is an uncommon skin disorder characterized by grouped erythematous, papulovesicular, vesicular, or bullous lesions arranged symmetrically. The disease has a predilection for the posterior axillary fold, the sacral region, the buttocks, and the forearms. Itching is often severe. Rarely, a pseudomembranous conjunctivitis occurs and may result in cicatrization resembling that seen in benign mucous membrane pemphigoid. The skin eruption and conjunctivitis usually respond readily to systemic sulfones or sulfapyridine.

7. EPIDERMOLYSIS BULLOSA

This is a rare hereditary disease characterized by vesicles, bullae, and epidermal cysts. The lesions occur chiefly on the extensor surfaces of the joints and other areas exposed to trauma. The severe dystrophic type that leads to scarring may also produce conjunctival scars similar to those seen in dermatitis herpetiformis and benign mucous membrane pemphigoid. No known treatment is satisfactory.

8. SUPERIOR LIMBIC KERATOCONJUNCTIVITIS

Superior limbic keratoconjunctivitis is usually bilateral and limited to the upper tarsus and upper limbus. The principal complaints are irritation and hyperemia. The signs are papillary hypertrophy of the upper tarsus, redness of the superior bulbar conjunctiva, thickening and keratinization of the superior limbus, epithelial keratitis, recurrent superior filaments, and superior micropannus. Rose bengal staining is a helpful diagnostic test. The keratinized epithelial cells and mucous debris pick up the stain. Scrapings from the upper limbus show keratinizing epithelial cells.

In about 50% of cases, the condition has been associated with abnormal function of the thyroid gland. Applying 0.5% or 1% silver nitrate to the upper palpebral conjunctiva and allowing the tarsus to drop back onto the upper limbus usually result in shedding of the keratinizing cells and relief of symptoms for 4–6 weeks. This treatment can be repeated. There are no complications, and the disease usually runs a course of 2–4 years.

In severe cases, one may consider 5-mm resection of the perilimbal superior conjunctiva.

9. LIGNEOUS CONJUNCTIVITIS

This is a rare bilateral, chronic or recurrent, pseudomembranous or membranous conjunctivitis that arises early in life, most commonly in young girls, and often persists for many years. Granulomas are often associated with it, and the lids may feel very hard. There is no satisfactory treatment.

10. REITER'S SYNDROME

A triad of disease manifestations—nonspecific urethritis, arthritis, and conjunctivitis or iritis—constitutes Reiter's syndrome. The disease occurs much more often in men than in women. The conjunctivitis is papillary in type and usually bilateral. Conjunctival scrapings contain polymorphonuclear cells. No bacteria grow in cultures. The arthritis usually affects the large weight-bearing joints. There is no satisfactory treatment. The disease has been found in association with HLA-B27.

11. MUCOCUTANEOUS LYMPH NODE SYNDROME (Kawasaki Disease)

This disease of unknown cause was first described in Japan in 1967. Conjunctivitis is one of its 6 diagnostic features. The others are (1) fever that fails to respond to antibiotics; (2) changes in the lips and oral cavity; (3) such changes in the extremities as erythema of the palms and soles, indurative edema, and membranous desquamation of the fingertips; (4) polymorphous exanthem of the trunk; and (5) acute nonpurulent swelling of the cervical lymph nodes.

The disease occurs almost exclusively in prepubertal children and carries a 1–2% mortality rate from cardiac failure. The conjunctivitis has not been severe, and no corneal lesions have been reported.

Treatment is supportive only.

CONJUNCTIVITIS ASSOCIATED WITH SYSTEMIC DISEASE

1. CONJUNCTIVITIS IN THYROID DISEASE

In orbital Graves' disease, the conjunctiva may be red and chemotic and the patient may complain of copious tearing. As the disease progresses the chemosis increases, and in advanced cases the chemotic conjunctiva may extrude between the lids.

Treatment is directed toward control of the thyroid disease, and every effort is made to protect the conjunctiva and cornea by bland ointment, lid adhesions if necessary, or even orbital decompression if the lids do not close enough to cover the cornea and conjunctiva.

2. GOUTY CONJUNCTIVITIS

Patients with gout often complain of a "hot eye" during their attacks. On examination, a mild conjunctivitis is found but is less severe than suggested by the symptoms. Gout may also be associated with episcleritis or scleritis, iridocyclitis, keratitis urica, vitreous opacities, and retinopathy. Treatment is aimed at controlling the gouty attack with colchicine and allopurinol.

3. CARCINOID CONJUNCTIVITIS

In carcinoid, the conjunctiva is sometimes congested and cyanotic as a result of the secretion of serotonin by the chromaffin cells of the gastrointestinal tract. The patient may complain of a "hot eye" during such attacks.

CONJUNCTIVITIS SECONDARY TO DACRYOCYSTITIS OR CANALICULITIS

1. CONJUNCTIVITIS SECONDARY TO DACRYOCYSTITIS

Both pneumococcal conjunctivitis (often unilateral and unresponsive to treatment) and beta-hemolytic streptococcal conjunctivitis (often hyperacute and purulent) may be secondary to chronic dacryocystitis. The nature and source of the conjunctivitis in both instances are often missed until the lacrimal system is investigated.

2. CONJUNCTIVITIS SECONDARY TO CANALICULITIS

Canaliculitis due to *A israelii* or *Candida* sp (or, very rarely, *Aspergillus* sp) may cause unilateral mucopurulent conjunctivitis, often chronic. The source of the condition is often missed unless the characteristic hyperemic, pouting punctum is noted. Expression of the canaliculus (upper or lower, whichever is involved) is curative provided the entire concretion is removed.

Conjunctival scrapings show a predominance of polymorphonuclear cells. Cultures (unless anaerobic) are usually negative. *Candida* grows readily on ordinary culture media, but almost all of the infections are caused by *A israelii*, which requires an anaerobic medium.

DEGENERATIVE DISEASES OF THE CONJUNCTIVA

PINGUECULA

Pinguecula is extremely common in adults. It appears as a yellow nodule on both sides of the cornea (more commonly on the nasal side) in the area of the lid fissure. The nodules, consisting of hyaline and yellow elastic tissue, rarely increase in size, but inflammation is common. In general, no treatment is required, but in certain cases of pingueculitis, weak topical steroids (eg, prednisolone 0.12%) may be given (Fig 5–24).

PTERYGIUM

Pterygium is a fleshy, bilateral, triangular encroachment of a pinguecula onto the cornea, usually on the nasal side (Fig 5–25). (Pterygiums are often referred to erroneously by patients as cataracts.) It is thought to be an irritative phenomenon due to ultraviolet light since it is common in farmers and sheepherders who spend much of their lives out of doors in sunny, dusty, or sandy, windblown areas. The pathologic findings in the conjunctiva are the same as those of pinguecula. In the cornea there is replacement of Bowman's layer by the hyaline and elastic tissue.

If the pterygium is enlarging and encroaches on the pupillary area, it should be removed surgically, along with a small portion of superficial clear cornea beyond the area of corneal encroachment. To prevent recurrences, particularly in people who work out of doors, protective glasses should be prescribed.

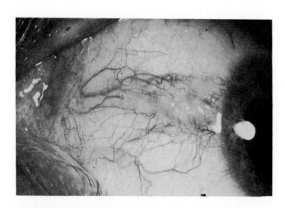

Figure 5–24. Pinguecula. (Courtesy of A Rosenberg.)

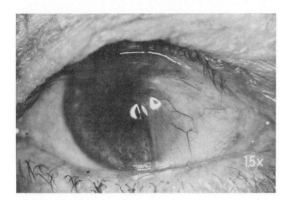

Figure 5–25. Pterygium encroaching on the cornea. (Courtesy of G Mintsioulis.)

CLIMATIC DROPLET KERATOPATHY
(Bietti's Band-Shaped Nodular Dystrophy, Labrador Keratopathy, Spheroidal Degeneration, Etc)

Climatic droplet keratopathy is a rare degenerative disorder of the cornea characterized by aggregates of yellowish-golden spherules that accumulate in the subepithelial layers. The cause is unknown, but certain factors such as exposure to ultraviolet light, aridity, and microtrauma are known predisposing factors. The deposits may result in elevation of the epithelium in a band-shaped configuration.

MISCELLANEOUS DISORDERS OF THE CONJUNCTIVA

LYMPHANGIECTASIS

Lymphangiectasis is characterized by small, clear, tortuous, localized dilatations in the conjunctiva. They are merely dilated lymph vessels, and no treatment is indicated unless they are irritating or cosmetically objectionable. They can then be cauterized or excised.

CONGENITAL CONJUNCTIVAL LYMPHEDEMA

This is a rare entity, unilateral or bilateral, and characterized by pinkish, fleshy edema of the bulbar conjunctiva. Usually observed as an isolated entity at birth, the condition is thought to be due to a congenital defect in the lymphatic drainage of the conjunctiva. It has been observed in chronic hereditary lymphedema of the lower extremities (Milroy's disease) and

is considered an ocular manifestation of this disease rather than an associated anomaly.

CYSTINOSIS

Cystinosis is a rare congenital disorder of amino acid metabolism characterized by a widespread intracellular deposition of cystine crystals in various body tissues, including the conjunctiva and cornea. Three types are recognized: childhood, adolescent, and adult. Life expectancy is reduced in the first 2 types.

SUBCONJUNCTIVAL HEMORRHAGE

This common disorder may occur spontaneously, usually in only one eye, in any age group. Its sudden onset and bright red appearance usually alarm the patient. The hemorrhage is caused by the rupture of a small conjunctival vessel, sometimes preceded by a bout of severe coughing or sneezing.

There is no treatment, and the hemorrhage usually absorbs in 2–3 weeks. The best treatment is reassurance.

In rare instances the hemorrhages are bilateral or recurrent; the possibility of blood dyscrasias should then be ruled out.

OPHTHALMIA NEONATORUM

Ophthalmia neonatorum in its broad sense refers to any infection of the newborn conjunctiva. In its narrow and commonly used sense, however, it refers to a conjunctival infection, chiefly gonococcal, that follows contamination of the baby's eyes during its passage through the mother's cervix and vagina. Since the newborn is a "compromised host," many opportunistic bacteria (and one virus: herpes simplex virus type 2) that are found in the female genital tract are capable of producing disease. For medicolegal reasons, the causes of all cases of ophthalmia neonatorum should be identified in smears of exudate, epithelial scrapings, and cultures.

The time of onset is important in clinical diagnosis since the 2 principal types, gonorrheal ophthalmia and inclusion blennorrhea, have widely differing incubation periods: gonococcal disease 2–3 days and chlamydial disease 5–12 days. The third important birth canal infection (herpes simplex virus type 2 keratoconjunctivitis) has a 2- to 3-day incubation period and is potentially extremely serious because of the possibility of systemic dissemination.

Credé 1% silver nitrate prophylaxis is effective for the prevention of gonorrheal ophthalmia. (Regrettably, it is not protective against inclusion blennorrhea or herpetic infection.) The slight chemical conjunctivitis induced by silver nitrate is minor and of short duration. Accidents with concentrated solutions can be avoided by using wax ampules specially prepared for Credé prophylaxis. Silver nitrate substitutes, including penicillin and other antibiotics, are under study, and erythromycin ointment appears to be especially promising.

OCULOGLANDULAR DISEASE
(Parinaud's Oculoglandular Syndrome)

This is a group of conjunctival diseases, usually unilateral, characterized by low-grade fever, grossly visible preauricular adenopathy, and one or more conjunctival granulomas (Fig 5–26). The commonest cause is cat-scratch disease, but there are many other causes, including *M tuberculosis, T pallidum, Francisella tularensis, Pasteurella (Yersinia) pseudotuberculosis, Chlamydia lymphogranulomatis,* and *Coccidioides immitis.*

Conjunctival Cat-Scratch Disease

This protracted but benign granulomatous conjunctivitis is found most commonly in children who have been in intimate contact with cats. The child often runs a low-grade fever and develops a reasonably enlarged preauricular node and one or more conjunctival granulomas. These may show focal necrosis and may sometimes ulcerate. The regional adenopathy does not suppurate. The clinical diagnosis is supported by a positive cat-scratch disease skin test.

The disease appears to be caused by a slender pleomorphic gram-negative bacillus, which grows in the walls of blood vessels. With special stains, this organism can be seen in biopsies of conjunctival tissue. Morphologically identical organisms have also been identified in lymph nodes from cases of nonocular cat-scratch disease, but isolation of the organism in culture has not yet been achieved. The organism closely resembles *Leptotrichia buccalis,* and the disease was previously known as leptotrichosis conjunctivae (Parinaud's conjunctivitis). *L buccalis* is commonly found

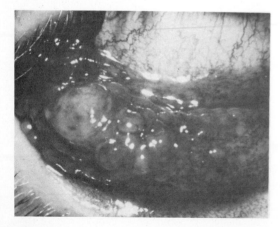

Figure 5–26. Conjunctival granuloma. (Courtesy of P Thygeson.)

in the mouth in humans and always in the mouth in cats. The eye may be contaminated by saliva on the child's fingers or by cat drool on the child's pillow.

The disease is self-limited (without corneal or other complications) and resolves in 2–3 months. The conjunctival nodule can be excised; in the case of a solitary granuloma, this may be curative. Systemic tetracyclines may shorten the course of the disease but should not be given to children under the age of 7.

Conjunctivitis Secondary to Neoplasms
(Masquerade Syndrome)

When examined superficially, a neoplasm of the conjunctiva or lid margin is often misdiagnosed as a chronic infectious conjunctivitis or keratoconjunctivitis. Since the underlying lesion is often not recognized, the condition has been referred to as masquerade syndrome. The masquerading neoplasms on record are conjunctival capillary carcinoma, conjunctival carcinoma in situ, molluscum contagiosum, infectious papilloma of the conjunctiva, and verruca. Verruca and molluscum tumors of the lid margin may desquamate toxic tumor material that produces a chronic conjunctivitis, keratoconjunctivitis, or (rarely) keratitis alone.

CONJUNCTIVAL TUMORS

J. Brooks Crawford, MD

PRIMARY BENIGN TUMORS OF THE CONJUNCTIVA

Nevus (Fig 5–27)

One-third of melanocytic nevi of the conjunctiva lack pigment. Over half have cystic epithelial inclusions that can be seen clinically.

Histologically, conjunctival nevi are composed of nests or sheets of typical nevus cells. Conjunctival nevi, like other nevi, rarely become malignant. Many are excised because they are disfiguring.

Papilloma

Conjunctival papillomas are not rare, occurring most frequently near the limbus, on the caruncle, or at the lid margins. Those on the caruncle and lid margin are usually soft and predunculated, with irregular surfaces. They frequently recur after removal.

Granuloma

Pyogenic granulomas are a variety of capillary hemangiomas. They frequently occur on the palpebral conjunctiva over chalazions or in an area of recent surgical incision.

Granulomatous inflammation occurs around foreign bodies and in association with diseases such as coccidioidomycosis and sarcoidosis. These inflam-

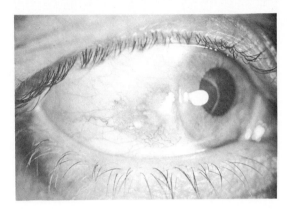

Figure 5–27. Conjunctival nevus. (Courtesy of A Irvine, Jr.)

matory foci may form elevated plaques or nodules in the skin or the conjunctiva of the eyelids.

Dermoid Tumor
(Fig 5–28)

This rare congenital tumor appears as a smooth, rounded, yellow elevated mass, frequently with hairs protruding. A dermoid tumor may remain quiescent, although it often increases in size during puberty. Removal is indicated only if cosmetic deformity is significant or if vision is impaired or threatened.

Dermolipoma

Dermolipoma is a common congenital tumor that usually appears as a smoothly rounded growth in the upper temporal quadrant of the bulbar conjunctiva near the lateral canthus. Treatment is usually not indicated, but at least partial removal may be indicated if the growth is enlarging or is cosmetically disfiguring. Posterior dissection must be undertaken with extreme care (if at all) since this lesion is frequently continuous with orbital fat; orbital derangement may cause scarring and complications far more serious than the original lesion.

Lymphoma & Lymphoid Hyperplasia

These are uncommon conjunctival lesions that may appear in adults without evidence of systemic disease or as part of the clinical picture of lymphosarcoma, lymphocytic leukemia, Hodgkin's disease, or other related conditions. Benign lymphoid hyperplasia can sometimes be distinguished by a pebbly appearance corresponding to follicle formation. However, the clinical appearance of benign lymphoid hyperplasia and malignant lymphoma can be similar; therefore, biopsy is essential to establish a diagnosis.

Treatment of both benign and malignant lesions is best accomplished with radiotherapy.

Fibroma

Fibromas are rare small, smooth, pedunculated, transparent growths that may appear anywhere in the conjunctival tissues but are most often seen in the lower fornix. Histologically, they consist of fibrous overgrowths covered by epithelium. Treatment is by excision.

Angioma

Conjunctival angiomas may occur as isolated, circumscribed capillary hemangiomas or as more diffuse vascular tumors, often associated with a more extensive lid or orbital capillary or cavernous hemangioma. Hemangiomas should be distinguished from telangiectases involving conjunctival capillaries. Telangiectases of the conjunctival vessels are not always associated with inflammatory disease; they occasionally occur over an underlying melanoma of the ciliary body.

PRIMARY MALIGNANT TUMORS OF THE BULBAR CONJUNCTIVA

Carcinoma

Carcinoma of the conjunctiva (Fig 5–29) arises most frequently at the limbus in the area of the palpebral

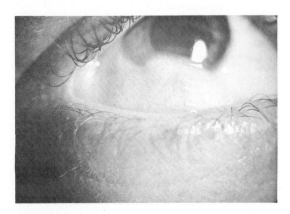

Figure 5–28. Dermoid tumor at the inferior limbus. (Courtesy of A Irvine, Jr.)

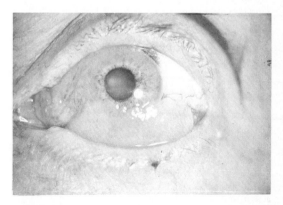

Figure 5–29. Intraepithelial epithelioma. (Courtesy of A Irvine, Jr.)

fissure and less often in nonexposed areas of the conjunctiva. Some of these tumors may resemble pterygiums. Most have a gelatinous surface; sometimes, abnormal keratinization of the epithelium produces leukoplakia. Growth is slow, and deep invasion and metastases are extremely rare; therefore, complete excision is effective treatment. Recurrences are common if the lesion is incompletely excised; treatment consists of reexcision.

Conjunctival dysplasia, a benign condition that occurs as an isolated lesion or sometimes over pterygiums and pingueculas, can resemble carcinoma in situ clinically and even histologically. Excisional biopsy will establish a diagnosis and result in cure of most of these lesions. The use of cryotherapy may help to prevent recurrences.

Malignant Melanoma

Malignant melanoma of the conjunctiva is rare. It may arise from a preexisting nevus, from an area of acquired melanosis, or de novo from formerly normal-appearing conjunctiva. Pigmentation may vary greatly, and the clinical course is often unpredictable.

Many tumors can be locally excised. More radical surgery (eg, exenteration of the orbit) does not usually improve the prognosis. The use of cryotherapy after excision of melanotic tumors may help to prevent recurrences.

Lymphosarcoma

Malignant lymphomas of the conjunctiva are much rarer than benign lymphoid hyperplasia. Many also involve the orbit, and a few are associated with systemic lymphoma. However, the conjunctival lesion may be the initial sign of a systemic problem.

REFERENCES

Allansmith MR et al: Giant papillary conjunctivitis in contact lens wearers. *Am J Ophthalmol* 1977;**83**:697.

Al-Mutlaq F, Byrne-Rhodes KA, Tabbara KF: *Neisseria meningitidis* conjunctivitis in children. *Am J Ophthalmol* 1987;**104**:280.

Andrew JW et al: Induction of conjunctival transdifferentiation on vascularized corneas by photothrombotic occlusion of corneal neovascularization. *Ophthalmology* 1988;**95**:228.

Coad CT, Osato MS, Wilhelmus KR: Bacterial contamination of eye drop dispensers. *Am J Ophthalmol* 1984;**98**:548.

Darougar S (editor): Chlamydial disease. *Br Med Bull* (April) 1983;**39**. [Entire issue.]

Darougar S, Wishart MS, Viswalingam ND: Epidemiological and clinical features of primary herpes simplex virus ocular infection. *Br J Ophthalmol* 1985;**69**:2.

Darougar S et al: Adenovirus serotypes isolated from ocular infections in London. *Br J Ophthalmol* 1983;**67**:111.

Dawson CR, Jones BR, Tarizzo ML: *Guide to Trachoma Control in Programmes for the Prevention of Blindness.* World Health Organization, 1981.

Dawson CR et al: Severe endemic trachoma in Tunisia. *Br J Ophthalmol* 1976:**60**:245.

Duane TD (editor): *Clinical Ophthalmology.* Harper & Row, 1985.

Foster CS: Evaluation of topical cromolyn sodium in the treatment of vernal keratoconjunctivitis. *Ophthalmology* 1988;**95**:194.

Fraunfelder FT et al: The role of cryosurgery in external ocular and periocular disease. *Trans Am Acad Ophthalmol Otolaryngol* 1977;**83**:713.

Jarvis VN, Levine R, Asbell PA: Ophthalmia neonatorum: Study of a decade of experience at the Mount Sinai Hospital. *Br J Ophthalmol* 1987;**71**:295.

Kersten RC, Shoukrey NM, Tabbara KF: Orbital myiasis. *Ophthalmology* 1986;**93**:1228.

Kiernan JP et al: Stevens-Johnson syndrome. *Am J Ophthalmol* 1981;**92**:543.

Lemp MA, Mahmood MA, Weiler HH: Association of rosacea and keratoconjunctivitis sicca. *Arch Ophthalmol* 1984;**102**:556.

Mondino BJ, Brown SI: Immunosuppressive therapy in ocular cicatricial pemphigoid. *Am J Ophthalmol* 1983;**96**:453.

Pfister RR: Chemical injuries of the eye. *Ophthalmology* 1983;**90**:1246.

Robbins JH et al: Xeroderma pigmentosum: An inherited disease with sun sensitivity, multiple cutaneous neoplasms, and abnormal DNA repair. *Ann Intern Med* 1974;**80**:221.

Salvaggio JE (editor): Primer on allergic and immunologic diseases. *JAMA* 1982;**248**:2579. [Special issue.]

Savino DF, Margo CE: Conjunctival rhinosporidiosis: Light and electron microscopic study. *Ophthalmology* 1983; **90**:1482.

Schachter J: Chlamydiae (psittacosis-lymphogranuloma venereum-trachoma group). Chap 85, pp 856–862, in: *Manual of Clinical Microbiology,* 4th ed. Lennette EH (editor). American Society for Microbiology, 1985.

Schwartz LK, Gelender H, Forster RK: Chronic conjunctivitis associated with "floppy eyelids." *Arch Ophthalmol* 1983;**101**:1884.

Sigelman J, Jakobiec FA: Lymphoid lesions of the conjunctiva: Relation of histopathology to clinical outcome. *Ophthalmology* 1978:**85**:818.

Singer TR, Isenberg SJ, Apt L: Conjunctival anaerobic and aerobic bacterial flora in paediatric versus adult subjects. *Brit J Ophthalmol* 1988;**72**:448.

Sjögren H: Keratoconjunctivitis sicca and the Sjögren syndrome. *Surv Ophthalmol* 1971;**16**:145.

Sklar VEF et al: Clinical findings and results of treatment in an outbreak of acute hemorrhagic conjunctivitis in southern Florida. *Am J Ophthalmol* 1983;**95**:45.

Sommer A: Effects of vitamin A deficiency on the ocular surface. *Ophthalmology* 1983;**90**:592.

Spencer WH (editor): *Ophthalmic Pathology,* 3rd ed. 3 vols. Saunders, 1985.

Tabbara KF et al: Metastatic squamous cell carcinoma of the conjunctiva. *Ophthalmology* 1988;**95**:318.

Tabbara KF, Hyndiuk RA: *Infections of the Eye.* Little, Brown, 1986.

Taylor PB, Tabbara KF, Burd EM: Effect of preoperative fusidic acid on the normal eyelid and conjunctival bacterial flora. *Br J Ophthalmol* 1988;**72:**206.

Thygeson P: Historical review of oculogenital disease. *Am J Ophthalmol* 1971;**71:**975.

Thygeson P: Observations on conjunctival neoplasms masquerading as chronic conjunctivitis or keratitis. *Trans Am Acad Ophthalmol Otolaryngol* 1969;**73:**969.

Wear DJ et al: Cat scratch disease bacilli in the conjunctiva of patients with Parinaud's oculoglandular syndrome. *Ophthalmology* 1985;**92:**1282.

Wishart PK et al: Prevalence of acute conjunctivitis caused by chlamydia, adenovirus, and herpes simplex virus in an ophthalmic casualty department. *Br J Ophthalmol* 1984;**68:**653.

Zaidman GW et al: Phlyctenular keratoconjunctivitis. *Am J Ophthalmol* 1981;**92:**178.

6

Cornea

Daniel Vaughan, MD

ANATOMY

The cornea is a transparent avascular tissue comparable in size and structure to the crystal of a small wristwatch. It is inserted into the sclera at the limbus. At the scleral junction there is a circumferential depression called the scleral sulcus. The cornea functions as a protective membrane and a "window" through which light rays pass en route to the retina.

The average adult cornea is 0.65 mm thick at the periphery and 0.54 mm thick in the center. From anterior to posterior, it has 5 distinct layers (Fig 6–1): the epithelium (which is continuous with the epithelium of the bulbar conjunctiva), Bowman's layer, the stroma, Descemet's membrane, and the endothelium. The epithelium has 5 or 6 layers of cells, the endothelium only one. Bowman's layer is a clear acellular layer, a modified portion of the stroma. Descemet's membrane is a clear elastic membrane that can be seen on electron microscopy to comprise many fine fibrils. The corneal stroma accounts for about 90% of the corneal thickness. It is composed of intertwining lamellar fibers about 1 μm wide that run almost the full diameter of the cornea. They run parallel to the surface of the cornea and by virtue of their size and periodicity are optically clear. Each lamella possesses a flattened nucleus.

Sources of nutrition for the cornea are the vessels of the limbus, the aqueous, and tears. The superficial cornea also gets most of its oxygen from the atmosphere. The sensory nerves of the cornea are supplied by the first division of the fifth (trigeminal) cranial nerve. In the corneal epithelium there is a rich network of nerve fibers with bare ends. Whenever they are exposed, they produce a sensation of pain. The large number of nerves and the location of their endings account for the severe pain that results from even minor abrasions of the corneal epithelium.

The transparency of the cornea is due to its uniform structure, avascularity, and deturgescence. Deturgescence, or the state of relative dehydration of the corneal tissue, is maintained by the active bicarbonate "pump" of the endothelium and the anatomic integrity of the endothelium and epithelium. The endothelium is more important than the epithelium in the mechanism of dehydration, and chemical or physical damage to the endothelium is far more serious than damage to the epithelium. Destruction of the endo-

thelial cells may cause marked swelling of the cornea and some loss of transparency. On the other hand, damage to the epithelium causes only slight transient, localized swelling of the corneal stroma that clears when the epithelial cells regenerate. Evaporation of water from the precorneal tear film produces slight hypertonicity of the film, which may be another factor in drawing water from the superficial corneal stroma, and helps to maintain the state of dehydration.

The penetration of the intact cornea by drugs is biphasic. Fat-soluble substances can pass through intact epithelium, and water-soluble substances can pass through intact stroma. To pass through the cornea, drugs must therefore have both a lipid-soluble and a water-soluble phase.

CORNEAL RESISTANCE TO INFECTION

The epithelium is a reliable barrier to the entrance of microorganisms into the cornea. Once the epithe-

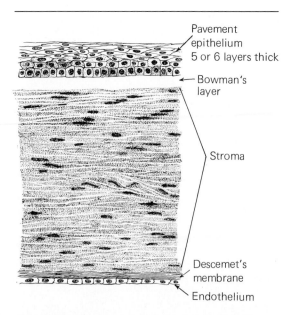

Figure 6–1. Transverse section of cornea. (Reproduced, with permission, from Wolff E: *Anatomy of the Eye and Orbit,* 4th ed. Blakiston-McGraw, 1954.)

Labels: Pavement epithelium 5 or 6 layers thick; Bowman's layer; Stroma; Descemet's membrane; Endothelium

lium is traumatized, however, the avascular stroma and Bowman's layer become excellent culture media for a variety of organisms, particularly *Pseudomonas aeruginosa*. Descemet's membrane resists most bacteria but is not a barrier to fungi. *Streptococcus pneumoniae* (the pneumococcus) is one of the true bacterial corneal pathogens; many other opportunistic pathogens require a heavy inoculum or a compromised host (eg, traumatized epithelium) to produce infection.

Since the advent of the corticosteroids in 1952, many opportunistic bacteria and fungi have become major causes of corneal ulcers. Local corticosteroid drops modify the immune reaction (the second line of defense against infection) and may allow opportunistic organisms to invade and flourish.

Moraxella liquefaciens, which occurs mainly in alcoholics (as a result of pyridoxine depletion), is a classic example of the bacterial opportunist, and in recent years a number of new bacterial corneal opportunists have been identified. Among them are *Serratia marcescens, Mycobacterium fortuitum, Streptococcus viridans, Staphylococcus epidermidis,* and various coliform and *Proteus* organisms.

PHYSIOLOGY OF SYMPTOMS

Since the cornea has many pain fibers, most corneal lesions, superficial or deep (corneal foreign body, corneal abrasion, phlyctenule, interstitial keratitis), cause pain and photophobia. The pain is worsened by movement of the lids (particularly the upper lid) over the cornea and usually persists until healing occurs. Since the cornea serves as the window of the eye and refracts light rays, corneal lesions usually blur vision somewhat, especially if centrally located.

Photophobia in corneal disease is the result of painful contraction of a hyperemic iris. Dilatation of iris vessels is a reflex phenomenon caused by irritation of the corneal nerve endings. Photophobia, severe in most corneal disease, is minimal in herpetic keratitis because of the hypesthesia associated with the disease, which is also a valuable diagnostic sign.

Although tearing and photophobia commonly accompany corneal disease, there is usually no discharge except in purulent bacterial ulcers.

INVESTIGATION OF CORNEAL DISEASE

Symptoms & Signs

The physician examines the cornea by inspecting it under adequate illumination. Examination is often facilitated by instillation of a local anesthetic. Fluorescein staining can outline a superficial epithelial lesion that might otherwise be impossible to see. The loupe and slit lamp are helpful but not absolutely essential aids; adequate illumination can be achieved with a hand flashlight. One should follow the course of the light reflex while moving the light carefully

over the entire cornea. Rough areas indicative of epithelial defects are demonstrated in this way.

The patient's history is important in corneal disease. A history of trauma can often be elicited—in fact, foreign bodies and abrasions are the 2 most common corneal lesions. A history of corneal disease may also be of value. The keratitis of herpes simplex infection is often recurrent, but since recurrent erosion is extremely painful and herpetic keratitis is not, these disorders can be differentiated by their symptoms. The patient's use of local medications should be investigated, since corticosteroids may have been used and may have predisposed to bacterial, fungal, or viral disease, especially herpes simplex keratitis. Immunosuppression also occurs with systemic diseases, such as diabetes and malignant disease, as well as with specific immunosuppressive therapy.

Laboratory Studies

To select the proper therapy for corneal infections, especially hypopyon ulceration, laboratory aid is essential. Bacterial and fungal ulcers, for example, require completely different medications. Since a few hours' delay in determining the cause may severely prejudice the ultimate visual result, scrapings from the ulcer should be stained by both Gram's and Giemsa's stains and the infecting organism identified presumptively while the patient waits. Appropriate therapy can then be instituted immediately. Cultures for bacteria and fungi should be started at the same time, but therapy should not be withheld while awaiting confirmation of the presumptive diagnosis.

Morphologic Diagnosis of Corneal Lesions

A. Subepithelial Keratitis: Table 6–1 lists a number of important types of subepithelial lesions. These are often secondary to epithelial keratitis (eg, the nummular lesions of epidemic keratoconjunctivitis, caused by adenoviruses 8 and 19). They can usually be observed grossly but may also be recognized in the course of biomicroscopic examination of epithelial keratitis.

B. Epithelial Keratitis: The corneal epithelium is involved in most types of conjuctivitis and keratitis and in rare cases may be the only tissue involved (eg, in superficial punctate keratitis). The epithelial changes vary widely from simple edema and vacuolation to minute erosions, filament formation, partial keratinization, etc. The lesions vary also in their location on the cornea. All of these variations have

Table 6–1. Subepithelial keratitis.

Types of keratitis with round, discrete, subepithelial opacities:
1. Nummular keratitis (Padi keratitis of the Orient).
2. Epidemic keratoconjunctivitis.
3. Nummular opacities in wearers of soft contact lenses.
4. Nummular opacities in herpes zoster, Epstein-Barr viral infections.
5. Nummular opacities in congenital syphilitic keratitis.

Table 6–2. Principal types of epithelial keratitis
(in order of frequency of occurrence).

Minute fluorescein-staining erosions; lower third of cornea affected predominantly.	Typically dendritic (occasionally round or oval) with edema and degeneration.	More diffuse than lesions of HSK; occasionally linear (pseudodendrites).
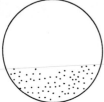	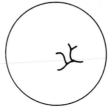	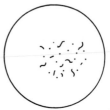
1. Staphylococcal keratitis	2. Herpetic keratitis (HSK)	3. Varicella-zoster keratitis
Minute fluorescein-staining erosions; diffuse but most conspicuous in pupillary area.	Minute pleomorphic, fluorescein-staining, damaged epithelium and erosions; epithelial and mucous filaments are typical; lower half of cornea affected predominantly.	Minute fluorescein-staining, irregular erosions; lower half of cornea affected predominantly.
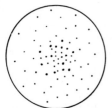	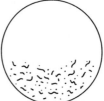	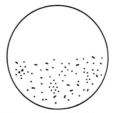
4. Adenovirus keratitis	5. Keratitis of Sjögren's syndrome	6. Exposure keratitis—due to lagophthalmos or exophthalmos
Blotchy gray, opaque, syncytiumlike lesions, most conspicuous in upper pupillary area. Sometimes a plaque of opaque epithelium forms.	Blotchy epithelial edema; diffuse but predominant in palpebral fissure, 9–3 o'clock.	Minute fluorescein-staining erosions with spotty cellular edema; highly characteristic picture.
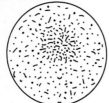	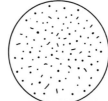	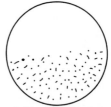
7. Vernal keratoconjunctivitis	8. Trophic keratitis—sequela of herpes simplex, herpes zoster, and gasserian ganglion destruction	9. Drug-induced keratitis—especially by broad-spectrum antibiotics
Foci of edematous epithelial cells, round or oval; elevated when disease is active.	Minute fluorescein-staining erosions of upper third of cornea; filaments during exacerbations; bulbar hyperemia, thickened limbus, micropannus.	Virus-type lesions like those of SPK; in pupillary area.
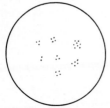	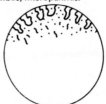	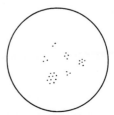
10. Superficial punctate keratitis (SPK)	11. Superior limbic keratoconjunctivitis	12. Rubeola, rubella, and mumps keratitis

Table 6–2 (cont'd).   Principal types of epithelial keratitis (in order of frequency of occurrence).

Minute fluorescein-staining epithelial erosions affecting upper third of cornea.	Spotty gray opacification of individual epithelial cells due to partial keratinization; associated with Bitot's spots.
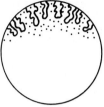	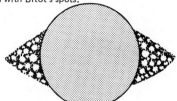
13. Trachoma	14. Vitamin A deficiency keratitis

incalculable diagnostic significance (Table 6–2), and biomicroscopic examination with and without fluorescein staining should be a part of every external eye examination.

CORNEAL ULCERATION

Cicatrization due to corneal ulceration is a major cause of blindness and impaired vision throughout the world. Most of this visual loss is preventable, but only if an etiologic diagnosis is made early and appropriate therpy instituted. Hypopyon ulcer, the most important type, was once caused almost exclusively by the pneumococcus (*S pneumoniae*). In recent years, however, as a result of the widespread use of compromising systemic and local medications (at least in the developed countries), opportunistic bacteria, fungi, and viruses have tended to cause more cases of corneal ulcer than the pneumococcus.

CENTRAL CORNEAL ULCERS (Hypopyon Ulcer)

Central ulcers are infectious ulcers that follow epithelial damage. The break in the epithelium may be peripheral, but the ulcer migrates toward the center of the cornea, away from the vascularized limbus. Hypopyon usually (not always) accompanies the ulcer. The pneumococcus, historically the chief cause of hypopyon ulcer, is pathogenic, even in small numbers, for an exposed corneal stroma.

BACTERIAL KERATITIS

Many types of bacterial corneal ulcer look alike and vary only in severity. This is especially true of ulcers caused by opportunistic bacteria (eg, alpha-hemolytic streptococci, *Staphylococcus aureus, Nocardia,* and *M fortuitum*), which cause indolent corneal ulcers that tend to spread slowly and superficially.

Pneumococcal Corneal Ulcer (Acute Serpiginous Ulcer)

The pneumococcus (*Streptococcus pneumoniae*) is still a common cause of bacterial corneal ulcer in many parts of the world. Before the popularization of dacryocystorhinostomy, pneumococcal ulcers often occurred in patients with obstructed nasolacrimal ducts. In trachoma-endemic areas, there is a high prevalence of nasolacrimal duct obstruction. Trachoma causes cicatrization of the lacrimal passages and leads to nasolacrimal duct obstruction. Such patients may develop chronic dacryocystitis.

Pneumococcal corneal ulcer usually occurs 24–48 hours after inoculation of an abraded cornea. It typically produces a gray, fairly well circumscribed ulcer that tends to spread erratically from the original site of infection toward the center of the cornea (Fig 6–2). The advancing border shows active ulceration and infiltration as the trailing border begins to heal. (This creeping effect suggested the term ''acute serpiginous ulcer.'') The superficial corneal layers become in-

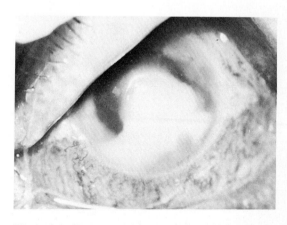

Figure 6–2. Pneumococcal corneal ulcer with hypopyon.

Table 6–3. Treatment of bacterial and fungal keratitis.

Organisms	Drug Route	First Choice	Recommended Drugs Second Choice	Third Choice
Gram-positive cocci: lancet-shaped with capsule = pneumococcus	Topical Subconjunctival Systemic[1]	Erythromycin Cefazolin Cefazolin	Bacitracin Penicillin G Penicillin G	Vancomycin Erythromycin or methicillin Oral: Erythromycin
Other gram-positive organisms: cocci and rods	Topical Subconjunctival	Bacitracin Cefazolin and gentamicin	Cefazolin Methicillin and gentamicin	Gentamicin or vancomycin Vancomycin and methicillin
Gram-negative cocci[2]	Topical Subconjunctival Systemic	Erythromycin Methicillin and gentamicin Penicillin G	Bacitracin Gentamicin and cefazolin Cefazolin	Gentamicin or vancomycin Erythromycin and methicillin Oral: Erythromycin
Gram-negative rods (thin = *Pseudomonas*)	Topical Subconjunctival Systemic	Tobramycin Tobramycin and carbenicillin . . .	Polymyxin B Gentamicin and carbenicillin . . .	Gentamicin and carbenicillin Polymyxin B . . .
Gram-negative rods: large, square-ended diplobacilli = *Moraxella*	Topical Subconjunctival Systemic	Gentamicin Rarely necessary . . .	Sodium sulfacetamide	Zinc sulfate or chloramphenicol . . . . . .
Other gram-negative rods	Topical Subconjunctival Systemic	Gentamicin Gentamicin and carbenicillin Ampicillin	Carbenicillin Gentamicin and cephaloridine Cefazolin	Chloramphenicol Carbenicillin and cephaloridine Carbenicillin
Gram-positive rods: slender and varying in length = *Mycobacterium fortuitum*, *Nocardia* sp, *Actinomyces* sp	Topical Subconjunctival Systemic	Amikacin Amikacin Oral: Sulfonamides[3]	Rifampin . . . Oral: Tetracycline[3]	Tetracycline . . . . . .
Yeastlike organisms = *Candida* sp[4]	Topical Subconjunctival Systemic	Amphotericin B and flucytosine Amphotericin B Oral: Flucytosine	Natamycin and flucytosine Miconazole Ketoconazole	Nystatin or miconazole . . . . . .
Hyphaelike organisms = fungal ulcer	Topical Subconjunctival Systemic	Natamycin Amphotericin B	Amphotericin B Miconazole Ketoconazole	Miconazole . . . . . .
No organisms identified; ulcer suggestive of bacterial type	Topical Subconjunctival Systemic	Gentamicin and cefazolin Gentamicin and cefazolin Penicillin G	Gentamicin and bacitracin Gentamicin and methicillin Nafcillin	Vancomycin Cephaloridine and polymyxin B Cefazolin
No organisms identified; ulcer suggestive of fungal type	Topical Subconjunctival Systemic	Natamycin Rarely necessary: Amphotericin B	Amphotericin B Miconazole . . .	Miconazole . . . . . .

[1] Intravenous unless otherwise stated; only when ulcer is severe.
[2] Ulcer associated with hyperacute conjunctivitis (eg, gonococcal conjunctivitis) should be treated with same drug used to treat the conjunctivitis.
[3] These 2 drugs often act synergistically.
[4] Rarely, *Pityrosporum ovale* or *Pityrosporum orbiculare* may be confused with *Candida* sp.

volved first and then the deep parenchyma. The cornea surrounding the ulcer is often clear.

A hypopyon of moderate size usually forms. Hypopyon is a collection of inflammatory cells, predominantly polymorphonuclear neutrophilic leukocytes with some mononuclear cells and macrophages, and is characteristic of both bacterial and fungal central corneal ulcers. Although hypopyon is sterile in bacterial corneal ulcers unless there has been a rupture of Descemet's membrane, in fungal ulcers it often contains fungal elements; this is because fungi can penetrate an intact Descemet membrane.

Scrapings from the leading edge of a pneumococcal corneal ulcer contain gram-positive lancet-shaped diplococci. Drugs recommended for use in treatment are listed in Tables 6–3 and 6–4. Concurrent dacryocystitis should also be treated.

Pseudomonas Corneal Ulcer

Pseudomonas corneal ulcer begins as a gray or yellow infiltrate at the site of break in the corneal epithelium (Fig 6–3). Severe pain usually accompanies it. The lesion tends to spread rapidly in all directions because of the proteolytic enzymes produced by the organisms. Although usually superficial at first, the ulcer may affect the entire cornea. There is often a large hypopyon that tends to increase in size as the ulcer progresses. The infiltrate and exudate may have a bluish-green color. This is due to a pigment produced by the organism and is pathognomonic of *P aeruginosa* infection.

Pseudomonas is a common cause of bacterial corneal ulcers. Cases of *Pseudomonas* corneal ulcer may follow minor corneal abrasion or the use of soft contact lenses—especially extended wear lenses. Some cases have been reported following the use of contaminated fluorescein solution or eye drops. It is mandatory that the clinician use sterile medications and sterile technique when caring for patients with corneal injuries.

Scrapings from the ulcer contain long, thin gram-negative rods that are often few in number. Drugs recommended for use in treatment are listed in Tables 6–3 and 6–4.

Table 6–4. Drug concentrations and dosages for treatment of bacterial or fungal ketatitis.

Drug	Topical[1]	Subconjunctival[1]	Systemic[1] (intravenous unless otherwise indicated)
Amikacin	10 mg/mL	25 mg/0.5 mL/dose	…
Amphotericin B	1.5–3 mg/mL	750 μg/0.5 mL/dose every other day	…
Ampicillin	…	…	150–200 mg/kg body wt/d in 4 doses
Bacitracin	10,000 units/mL	…	…
Carbenicillin	4 mg/mL	125 mg/0.5 mL/dose	100–200 mg/kg body wt/d in 4 doses
Cefazolin	50 mg/mL	100 mg/0.5 mL/dose	15 mg/kg body wt/d in 4 doses
Chloramphenicol	5 mg/mL	…	…
Erythromycin	5 mg/g (ointment)	100 mg/0.5 mL/dose	Oral: first dose 1 g; then 0.5 g every 6 h
Flucytosine	1% solution	…	Oral: 50–150 mg/kg body wt/d in 4 doses
Gentamicin	3–10 mg/mL	20 mg/0.5 mL/dose	…
Methicillin	…	100 mg/mL; dose: 0.5–1 mL	
Miconazole	1% solution or 2% ointment	5 mg/0.5 mL/dose	…
Nafcillin	…	…	1 g every 4–6 h
Natamycin (pimaricin)	5% suspension	…	…
Nystatin	100,000 units/g (ointment)	…	…
Penicillin G	10,000–20,000 units/mL	1 million units/mL/dose	40,000–50,000 units/kg body wt/d in 4 doses or continuously
Polymyxin B	10,000–25,000 units/mL	10,000 units/mL/dose	…
Rifampin	1% ointment	…	Oral: 600 mg/d
Sodium sulfacetamide	10–15% solution	…	…
Tetracycline	5 mg/mL	…	Oral: 1.5 g/d in 4 doses for patients under 70 kg; 2 g/d if over 70 kg
Tobramycin	3–15 mg/mL	20 mg/0.5 mL/dose	…
Vancomycin	50 mg/mL	100 mg/mL; dose: 0.25 mL	…
Zinc sulfate	0.5 mg/mL	…	…

[1] Treatment schedule: Topical: Every hour during day, every 2 hours during night, for 5 days. Subconjunctival: One injection daily for 4 days unless otherwise stated; in exceptionally severe cases, initial dose sometimes repeated after 12 hours. Systemic, intravenous, or oral: One dose daily for 5 days.

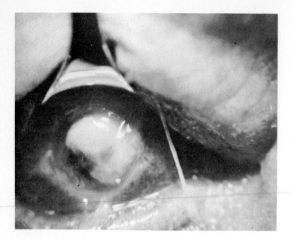

Figure 6–3. *Pseudomonas* corneal ulcer of right eye. Evisceration was done.

Moraxella liquefaciens Corneal Ulcer

M liquefaciens (diplobacillus of Petit) causes an indolent oval ulcer that usually affects the inferior cornea and progresses into the deep stroma over a period of days. There is usually no hypopyon or only a small one, and the surrounding cornea is usually clear. *M liquefaciens* ulcer almost always occurs in a patient with alcoholism, diabetes, or other immunosuppressing disease. Scrapings contain large, square-ended gram-negative diplobacilli. Drugs recommended for use in treatment are listed in Tables 6–3 and 6–4.

Streptococcus pyogenes Corneal Ulcer

Central corneal ulcers caused by beta-hemolytic streptococci have no identifying features. The surrounding corneal stroma is often infiltrated and edematous, and there is usually a moderately large hypopyon. Scrapings contain gram-positive cocci in chains. Drugs recommended for use in treatment are listed in Tables 6–3 and 6–4.

Klebsiella pneumoniae Corneal Ulcer

The corneal ulcer caused by *K pneumoniae* is usually indolent and often without a hypopyon. There may be edema of the surrounding stroma, and scrapings contain gram-negative rods with capsules. Drugs recommended for use in treatment are listed in Tables 6–3 and 6–4.

Staphylococcus aureus, Staphylococcus epidermidis, & Streptococcus viridans Corneal Ulcers

Central corneal ulcers caused by these organisms are now being seen more often than formerly, most of them in corneas compromised by topical corticosteroids. The ulcers are often indolent but may be associated with hypopyon and some surrounding corneal infiltration. They are often superficial, and the ulcer bed feels firm when scraped. Scrapings contain gram-positive cocci—singly, in pairs, or in chains. Tables 6–3 and 6–4 show recommended drug regimens.

Mycobacterium fortuitum & Nocardia Corneal Ulcers

Ulcers due to *M fortuitum* and *Nocardia* are rare. They often follow trauma and are often associated with contact with soil. The ulcers are indolent, and the bed of the ulcer often has radiating lines that make it look like a cracked windshield. Hypopyon may or may not be present. Scraping may contain acid-fast slender rods (*M fortuitum*) or gram-positive filamentous, often branching organisms (*Nocardia*). See Tables 6–3 and 6–4 for recommended drug regimens.

FUNGAL KERATITIS

Fungal corneal ulcers, once seen most commonly in agricultural workers, have become relatively common in the urban population since the introduction of the corticosteroid drugs for use in ophthalmology and the advent of soft contact lenses. Before the corticosteroid era, fungal corneal ulcers occurred only if an overwhelming inoculum of organisms was introduced into the corneal stroma—an event that can still take place in an agricultural setting. The uncompromised cornea seems to be able to handle the small inocula to which urban residents are ordinarily subjected.

Fungal ulcers are indolent and have a gray infiltrate, often a hypopyon, marked inflammation of the globe, superficial ulceration, and satellite lesions (usually infiltrates at sites distant from the main area of ulceration) (Fig 6–4). The principal lesion—and often the satellite lesions as well—is an endothelial plaque with irregular edges underlying the principal corneal

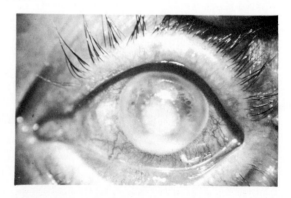

Figure 6–4. Corneal ulcer caused by *Candida albicans*. (Courtesy of P Thygeson.)

lesions, associated with a severe anterior chamber reaction and a corneal abscess.

Most fungal ulcers are caused by opportunists such as *Candida, Fusarium, Aspergillus, Penicillium, Cephalosporium,* and others. There are no identifying features that help to differentiate one type of fungal ulcer from another.

Scrapings from fungal corneal ulcers, except those caused by *Candida,* contain hyphal elements; scrapings from *Candida* ulcers usually contain pseudohyphae or yeast forms that show characteristic budding. Tables 6–3 and 6–4 list the drugs recommended for the treatment of fungal ulcers.

VIRAL KERATITIS

Herpes Simplex Keratitis

Herpes simplex virus (HSV) keratitis is the commonest cause of corneal ulceration in the USA. It occurs in 2 forms: primary and recurrent. The primary disease is a rare keratoconjunctivitis in young children, and the recurrent disease a common ulcerative keratitis, usually but not always dendritic. Most HSV infections of the cornea are still caused by HSV type 1 (the cause of labial herpes), but in both infants and adults a few cases caused by HSV type 2 (the cause of genital herpes) have been reported. The corneal lesions caused by the 2 types are indistinguishable.

Herpetic keratitis is the ocular counterpart of labial herpes, and the dendritic lesion resembles the fever blister immunologically, pathologically, and in clinical course. The only difference is that the clinical course of the keratitis may be slightly prolonged because of the avascularity of the corneal stroma, which retards the migration of lymphocytes and macrophages to the lesion. HSV ocular infection is self-limited and benign in the immunocompetent host, but in the immunologically compromised host its course can be chronic and damaging.

Scrapings of the epithelial lesions of HSV keratitis contain multinucleated giant cells. The virus can be cultivated on the chorioallantoic membrane of embryonated hens' eggs and in many tissue cell lines— eg, HeLa cells, on which it produces characteristic plaques. In the majority of cases, however, diagnosis can be made clinically on the basis of typical dendritic or geographic ulcers and greatly reduced or absent corneal sensation.

A. Clinical Findings: Attacks of the common recurrent type of herpetic keratitis (Fig 6–5) are triggered by fever, overexposure to ultraviolet light, trauma, psychic stress (especially anger), the onset of menstruation, or some other local or systemic source of immunosuppression. Unilaterality is the rule, but bilateral lesions develop in 4–6% of cases and are seen most often in atopic patients.

1. Symptoms–The first symptoms are usually irritation, photophobia, and tearing. When the central cornea is affected, there is also some reduction in vision. Since corneal anesthesia usually occurs early

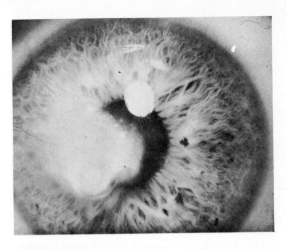

Figure 6–5. Corneal scar caused by recurrent herpes simplex keratitis. (Courtesy of A Rosenberg.)

in the course of the infection, the symptoms may be minimal and the patient may not seek medical advice. There is often a history of fever blisters or other herpetic infection, but corneal ulceration can occasionally be the only sign of a recurrent herpetic infection.

2. Lesions–The most characteristic lesion is the **dendritic ulcer.** It occurs in the corneal epithelium, has a typical linear pattern with a tendency to branch, and has terminal bulbs at its ends (Fig 6–6). Fluorescein staining makes the dendrite very easy to identify, but unfortunately herpetic keratitis can also simulate almost any corneal infection and must be considered in the differential diagnosis of many corneal lesions.

Other corneal epithelial lesions that may be caused by HSV are a blotchy epithelial keratitis, stellate epithelial keratitis, and filamentary keratitis. All of these are usually transitory, however, and often become typical dendrites within a day or two.

Subepithelial opacities can be caused by HSV infection. A ghostlike image, corresponding in shape to the original epithelial defect but slightly larger, can

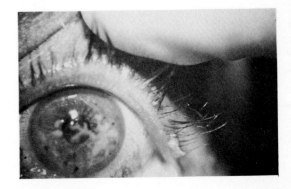

Figure 6–6. Dendritic figures seen in herpes simplex keratitis.

be seen in the area immediately underlying the epithelial lesion. The "ghost" remains superficial but is often enlarged by the use of antiviral drugs, especially idoxuridine. As a rule, these subepithelial lesions do not persist for more than a year.

Disciform keratitis is the commonest complication of HSV infection. This round lesion is associated with moderate or severe edema of the affected stroma. Small or medium-sized white keratic precipitates sometimes lie directly under the lesions, and there may be folds in Descemet's membrane. Disciform keratitis is usually associated with local or systemic immunosuppression. Local immunosuppression is commonly produced by topical corticosteroids.

Like all herpetic lesions in immunocompetent individuals, disciform keratitis is normally self-limited, lasting from several weeks to several months. Edema is the prominent sign, and healing occurs with minimal scarring and vascularization. But when immunosuppression, local or systemic, is severe, the lesion becomes chronic and may persist for years. In that event, the stroma often becomes necrotic, and an accompanying iridocyclitis may be severe. Hypopyon is rare and usually indicates secondary bacterial or fungal infection. In exceptional cases, however, it may be due to the pyogenic properties of necrotic tissue. Corneal perforation in disciform keratitis was virtually unknown prior to 1952, when the topical corticosteroids were first introduced; unfortunately, perforation has become less rare since that time.

If perforation has occurred or is imminent, immediate corneal transplantation should be considered. Alternative procedures are the application of a thin conjunctival flap, sealing the perforation with tissue glues, or protecting the eye with soft corneal contact lenses while healing takes place.

Focal avascular interstitial keratitis can also occur in HSV infection and—like stromal necrosis—is almost always associated with the use of corticosteroids. Small areas of focal infiltration and edema are surrounded by clear areas. There is no sign of vascularization, and the lesions may affect any level of the cornea. If they are examined by retroillumination at the slit lamp, their pattern often suggests a previous disciform lesion.

Peripheral lesions of the cornea can also be caused by HSV. They are usually linear and show a loss of epithelium before the underlying corneal stroma becomes infiltrated. (This is in sharp contrast to the marginal ulcer associated with bacterial hypersensitivity—eg, to S aureus in staphylococcal blepharitis, in which the infiltration precedes the loss of the overlying epithelium.) Corneal sensation is usually absent or so diminished that the patient is far less photophobic than patients with nonherpetic corneal infiltrates and ulceration usually are.

B. Treatment: The treatment of HSV keratitis should be directed toward elimination of the virus from the cornea. In the immunocompetent patient, the infection is self-limited and scarring minimal. Regrettably, the clinician sometimes immunosuppresses the patient by using corticosteroids in eagerness to reduce local inflammation. This is of course based on a misconception that reducing inflammation reduces disease.

1. Denudation—The best way to treat dendritic keratitis is by denudation of the corneal epithelium, which is where the virus is established. Treatment with topical drugs (see below) is less effective and involves a hazard of drug toxicity. Healthy epithelium adheres tightly to the cornea, but infected epithelium is easy to remove.

Denudation is accomplished with a tightly wound cotton-tipped applicator. Topical iodine or ether has no value and can cause chemical keratitis. A cycloplegic such as atropine 1% or homatropine 5% is then instilled into the conjunctival sac, and a pressure dressing is applied. The patient should be examined daily and the dressing changed until the corneal defect has healed—usually within 72 hours.

2. Drug therapy—Topical drug therapy offers the advantage of not requiring patching but is less effective than debridement. The drugs used are idoxuridine (Herplex, Stoxil), trifluridine (Viroptic), vidarabine (Vira-A), and acyclovir (Zovirax). Idoxuridine is a cytotoxic drug and can be locally immunosuppressive.

Corticosteroid therapy is contraindicated at all stages of HSV disease for the following reasons: (1) The corticosteroids increase the destructive action of collagenase (produced by the damaged corneal epithelial cells or polymorphonuclear cells) on the corneal stroma; and (2) their immunosuppressive activity increases (a) the activity of the virus and (b) the susceptibility of the HSV-infected host to secondary infections with opportunistic organisms, especially fungi and such bacteria as S viridans and S epidermidis. Unfortunately, steroids are still widely used because of their anti-inflammatory effect and their temporary but dramatically beneficial effect on symptoms.

3. Control of trigger mechanisms that reactivate HSV infection—Recurrent HSV infections of the eye are common, occurring in about one-third of cases within 2 years of the first attack. A trigger mechanism can often be discovered by careful questioning of the patient. Once identified, the trigger can often be avoided. Aspirin can be used to avoid fever, excessive exposure to the sun or ultraviolet light can be avoided, situations that might cause psychic stress can be minimized, and aspirin can be taken just prior to the onset of menstruation.

Varicella-Zoster Viral Keratitis

Varicella-zoster virus (VZV) infection occurs in 2 forms: primary (varicella) and recurrent (zoster). Ocular manifestations are uncommon in varicella but common in ophthalmic zoster. In varicella (chickenpox), the usual eye lesions are pocks on the lids and lid margins. Rarely, keratitis occurs (typically a phlyctenulelike lesion at the limbus), and still more rarely epithelial keratitis with or without pseudodendrites. Disciform keratitis, with uveitis of short duration, has been reported.

In contrast to the rare and benign corneal lesions of varicella, the relatively frequent ophthalmic zoster is often accompanied by keratouveitis that varies in severity according to the immune status of the patient. Thus, although children with zoster keratouveitis usually have benign disease, the aged have severe and sometimes blinding disease. Corneal complications in ophthalmic zoster can be anticipated if there is a skin eruption along the branches of the nasociliary nerve.

Unlike recurrent HSV keratitis that affects only the epithelium, VZV keratitis affects the stroma and anterior uvea at onset. The epithelial lesions are blotchy and amorphous except for an occasional linear pseudodendrite that only vaguely resembles the true dendrites of HSV keratitis. Stromal opacities are prominent, characteristically nummular in shape, and largely but not exclusively subepithelial. A disciform keratitis sometimes develops and resembles HSV disciform keratitis. Loss of corneal sensation is always a prominent feature and often persists for months after the corneal lesion appears to have healed. The associated uveitis tends to persist for weeks or months, but unless corticosteroid preparations have been used it eventually heals.

In clinical trials and outside the USA, intravenous and oral forms of acyclovir have been used successfully for the treatment of herpes zoster ophthalmicus. Acyclovir (Zovirax) may be given intravenously, orally, and topically to immunocompromised patients who develop herpes zoster infections. Corticosteroid preparations, although they do provide temporary relief, may prolong the course of the disease and worsen its prognosis. Of the various complications, postherpetic neuralgia, which is particularly severe in elderly patients, is the most troublesome. Fortunately it is self-limited, and reassurance can be helpful as a supplement to analgesics.

Since zoster is a disease of immunosuppression, the restoration of immunocompetence by immunopotentiators is logical and can be looked upon as the hope of the future. The early results of the study of a number of immunopotentiating procedures are definitely encouraging.

Variola Virus Keratitis

Variola virus corneal ulcers were once a common cause of corneal scarring and blindness in developing countries. The lesions usually involved the pupillary area, and perforations with resultant adherent leukomas were common. This is one ocular disease that will be seen no more, however, for according to the World Health Organization, smallpox is now extinct.

Vaccinial Keratitis

Vaccinial keratitis used to occur on rare occasions as a complication of vaccination for the prevention of smallpox. It was either a blotchy epithelial keratitis or a true corneal ulcer and was usually associated with lesions on the lid margin. Atypically, disciform ker-

atitis sometimes occurred. Topical rifampin was apparently sometimes beneficial. Of academic interest (since vaccinial keratitis, like variolar keratitis, is no longer a problem) is the fact that intramuscular vaccinia immune globulin sometimes increased the severity of the disciform lesion.

Adenovirus Keratitis

Keratitis usually accompanies all types of adenoviral conjunctivitis, reaching its peak 5–7 days after onset of the conjunctivitis. It is a fine epithelial keratitis best seen with the slit lamp after instillation of fluorescein. The minute lesions may group together to make up larger ones.

The epithelial keratitis is often followed by subepithelial opacities. In epidemic keratoconjunctivitis (EKC), which is due to adenovirus types 8 and 19, the subepithelial lesions are round and grossly visible. They appear 8–15 days after onset of the conjunctivitis and may persist for months or even (rarely) for several years. Similar lesions occur very exceptionally in other adenoviral infections, eg, those caused by types 3, 4, and 7, but tend to be transitory and mild, lasting a few weeks at most.

Although the corneal opacities of adenoviral keratoconjunctivitis tend to fade temporarily with the use of topical corticosteroids, and although the patient is often made temporarily more comfortable thereby, corticosteroid therapy prolongs the disease and is therefore not recommended. No medication is needed.

Other Viral Keratitides

A fine epithelial keratitis may be seen in other viral infections such as measles (in which the central cornea is affected predominantly), rubella, mumps, infectious mononucleosis, acute hemorrhagic conjunctivitis, Newcastle disease conjunctivitis, and verruca of the lid margin. A superior epithelial keratitis and pannus often accompany molluscum contagiosum nodules on the lid margin. Rare cases of orf virus keratitis have been seen in sheepherders in California and Nevada. The corneal lesions resembled those of the now extinct vaccinial keratitis.

CHLAMYDIAL KERATITIS

All 5 principal types of chlamydial conjunctivitis (trachoma, inclusion conjunctivitis, primary ocular lymphogranuloma venereum, parakeet or psittacosis conjunctivitis, and feline pneumonitis conjunctivitis) are accompanied by corneal lesions. Only in trachoma and lymphogranuloma venereum, however, have they been blinding or visually damaging. The corneal lesions of trachoma have been the most studied and are of great diagnostic importance. In order of appearance they consist of (1) epithelial microerosions affecting the upper third of the cornea; (2) micropannus; (3) subepithelial round opacities, commonly called trachoma pustules; (4) limbal follicles and their cicatricial remains, known as Herbert's peripheral pits; (5)

gross pannus; and (6) extensive, diffuse, subepithelial cicatrization. Mild cases of trachoma may show only epithelial keratitis and micropannus and may heal without impairing vision.

The rare cases of lymphogranuloma venereum have shown fewer characteristic changes but are known to have caused blindness by diffuse corneal scarring and total pannus. The remaining types of chlamydial infection cause only micropannus, epithelial keratitis, and rare subepithelial opacities not visually significant.

Chlamydial keratoconjunctivitis responds to treatment with the sulfonamides (except for the rare *C psittaci* infections, which are sulfonamide-resistant) and to tetracyclines and erythromycin.

ACANTHAMOEBA KERATITIS

Acanthamoeba is a free-living protozoan that thrives in polluted water containing bacteria and organic material. It has been reported recently in association with soft contact lens wear. There is usually a history of exposure to homemade saline solution or contaminated water or soil.

The initial symptoms are pain out of proportion to the clinical findings, redness, and photophobia. The clinical findings include corneal ulceration with a corneal ring infiltrate and corneal neuritis. The keratitis is indolent.

The diagnosis is confirmed by corneal scrapings and by culturing on specially prepared media. Histopathologic sections reveal the presence of amebic forms (trophozoites or cysts).

The differential diagnosis includes fungal keratitis, herpetic keratitis, mycobacterial keratitis, and *Nocardia* infection of the cornea.

Treatment requires superficial debridement. Medical treatment is with topical propamidine eyedrops every $\frac{1}{2}$–1 hour and dibromopropamidine ointment at bedtime. Neomycin drops, 3 mg/mL, may be given. Topical imidazoles (miconazole, 10 mg/mL, or clotrimazole, 10 mg/mL) have also been found to be effective. Imidazoles may be reserved for patients who do not respond to propamidine. Topical corticosteroids should be avoided because they compromise host defenses and aggravate the disease.

Severe cases may require therapeutic keratoplasty.

DRUG-INDUCED EPITHELIAL KERATITIS

Epithelial keratitis is not uncommonly seen in patients using antiviral medications (idoxuridine and vidarabine) and the broad-spectrum and medium-spectrum antibiotics. It is usually a blotchy keratitis affecting predominantly the lower half of the cornea and interpalpebral fissure.

KERATOCONJUNCTIVITIS SICCA (Sjögren's Syndrome)

Epithelial filaments in the lower quadrants of the cornea are the cardinal signs of this autoimmune disease in which secretion of the lacrimal and accessory lacrimal glands is diminished or eliminated. There is also a blotchy epithelial keratitis that affects mainly the lower quadrants. Severe cases show mucous pseudofilaments that stick to the dry corneal epithelium.

This keratitis of Sjögren's syndrome must be distinguished from the keratitis sicca of such cicatrizing diseases as trachoma and pemphigoid, in which the goblet cells of the conjunctiva have been destroyed. Such cases sometimes still produce tears, but without mucus the corneal epithelium sheds the tears and continues to be dry.

Treatment of keratoconjunctivitis sicca calls for the frequent use of tear substitutes, of which there are many commercial preparations. When goblet cells have been destroyed, as in the cicatricial conjunctivitides, mucus substitutes must be used in addition to artificial tears. Topical vitamin A may help to reverse the epithelial keratinization.

PERIPHERAL CORNEAL ULCERS

Marginal Infiltrates & Ulcers

The majority of marginal corneal ulcers are benign but extremely painful. They are secondary to acute or chronic bacterial conjunctivitis, particularly staphylococcal blepharoconjunctivitis and less often Koch-Weeks (*Haemophilus aegyptius*) conjunctivitis. They are not an infectious process, however, and scrapings do not contain the causal bacteria. They are the result of sensitization to bacterial products, antibody from the limbus vessels reacting with antigen that has diffused through the corneal epithelium.

Marginal infiltrates and ulcers (Fig 6–7) start as

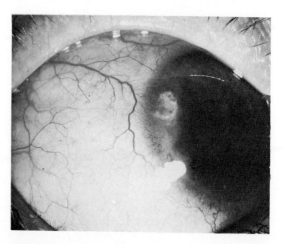

Figure 6–7. Marginal ulcer of temporal cornea, right eye. (Courtesy of P Thygeson.)

oval or linear infiltrates, separated from the limbus by a lucid interval, and only later may ulcerate and vascularize. They are self-limited, usually lasting from 7 to 10 days, but those associated with staphylococcal blepharoconjunctivitis usually recur. Topical corticosteroid preparations shorten their course and relieve symptoms, which are often severe, but treatment of the underlying conjunctivitis is essential if recurrences are to be prevented. Before starting corticosteroid therapy, great care must be taken to distinguish this entity, formerly known as "catarrhal corneal ulceration," from marginal herpetic keratitis. Since marginal herpetic keratitis is usually almost symptomless because of corneal anesthesia, differentiating it from the painful, hypersensitivity-type marginal ulcer is not difficult.

Ring Ulcers
(Fig 6–8)

Ring ulcers are rare but more destructive than marginal ulcers. They occasionally result from the confluence of multiple marginal ulcers secondary to conjunctivitis but are more often associated with systemic disease. They have been seen in the convalescent period of such infectious diseases as influenza and bacillary dysentery but can also be a complication of autoimmune disease. A few ring ulcers have been seen in ocular diphtheria, in severe beta-hemolytic streptococcal conjunctival infection, and (more often) in gonococcal conjunctivitis. They may also occur as a secondary manifestation of infectious endophthalmitis; in this event, the ulceration is preceded by a massive infiltration of neutrophils.

Treatment—often unsatisfactory—depends on identification of the underlying cause. Infectious ring ulcer may respond to appropriate systemic and topical antibiotics and the hypersensitivity types to topical corticosteroid therapy.

Mooren's Ulcer
(Fig 6–9)

The cause of Mooren's ulcer is still unknown, but an autoimmune origin is suspected. It is a marginal

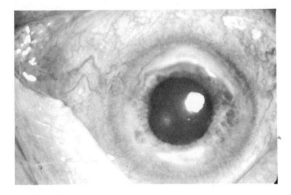

Figure 6–8. Ring ulcer of the cornea. (Courtesy of M Hogan.)

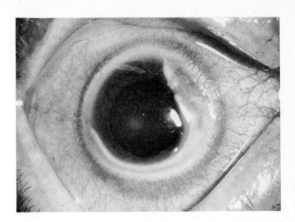

Figure 6–9. Mooren's ulcer. (Courtesy of M Hogan.)

ulcer, unilateral in 60–80% of cases and characterized by painful, progressive excavation of the limbus and peripheral cornea that often leads to loss of the eye. It occurs most commonly in old age but does not seem to be related to any of the systemic diseases that most often afflict the aged. It is unresponsive to both antibiotics and corticosteroids. Surgical excision of the limbal conjunctiva in an effort to remove sensitizing substances has recently been advocated. Past generations of ophthalmologists used repeated paracentesis with some success.

Phlyctenular Keratoconjunctivitis

This hypersensitivity disease (due to delayed hypersensitivity to bacterial products, mainly of the human tubercle bacillus) was formerly a major cause of visual loss in the USA, particularly among the Eskimos and Native Americans. Phlyctenules are localized accumulations of lymphocytes, monocytes, macrophages, and finally neutrophils. They appear first at the limbus, but in recurrent attacks they may involve the bulbar conjunctiva and cornea. Corneal phlyctenules, usually bilateral, cicatrize and vascularize, but conjunctival phlyctenules leave no trace.

Most cases of phlyctenular keratoconjunctivitis in the USA today are caused by delayed hypersensitivity to *S aureus*. The antigen is released locally from staphylococci that proliferate on the lid margin in staphylococcal blepharitis. Rare phlyctenules have occurred in San Joaquin Valley fever, a result of hypersensitivity to a primary infection with *Coccidioides immitis*. In this disease they are not visually important, however.

In the tuberculous type, the attack may be triggered by an acute bacterial conjunctivitis but is associated typically with a transient increase in the activity of a childhood tuberculosis. Untreated phlyctenules run a course to healing in 10–14 days, but topical therapy with corticosteroid preparations dramatically shortens the course to a day or two. The corticosteroid response in the staphylococcal type is poor, however, and treatment consists essentially of eliminating the causal bacterial infection. In resistant staphylococcal cases, desensitization with *Staphylococcus* toxoid or Staphage Lysate has been useful.

Marginal Keratitis in Autoimmune Disease

The corneal periphery receives its nourishment from the aqueous humor, the limbal capillaries, and the tear film. It is contiguous with the subconjunctival lymphoid tissue and the lymphatic arcades at the limbus. The perilimbal conjunctiva appears to play an important role in the pathogenesis of corneal lesions that arise both from local ocular disease and from systemic disorders, particularly those of autoimmune origin. There is a striking similarity between the limbal capillary network and the renal glomerular capillary network: On the endothelial basement membranes of the capillaries of both networks, immune complexes are deposited and immunologic disease results. Thus, the peripheral cornea often participates in such autoimmune diseases as rheumatoid arthritis, polyarteritis nodosa, systemic lupus erythematosus, scleroderma, midline lethal and Wegener's granulomatosis, ulcerative colitis, Crohn's disease, relapsing polychondritis, and Reiter's syndrome. These diseases are characteristically associated with infiltration, ulceration, thinning, and (rarely) perforation of the peripheral cornea. The corneal lesions range in severity from benign and even self-limited changes to perforation and loss of the eye. Treatment is directed toward the control of the underlying disease but is for the most part unsatisfactory.

CORNEAL ULCER DUE TO VITAMIN A DEFICIENCY

The typical corneal ulcer associated with avitaminosis A is centrally located and bilateral, gray and indolent, with a definite lack of corneal luster in the surrounding area (Fig 6–10). The cornea becomes soft and necrotic (hence the term, "keratomalacia"), and perforation is common. The epithelium of the conjunctiva is keratinized, as evidenced by the presence of a Bitot spot. This is a foamy, wedge-shaped area in the conjunctiva, usually on the temporal side, with the base of the wedge at the limbus and the apex extending toward the lateral canthus. Within the triangle the conjunctiva is furrowed concentrically with the limbus, and dry flaky material can be seen falling from the area into the inferior cul-de-sac. A stained conjunctival scraping from a Bitot spot will show many saprophytic xerosis bacilli (*Corynebacterium xerosis;* small curved rods) and keratinized epithelial cells.

Avitaminosis A corneal ulceration results from dietary lack of vitamin A or impaired absorption from the gastrointestinal tract and impaired utilization by the body. It may develop in an infant who has a feeding problem; in an adult who is on a restricted or generally inadequate diet; or in any person with a biliary ob-

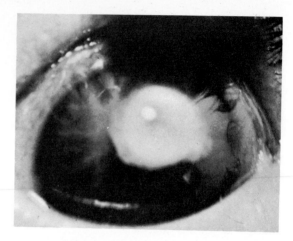

Figure 6–10. Keratomalacia with ulceration associated with xerophthalmia (dietary) in an infant. (Photo by Diane Beeston.)

struction since bile in the gastrointestinal tract is necessary for the absorption of vitamin A. Lack of vitamin A causes a generalized keratinization of the epithelium throughout the body. The conjunctival and corneal changes together are known as **xerophthalmia.** Since the epithelium of the air passages is affected, many patients, if not treated, will die of pneumonia. Avitaminosis A also causes a generalized retardation of osseous growth. This is extremely important in infants; for example, if the skull bones do not grow and the brain continues to grow, increased intracranial pressure and papilledema can result.

Vitamin A should be administered in a dosage of at least 20,000 IU/d intramuscularly. Sulfonamide or antibiotic ointment can be used locally in the eye to prevent secondary bacterial infection. The average daily requirement of vitamin A is 1500–5000 IU for children, according to age, and 5000 IU for adults.

NEUROTROPHIC CORNEAL ULCERS

If the trigeminal nerve, which supplies the cornea, is interrupted by trauma, surgery, tumor, inflammation, or in any other way, the cornea loses its sensitivity and one of its best defenses against degeneration, ulceration, and infection. In the early stages of a typical neurotrophic ulcer, fluorescein solution will produce punctate staining of the superficial epithelium. As this process progresses, patchy areas of denudation appear. Occasionally the epithelium may be absent from a large area of the cornea.

The progress of the condition depends on the treatment. Without treatment, the denuded areas become infected. The integrity of the cornea can be maintained as long as the corneal surface is kept moist by wearing a Buller shield,* by suturing the lids together, by using a conjunctival flap, or by using a therapeutic soft contact lens. Artificial tears may be of benefit. Under the best conditions, however, the prognosis is poor, and repeated epithelial breakdown often occurs.

EXPOSURE KERATITIS

Exposure keratitis may develop in any situation in which the cornea is not properly moistened and covered by the eyelids. Examples include exophthalmos from any cause, ectropion, the absence of part of an eyelid as a result of trauma, and inability to close the lids properly, as in Bell's palsy. The 2 factors at work are the drying of the cornea and its exposure to minor trauma. The uncovered cornea is particularly subject to drying during sleeping hours. If an ulcer develops it usually follows minor trauma and occurs in the inferior third of the cornea.

This type of keratitis will be sterile unless it is secondarily infected, and the therapeutic objective is to provide protection and moisture for the entire corneal surface. The method depends upon the underlying condition: a plastic procedure on the eyelids, a Buller shield,* soft lens, or surgical relief of exophthalmos.

DEGENERATIVE CORNEAL CONDITIONS

KERATOCONUS

Keratoconus is an uncommon degenerative bilateral disease that may be inherited as an autosomal recessive or autosomal dominant trait. Unilateral cases of unknown cause occur rarely. Symptoms appear in the second decade of life. The disease affects all races. Keratoconus has been associated with a number of diseases, including Down's syndrome, atopic dermatitis, retinitis pigmentosa, aniridia, vernal catarrh, Marfan's syndrome, Apert's syndrome, and Ehlers-Danlos syndrome. Pathologically, there are generalized thinning and anterior protrusion of the central cornea, ruptures in Descemet's membrane, and irregular, superficial linear scars at the apex of the cone that is formed.

Acute hydrops of the cornea may occur, in which there is sudden diminution of vision associated with central corneal edema. This usually arises as a consequence of rupture of Descemet's membrane and may be triggered by the patient rubbing the eye. Acute hydrops usually clears gradually without treatment.

Blurred vision is the only symptom. Signs include cone-shaped cornea (Fig 6–11), indentation of the

*The Buller shield is a watertight cone of exposed x-ray film secured to the surrounding skin with adhesive tape.

lower lid by the cornea when the patient looks down (Munson's sign), an irregular shadow on retinoscopy, and a distorted corneal reflection with Placido's disk or the keratoscope. The fundi cannot be clearly seen because of corneal distortion.

Corneal perforation may occur in advanced cases. When this happens, the eye should be bandaged and the dressing changed daily until a corneal scar seals the wound. Corneal transplantation may be necessary. Keratoconus is one of the most common indications for keratoplasty.

Contact lenses improve visual acuity in the early stages. A corneal transplant is indicated when the corrected visual acuity decreases to the point where it interferes with the patient's normal activities.

Keratoconus is often slowly progressive between the ages of 20 and 60, although an arrest in progression of the keratoconus may occur at any time. If a corneal transplant is done before extreme corneal thinning occurs, the prognosis is excellent; about 80–95% obtain reading vision.

CORNEAL DEGENERATION

The corneal degenerations are a rare group of slowly progressive, bilateral, degenerative disorders that usually appear in the second or third decades of life. Some are hereditary. Other cases follow ocular inflammatory disease, and some are of unknown cause.

Fatty or Lipoid Degeneration

This disorder may begin in infancy or adulthood. The cause is not known. There is a generalized deposition of lipid material within the corneal stroma, replacement of Bowman's layer by macrophages, and thickening of the epithelium with some infiltration of lipid material. Clinical findings include blurred vision and haziness and thickening of the cornea, particularly in the central zone.

Symptoms and signs are slowly progressive until useful vision is lost. Corneal transplant improves vision significantly in most cases.

Marginal Degeneration of the Cornea (Terrien's Disease)

This is a rare bilateral symmetric degeneration characterized by marginal thinning of the upper nasal quadrants of the cornea. Males are more commonly affected than females, and the condition occurs more frequently in the third and fourth decades. There are no symptoms except for mild irritation, and the condition is slowly progressive. The clinical picture consists of marginal thinning, arcuate opacity distal to the thinned area simulating arcus senilis, and vascularization. Perforation is a known complication of this condition and may lead to iris prolapse. Histopathologic studies of affected corneas have revealed vascularized connective tissue with fibrillary degeneration and fatty infiltration of collagen fibers.

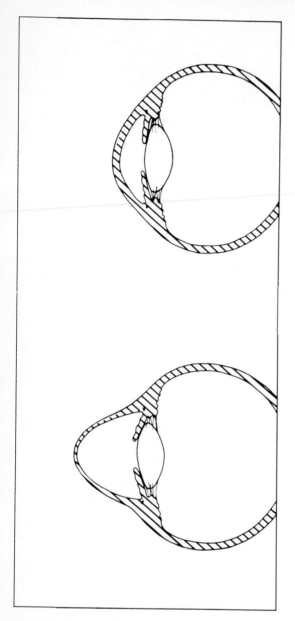

Figure 6–11. *Top:* Side view of normal cornea. *Bottom:* Keratoconus.

in the basement membrane, Bowman's layer, and anterior stromal lamellas. A clear margin separates the calcific band from the limbus, and clear holes may be seen in the band, giving the Swiss cheese appearance. Symptoms include irritation, injection, and blurring of vision.

Calcific band keratopathy has been described in a number of inflammatory, metabolic, and degenerative conditions. It is characteristically associated with juvenile rheumatoid arthritis. It has been described in long-standing inflammatory conditions of the eye, glaucoma, and chronic cyclitis. Band keratopathy may also be associated with hyperparathyroidism, vitamin D intoxication, sarcoidosis, and leprosy. Treatment consists of ablation of the corneal epithelium by curettage under topical anesthesia followed by irrigation of the cornea with a sterile 0.01-molar solution of ethylenediaminetetraacetic acid (EDTA) or application of EDTA with a cotton applicator.

Climatic Droplet Keratopathy (Pearl Diver's Keratopathy, Bietti's Keratopathy, Labrador Keratopathy, Spheroid Degeneration of the Cornea) (Fig 6–13)

Climatic droplet keratopathy affects mainly men who work out of doors. The corneal degeneration is thought to be caused by exposure to ultraviolet light and is characterized in the early stages by fine subepithelial yellow droplets in the peripheral cornea. As the disease advances, the droplets become central, with subsequent corneal clouding causing blurred vi-

Because the course of progression is slow and the central cornea is spared, the prognosis is good.

Calcific Band Keratopathy (Fig 6–12)

This disorder is characterized by the deposition of calcium salts in the anterior layers of the cornea. The keratopathy is usually limited to the interpalpebral area and appears as a band. The calcium deposits are noted

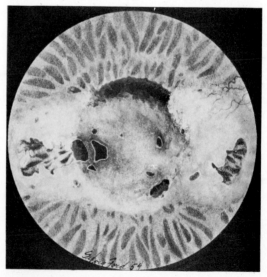

Figure 6–12. Calcific band keratopathy. (Courtesy of M Hogan.)

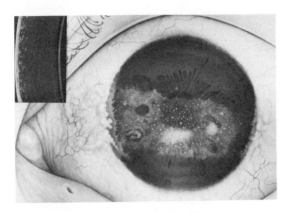

Figure 6–13. Climatic droplet keratopathy. Inset shows slip lamp view. (Courtesy of A Ahmad.)

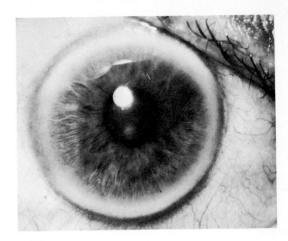

Figure 6–14. Arcus senilis. (Photo by Diane Beeston.)

sion. Treatment in advanced cases is by corneal transplantation.

Salzmann's Nodular Degeneration

This disorder is always preceded by corneal inflammation, particularly phlyctenular keratoconjunctivitis or trachoma. Symptoms include redness, irritation, and blurring of vision. There is degeneration of the superficial cornea that involves the stroma, Bowman's layer, and epithelium with superficial whitish-gray elevated nodules sometimes occurring in chains.

Corneal transplantation will significantly improve visual acuity in most cases.

ARCUS SENILIS (Corneal Annulus, Anterior Embryotoxon)

Arcus senilis is an extremely common, bilateral, benign peripheral corneal degeneration that may occur at any age but is far more common in elderly people as part of the aging process. Arcus senilis in people under age 50 is usually associated with hypercholesterolemia.

Pathologically, lipid droplets involve the entire corneal thickness but are more concentrated in the superficial and deep layers, being relatively sparse in the corneal stroma.

There are no symptoms. Clinically, arcus senilis appears as a hazy gray ring about 2 mm in width and with a clear space between it and the limbus (Fig 6–14). No treatment is necessary, and there are no complications. Since arcus senilis causes no visual defect, it is not always classified with the corneal dystrophies.

HEREDITARY CORNEAL DYSTROPHIES

This is a group of rare hereditary disorders of the cornea of unknown cause characterized by bilateral abnormal deposition of substances and associated with alteration in the normal corneal architecture that may or may not interfere with vision. These corneal dystrophies usually manifest themselves during the first or second decade but sometimes later. They may be stationary or slowly progressive throughout life. Corneal transplantation improves vision in most patients with hereditary corneal dystrophy.

Anatomically, corneal dystrophies may be classified as anterior limiting membrane, stromal, and posterior limiting membrane dystrophies.

Anterior Limiting Membrane Corneal Dystrophies

A. Meesman's Dystrophy: This slowly progressive disorder is characterized by microcystic areas in the epithelium. The onset is in early childhood (first 1–2 years of life). The main symptom is slight irritation, and vision is slightly affected. The inheritance is autosomal dominant.

B. Cogan's Dystrophy: This condition is characterized by discrete comma-shaped or rounded, gray-white intraepithelial opacities located in the pupillary area. Fingerprint or maplike fine opacities may be seen at the level of the basement membrane. The disease is more common in females. Patients may develop recurrent erosion. Visual acuity is affected very slightly.

C. Fingerprint Dystrophy: This entity refers to fine wavy concentric lines located anterior to Bowman's layer that can be seen best by retroillumination with the slit lamp. These lines may be associated with a map- or dotlike pattern. The condition is asymptomatic but may be associated with recurrent erosion. The findings are noted during routine examination.

D. Recurrent Corneal Erosion: See p 121.

E. Others: Reis-Bücklers dystrophy is a dominantly inherited dystrophy affecting primarily Bowman's layer. The disease begins within the first decade of life with symptoms of recurrent erosion. Opacification of Bowman's layer gradually occurs and the epithelium is irregular. No vascularization is usually noted. Vision may be markedly reduced.

Vortex dystrophy, or cornea verticillata, is characterized by pigmented lines occurring in Bowman's layer or the underlying stroma and spreading over the entire corneal surface. Visual acuity is not markedly affected. Such a pattern of radiating pigmented lines may also be seen in patients suffering from chlorpromazine, chloroquine, or indomethacin toxicity as well as Fabry's disease.

Stromal Corneal Dystrophies

There are 3 types of stromal corneal dystrophies:

A. Granular Dystrophy: This usually asymptomatic, slowly progressive corneal dystrophy most often begins in early childhood. The lesions consist of central, fine, whitish "granular" lesions in the stroma of the cornea. The epithelium and Bowman's layer may be affected late in the disease. Visual acuity is slightly reduced. Histologically, the cornea shows uniform deposition of hyaline material. Corneal transplant is not needed except in very severe and late cases. The inheritance is autosomal dominant.

B. Macular Dystrophy: This type of stromal corneal dystrophy is manifested by a dense gray central opacity that starts in Bowman's layer. The opacity tends to spread toward the periphery and later involves the deeper stromal layers. Recurrent corneal erosion may occur, and vision is severely impaired. Histologic examination shows deposition of acid mucopolysaccharide in the stroma and degeneration of Bowman's layer.

The inheritance is autosomal recessive.

C. Lattice Dystrophy: Lattice dystrophy starts as fine, branching linear opacities in Bowman's layer in the central area and spreads to the periphery. The deep stroma may become involved, but the process does not reach Descemet's membrane. Recurrent erosion may occur. Histologic examination reveals amyloid deposits in the collagen fibers.

Posterior Limiting Membrane Corneal Dystrophies

A. Fuchs's Dystrophy: This disorder begins in the third or fourth decade and is slowly progressive throughout life. Women are more commonly affected than men. There are central wartlike deposits on Descemet's membrane, thickening of Descemet's membrane, and defects in the endothelium. Decompensation of the endothelium occurs and leads to edema of the corneal stroma and epithelium, causing blurring of vision. The cornea becomes progressively more opaque. Glaucoma or iris atrophy may be associated with this disorder. Histologic examination of the cornea reveals the wartlike excrescences over Descemet's membrane that are secreted by the endothelial cells. Thinning and pigmentation of the endothelium and thickening of Descemet's membrane are characteristics.

B. Posterior Polymorphous Dystrophy: This

is a common disorder with onset in early childhood. Polymorphous plaques of calcium crystals are observed in the deep stromal layers. Vesicular lesions may be seen in the endothelium. Edema occurs in the deep stroma. The condition is asymptomatic in most cases, but in severe cases epithelial and total stromal edema may occur. The inheritance is autosomal dominant.

MISCELLANEOUS CORNEAL DISORDERS

SCLEROKERATITIS (Sclerosing Keratitis)

Sclerokeratitis is an uncommon, unilateral, localized inflammation of the sclera and cornea. The cause is not known, but tuberculosis was formerly implicated. However, antituberculosis therapy is not effective. Pathologically, there are many chronic inflammatory cells (small round cells) in the involved portion of both structures. Fibrosis occurs in the later stages (Fig 6–15). The patient complains of pain, photophobia, and irritation, but there is no discharge. A moderately severe iritis (anterior nongranulomatous uveitis) is usually associated. The disease may be seen in patients with herpes zoster infections.

No specific treatment is available. The pupil should be kept dilated with atropine, 1%, 2 drops once daily. Warm compresses and local corticosteroid drops are used to relieve the discomfort. Although the process starts as a small area of infiltration, it may progress to total corneal opacification. It may, however, subside after months or years.

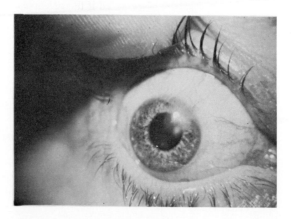

Figure 6–15. Sclerokeratitis. Note fibrovascular scar in upper nasal quadrant of cornea.

THYGESON'S SUPERFICIAL PUNCTATE KERATITIS

Superficial punctate keratitis is an uncommon chronic and recurrent bilateral disorder without regard to sex or age. It is characterized by discrete and elevated oval epithelial opacities that show punctate staining with fluorescein, mainly in the pupillary area. The opacities are not visible grossly but can be easily seen with the slit lamp or loupe. Subepithelial opacities underlying the epithelial lesions (ghosts) are often observed in patients who have been misdiagnosed as having herpes simplex keratitis and treated with topical idoxuridine.

No causative organism has been identified, but a virus is suspected. A varicella-zoster virus has been isolated from the corneal scrapings of one case.

Mild irritation, slight blurring of vision, and photophobia are the only symptoms. The conjunctiva is not involved.

Epithelial keratitis secondary to staphylococcal blepharoconjunctivitis is differentiated from superficial punctate keratitis by its involvement of the lower third of the cornea. Epithelial keratitis in trachoma is ruled out by its location in the upper third of the cornea and the presence of pannus. Many other forms of keratitis involving the superficial cornea are unilateral or are eliminated by their histories.

Short-term instillation of corticosteroid drops will often cause disappearance of the opacities and subjective improvement, but recurrences are the rule. The ultimate prognosis is good since there is no scarring or vascularization of the cornea. Untreated, the disease runs a protracted course of 1–3 years. Long-term treatment with topical corticosteroids may prolong the course of the disease for many years and lead to steroid-induced cataract and glaucoma.

RECURRENT CORNEAL EROSION

This is a fairly common and serious mechanical corneal disorder that presents some classic signs and symptoms but may be easily missed if the physician does not look for it specifically. The patient is usually awakened during the early morning hours by a pain in the affected eye. The pain is continuous, and the eye becomes red, irritated, and photophobic. When the patient attempts to open the eyes in the morning, the lid pulls off the loose epithelium, resulting in pain and redness.

Three types of recurrent corneal erosions can be recognized:

(1) Acquired recurrent erosion (traumatic): The patient usually gives a history of previous corneal injury. It is unilateral, occurs with equal frequency in males and females, and the family history is negative. The recurrent erosion occurs most frequently in the center below the pupil no matter where the site of the previous corneal injury was.

(2) Familial recurrent erosion: This condition is bilateral and occurs more frequently in women. Patients give a family history of similar cases. There is usually no history of trauma.

(3) Recurrent erosion associated with corneal dystrophies: (See above.) Recurrent erosions of the cornea may be observed in patients with Cogan's microcystic corneal dystrophy, fingerprint dystrophy, and Reis-Bücklers corneal dystrophy.

Recurrent corneal erosion is due to a defect in the basement membrane of the corneal epithelium. The hemidesmosomes of the basal layer of the corneal epithelium fail to adhere to the basement membrane, and the corneal epithelium remains loose over the basement membrane with very slight subepithelial edema. The loose epithelial layers are vulnerable to separation and erosion.

Instillation of a local anesthetic relieves the symptoms immediately, and fluorescein staining will show the eroded area. This is typically a small area in the lower central cornea.

Treatment consists of a pressure bandage on the eye to promote healing. Mechanical denuding of the corneal epithelium may be necessary. The other eye should be kept closed most of the time to minimize movement of the lid over the affected eye. Bed rest is desirable for 24 hours. The cornea usually heals in 2–3 days. To prevent recurrence and to promote continued healing, it is important for these patients to use a bland ointment (eg, boric acid or other ocular lubricant) at bedtime for several months. In more severe cases, artificial tears are instilled during the day. The use of hypertonic ointment (glucose 40%) or 5% saline drops (Adsorbonac 5%) is often of value.

Rare instances of bilateral atraumatic dystrophic recurrent corneal erosion with a poor prognosis have also been reported.

INTERSTITIAL KERATITIS DUE TO CONGENITAL SYPHILIS

This self-limited inflammatory disease of the cornea is a late manifestation of congenital syphilis. There has been a sharp decrease in the incidence of the disease in recent years—almost to the point of extinction in some parts of the USA. It occasionally starts unilaterally but almost always becomes bilateral weeks to months later. It affects all races and is more common in females than males. Symptoms appear between the ages of 5 and 20. Pathologic findings include edema, lymphocytic infiltration, and vascularization of the corneal stroma.

Interstitial keratitis may be allergic in nature since *Treponema pallidum* is not found in the cornea during the acute phase. It has been postulated that these organisms enter the cornea at birth and that later in life there is a violent allergic reaction in the cornea to the organisms circulating in the bloodstream.

Clinical Findings

A. Symptoms and Signs: Other signs of congenital syphilis may be present, such as saddle nose and Hutchinson's triad (interstitial keratitis, deafness, and notched upper central incisors). The patient complains of pain, photophobia, and blurring of vision. Physical signs include conjunctival injection, corneal edema, vascularization of the deeper corneal layers, and miosis. There is an associated severe anterior granulomatous uveitis and blepharospasm due to photophobia. The grayish-pink appearance of the cornea (due to edema and vascularization) that occurs in the acute phase is sometimes referred to as a "salmon patch."

B. Laboratory Findings: Serologic tests for syphilis are positive.

Complications & Sequelae

Corneal scarring occurs if the process has been particularly severe and prolonged. Secondary glaucoma may result from the uveitis.

Treatment

There are no specific measures. Treatment is aimed at preventing the development of posterior synechiae, which will occur if the pupil is not dilated.

Both eyes should be dilated with frequent instillation of 2% atropine solution. Corticosteroid drops often relieve the symptoms dramatically but must be continued for long periods to prevent recurrence of symptoms. Dark glasses and a darkened room may be necessary if photophobia is severe. Treatment should be given for systemic syphilis, even though this usually has little effect on the ocular condition.

Corneal scarring may necessitate corneal transplant, and glaucoma, if present, may be difficult to control.

Course & Prognosis

The corneal disease process itself is not affected by treatment, which is aimed at prevention of complications. The inflammatory phase lasts 3 or 4 weeks. The corneas then gradually clear, leaving ghost vessels and scars in the corneal stroma.

INTERSTITIAL KERATITIS DUE TO OTHER CAUSES

Although congenital syphilis is no longer a common cause of interstitial keratitis, the disease still occurs as a complication of other granulomatous diseases, eg, tuberculosis and leprosy. Treatment is usually symptomatic, but it is important to establish the cause.

Cogan's syndrome is a rare disorder generally believed to be a vascular hypersensitivity reaction of unknown origin. It is a disease of young adults and is characterized by nonsyphilitic interstitial keratitis and a vestibuloauditory difficulty. Corticosteroids are reputed to be of value, but some degree of visual impairment and complete nerve deafness, with unresponsive labyrinths, usually supervene.

CORNEAL PIGMENTATION

Pigmentation of the cornea may occur with or without ocular or systemic disease. There are several distinct varieties.

Krukenberg's Spindle

In this disorder, brown uveal pigment is deposited bilaterally upon the central endothelial surface in a vertical spindle-shaped fashion. It occurs in a small percentage of people over age 20, usually in myopic women. It can be seen grossly but is best observed with the loupe or slit lamp. The visual acuity is only slightly affected, and the progression is extremely slow. Pigmentary glaucoma should be ruled out.

Blood Staining

This disorder occurs occasionally as a complication of traumatic hyphema and is due to hemosiderin in the corneal stroma. The cornea is golden brown, and vision is blurred. In most cases the cornea gradually clears in 1–2 years.

Kayser-Fleischer Ring

This is a pigmented ring whose color varies widely from ruby red to bright green, blue, yellow, or brown. The ring is 1–3 mm is diameter and located just inside the limbus posteriorly. In exceptional cases there is a second ring. The pigment is composed of fine granules immediately below the endothelium. It involves Descemet's membrane, rarely the stroma. Electron microscopic studies suggest that the pigment is a copper compound. The intensity of the pigmentation can be reduced markedly by the use of chelating agents.

These rings, which were long considered to be pathognomonic of hepatolenticular degeneration (Wilson's disease), have recently been described in 3 nonwilsonian patients with chronic hepatobiliary disease and in one patient with chronic cholestatic jaundice. Recognition of the Kayser-Fleischer rings, however, remains important, since they call attention to the possibilty that the patient has Wilson's disease. Specific medical treatment with the copper chelating agent penicillamine may dramatically improve a disease that would otherwise inevitably be fatal.

Iron Lines (Hudson-Stähli Line, Fleischer's Ring, Stocker's Line, Ferry's Line)

Localized deposits of iron within the corneal epithelium may occur in sufficient quantity to become visible clinically. The Hudson-Stähli line is a horizontal line at the junction of the middle and lower thirds of the cornea, corresponding to the line of lid closure, in otherwise normal elderly patients. Fleischer's ring surrounds the base of the cone in keratoconus. Stocker's line is a vertical line associated with pterygia, and Ferry's line develops adjacent to limbal filtering blebs. Similar iron deposits are seen at the site of corneal scars.

CORNEAL TRANSPLANTATION

Corneal transplantation (keratoplasty) is indicated for a number of serious corneal conditions, eg, scarring, edema, thinning, and distortion. The term penetrating keratoplasty denotes full-thickness corneal replacement; lamellar keratoplasty denotes a partial-thickness procedure.

Young donors are preferred for penetrating keratoplasties; there is a direct relationship between age and the health of the endothelial cells. Because of the rapid endothelial cell death rate, the eyes should be enucleated soon after death and should be used within 48 hours, preferably within 24 hours.

For lamellar keratoplasty, corneas can be frozen, dehydrated, or refrigerated for several weeks; the endothelial cells are not important in this partial-thickness procedure.

Technique

The recipient eye is prepared by a partial-thickness cutting of a circle of diseased cornea with a trephine (cookie cutter action) (Fig 6–16) and full-thickness removal with scissors or partial-thickness removal with dissection.

The donor eye is prepared in 2 ways. For penetrating keratoplasty, the entire cornea is placed endothelium up on a Teflon block; the trephine is pressed down into the cornea, and a full-thickness button is punched out. In lamellar keratoplasty, a partial-thickness trephine incision is made in the cornea and the lamellar button is dissected free. Certain refinements in technique, such as free hand grafts, may be necessary.

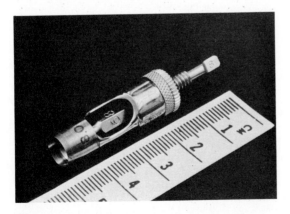

Figure 6–16. Eight-millimeter Castroviejo disposable trephine. (Courtesy of R Biswell and T King.)

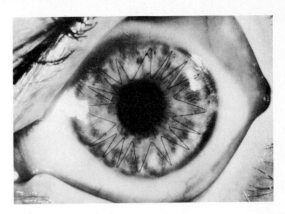

Figure 6–17. Penetrating keratoplasty with 10-0 nylon running suture, 3 months after operation. (Courtesy of R Biswell and T King.)

In recent years, refined sutures (Fig 6–17) and instruments and sophisticated operating microscopes and illuminating systems have significantly improved the prognosis in all patients requiring corneal transplants.

REFRACTIVE CORNEAL SURGERY

Roderick Biswell, MD

Spectacles are considered inconvenient or unattractive by many wearers. Corneal contact lenses, invented by Kalt and improved by Tuohy, have solved many optical and cosmetic problems but have introduced other complications, and the search for an alternative solution to the correction of refractive errors continues. Results and technique for most refractive surgery continue to change; complications may cause visual loss, and the various procedures have not gained general acceptance in ophthalmology.

Radial Keratotomy

In the late 1940s, Sato of Japan created anterior and posterior corneal incisions to alter the curvature of the cornea. Results were poor, and endothelial decompensation with corneal edema occurred frequently. In 1972, Fyodorov of the USSR began to use anterior corneal cuts only. Currently, the operation consists of radial incisions involving 90% of the corneal thickness and extending from a clear optical zone (usually the central 3 mm or more of the cornea) toward but not reaching the limbus. The amount of correction achieved is modified by the size of the optical zone and the number and depth of the incisions.

Various formulas and computer programs are used to determine the value of these parameters in each case.

There is general agreement that radial keratotomy does reduce the degree of myopia and is most effective for myopia in the lower range (−2 to −4 diopters). There is a significant degree of unpredictability in the final result, with under- or overcorrection or even progressive hyperopia. Glare and fluctuations of vision during the day are commonly reported side effects. Delayed healing of corneal incisions, with corneal infections occurring up to 2 years after the procedure, have been reported. Endophthalmitis, traumatic cataract, and endothelial cell loss are rare but have been reported. Agreement on whether the procedure should be done at all has not been reached.

Keratomileusis

In 1961, Barraquer of Colombia reported on the technique of myopic keratomileusis for the correction of high degrees of myopia. The procedure has been performed in other countries but by relatively few surgeons. A deep lamellar corneal autograft is cut; the tissue is frozen and then reshaped with a cryolathe to obtain a flatter curvature after thawing; and the autograft is then sutured back into position. Expensive cryolathe and microkeratome equipment is required. The procedure has also been used for hyperopia.

Complications of keratomileusis include improper depth of the lamellar bed, delayed epithelialization over the resutured tissue, interface epithelial growth and opacity, and irregular astigmatism.

Keratophakia

In keratophakia, a cryolathe is used to shape a donor cornea into a lens, which is then inserted into a lamellar bed. The outer disk of the recipient cornea, which was removed prior to placement of the donor lenticule, is sutured back into position, thus thickening and steepening the cornea. Up to +15 diopters can be corrected. The procedure has been recommended for young aphakic patients who cannot tolerate contact lenses and are poor candidates for secondary lens implantation. The operation has also been performed at the time of cataract extraction. Complications have included interface opacities and astigmatism, both of which may take many months to stabilize or may never do so.

Epikeratophakia

In epikeratophakia, an epigraft of homologous tissue is sutured to a peripheral circular groove formed in the superficial corneal stroma, following removal of the host corneal epithelium. The donor lens is precut on a cryolathe and lyophilized. The procedure has been described by Kaufman and others as useful for myopia, hypermetropia, keratoconus, and even astigmatism (toric epigraft). Epikeratophakia has been used in adult aphakia when contact lenses have failed and a secondary lens implant is contraindicated. Childhood aphakia has been mentioned prominently as an indication, since contact lenses are difficult for children to use and intraocular lens implants may result in long-term complications in children. Epikeratophakia has also been used on scarred corneas and on corneas affected with endothelial dystrophy. It has been described as having few complications because the graft can be removed at any time, but the procedure is still in the developmental stage.

Operation to Correct Astigmatism

Various patterns of keratotomy have been described to correct corneal astigmatism. These cuts can be used alone or with radial keratotomy. Irregular astigmatism continues to be a serious problem following most corneal operations, including radial keratotomy and penetrating keratoplasty, and after cataract surgery. Troutman and others have described relaxing incisions and wedge resections for postkeratoplasty astigmatism, utilizing a surgical keratometer. Various techniques for cataract incision, such as scleral "pocket" incisions, have been reported as useful in preventing postoperative astigmatism after cataract surgery.

Alloplastic Corneal Implants

Disks of many different materials have been inserted into corneal stromal pockets, initially to control corneal edema but more recently to correct refractive errors. In most cases, the corneal tissue anterior to the implant undergoes necrosis. Hydrogel and polysulfone lenses have been more successful than other types of lenses tried so far. Use of alloplastic corneal implants would remove the need to rely on autologous or homologous material in refractive surgery.

Clear Lens Removal

A few surgeons around the world have advocated the removal of clear lenses in high degrees of myopia, suggesting that the risk of doing so is minimal owing to the safety of extracapsular lens extraction. The procedure is controversial because of a significant risk of retinal detachment in high myopes.

REFERENCES

Acanthamoeba keratitis (editorial). *Arch Ophthalmol* 1988;**106**:1181.

Angell LK et al: Visual prognosis in patients with ruptures in Descemet's membrane due to forceps injuries. *Arch Ophthalmol* 1981;**99**:2137.

Baum J, Barza M: Topical vs subconjunctival treatment of bacterial corneal ulcers. *Ophthalmology* 1983;**90**:162.

Baum J et al: Bilateral keratitis as a manifestation of Lyme disease. *Am J Ophthalmol* 1988;**105**:75.

Bloomfield SE, Jakobiec FA, Theodore FH: Contact lens

induced keratopathy: A severe complication extending the spectrum of keratoconjunctivitis in contact lens wearers. *Ophthalmology* 1984;**91**:290.

Boger WP III et al: Keratoconus and acute hydrops. *Am J Ophthalmol* 1981;**91**:231.

Boisjoly HM et al: Superinfections in herpes simplex keratitis. *Am J Ophthalmol* 1983;**96**:354.

Boyd BF: Does refractive surgery have a significant future? *Highlights of Ophthalmology* 1985;**13(12)**:1. [Entire issue.]

Carlson KH, Bourne WM, Brubaker RF: Effect of long-term contact lens wear on corneal endothelial cell morphology and function. *Invest Ophthalmol* 1988;**29**:185.

Cole EL et al: Herpes zoster ophthalmicus and acquired immune deficiency syndrome. *Arch Ophthalmol* 1984;**102**:1027.

Cole MD, Smerdon D: Perforating eye injuries caused by darts. *Br J Ophthalmol* 1988;**72**:511.

Del Priore LV, Robin AL, Pollack IP: Neodymium:YAG and argon laser iridotomy. *Ophthalmology* 1988;**95**:1207.

DeLuise VP, Tabbara KF: *Peripheral Corneal Disorders.* Little, Brown, 1986.

Donzis PB, Mondino BJ, Weissman BA: *Bacillus* keratitis associated with contaminated contact lens care systems. *Am J Ophthalmol* 1988;**105**:195.

Facheson J, Joseph J, Spalton DJ: Use of soft contact lenses in an eye casualty department for the primary treatment of traumatic corneal abrasions. *Br J Ophthalmol* 1987; **71**:285.

Falcon MG: Rational acyclovir therapy in herpetic eye disease. *Br J Ophthalmol* 1987;**71**:102.

Foster A, Sommer A: Corneal ulceration, measles, and childhood blindness in Tanzania. *Br J Ophthalmol* 1987;**71**:331.

Foster CS: Evaluation of topical cromolyn sodium in the treatment of vernal keratoconjunctivitis. (From the Cromolyn Sodium Collaborative Study Group.) *Ophthalmology* 1988;**95**:194.

Jaros PA, DeLuise VP: Pingueculae and pterygia. *Surv Ophthalmol* 1988;**33**:41.

Jarvis VN, Levine R, Asbell PA: Ophthalmia neonatorum: Study of a decade of experience at the Mount Sinai Hospital. *Br J Ophthalmol* 1987;**71**:295.

Johns KJ, O'Day DM: *Pseudomonas* corneal ulcer with colored cosmetic contact lenses in an emmetropic individual. *Am J Ophthalmol* 1988;**105**:210.

Kaufman HE: The correction of aphakia. *Am J Ophthalmol* 1980;**89**:1.

Kaufman HE, Centifanto-Fitzgerald YM, Varnell ED: Herpes simplex keratitis. *Ophthalmology* 1983;**90**:700.

Kelly SP: Serious eye injury in badminton players. *Br J Ophthalmol* 1987;**71**:746.

Kenyon KR: Decision-making in the therapy of external eye disease: Noninfected corneal ulcers. *Ophthalmology* 1982;**89**:44.

Kim KJ, Ostler HB: Marginal corneal ulcer due to β-streptococcus. *Arch Ophthalmol* 1977;**95**:454.

Klintworth GK et al: Recurrence of lattice corneal dystrophy type 1 in the corneal grafts of two siblings. *Am J Ophthalmol* 1982;**94**:540.

Lemp MA et al: Gram-negative corneal ulcers in elderly aphakic eyes with extended-wear lenses. *Ophthalmology* 1984;**91**:60.

Leopold IH: Update on antibiotics in ocular infections. *Am J Ophthalmol* 1985;**100**:134.

Lindquist TD, Sher NA, Doughman DJ: Clinical signs and medical therapy of early *Acanthamoeba* keratitis. *Arch Ophthalmol* 1988;**106**:73.

Macewen CJ: Sport associated eye injury: A casualty department survey. *Br J Ophthalmol* 1987;**71**:701.

Malbran ES: Corneal dystrophies: A clinical, pathological, and surgical approach: The 28th Edward Jackson Memorial Lecture. *Am J Ophthalmol* 1972;**74**:771.

Matsuda M et al: Corneal endothelial changes associated with aphakic extended contact lens wear. *Arch Ophthalmol* 1988;**106**:70.

McDonald MB et al: Epikeratophakia for keratoconus. *Arch Ophthalmol* 1986;**104**:1294.

McDonald MB et al: The nationwide study of epikeratophakia for aphakia in adults. *Am J Ophthalmol* 1987; **103**:358.

Meisler DM, Friedlander MH, Okumoto M: *Mycobacterium chelonei* keratitis. *Am J Ophthalmol* 1982; **92**:398.

Morgan KS et al: The nationwide study of epikeratophakia for aphakia in older children. *Ophthalmology* 1988;**95**:526.

Morgan SJ: Chemical burns of the eye: Causes and management. *Br J Ophthalmol* 1987;**71**:854.

Murray PI, Rahi AHS: Pathogenesis of Mooren's ulcer: Some new concepts. *Br J Ophthalmol* 1984;**68**:182.

Olson R (editor): Common corneal problems. *Int Ophthalmol Clin* (Summer) 1984;**24**. [Entire issue.]

Penna EP, Tabbara KF: Oxybuprocaine keratopathy: A preventable disease. *Br J Ophthalmol* 1986;**70**:202.

Schein OD et al: Microbial keratitis associated with contaminated ocular medications. *Am J Ophthalmol* 1988; **105**:361.

Schwab IR: Oral acyclovir in the management of herpes simplex ocular infections. *Ophthalmology* 1988; **95**:423.

Seiler T et al: Excimer laser keratectomy for correction of astigmatism. *Am J Ophthalmol* 1988;**105**:117.

Smolin G, Thoft RA: *The Cornea,* 2nd ed. Little, Brown, 1987.

Sommer A: Effects of vitamin A deficiency on the ocular surface. *Ophthalmology* 1983;**90**:592.

Sommer A: Treatment of corneal xerophthalmia with topical retinoic acid. *Am J Ophthalmol* 1983;**95**:349.

Spencer WH (editor): *Ophthalmic Pathology,* 3rd ed. 3 vols. Saunders, 1985.

Stern GA: Update on the medical management of corneal and external eye diseases, corneal transplantation, and keratorefractive surgery. (Subspecialty synopsis.) *Ophthalmology* 1988;**95**:842.

Tabbara KF, Shammas HF: Bilateral corneal perforations in Stevens-Johnson syndrome. *Can J Ophthalmol* 1975; **10**:514.

Tabbara KF et al: Thygeson's superficial punctate keratitis. *Ophthalmology* 1981;**88**:75.

Thygeson P: Clinical and laboratory observations on superficial punctate keratitis. *Am J Ophthalmol* 1960;**61**:1344.

Thygeson P, Okumoto M: Keratomycosis: A preventable disease. *Trans Am Acad Ophthalmol Otolaryngol* 1974; **78**:433.

Torres MA et al: Topical ketoconazole for fungal keratitis. *Am J Ophthalmol* 1985;**100**:293.

Waring GO III et al: The corneal endothelium: Normal and pathologic structure and function. *Ophthalmology* 1982; **89**:531.

Wilson LA, Schlitzer RL, Ahearn DG: *Pseudomonas* corneal ulcers associated with soft contact-lens wear. *Am J Ophthalmol* 1981;**92**:546.

7

Sclera

Khalid F. Tabbara, MD

ANATOMY & FUNCTION

The sclera is the fibrous outer protective coating of the eye. It is dense and white and continuous with the cornea anteriorly and with the dural sheath of the optic nerve posteriorly. At the insertion of the rectus muscles, it is about 0.3 mm thick; elsewhere, about 1 mm thick. A few strands of scleral tissue pass over the optic disk. This sievelike structure is known as the lamina cribrosa. Around the optic nerve, the sclera is penetrated by the long and short posterior ciliary arteries and the long and short ciliary nerves. Slightly posterior to the equator, the 4 vortex veins exit through the sclera, usually one in each quadrant. About 4 mm posterior to the limbus, the 4 anterior ciliary arteries and veins penetrate the sclera. Each set penetrates slightly anterior to the insertion of a rectus muscle.

The outer surface of the sclera is covered by a thin layer of fine elastic tissue, the episclera, containing numerous blood vessels that nourish the sclera. The brown pigment layer on the inner surface is the lamina fusca, which is continuous with the sclera and the choroid. On the inner surface at 180 degrees (in a horizontal plane through 9 and 3 o'clock), there is a shallow groove from the optic nerve to the ciliary body in which are embedded the long posterior ciliary artery and the long ciliary nerve. The nerve supply to the sclera is from the ciliary nerves.

Histologically, the sclera consists of many dense bands of parallel and interlacing fibrous tissue bundles each of which is 10–16 μm thick and 100–140 μm wide. The histologic structure of the sclera is remarkably similar to that of the cornea; this raises the question why the cornea is transparent and the sclera opaque. The apparent physiologic reason is the relative deturgescence of the cornea and the less uniform structure of the sclera. The cornea has the ability to absorb a great deal of water, whereupon it becomes opaque; the sclera is almost completely hydrated in its normal state.

DISEASES & DISORDERS OF THE SCLERA

BLUE SCLERAS

The normal sclera is white and opaque, so that the underlying uveal structures are not visible. Structural changes of the scleral collagen fibers and thinning of the sclera may allow the underlying uveal pigment to be seen, giving the sclera a bluish discoloration. Blue sclera occurs in several disorders that lead to disturbances in the connective tissues, particularly the collagen fibers. Blue scleras are part of the clinical picture in osteogenesis imperfecta, Ehlers-Danlos syndrome, pseudoxanthoma elasticum, Marfan's syndrome, and pseudohypoparathyroidism and may occur with prolonged use of corticosteroids. Blue scleras are sometimes noted in normal newborn infants, in keratoconus, and in keratoglobus.

SCLERAL ECTASIA

Prolonged elevation of intraocular pressure early in infancy, such as occurs in cases of congenital glaucoma, may lead to stretching and ectasia of the sclera. Scleral ectasia may occur as a congenital anomaly surrounding the disk or occasionally in the macular area. It may also follow inflammation or injury of the sclera.

STAPHYLOMA

Staphyloma results from bulging of the uvea into a thinned and stretched sclera. Staphylomas can be characterized as ectatic dark blue, bulging areas involving a localized segment of the eyeball. The staphyloma may be anterior, equatorial, or posterior. Anterior staphylomas are generally located over the ciliary body (ciliary staphyloma) (Fig 7–1) or between the ciliary body and the limbus (intercalary staphyloma). Equatorial staphylomas are located at the equator and posterior staphylomas posterior to the equator. Posterior staphylomas are most commonly seen at the optic nerve head. They affect the lamina cribrosa and may follow extreme myopia. Large congenital posterior staphylomas associated with poor vision have been observed. Patients having such conditions are generally extremely myopic. Cases of congenital peripapillary staphylomas in patients with normal or nearly normal vision have been reported. Posterior staphyloma is usually associated with areas of pronounced choroidal atrophy.

Staphyloma must be differentiated from extreme myopia and scleral ectasia in a coloboma of the optic nerve head.

INTRASCLERAL NERVE LOOPS OF AXENFELD

The intrascleral nerve loops are sites of branches of the long ciliary nerves. They enter the sclera close to the ciliary body and about 3.5 mm from the limbus. They are more commonly seen nasally. They may be pigmented and are usually accompanied by the small anterior ciliary artery in its inward course.

INFLAMMATION OF THE SCLERA & EPISCLERA

Inflammation involving the episclera, the thin layer of vascular elastic tissue overlying the sclera, is referred to as **episcleritis. Scleritis** is inflammation of the sclera itself, with or without inflammation of the

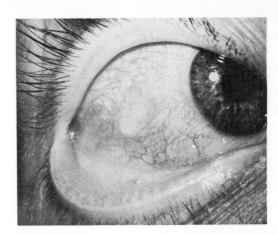

Figure 7–2. Nodular episcleritis, right eye. (Photo by Diane Beeston.)

episclera. The 2 diseases are considered distinct clinical entities and will be considered separately.

Episcleritis

This is a relatively common localized inflammation of the episclera. It is unilateral in about two-thirds of cases, and the sex incidence is equal. It may recur at the same or adjacent sites in the palpebral fissure.

The cause is not known, but hypersensitivity reactions may play a role. Certain systemic diseases such as rheumatoid arthritis, Sjögren's syndrome, coccidioidomycosis, syphilis, herpes zoster, and tuberculosis have been associated with episcleritis.

Symptoms of episcleritis include redness, pain, photophobia, tenderness, and lacrimation. Ocular examination reveals localized hyperemia that gives the eyeball a pink or purple color. There is also infiltration, congestion, and edema of the episclera, the overlying conjunctiva, and the underlying Tenon capsule. Two types of episcleritis are recognized: simple and nodular (Fig 7–2). The sclera itself is not involved. About 15% of patients with episcleritis develop mild iritis.

Conjunctivitis is ruled out by the localized nature of episcleritis and the lack of palpebral conjunctival involvement.

The condition is benign, and the course is generally self-limited in 1–2 weeks. However, recurrences may torment the patient for years. Topical therapy with corticosteroids (dexamethasone 0.1%) resolves the inflammatory changes in 3 or 4 days. Corticosteroids are more effective in simple episcleritis than in nodular episcleritis.

Scleritis

The eyes and the joints have certain anatomic and biochemical similarities. The sclera is composed of collagen and is relatively avascular, and many of the conditions that affect the sclera and episclera can simultaneously involve the joints. The sclera and ep-

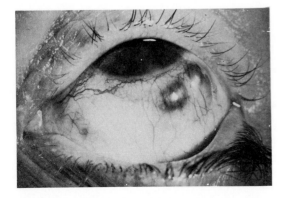

Figure 7–1. Ciliary staphyloma. (Courtesy of P Thygeson.)

isclera may therefore be involved by a number of autoimmune, infectious, degenerative, metabolic, and hypersensitivity disorders that may also affect the joints (Table 7–1). Diseases of the sclera may represent local manifestations of systemic disorders. Laboratory studies may help identify these entities (Table 7–2).

Scleritis may be unilateral or bilateral, of sudden or insidious onset, and may occur as a single episode or may be recurrent. Women are more commonly affected than men. Patients with scleritis almost always complain of pain. A decrease in visual acuity is usually associated with an anterior chamber reaction or evidence of infectious scleritis and cyclitis. Patients with scleritis have violaceous discoloration of the eye and diffuse redness and tenderness.

Visual acuity may be slightly reduced. Tenderness and pain are typical of scleritis. Examination in daylight rather than with artificial illumination helps in observation of the deep violaceous discoloration. Slit lamp examination helps in assessing the depth and nature of the scleral and episcleral conditions and in identifying corneal disease. The use of epinephrine 1:1000 helps in constricting the conjunctival vessels, but the deep scleral vessels are not affected by these drops. If the patient has conjunctivitis, the eye will become white following instillation of epinephrine, but if there is deep scleritis the use of topical decongestants will cause the deep violaceous discoloration to become more prominent. Use of a green filter in the slit lamp may help in confirming areas of maximal congestion and in assessing the depth of the blood vessels.

Table 7–1. Causes of scleritis.

Autoimmune diseases
  Ankylosing spondylitis
  Rheumatoid arthritis
  Polyarteritis nodosa
  Relapsing polychondritis
  Wegener's granulomatosis
  Systemic lupus erythematosus
  Pyoderma gangrenosum
  Ulcerative colitis
  IgA nephropathy
  Psoriatic arthritis
Granulomatous diseases
  Tuberculosis
  Syphilis
  Sarcoidosis
  Leprosy
  Vogt-Koyanagi-Harada syndrome (rare)
Metabolic disorders: Gout, thyrotoxicosis, active rheumatic heart disease
Infections: Onchocerciasis, herpes zoster, herpes simplex, infections with *Pseudomonas, Aspergillus, Streptococcus, Staphylococcus*
Others
  Physical (irradiation, thermal burns)
  Chemical (alkali or acid burns)
  Mechanical (penetrating injuries)
  Lymphoma
  Rosacea
  Post cataract extraction
Unknown

Table 7–2. Laboratory workup for scleritis.

Complete blood count and sedimentation rate
Serum complement (C3) level
Serum rheumatoid factor
Serum antinuclear antibodies
PPD, chest x-ray
Serum FTA-ABS, VDRL
X-ray of the orbit to rule out foreign body, especially in patients with nodular scleritis
X-ray of the sinuses
Serum levels of uric acid
Urinalysis

Posterior scleritis may be associated with periorbital edema and slight proptosis. Inflammation of the sclera is less common than episcleritis and is frequently associated with systemic diseases.

Scleritis is classified according to its clinical and pathologic features. Two types are recognized: anterior and posterior. Anterior scleritis may be subdivided into diffuse nodular or necrotizing scleritis with or without adjacent inflammation.

Areas of avascularity suggest occlusive vasculitis and imply a grave prognosis. Elevated nodules are noted in nodular scleritis associated with rheumatoid arthritis.

A. Necrotizing Scleritis: The most severe form of scleritis is necrotizing scleritis with adjacent inflammation, otherwise known as **brawny scleritis.** This disorder is characterized by an acute, painful, tender area of localized congestion and necrosis that leads to thinning and destruction of the scleral collagen fibers. There may be an avascular area in the overlying episcleral tissue. The disease may remain localized or may progress to involve the entire anterior sclera, allowing visualization of the underlying uvea. Elevation of the intraocular pressure may exacerbate scleral ectasia. Corticosteroids may exacerbate both scleral thinning and destruction of collagen fibers.

B. Necrotizing Scleromalacia (Scleromalacia Perforans): This is a rare scleral disease characterized by thinning and melting of the scleral tissue, leading to areas of dehiscence without any history or

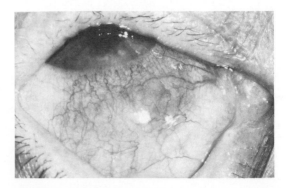

Figure 7–3. Nodular scleritis, left eye, associated with rheumatoid arthritis. (Courtesy of GR O'Connor.)

clinical evidence of inflammation of the sclera. This form of "scleral melting" is usually associated with severe forms of rheumatoid arthritis. As is true also of necrotizing scleritis, uveal pigment may be visualized through the areas of scleral thinning. Such thinning may lead to bulging. Rupture of the globe secondary to minor trauma may occur, but this is rare. The prognosis depends on the area of the globe affected but is in general poor. Corticosteroids are contraindicated. In cases of perforation or impending perforation, treatment may consist of repair of the dehiscence with a segment of homologous preserved sclera.

C. Posterior Scleritis: This is an uncommon disorder and is difficult to diagnose because of the absence of signs in the anterior segment. CT scan with contrast medium is valuable in making the diagnosis. The disease should be suspected in patients with pain, proptosis, papilledema, and exudative retinal detachment. The disease is unilateral and is associated with severe pain, a decrease in visual acuity, diplopia, and limitation of ocular movements. Posterior scleritis is usually associated with severe rheumatoid arthritis. Recurrences may lead to extreme thinning of the sclera, giving rise to posterior staphyloma or perforation, especially when intraocular pressure is elevated. Ocular complications other than perforation include keratitis, uveitis, cataract, and glaucoma.

Scleritis is generally resistant to treatment. Topical corticosteroids should be used only with extreme caution because of their potential thinning effects on the scleral tissue and because of the possibility of increasing the intraocular pressure in certain patients.

Systemic nonsteroidal anti-inflammatory agents such as salicylates, indomethacin, or ibuprofen appear to be effective in some patients. Systemic immunosuppressive agents are rarely indicated for the treatment of severe resistant forms of scleritis.

INJURIES OF THE SCLERA

The most frequently encountered injuries of the sclera are trauma (penetrating and blunt), physical damage (irradiation, thermal burns), and chemical injuries (alkali and acid burns).

Scleral wounds (lacerations) may result either from blunt trauma or from penetrating trauma caused by sharp instruments or flying objects. Scleral lacerations may be associated with intraocular hemorrhage and injury to other ocular structures. The management of scleral lacerations includes microbiologic control (surface antisepsis and the preparation of a sterile field), suturing of the wound, and excision of any prolapsed uveal tissue. Lacerations of the conjunctiva and Tenon's capsule must be approximated over the scleral wound.

HYALINE DEGENERATION

Hyaline degeneration is a fairly frequent finding in the scleras of persons over age 60. It is manifested by small, round, translucent gray areas that are usually about 2–3 mm in diameter and are located anterior to the insertion of the rectus muscles. They cause no symptoms or complications.

REFERENCES

Cobo M: Inflammation of the sclera. *Int Ophthalmol Clin* 1983;**23**:159.
Foster CS, Forstot SL, Wilson LA: Mortality rate in rheumatoid arthritis patients developing necrotizing scleritis or peripheral ulcerative keratitis: Effects of systemic immunosuppression. *Ophthalmology* 1984; **91**:1253.
Koenig SB, Kaufman HE: The treatment of necrotizing scleritis with an autogenous periosteal graft. *Ophthalmic Surg* 1983;**14**:1029.
Tabbara KF: Scleromalacia associated with Vogt-Koya-nagi-Harada syndrome. *Am J Ophthalmol* 1988; **105**:694.
Watson PG, Bovey E: Anterior segment fluorescein angiography in the diagnosis of scleral inflammation. *Ophthalmology* 1985;**92**:1.
Wilhelmus KR, Yokoyama CM: Syphilitic episcleritis and scleritis. *Am J Ophthalmol* 1987;**104**:595.
Young RD, Watson PG: Microscopical studies of necrotising scleritis. 1. Cellular aspects. 2. Collagen degradation in the scleral stroma. *Br J Ophthalmol* 1984;**68**:770, 781.

Uveal Tract

Taylor Asbury, MD and Khalid F. Tabbara, MD

ANATOMY & FUNCTION

The uveal tract is composed of 3 parts: the iris, the ciliary body, and the choroid. It is the middle, vascular layer of the eye, protected externally by the cornea and sclera. It contributes to the blood supply of the retina.

Anatomy of the Iris

The iris is the anterior extension of the ciliary body. It presents a relatively flat surface with a round aperture in the middle called the pupil, which varies in size and has the same form and function as the aperture of a camera. The sphincter and dilator muscles, which serve to constrict and dilate the pupil, are in the iris stroma. The iris lies in contact with the lens and divides the anterior chamber from the posterior chamber, each of which contains aqueous humor.

Because of the presence of a thick collagenous adventitia, normal iris vessels have the histologic appearance of being quite sclerotic. The iris capillaries have an unfenestrated endothelium and hence do not normally leak intravenously injected fluorescein. The 2 layers of epithelium on the posterior surface are heavily pigmented and represent the anterior extension of the pigmented epithelium of the retina as well as the retina proper. The blood supply is from the major circle of the iris (see Fig 1–7). The nerve supply is described in Chapter 15.

When the iris is cut, as in doing a small peripheral iridectomy for acute angle-closure glaucoma, it seldom bleeds, and the wound remains permanently with no tendency to heal. Pain fibers are present, as is shown by the pain caused by traction on the iris during surgery.

Anatomy of the Ciliary Body

The ciliary body, roughly triangular in cross section, extends forward from the anterior termination of the choroid to the root of the iris, a distance of about 6 mm. Grossly it consists of 2 zones: the pars plicata, the corrugated anterior 2 mm; and the pars plana, the smoother and flatter posterior 4 mm. The surface of the corona ciliaris consists of many elevations and depressions.

There are 2 layers of ciliary epithelium, the external pigmented and the internal nonpigmented, both of which continue as pigmented layers over the posterior surface of the iris. The pigment epithelium represents the forward extension of the pigment epithelium of the retina.

The ciliary muscle consists of longitudinal, radial, and circular portions. Its function is to contract and relax the zonular fibers. This results in altered tension on the capsule of the lens, which gives the lens variable focus for both near and distant objects. The ciliary processes themselves are composed mainly of capillaries and veins that drain through vortex veins. The capillaries are large and fenestrated and hence leak intravenously injected fluorescein.

The pars plana consists of a thin layer of ciliary muscle and vessels covered by ciliary epithelium. The zonular fibers, which hold the lens in place, originate in the valleys between the ciliary processes (Fig 8–

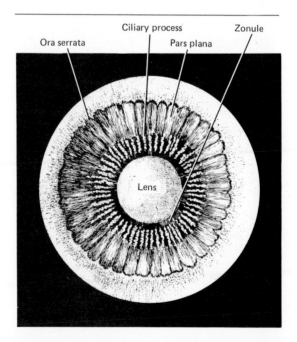

Figure 8–1. Posterior view of ciliary body, zonule, lens, and ora serrata. (Redrawn and reproduced, with permission, from Wolff E: *Anatomy of the Eye and Orbit,* 4th ed. Blakiston-McGraw, 1954.)

1). The blood vessels to the ciliary body come from the major circle of the iris (see Fig 1–7). The sensory nerve supply is through the ciliary nerves.

Anatomy of the Choroid
(Fig 8–2)

The choroid (the posterior portion of the uveal tract and the middle coat of the eye) lies between the retina and the sclera. It is largely composed of blood vessels. The choroidal vessels are bounded by Bruch's membrane internally and the suprachoroid externally. The avascular suprachoroid is composed of lamellas of collagenous and elastic tissue. Bruch's membrane can be divided into 3 portions: an outer elastic sheath, a middle collagenous sheath, and an inner cuticular sheath. (The latter is actually the basement membrane of the retinal pigment epithelium.)

The lumens of the blood vessels increase the deeper they are located in the choroid. There are 3 layers of blood vessels: large, medium, and small. The innermost layer of small blood vessels is known as the choriocapillaris and consists of large capillaries that nourish the outer portion of the retina. The endothelium of these capillaries is fenestrated and hence leaks intravenously injected fluorescein. Most of the large vessels consist of veins. These coalesce and leave the eye as the 4 vortex veins, one in each of the 4 posterior quadrants. The vessel layers of the choroid also contain some elastic fibers and chromatophores.

The choroid is firmly attached to the margin of the optic nerve posteriorly and extends to the ora serrata anteriorly, where it joins the ciliary body.

Functions of Uveal Structures

The function of the iris is to control the amount of light that enters the eye. This occurs by reflex constriction of the pupil under the stimulus of light and dilatation of the pupil in darkness. The ciliary body forms the root of the iris and serves, through the zonular fibers, to govern the size of the lens in accommodation. Aqueous humor is secreted by the ciliary processes into the posterior chamber. The choroid consists of abundant blood vessels; its function is to nourish the outer portion of the underlying retina.

Physiology of Symptoms

Symptoms of uveal tract disorders depend upon the site of the disease process. For example, since there are pain fibers in the iris, the patient with iritis will complain of moderate pain and photophobia. Inflammation of the iris itself does not cause blurring of vision unless the process is severe or advanced enough to cause clouding of the aqueous humor, cornea, or lens. Choroidal disease itself does not cause pain or blurred vision. Because of the close contact of the choroid with the retina, choroidal disease almost always affects the retina (eg, chorioretinitis). If the macular area of the retina is involved, central vision will be impaired.

The vitreous may also become cloudy as a result of posterior uveitis. The impairment of vision is in proportion to the density of vitreous opacity and is reversible as the inflammation subsides and the vitreous haze clears.

The physician examines for disease of the anterior uveal tract with the flashlight and loupe or slit lamp, and disease of the posterior uveal tract with the ophthalmoscope.

UVEITIS*

Inflammation of the uveal tract has many causes and may involve one or all 3 portions simultaneously. The most frequent form of uveitis is acute anterior uveitis (iritis), usually unilateral and characterized by a history of pain, photophobia, and blurring of vision; a red eye (circumcorneal flush) without purulent discharge; and a small pupil. It is important to make the diagnosis early and to dilate the pupil to prevent the formation of permanent posterior synechiae.

Inflammatory disorders of the uveal tract, usually unilateral, are common principally in the young and middle age groups. In most cases the cause is not known. In posterior uveitis the retina is almost always secondarily affected. This is known as chorioretinitis.

Two major types of uveitis may be distinguished upon clinical as well as pathologic grounds: nongranulomatous (more common) and granulomatous (Table 8–1). Because pathogenic organisms have not been found in the nongranulomatous type and because it responds to corticosteroid therapy, it is thought to be a hypersensitivity phenomenon. Granulomatous uveitis usually follows active microbial invasion of the tissues by the causative organism (eg, *Mycobacterium tuberculosis* or *Toxoplasma gondii*). However, these pathogens are rarely recovered, and a definite etiologic diagnosis is seldom possible. The possibilities can often be narrowed down by clinical and laboratory examination.

Nongranulomatous uveitis occurs mainly in the anterior portion of the tract, ie, the iris and ciliary body. There is an inflammatory reaction, as evidenced by the cellular infiltration of lymphocytes and plasma cells in significant numbers and an occasional mononuclear cell. In severe cases, a large fibrin clot or a hypopyon may form in the anterior chamber.

Granulomatous uveitis may involve any portion of the uveal tract but has a predilection for the posterior uvea. Nodular collections of epithelioid cells and giant

---

* "Uveitis" is a general term for inflammatory disorders of the uveal tract. "Anterior uveitis" is the preferred general term for iritis and iridocyclitis. "Posterior uveitis" is the preferred term for choroiditis and chorioretinitis. The term "iritis," used above, means acute anterior nongranulomatous uveitis.

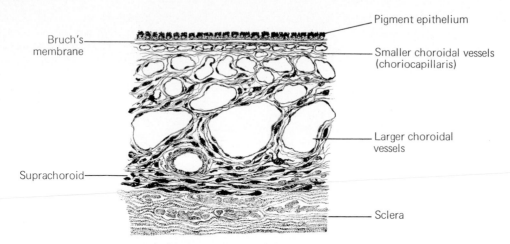

Figure 8–2. Cross section of choroid. (Redrawn and reproduced, with permission, from Wolff E: *Anatomy of the Eye and Orbit,* 4th ed. Blakiston-McGraw, 1954.)

cells surrounded by lymphocytes are present in the affected areas. Inflammatory deposits on the posterior surface of the cornea are composed mainly of macrophages and epithelioid cells. It is possible to make a specific etiologic diagnosis histologically in an enucleated eye by identifying the cysts of *Toxoplasma,* the acid-fast bacillus of tuberculosis, the spirochete of syphilis, the distinctive granulomatous appearance of sarcoidosis and sympathetic ophthalmia, and a few other rare specific causes.

Clinical Findings

A. Symptoms and Signs: In the nongranulomatous form, the onset is characteristically acute, with

pain, injection, photophobia, and blurred vision. There is a circumcorneal flush caused by dilated limbal blood vessels. Fine white deposits (keratic precipitates, ''KPs'') on the posterior surface of the cornea can be seen with the slit lamp or with a loupe. The pupil is small, and there may be a collection of fibrin with cells in the anterior chamber. If posterior synechiae are present, the pupil will be irregular in shape (Figs 8–3 to 8–6). Posterior uveitis is generally classified as granulomatous.

The patient should be asked about previous episodes of arthritis and possible exposure to toxoplasmosis, histoplasmosis, tuberculosis, and syphilis. The remote possibility of a focus of infection elsewhere in the body should also be investigated.

In granulomatous uveitis (which may cause anterior

Table 8–1. Differentiation of granulomatous and nongranulomatous uveitis.

	Nongranulomatous	Granulomatous
Onset	Acute	Insidious
Pain	Marked	None or minimal
Photophobia	Marked	Slight
Blurred vision	Moderate	Marked
Circumcorneal flush	Marked	Slight
Keratic precipitates	Fine white	Large gray (''mutton fat'')
Pupil	Small and irregular	Small and irregular (variable)
Posterior synechiae	Sometimes	Sometimes
Iris nodules	Sometimes	Sometimes
Site	Anterior uvea	Posterior uvea and anterior uvea
Course	Acute	Chronic
Recurrence	Common	Sometimes

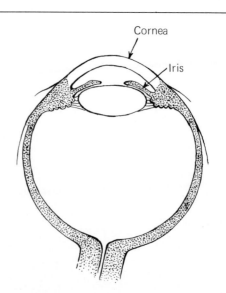

Figure 8–3. Normal anterior chamber.

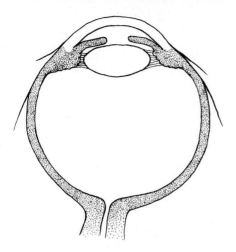

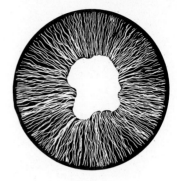

Figure 8–6. Posterior synechiae (anterior view). The iris is adherent to the lens in several places as a result of previous inflammation, causing an irregular fixed pupil.

Figure 8–4. Anterior synechiae (adhesions). The peripheral iris adheres to the cornea.

uveitis, posterior uveitis, or both), the onset is usually insidious. Vision gradually becomes blurred, and the affected eye becomes diffusely red with circumcorneal flush. Pain is minimal, and photophobia is less marked than in the nongranulomatous form. The pupil is often constricted and becomes irregular as posterior synechiae form. Large "mutton fat" KPs on the posterior surface of the cornea may be seen with the slit lamp. Flare and cells are seen in the anterior chamber, and nodules consisting of clusters of white cells are seen on the pupillary margin of the iris (Koeppe nodules). These nodules are the equivalent of mutton fat KPs.

Fresh active lesions of the choroid and retina appear as yellowish-white patches seen hazily with the ophthalmoscope through the cloudy vitreous body. Such posterior cases are generally classified as granulomatous disease. Because of the intimate relationship of the choroid and retina, the retina is nearly always involved (chorioretinitis). As healing progresses, the vitreous haze lessens, and pigmentation occurs gradually at the edges of the yellowish-white spots. In the healed stage, there is usually considerable pigment deposition. If the macula has not been involved, recovery of central vision is complete. The patient is usually not aware of the scotoma in the peripheral field corresponding to the scarred area.

B. Laboratory Findings: Extensive laboratory investigation is usually not indicated in anterior uveitis, particularly if it is nongranulomatous or is readily responsive to nonspecific treatment. In persistent nonresponsive anterior or posterior uveitis, an attempt should be made to arrive at an etiologic diagnosis. Skin tests for tuberculosis and histoplasmosis may be helpful, as well as complement fixation tests and methylene blue dye tests (toxoplasmosis). On the basis of these tests and the clinical appearance, it is often possible to make an etiologic diagnosis.

Differential Diagnosis

In conjunctivitis, vision is not blurred, pupillary responses are normal, a discharge is present, and there is usually no pain, photophobia, or ciliary injection.

In keratitis or keratoconjunctivitis, vision may be blurred and pain and photophobia may be present. Some causes of keratitis such as herpes simplex and herpes zoster may be associated with a true anterior uveitis.

In acute glaucoma the pupil is dilated, there are no posterior synechiae, and the cornea is steamy.

After repeated attacks, nongranulomatous uveitis may acquire the characteristics of granulomatous uveitis. In recent years there has been less emphasis on this differentiation, and some authorities are disregarding it completely. Nevertheless, the differentiation is still of value as a guide to treatment and prognosis.

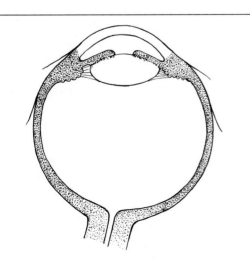

Figure 8–5. Posterior synechiae. The iris adheres to the lens.

Table 8–2. Treatment of granulomatous uveitis.

	Anti-infective Chemotherapy	Use of Corticosteroids
Toxoplasmosis	If central vision is threatened, give pyrimethamine (Daraprim), 75 mg orally as a loading dose for 2 days followed by 25 mg once daily for 4 weeks, in combination with trisulfapyrimidines (sulfadiazine, sulfamerazine, and sulfamethazine, 0.167 g of each per tablet), 2 g orally as loading dose followed by 0.5 g 4 times daily for 4 weeks. If a fall in the white or platelet count occurs during therapy, give folinic acid (leucovorin), 1 mL IM twice weekly or 3 mg orally 3 times a week. Alternative chemotherapeutic approach for ocular toxoplasmosis: Clindamycin, 300 mg orally 4 times a day with sulfonamides (as above), or minocycline (investigational), 100 mg orally daily for 3–4 weeks.	If the response is not favorable after 2 weeks, continue anti-infective therapy and give systemic corticosteroids, eg, prednisolone, 20–25 mg 4 times a day for 1 week, followed by 60–120 mg every other day thereafter,[1] to protect the macula. Corticosteroids may activate the organisms of toxoplasmosis and tuberculosis but are given as a calculated risk to control the inflammatory response when it threatens vision.
Tuberculosis	Isoniazid, 300 mg orally daily; ethambutol, 400 mg orally twice daily; pyridoxine, 50 mg orally daily. Continue treatment for 6 months.	If a favorable response does not occur in 6 weeks, continue antimycobacterial therapy and give systemic corticosteroids, eg, prednisolone, 40–80 mg every other day for 2 months.[1]
Sarcoidosis	Treat with local corticosteroids and mydriatics and, during active stages, with systemic corticosteroids such as prednisolone, 40–80 mg every other day.[1] Give supplemental potassium chloride, 2 g 3 times daily. The usual contraindications to systemic corticosteroid therapy apply.	
Sympathetic ophthalmia	Treat with local cortisteroids and mydriatics and systemic corticosteroids in high doses, eg, prednisone, 40–120 mg every other day.[1] The usual contraindications to systemic corticosteroid therapy apply, and the drugs may be needed in higher doses and for a longer time. Therefore, management of the side effects is often more difficult. Azathioprine may be helpful in reducing the required dose of corticosteroids. In severe cases that fail to respond to corticosteroids, treatment with cytotoxic agents such as chlorambucil and cyclophosphamide or other immunosuppressants such as cyclosporine has met with some success. *Caution:* White blood counts and platelets must be monitored very carefully in these patients, and these drugs should not be used without careful consideration.	

[1] Administration every other day has been advocated to minimize the effects of stress and make drug withdrawal easier and safer.

Complications & Sequelae

Anterior uveitis may produce peripheral anterior synechiae (Fig 8–4), which impede aqueous outflow at the anterior chamber angle and cause glaucoma. Posterior synechiae can cause glaucoma by impeding the flow of aqueous from the posterior to the anterior chamber. Early and constant pupillary dilatation lessens the likelihood of posterior synechiae. Interference with lens metabolism may cause cataract. Retinal detachment occasionally occurs as a result of traction on the retina by vitreous strands. Cystoid macular edema and degeneration can result from long-standing anterior uveitis.

Treatment

A. Nongranulomatous Uveitis: Systemic analgesics as necessary for pain, and dark glasses for photophobia. The pupil must be kept dilated. Atropine is unrivaled in its ability to relieve ciliary spasm. Once relief has been achieved, short-acting dilators such as cyclopentolate (Cyclogyl 1%) should be used to prevent spasm and posterior synechia formation. Local steroid drops are usually quite effective for their anti-inflammatory action. In severe and unresponsive cases, systemic steroids are given also.

B. Granulomatous Uveitis: If the process includes the anterior segment, pupillary dilatation with atropine, 2%, is indicated. Since it is often possible to make a tentative or likely diagnosis of the cause, an attempt at specific therapy is indicated as outlined in Table 8–2.

C. Treatment of Complications: Glaucoma is a common complication. Treatment of the uveitis is of primary importance, particularly dilating the pupil with atropine (not constricting the pupil, as with all forms of primary glaucoma). Carbonic anhydrase inhibitors often effectively reduce intraocular tension by depressing aqueous production. Epinephrine also lowers intraocular pressure by reducing ciliary body secretion of aqueous, and topical timolol maleate (Timoptic), 0.5% solution, 1 drop twice daily, is frequently helpful.

Cataract frequently develops in chronic uveitis. The eye tolerates removal of such cataracts very poorly; but if vision is poor enough, cataract surgery may be essential. Retinal detachment is also very difficult to treat successfully surgically when it occurs in association with uveitis.

Course & Prognosis

With treatment, an attack of nongranulomatous uveitis usually lasts a few days to weeks. Recurrences are common.

Granulomatous uveitis lasts months to years, sometimes with remissions and exacerbations, and may cause permanent damage with marked visual loss despite the best treatment. The prognosis for a focal peripheral chorioretinal lesion is considerably better, often healing well with no significant visual loss.

ANTERIOR UVEITIS
(Table 8–3)

1. UVEITIS ASSOCIATED WITH JOINT DISEASE

About 20% of children with the pauciarticular form of **juvenile rheumatoid arthritis** develop a chronic bilateral nongranulomatous iridocyclitis. Females are far more commonly affected than males (4:1). The average age at which the uveitis is detected is $5\frac{1}{2}$ years. In most cases the onset is insidious, the disease being discovered only when the child is noted to have a difference in the color of the 2 eyes, a difference in the size or shape of the pupil, or the onset of strabismus. There is no correlation between the onset of the arthritis and that of the uveitis. The uveitis may precede the arthritis by 3–10 years. The knee is the most common joint involved. The cardinal signs of the disease are calcific band keratopathy, cells and flare in the anterior chamber, small to medium-sized white KPs with or without flecks of fibrin on the endothelium, posterior synechiae, often progressing to seclusion of the pupil, complicated cataract, variable secondary glaucoma, and macular edema.

Corticosteroids and mydriatics are of value, especially in acute exacerbations, but their long-term effect seems merely to delay the inevitable, ie, severe visual impairment or phthisis bulbi. The prognosis is very poor because of the relentless and progressive char-

Table 8–3. Causes of anterior uveitis.

Autoimmune
Juvenile rheumatoid arthritis
Ankylosing spondylitis
Reiter's syndrome
Ulcerative colitis
Lens-induced uveitis
Crohn's disease
Psoriasis

Infections
Syphilis
Tuberculosis
Herpes zoster
Herpes simplex
Onchocerciasis
Adenovirus

Malignancy
Masquerade syndrome
Retinoblastoma
Leukemia
Lymphoma
Malignant melanoma

Other
Traumatic uveitis
Retinal detachment
Fuchs' heterochromic iridocyclitis
Gout
Glaucomatocyclitic crisis
Idiopathic

acter of the disease, which leads to serious complications. These patients tend to do poorly after surgery.

Iridocyclitis occurring in association with adult peripheral rheumatoid arthritis is strictly coincidental. The adult group is more likely to develop scleritis and sclero-uveitis. It is unfortunate that the associated cells and flare in the aqueous humor that accompany the scleritis have been misinterpreted as "iridocyclitis."

About 10–60% of patients with **Marie-Strümpell ankylosing spondylitis** develop an anterior uveitis. There is a marked preponderance in males. The uveitis presents as a mild to fairly severe nongranulomatous type of iridocyclitis with moderate to severe ciliary injection, pain, blurred vision, and photophobia. It is usually recurrent and eventually may lead to permanent damage if not adequately treated. Histocompatibility antigen HLA-B27 is present in approximately 90% of patients with ankylosing spondylitis.

Ocular examination shows ciliary injection, moderate cells and flare in the anterior chamber, and fine white keratic precipitates located mostly on the inferior cornea. Posterior synechiae, peripheral anterior synechiae, cataracts, and glaucoma are common complications after hyperacute attacks of inflammation. Macular edema occurs in 1% of cases with severe anterior iridocyclitis, which, if persistent, leads to cystoid degeneration and loss of central vision.

Confirmation of the diagnosis is by x-rays of the lumbosacral spine. In about 50% of patients, clinical signs and symptoms may all be absent so that the diagnosis may be made only by the radiologist.

The erythrocyte sedimentation rate, although nonspecific and sometimes normal in mild cases, is elevated in most patients, indicating active disease. The rheumatoid factor test, however, is negative in all but 5% of patients with this disease.

2. HETEROCHROMIC UVEITIS (Fuchs's Heterochromic Iridocyclitis)

This disease of unknown cause accounts for about 3% of all cases of uveitis. It is essentially a quiet cyclitis associated with depigmentation of the iris in the affected eye. Pathologically, the iris and ciliary body show moderate atrophy, patchy depigmentation of the pigment layer, and diffuse infiltration of lymphocytes and plasma cells. Involvement is typically unilateral but may be bilateral, and the irises become different colors. Early in the course of the disease, the difference in color may not be readily apparent and is best noted in daylight.

The onset is insidious in the third or fourth decade, with no redness, pain, or photophobia; the patient is often unaware of the disorder until cataract formation results in blurred vision.

With the slit lamp (or loupe) one sees fine white crenated deposits on the posterior corneal surface, flare and cells in the anterior chamber, and a slightly atrophic iris. Anterior vitreous floaters may be evident with the ophthalmoscope or slit lamp.

Cataract develops within a few years in about 15% of cases. Glaucoma occurs in 10–15% of cases. It is usually not necessary to dilate the pupil, as this is one type of uveitis in which posterior synechiae rarely form. The disease does not subside spontaneously, but the visual prognosis is good since the cataract can usually be removed safely despite the low-grade active uveitis.

3. LENS-INDUCED UVEITIS

There are no data at present to substantiate the implication that lens material per se is toxic, so that the term phacotoxic uveitis should no longer be used to describe lens-induced uveitis. The terms phacogenic or lens-induced uveitis are more appropriate when referring to an autoimmune disease secondary to lens antigen. The classic case of lens-induced uveitis occurs when the lens develops a hypermature cataract. The lens capsule leaks and lens material passes into the anterior chamber, causing an inflammatory reaction characterized by the accumulation of plasma cells, mononuclear phagocytes, and a few polymorphonuclear cells. The eye becomes red and moderately painful; the pupil is small; and vision is markedly reduced (at times to light perception only). Lens-induced uveitis may also occur following traumatic cataracts.

Endophthalmitis phaco-anaphylactica, the term used for the more severe form of lens-induced uveitis, occurs following an extracapsular lens extraction when the same operation has already been performed on the fellow eye and the patient has been sensitized to his or her own lens material. Many polymorphonuclear leukocytes and mononuclear phagocytes appear in the anterior chamber. The eye becomes red and painful, and vision is blurred. Since most of the lens material has already been removed, treatment is conservative, consisting of corticosteroids locally and systemically plus atropine drops to keep the pupil dilated. If this is ineffective, the cataract incision must be opened and the anterior chamber irrigated.

Glaucoma (phacolytic glaucoma) is a common complication of lens-induced uveitis. Treatment consists of lens extraction after intraocular pressure has been brought under control. If this is done, both the uveitis and the glaucoma are cured, and the visual prognosis is good if the process has not been present for more than 1–2 weeks.

INTERMEDIATE UVEITIS (Pars Planitis, Chronic Cyclitis)

The usual patient with pars planitis is a young adult presenting with "floating spots" in the field of vision as the chief complaint. In the majority of cases, both eyes are affected. The sex distribution is equal. Pain, redness, and photophobia do not occur. The patient may be unaware of any ocular problem, but the physician detects vitreous opacities with the ophthalmoscope.

There are few, if any, signs of anterior uveitis. A few cells may occasionally be seen in the anterior chamber; rarely, anterior or posterior synechiae occur. Inflammatory cells are more likely to be seen in the retrolental space or in the anterior vitreous on slit lamp examination. Posterior subcapsular cataract occurs frequently.

Indirect ophthalmoscopy often reveals soft, round, white opacities over the peripheral retina. These cellular exudates may be confluent, often overlying the pars plana. Some of these patients may also have vasculitis, as shown by perivascular sheathing of retinal vessels.

In most patients, the disease remains stationary or gradually improves over a 5- to 10-year period. Some patients develop cystoid macular edema and permanent macular scarring as well as posterior subcapsular cataracts. In severe cases, cyclitic membranes and retinal detachments may occur. Secondary glaucoma is a rare complication.

The cause is unknown. Corticosteroids constitute the only helpful treatment and should only be used in more severe cases, especially when there is decreased vision secondary to macular edema. Topical corticosteroids are used first; if they fail, sub-Tenon or retrobulbar injections of corticosteroids may be effective. Such treatment increases the risk of cataract development. Fortunately, these patients do well following cataract surgery.

POSTERIOR UVEITIS
(Table 8–4)

Differential Diagnosis

The retina and choroid are affected by a variety of infectious and noninfectious disorders. Table 8–1 lists disorders that might involve the posterior segment of the eye.

Most cases of posterior uveitis are associated with some form of systemic disease. The cause of posterior uveitis can often be established on the basis of (1) the morphology of the lesions, (2) the mode of onset and course of the disease, or (3) the association with systemic disease. Other considerations are the age of the patient and whether involvement is unilateral or bilateral. Laboratory tests are of help in confirmation.

Lesions of the posterior segment of the eye can be focal, geographic, or diffuse. Those that cause clouding of the overlying vitreous should be differentiated from those that never give rise to vitreous cells. The type and distribution of vitreous opacities must be described.

Inflammatory lesions of the posterior segment are generally insidious in onset, but some may be accompanied by abrupt development of vitreous clouding and visual loss. Such diseases are usually accompanied by anterior uveitis, which in turn is sometimes associated with a form of secondary glaucoma.

Table 8–4. Causes of posterior uveitis.

Infectious disorders
  Viruses
    CMV, herpes simplex, herpes zoster, rubella, rubeola, human immune deficiency virus, Epstein-Barr virus, coxsackie virus. Probable viral etiology: Acute retinal necrosis.
  Bacteria
    Mycobacterius tuberculosis, brucellosis, sporadic and endemic syphilis, *Nocardia*, *Neisseria meningitidis*, *Mycobacterium avium*, *Yersinia*, and *Borrelia* (cause of Lyme disease).
  Fungi
    Candida, *Histoplasma*, *Cryptococcus*, and *Aspergillus*.
  Parasites
    Toxoplasma, *Toxocara*, *Cysticercus*, and *Onchocerca*.

Noninfectious disorders
  Autoimmune
    Behçet's disease
    Vogt-Koyanagi-Harada syndrome
    Periarteritis nodosa
    Sympathetic ophthalmia
    Retinal vasculitis
  Malignancy
    Reticulum cell sarcoma
    Leukemia
    Metastatic lesions
  Unknown etiology
    Sarcoidosis
    Geographic choroiditis
    Acute multifocal placoid pigment epitheliopathy
    Birdshot retinopathy
    Retinal pigment epitheliopathy

In western United States, the most common causes of posterior uveitis are toxoplasmosis, Behçet's disease, and Vogt-Koyanagi-Harada disease.

In the following paragraphs, clues to the diagnosis and some characteristic clinical features of posterior uveitis are described.

A. Age of the Patient: Posterior uveitis in patients up to 3 years of age may be caused by a masquerade syndrome, such as retinoblastoma or leukemia. Infectious causes of posterior uveitis in this age group include cytomegalovirus (CMV) infection, toxoplasmosis, syphilis, herpetic retinitis, and rubella infection.

In the age group from 4 to 15 years, the causes of posterior uveitis may include toxocariasis, toxoplasmosis, intermediate uveitis, CMV infection, masquerade syndrome, subacute sclerosing panencephalitis, and, less frequently, bacterial or fungal infections of the posterior segment.

In the age group from 16 to 40 years, the differential diagnosis includes toxoplasmosis, Behçet's disease, Vogt-Koyanagi-Harada syndrome, syphilis, candidal endophthalmitis, and, less frequently, endogenous bacterial infection, eg, meningococcal meningitis.

Patients who present with posterior uveitis and are over age 40 years may have acute retinal necrosis syndrome, toxoplasmosis, CMV infection, retinitis, reticulum cell sarcoma, or cryptococcosis.

B. Laterality: Unilateral involvement favors a diagnosis of uveitis due to toxoplasmosis, candidiasis, toxocariasis, acute retinal necrosis syndrome, CMV infection, or endogenous bacterial infection.

C. Symptoms:

1. Reduced vision–Reduced visual acuity is present in all types of posterior uveitis and so is not useful in differential diagnosis.

2. Ocular injection–Redness of the eye occurs in diffuse uveitis and thus is not present with toxoplasmosis or histoplasmosis.

3. Pain–Pain occurs in patients with acute retinal necrosis syndrome, syphilis, endogenous bacterial infection, and posterior scleritis and in conditions involving the optic nerve. Patients with toxoplasmosis, toxocariasis, and CMV retinitis who do not have evidence of glaucoma usually present with no pain in the eye. Other noninfectious posterior segment diseases typically not associated with pain include acute multifocal placoid pigment epitheliopathy, geographic choroiditis, and Vogt-Koyanagi-Harada syndrome.

D. Signs: Signs important in the diagnosis of posterior uveitis include hypopyon, granuloma formation, glaucoma, vitritis, morphology of the lesions, vasculitis, retinal hemorrhages, and old scars.

1. Hypopyon–Disorders of the posterior segment that may present with inflammatory changes in the anterior uvea associated with hypopyon include leukemia, Behçet's disease, syphilis, toxocariasis, and endogenous bacterial infections.

2. Type of uveitis–Anterior granulomatous uveitis may be associated with conditions that affect the posterior retina and choroid. Sarcoidosis, tuberculosis, toxoplasmosis, syphilis, Vogt-Koyanagi-Harada syndrome, and sympathetic ophthalmia may lead to inflammatory changes in the posterior segment of the eye and are usually associated with mutton fat KPs. On the other hand, nongranulomatous anterior uveitis may be associated with Behçet's disease, acute multifocal placoid pigment epitheliopathy, brucellosis, reticulum cell sarcoma, and acute retinal necrosis syndrome.

3. Glaucoma–Secondary glaucoma may be observed in patients with acute retinal necrosis syndrome, toxoplasmosis, tuberculosis, or sarcoidosis.

4. Vitritis–Inflammation of the vitreous body may be associated with posterior uveitis. The inflammatory changes in the vitreous are due to spillover from inflammatory foci in the posterior segment of the eye due to active invasion by infectious agents into the vitreous. Inflammatory changes in the vitreous are not observed in patients with geographic choroiditis or histoplasmosis. Minimal inflammatory cells in the vitreous may be observed in patients with reticulum cell sarcoma, CMV infection, and rubella and in some cases of toxoplasmosis in which small foci of infection are seen in the retina. On the other hand, severe inflammatory changes in the vitreous associated with many cells and large exudates may be seen in tuberculosis, toxocariasis, syphilis, Behçet's disease, nocardiosis, and toxoplasmosis and in patients with endogenous candidal or bacterial endophthalmitis.

5. Morphology and location of lesions–

a. Retina–The retina is the primary target of many types of infectious agents. Toxoplasmosis is a typical example, causing chiefly retinitis and evidence of necrotizing retinitis with inflammation of subjacent choroid. Furthermore, infections with CMV, herpesviruses, rubella virus, and rubeola virus usually involve the retina primarily and cause more retinitis than choroiditis.

Each of these known entities affects the retina more prominently than any other structure in the posterior segment of the eye, and the clinical pictures are fairly characteristic. The active lesion of toxoplasmosis is generally seen in the company of old healed scars of retinochoroiditis that may be heavily pigmented. The lesions may appear in juxtapapillary location and often give rise to retinal vasculitis. The vitreous is generally clouded when large lesions are present. The lesions of CMV infection affect the retina of immunologically compromised hosts. On the other hand, the choroid (see below) is the primary target of insults by a variety of disorders.

b. Choroid–In patients with tuberculosis, the choroid is the primary target of a granulomatous process also affecting the retina. Patients with tuberculosis may present with geographic choroiditis. By contrast, patients with presumed ocular histoplasmosis syndrome have multiple small coinlike lesions that never cloud the overlying vitreous. There is often evidence of certain peripapillary scarring and macular lesions leading to subretinal neovascular nets. In general, there are no signs of systemic disease in patients with presumed ocular histoplasmosis syndrome; but x-rays of the chest may show evidence of dissemination and calcific changes in the periphery of the lung fields. Patients with geographic choroiditis develop predominant involvement of the choroid with little or no affection of the retina and have no systemic disease. The choroid, on the other hand, is primarily involved in sympathetic ophthalmia and Lyme disease.

c. Morphologic features–Active lesions in the various disorders causing posterior uveitis may vary in shape—some geographic and others punctate or nummular. Geographic lesions are seen in CMV retinitis, tuberculosis, toxocariasis, and geographic choroiditis in acute retinal necrosis syndrome. Nummular or punctate lesions are seen in patients with Epstein-Barr viral infection, rubella, rubeola, Behçet's disease, acute multifocal placoid pigment epitheliopathy (AMPPE), and toxoplasmosis. In Vogt-Koyanagi-Harada syndrome and sympathetic ophthalmia, Dalen-Fuchs nodules are seen. Sarcoidosis affects any tissue in the eye and may show geographic lesions, retinal vasculitis, and candle wax drippings. In patients with CMV infection, herpes simplex, rubella, rubeola, and acute retinal necrosis syndrome, the lesions are strictly retinal, with minimal or no inflammatory changes in the subjacent tissue. In patients with Epstein-Barr viral infection, histoplasmosis, tuberculosis, syphilis, nonendemic syphilis, and cryptococcosis, the inflammatory lesions are deep and choroidal and multifocal. On the other hand, in patients with Vogt-Koyanagi-

Harada syndrome and AMPPE, the lesions are at the level of the retinal pigment epithelium. Elevated necrotic whitish lesions are seen in patients with candidal retinitis and toxoplasmosis. In addition, patients with candidal retinitis may also show the "string of pearls" appearance in the vitreous as well as snowball-like lesions floating in the vitreous. Exudative retinal detachment is typically seen in patients with Vogt-Koyanagi-Harada syndrome and Lyme disease. Diffuse choroiditis is seen in Vogt-Koyanagi-Harada syndrome, sympathetic ophthalmia, leukemia, and Lyme disease.

E. Trauma: A history of trauma is important to rule out intraocular foreign body or sympathetic ophthalmia in patients with uveitis.

F. Mode of Onset: The onset of posterior uveitis may be acute and sudden or chronic and insidious. Diseases of the posterior segment of the eye that may present with sudden onset include toxoplasmic retinitis, CMV retinitis, acute retinal necrosis, and bacterial infections. Most other causes of posterior uveitis present with chronic and insidious onset.

1. OCULAR TOXOPLASMOSIS

Toxoplasmosis is caused by *Toxoplasma gondii*, an obligate intracellular protozoan. The ocular lesions may be acquired in utero or may occur following an episode of acute systemic infection. Clinical manifestations range from subclinical to generalized disease with fatal outcome. Toxoplasmosis is the most common current cause of retinochoroiditis in humans and accounts for 28% of cases of posterior uveitis.

The domestic cat and other feline species serve as definitive hosts for the parasite. Susceptible women who acquire the disease during pregnancy may transmit the disease to the fetus. Sources of human infection include öocysts in soil or airborne in dust, undercooked meat containing bradyzoites (encysted forms of the parasite), and tachyzoites (proliferative form) via transplacental transmission.

Clinical Findings
(Fig 8–7)
A. Symptoms and Signs: Patients with toxoplasmic retinochoroiditis present with a history of seeing floaters, blurring of vision, or photophobia. The ocular lesions consist of fluffy-white areas of necrotic focal retinochoroiditis that may be small or large and single or multiple. Active lesions may be adjacent to healed punched-out retinal scars surrounded by retinal edema. Retinal vasculitis may occur, leading to retinal hemorrhages. The inflammation gives rise to vitreous cells and exudations. Cystoid macular edema may occur.

Iridocyclitis is frequently seen in patients with toxoplasmic retinochoroiditis. Healing of retinochoroiditis is associated with decrease in the inflammatory reactions of the iris, ciliary body, and vitreous. The

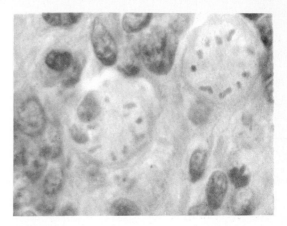

Figure 8–7. *Toxoplasma* cysts in the retina. (Courtesy of K Tabbara.)

retinal lesion develops sharp borders with pigment proliferations.

B. Laboratory Findings: *Toxoplasma* antibodies can be detected in the serum by the Sabin-Feldman dye test, the indirect immunofluorescent antibody test, the hemagglutination test, or ELISA. A finding of a positive serologic test for *Toxoplasma* with consistent clinical signs is considered diagnostically significant. No increase in antibody titer is detected during the recurrences of retinochoroiditis.

Treatment
Small lesions in the periphery of the retina that are not associated with significant vitreous cells may be left without treatment. Treatment of toxoplasmic retinochoroiditis can be initiated by the simultaneous administration of pyrimethamine, 25 mg orally daily, and sulfadiazine, 0.5–1 g orally 4 times daily for 4 weeks. A loading dose of 75 mg of pyrimethamine and 2 g of sulfadiazine may be given at initiation of therapy. In addition, patients are given 3 mg of leucovorin calcium orally twice weekly, and the urine should be kept alkaline by daily intake of 1 tsp of sodium bicarbonate. Because pyrimethamine may cause bone marrow depression, hematopoietic function must be monitored (Table 8–2).

An alternative approach for ocular toxoplasmosis consists of administration of clindamycin, 300 mg orally 4 times daily, with sulfadiazine, 0.5–1 g orally 4 times daily. Clindamycin may cause pseudomembranous colitis in 10–15% of patients. Minocycline has been shown to be effective in the treatment of experimental ocular toxoplasmosis.

Other antibiotics that have been shown to be effective in ocular toxoplasmosis include spiramycin and minocycline. Photocoagulation and cryotherapy have been advocated, but these ablative procedures may lead to complications such as retinal hemorrhages or retinal detachment. Certain retinal neovascular membranes caused by toxoplasmosis may be treated by photocoagulation.

Anterior uveitis associated with ocular toxoplasmosis may be treated with 1% prednisolone eye drops 3–4 times daily and 5% homatropine eye drops twice daily. Timolol maleate (0.25% eye drops) may be added if intraocular pressure is increased. Periocular steroid are contraindicated. Systemic corticosteroids in conjunction with antimicrobial therapy may be administered for vision-threatening inflammatory lesions. Corticosteroids should not be given without appropriate antimicrobial coverage.

2. HISTOPLASMOSIS

In some areas of the USA where histoplasmosis is endemic (eg, Cincinnati, Baltimore), the diagnosis of choroiditis presumably due to histoplasmosis is being made with increasing frequency. The patient usually has a positive skin test to histoplasmin and demonstrates "punched-out" spots in the peripheral fundus. These spots are small, irregularly round or oval, depigmented areas, sometimes with a fine pigmented border. They are smaller and have less pigment than the usual healed chorioretinal lesion. Peripapillary atrophy and hyperpigmentation are usually present. Macular lesions that begin as small edematous areas and may progress to hemorrhagic detachments are the most visually threatening feature of the disease. Vitreous haze does not occur.

It has been postulated that in areas where histoplasmosis is endemic, many persons develop a benign form of asymptomatic peripheral chorioretinitis. These lesions soon heal, leaving "histo" spots. This exposure sensitizes the choroid. A later antigenic insult to the choroid results in the observed macular changes. This hypothesis has not been verified, but it has stood the test of time since first postulated by Woods in 1959.

Many types of treatment have been advocated, including systemic corticosteroids, amphotericin B (Fungizone), antihistamines, intradermal desensitization with histoplasmin. The results have been questionable in all cases, and treatment with amphotericin B is now contraindicated.

Blue-green argon laser photocoagulation has been shown to be effective in the treatment of those paramacular lesions that cause leaks demonstrable by fluorescein angiography. This form of treatment has limited application since most lesions involve the macula directly and are thus not suitable for coagulation.

3. OCULAR TOXOCARIASIS

Toxocariasis is infection with *Toxocara cati* (an intestinal parasite of cats) or *Toxocara cani* (of dogs). Visceral larva migrans is a disseminated systemic infection occurring in a young child (Table 8–5). Ocular involvement does not occur in visceral larva migrans.

Ocular toxocariasis may occur without systemic manifestations. Children acquire the disease by close association with pets and by eating dirt contaminated with *Toxocara* ova. The ingested ova form larvae that penetrate the intestinal mucosa and gain access to the systemic circulation and finally to the eye. The parasite does not infect the intestinal tract of humans.

Clinical Findings

A. Symptoms and Signs: The disease is usually unilateral. *Toxocara* larvae lodge in the retina and die, leading to a marked inflammatory reaction and local production of *Toxocara* antibodies. Children are brought to the ophthalmologist because of redness, blurred vision, or a whitish pupil or after failing a screening vision test at school.

The ocular findings consist of a peripheral focal whitish granuloma. The granuloma may occur anywhere in the posterior pole. Death of the larva is associated with a severe uveitis that may lead to diffuse endophthalmitis. Whitish exudates and fibrosis may occur in the vitreous. Iridocyclitis and cataract may complicate the course of the disease.

Table 8–5. Comparison between visceral and ocular larva migrans.

	Visceral Larva Migrans	Ocular Larva Migrans[1]
Average age at onset	2 years	7 years
Fever	+	−
Abdominal symptoms (pain, nausea, diarrhea)	+	−
Nonspecific pulmonary disease	+	−
Hepatosplenomegaly	+	−
Eosinophilia	+	−
Hypergammaglobulinemia	+	−
ELISA (serum anti-*Toxocara* antibodies)	+	±
ELISA (aqueous anti-*Toxocara* antibodies)	−	+
Ocular findings[1]	−	+

[1] Ocular findings of ocular larva migrans: diffuse chronic panuveitis, posterior pole granuloma, or peripheral granuloma.

B. Laboratory Findings: The enzyme-linked immunosorbent assay (ELISA) for *T canis* antibody has helped in the diagnosis of toxocariasis. A positive test for ocular toxocariasis is a titer of 1:8. The antibody titer of the ocular fluids of patients with ocular toxocariasis is elevated and is higher than that in serum, suggesting local antibody production. Aqueous and vitreous specimens subjected to ELISA are therefore helpful in the diagnosis of ocular toxocariasis.

Treatment

Systemic or periocular injections of corticosteroids should be given when there is evidence of an intraocular inflammatory reaction. Vitrectomy may have to be considered in patients with marked vitreous fibrosis. Thiobendazole has been used for the treatment of toxocariasis, but no anthelmintic has been shown to be effective in ocular toxocariasis, and the intraocular inflammation is aggravated by the death and disintegration of the parasite. Corticosteroids help to prevent ocular damage from the inflammatory reactions.

4. ACQUIRED IMMUNODEFICIENCY SYNDROME

Posterior uveitis may be seen in patients with AIDS. Ophthalmic manifestations in this disease are frequent and may have both prognostic and diagnostic significance. Clinical and histopathologic studies have led to a better understanding of ophthalmic disorders associated with AIDS.

Ocular manifestations include cotton-wool spots, retinal hemorrhages, Kaposi's sarcoma of the ocular surface and adnexa, and neuro-ophthalmologic abnormalities associated with intracranial disease.

In addition, patients with AIDS frequently develop infections by opportunistic organisms. Cytomegalovirus retinopathy is a blinding disease and is the most common ocular infection in patients with AIDS. Other infections that may cause ocular manifestations in patients with AIDS include *Pneumocystis carinii*, *Candida* species, *Toxoplasma gondii*, *Mycobacterium avium-intracellulare*, and *Cryptococcus*.

DIFFUSE UVEITIS (Table 8–6)

1. SYMPATHETIC OPHTHALMIA (Sympathetic Uveitis)

Sympathetic ophthalmia is a rare but devastating granulomatous bilateral uveitis that comes on 10 days to many years following a perforating eye injury in the region of the ciliary body, or following retained foreign body. The cause is not known, but the disease is probably related to hypersensitivity to some element of the pigment-bearing cells in the uvea. It very rarely occurs following uncomplicated intraocular surgery for cataract or glaucoma.

Table 8–6. Causes of diffuse uveitis.

Sarcoidosis
Tuberculosis
Syphilis
Brucellosis
Sympathetic ophthalmia
Behçet's disease
Vogt-Koyanagi-Harada syndrome
Amyloidosis
Masquerade syndrome: Retinoblastoma, leukemia
Retained intraocular foreign body

The injured (exciting) eye becomes inflamed first and the fellow (sympathizing) eye second. Pathologically, there is a diffuse granulomatous uveitis. The epithelioid cells, together with giant cells and lymphocytes (Fig 8–8), form noncaseating tubercles. From the uveal tract the inflammatory process spreads to the optic nerve and to the pia and arachnoid surrounding the optic nerve.

The patient complains of photophobia, redness, and blurring of vision. If a history of trauma is obtained, look for a scar representing the wound of entry in the exciting eye. With the slit lamp or loupe one sees KPs and a flare in the anterior chamber of both eyes. Iris nodules may be present.

Sympathetic ophthalmia may be differentiated from other granulomatous uveitides by the history of trauma or ocular surgery and by the fact that it is bilateral, diffuse, and (usually) acute rather than unilateral, localized, and chronic.

The recommended treatment of a severely injured sightless eye (eg, a penetrating injury through the sclera, ciliary body, and lens, with loss of vitreous) is immediate enucleation to prevent sympathetic ophthalmia, and every effort must be made to secure the patient's informed consent to the operation. If enucleation can be performed within 10 days after injury,

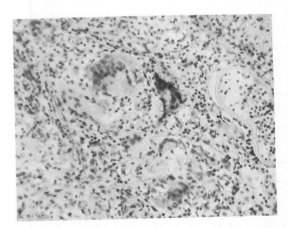

Figure 8–8. Microscopic section of giant cells and lymphocytes in sympathetic ophthalmia involving the choroid. (Courtesy of R Carriker.)

there is almost no chance that sympathetic ophthalmia will develop. However, when the inflammation in the sympathizing eye is advanced, it is wise not to enucleate the injured eye, since it may eventually prove to be the better of 2 very bad eyes.

If inflammation appears in the sympathizing eye, treat at once with local corticosteroids and atropine. Systemic corticosteroids or cytotoxic drugs may be required. Cyclosporine has also proved useful in intractable cases. (See Table 8–2.)

Without treatment, the disease progresses slowly but relentlessly over a period of months or years to complete bilateral blindness.

2. TUBERCULOUS UVEITIS

Tuberculosis causes a granulomatous type of uveitis if the patient is not receiving topical steroids. Tuberculous uveitis is diagnosed clinically far more often than the disease can be proved by positive identification of tubercle bacilli in the tissues. Although the infection is said to be transmitted from a primary focus elsewhere in the body, uveal tuberculosis is rare in patients with active pulmonary tuberculosis.

Tuberculous uveitis may be diffuse but is characteristically localized in the form of a severe caseating granulomatous chorioretinitis. The tubercle itself consists of giant cells and epithelioid cells. Caseation necrosis commonly occurs.

The patient complains of blurred vision, and the eye is moderately injected. If the anterior segment is involved, iris nodules and "mutton fat" KPs are visible on slit lamp examination. If the choroid and retina are primarily affected, one can see a localized yellowish mass partially obscured by a hazy vitreous.

The nodules and the localized nature of tuberculous uveitis help to make a clinical differentiation from sympathetic ophthalmia, and the caseation necrosis differentiates it pathologically from sympathetic ophthalmia and Boeck's sarcoid.

The pupil should be kept dilated with atropine, 1%, 1 drop 2–3 times daily. Antituberculosis drugs should be prescribed systemically if a reasonably certain clinical diagnosis can be made. (See Table 8–2.)

After a prolonged course of several months, the disease usually resolves, leaving permanently damaged tissue and blurred vision because of scarring of the retina.

3. SARCOIDOSIS

Sarcoidosis is a chronic granulomatous disease of unknown cause characterized by multiple cutaneous and subcutaneous nodules, with similar invasions in the viscera and bones, and periodic exacerbations and remissions. The onset is usually in the third decade. The tissue reaction is much less severe than in tuberculous uveitis, and caseation does not occur. The

tuberculin skin test is usually negative or only faintly positive. When the parotid glands are involved, the disease is called uveoparotid fever (Heerfordt's disease); when the lacrimal glands are involved, it is called Mikulicz's syndrome.

Thirty percent of cases are complicated by chronic bilateral anterior uveitis, whereas posterior uveitis is far less common. Anterior uveitis is nodular, and in prolonged cases it may lead to severe visual impairment due to cataract and secondary glaucoma. Posterior uveitis is characterized by multiple whitish-yellow retinal and periretinal exudates (candle wax drippings) along with perivasculitis.

Diagnosis should be supported by biopsy of the cutaneous nodules. In a small number of cases, typical nodules were also found on the tarsal or bulbar conjunctiva. Chest x-ray may show prominent hilar adenopathy, while serum angiotensin converting enzyme or serum lysozyme concentrations may be elevated.

Corticosteroid therapy (Table 8–2) given early in the disease may be effective, but recurrences are common and the long-term visual prognosis is poor.

4. ONCHOCERCIASIS

Onchocerciasis is caused by *Onchocerca volvulus*. The disease afflicts about 30 million people in Africa and Central America and is a major cause of blindness. It is transmitted by *Simulium damnosum*, a black fly that breeds in areas of rapidly flowing streams—thus the term river blindness. Microfilariae picked up from the skin by the fly mature into larvae that become adult worms in 1 year. The parasite produces cutaneous nodules 5–25 mm in diameter on the trunk, thighs, arms, head, and shoulders. Microfilariae cause itching, and healing of skin lesions may lead to loss of skin elasticity and areas of depigmentation. Lymphedema may occur secondary to lymphatic involvement.

Clinical Findings

A. Symptoms and Signs: Skin nodules may be seen. The cornea reveals nummular keratitis and sclerosing keratitis. Microfilariae swimming actively in the anterior chamber look like silver threads. Death of the microfilariae causes an intense inflammatory reaction and severe uveitis, vitritis, and retinitis. Focal retinochoroiditis may be seen. Optic atrophy may develop secondary to glucoma.

B. Laboratory Findings: The diagnosis of onchocerciasis is made by a snip skin biopsy and microscopic examination looking for live microfilariae.

Treatment

The preferred treatment for onchocerciasis is with nodulectomy and ivermectin. Diethylcarbamazine and suramin have significant toxicity and should be used only when ivermectin is not available. For dosages and other comments pertaining to those drugs, see the eleventh edition (1986) of this book.

The great advantage of ivermectin over diethylcarbamazine is that a single oral dose of 100 or 200 µg/kg reduces the worm burden in the skin and anterior chamber more slowly and therefore with a significant reduction in systemic and ocular reactions. The reduction also persists longer.

The minimum effective dose remains to be determined. A dose of 100 µg/kg may be as effective as 200 µg/kg and is associated with fewer of the mild and transient side effects: fever, headache, etc. Treatment is repeated at 6 or 12 months.

Ivermectin is not marketed in the USA, but the drug is available on a compassionate basis from the manufacturer, Merck Sharp & Dohme.

Topical therapy with corticosteroids and cycloplegics is helpful for uveitis.

5. CYSTICERCOSIS

Cysticercosis is a common cause of serious ocular morbidity. The disease is endemic in Mexico and other Central and South American countries. It is caused either by the ingestion of eggs of *Taenia solium* or by reverse peristalsis in cases of intestinal obstruction caused by adult tape worms. Eggs mature and embryos penetrate intestinal mucosa, thus gaining access to the circulation. The larva (*Cysticercus cellulosae*) is the most common tapeworm that invades the human eye.

Clinical Findings

The larvae may reach the subretinal space and can migrate under the retina. Larvae may live in the eye for as long as 2 years. Death of the larvae inside the eye leads to a severe inflammatory reaction.

Movements of larvae within the ocular tissue may stimulate a chronic inflammatory reaction and fibrosis.

In rare instances, the larva may be seen in the anterior chamber. Involvement of the brain is a cause of convulsions. Calcification may be seen in the subcutaneous tissue by x-ray.

Treatment

Treatment of cysticercosis is by surgical removal. Subretinal cysticerci can be removed by localized sclerotomy or destroyed by photocoagulation.

REFERENCES

Aaberg TM, Obrien WJ: Expanding ophthalmologic recognition of Epstein-Barr infections. *Am J Ophthalmol* 1987;**104**:420.

Bialasiewicz AA et al: Bilateral diffuse choroiditis and exudative retinal detachments with evidence of Lyme disease. *Am J Ophthalmol* 1988;**105**:419.

Canning CR, Hungerford J: Familial uveal melanoma. *Br J Ophthalmol* 1988;**72**:241.

de Souza EC et al: Unusual central chorioretinitis as the first manifestation of early secondary syphilis. *Am J Ophthalmol* 1988;**105**:271.

Gass JD: Sympathetic ophthalmia following vitrectomy. *Am J Ophthalmol* 1982;**93**:552.

Henderly DE et al: Changing patterns of uveitis. *Am J Ophthalmol* 1987;**103**:131.

Hoover DL, Khan JA, Giangiacomo J: Pediatric ocular sarcoidosis. *Surv Ophthalmol* 1986;**30**:215.

Kaplan HJ, Waldrep JC: Immunologic insights into uveitis and retinitis: The immunoregulatory circuit. *Ophthalmology* 1984;**91**:655.

Kraus-Mackiw E, O'Connor GR: *Uveitis: Pathophysiology and Therapy.* Thieme-Stratton, 1983.

Lakhanpal V, Schocket SS, Nirankari VS: Clindamycin in the treatment of toxoplasmic retinochoroiditis. *Am J Ophthalmol* 1983;**95**:605.

Macular Photocoagulation Study Group: Argon laser photocoagulation for ocular histoplasmosis: Results of a randomized clinical trial. *Arch Ophthalmol* 1983; **101**:1347.

Meredith TA, Wilson LA, Kaplan HJ: Role of vitrectomy in Staphylococcus epidermidis endophthalmitis. *Br J Ophthalmol* 1988;**72**:321.

Newman PE et al: The role of hypersensitivity reactions to *Toxoplasma* antigens in experimental ocular toxoplasmosis in nonhuman primates. *Am J Ophthalmol* 1982;**94**:159.

Noble KG, Carr RE: Toxoplasma retinochoroiditis. *Ophthalmology* 1982;**89**:1289.

Nussenblatt RB et al: Treatment of intraocular inflammatory disease with cyclosporin A. *Lancet* 1983;**2**:235.

O'Connor GR: Factors related to the initiation and recurrence of uveitis. *Am J Ophthalmol* 1983;**96**:577.

Passo MS, Rosenbaum JT: Ocular syphilis in patients with human immunodeficiency virus infection. *Am J Ophthalmol* 1988;**106**:1.

Rothova A et al: Clinical features of acute anterior uveitis. *Am J Ophthalmol* 1987;**103**:137.

Shields JA et al: The differential diagnosis of posterior uveal melanoma. *Ophthalmology* 1980;**87**:518.

Smith RE, Nozik RM: *Uveitis: A Clinical Approach to Diagnosis and Management.* Williams & Wilkins, 1983.

Smith RE, O'Connor GR: Cataract extraction in Fuchs' syndrome. *Arch Ophthalmol* 1974;**91**:39.

Tabbara KF: Chlorambucil in Behçet's disease: A reappraisal. *Ophthalmology* 1983;**90**:906.

Tabbara KF: Management of ocular toxoplasmosis. *Trans Pac Coast Oto-Ophthalmol Soc* 1982;**63**:23.

Tabbara KF: Ocular toxoplasmosis. Pages 1–23 in: *Clinical Ophthalmology.* Duane TD (editor). Harper & Row, 1987.

Tiedman JS: Epstein-Barr viral antibodies in multifocal choroiditis and pan uveitis. *Am J Ophthalmol* 1987;103:**659**.

Wilson CA, Choromokos EA, Sheppard R: Acute posterior multifocal placoid pigment epitheliopathy and cerebral vasculitis. *Arch Ophthalmol* 1988;**106**:796.

9

Lens

John P. Shock, MD

ANATOMY & FUNCTION

The lens is a biconvex, avascular, colorless and almost completely transparent structure, about 4 mm thick and 9 mm in diameter. It is suspended behind the iris by the zonule, which connects it with the ciliary body. Anterior to the lens is the aqueous; posterior to it, the vitreous. The lens capsule (see below) is a semipermeable membrane (slightly more permeable than a capillary wall) that will admit water and electrolytes.

A subcapsular epithelium is present anteriorly (Fig 9–1). The lens nucleus is harder than the cortex. With age, subepithelial lamellar fibers are continuously produced, so that the lens gradually becomes larger and less elastic throughout life. The nucleus and cortex are made up of long concentric lamellas. The suture lines formed by the end-to-end joining of these lamellar fibers are Y-shaped when viewed with the slit lamp (Fig 9–2). The Y is erect anteriorly and inverted posteriorly.

Each lamellar fiber contains a flattened nucleus. These nuclei are evident microscopically in the peripheral portion of the lens near the equator and are continuous with the subcapsular epithelium.

The lens is held in place by a suspensory ligament known as the zonule (zonule of Zinn). This is composed of numerous fibrils that arise from the surface of the ciliary body and insert into the lens equator.

The primary function of the lens is to focus light rays upon the retina. In order to focus light from a distant object, the ciliary muscle relaxes, tautening the zonular fibers and reducing the anteroposterior diameter of the lens to its minimal dimension; in this position the refractive power of the lens is minimized, and parallel rays are thus focused upon the retina. In order to focus light from a near object, the ciliary muscle contracts, pulling the choroid forward and releasing the tension on the zonules. The elastic lens capsule then molds the lens into a more spherical body with correspondingly greater refractive power. The physiologic interplay of the ciliary body, zonule, and

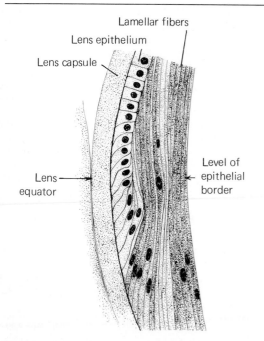

Figure 9–1. Magnified view of lens showing termination of subcapsular epithelium (vertical section).

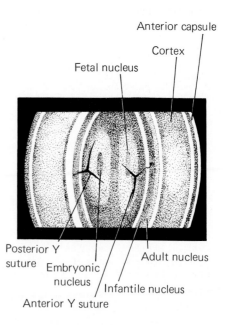

Figure 9–2. Zones of lens showing Y sutures.

[Figs 9–1 and 9–2 are redrawn from Duke-Elder WS: *Textbook of Ophthalmology.* Vol 1. Mosby, 1942. Drawings first appeared in Salzmann M: *Anatomy and History of the Human Eyeball in the Normal State.* Univ of Chicago Press, 1912.]

lens that results in focusing near objects upon the retina is known as **accommodation.** As the lens ages, its accommodative power is gradually reduced.

Composition

The lens consists of about 65% water, about 35% protein (the highest protein content of any tissue of the body), and a trace of minerals common to other body tissues. Potassium is more concentrated in the lens than in most tissues. Ascorbic acid and glutathione are present in both the oxidized and reduced forms.

There are no pain fibers, blood vessels, or nerves in the lens.

Physiology of Symptoms

Disorders of the lens include opacification, distortion, dislocation, and geometric anomalies. Patients with these conditions have blurred vision without pain. Examination for diseases of the lens is by visual acuity testing and by viewing the lens with a slit lamp, ophthalmoscope, hand flashlight, or loupe, preferably through a dilated pupil.

CATARACT

A cataract is a lens opacity. Cataracts vary markedly in degree of density and may be due to a variety of causes but are usually associated with aging. Some degree of cataract formation is to be expected in persons over age 70. Most are bilateral, although the rate of progression in each eye is seldom equal. Traumatic cataract, congenital cataract, and other types are less common.

Cataractous lenses are characterized by lens edema, protein alteration, necrosis, and disruption of the normal continuity of the lens fibers. In general, lens edema varies directly with the stage of cataract development. The immature (incipient) cataract is only slightly opaque. A completely opaque mature (moderately advanced) cataractous lens is somewhat edematous. If the water content is maximal and the lens capsule is stretched, the cataract is called intumescent (swollen). In the hypermature (far-advanced) cataract, water has escaped from the lens, leaving a relatively dehydrated, very opaque lens and a wrinkled capsule.

Most cataracts are not visible to the casual observer until they become dense enough (mature or hypermature) to cause blindness. However, a cataract in its earliest stages of development can be observed through a well-dilated pupil with an ophthalmoscope, loupe, or slit lamp.

The ocular fundus becomes increasingly more difficult to visualize as the lens opacity becomes denser, until the fundus reflection is completely absent. At this stage the cataract is usually mature and the pupil may be white.

The clinical degree of cataract formation, assuming that no other eye disease is present, is judged primarily by the visual acuity. Generally speaking, the decrease in visual acuity is directly proportionate to the density of the cataract. However, some individuals who have clinically significant cataracts when examined with the ophthalmoscope or slit lamp see well enough to carry on with their normal activities. Others have a decrease in visual acuity out of proportion to the degree of lens opacification. This is due to distortion of the image by the partially opaque lens.

Cataract formation is characterized chemically by a reduction in oxygen uptake and an initial increase in water content followed by dehydration. Sodium and calcium content is increased; potassium, ascorbic acid, and protein content is decreased. Glutathione is not present in cataractous lenses. Attempts to accelerate or retard these chemical changes by medical treatment have not been successful, and their causes and implications are not known.

During the past few years, there has been increasing evidence implicating ultraviolet radiation as a significant factor in the occurrence of senile cataracts. Epidemiologic investigations have shown that for persons age 65 years or older there is an increased incidence of cataracts in geographic areas where there are long periods of strong sunlight. Further investigation of the effects of ultraviolet light on the lens is warranted.

AGE-RELATED CATARACT
(Senile Cataract)

Age-related cataract (Figs 9–3 to 9–5) is by far the most common type of cataract. Increasingly blurred vision and visual distortion are the only symptoms. Paradoxically, although distant vision is blurred in the incipient stage of cataract formation, near vision may improve slightly, so the patient will read better without glasses ("second sight"). This artificial myopia is due to the greater convexity of the lens in the incipient stage.

There is no medical treatment for cataract. Lens extraction (see Cataract Surgery, below) is indicated when visual impairment interferes with the patient's normal activities. If glaucoma secondary to lens swelling (intumescent lens) occurs, surgical extraction of the lens is indicated.

Glaucoma and lens-induced uveitis are uncommon complications. Lens-induced uveitis requires surgical extraction of the lens to remove the source of the offending lens products.

Senile cataract is usually slowly progressive over years, and death may occur before surgery becomes necessary. If surgery is indicated, lens extraction definitely improves visual acuity in well over 90% of cases. The remainder of patients either have preexisting retinal damage or develop serious postsurgical complications such as glaucoma, retinal detachment, vitreous hemorrhage, infection, or epithelial down-

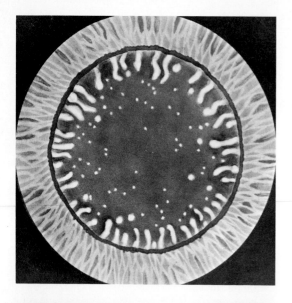

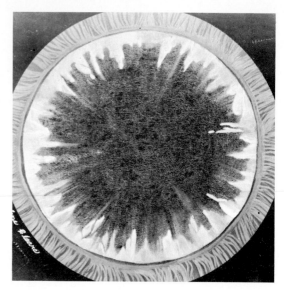

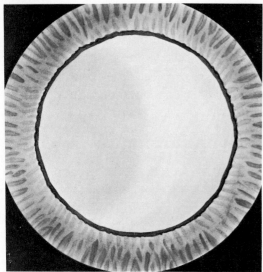

Figure 9–3. Cataract types. **Above, left:** senile cataract, "coronary" type: club-shaped peripheral opacities with clear central lens; slowly progressive. **Above, right:** Senile cataract, "cuneiform" type: peripheral spicules and central clear lens; slowly progressive. **Left:** Senile cataract, "morgagnian" type (hypermature lens); the entire lens is opaque, and the lens nucleus has fallen inferiorly. (Reproduced, with permission, from Cordes FC: *Cataract Types,* 3rd ed. American Academy of Ophthalmology and Otolaryngology, 1954.)

growth into the anterior chamber, which prevent significant visual improvement.

Intraocular lenses and corneal contact lenses have made adjustment following cataract operation much easier than was the rule when only thick cataract glasses were available.

CHILDHOOD CATARACT
(Figs 9–6 and 9–7)

Childhood cataracts are divided into 2 groups: congenital (infantile) cataracts, which are present at birth

or appear shortly thereafter; and acquired cataracts, which occur later and are usually related to a specific cause. Either type may be unilateral or bilateral and partial or complete.

Many congenital cataracts are of unknown cause though probably genetically determined; others are secondary to metabolic or infectious diseases or associated with a variety of syndromes. A search for a cause is appropriate, but in most cases none can be identified.

Acquired cataracts arise most commonly from trauma, either blunt or penetrating. Other causes in-

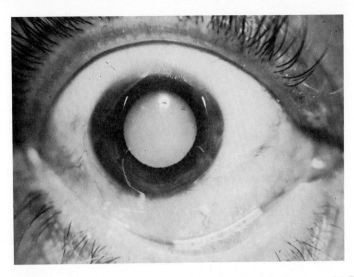

Figure 9–4. Mature senile cataract viewed through a dilated pupil. (Courtesy of A Rosenberg.)

clude uveitis, acquired ocular infections, diabetes, and drugs.

Clinical Findings

A. Congenital Cataract: Congenital lens opacities are common and often visually insignificant. A partial opacification or one out of the visual axis—or not dense enough to interfere significantly with light transmission—requires no treatment other than observation for progression. Dense central congenital cataracts require surgery.

Congenital cataracts that cause significant visual loss must be detected early—preferably in the newborn nursery by the pediatrician or family physician. Large, dense white cataracts may present as leukocoria noticeable by parents, but many dense cataracts cannot be seen by the parents. Unilateral infantile cataracts that are dense, central, and larger than 2 mm in diameter will cause permanent deprivation amblyopia

if not treated within the first 2 months of life and thus require surgical management on an urgent basis. Symmetric bilateral cataracts demand less urgent management, but bilateral deprivation amblyopia can result from unwarranted delay.

B. Acquired Cataract: Acquired cataracts do not require the same urgent care (aimed at preventing amblyopia) as infantile cataracts, because the children are older and the visual system more mature. Surgical assessment is based on the location, size, and density of the cataract, but a period of observation along with subjective visual acuity testing can be part of the decision process. Because unilateral cataracts in children will not produce any symptoms or signs parents would routinely notice, screening programs are important for case finding.

Treatment

Surgical treatment of infantile and early childhood

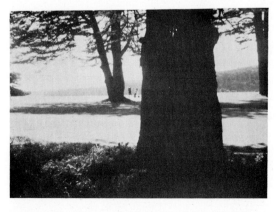 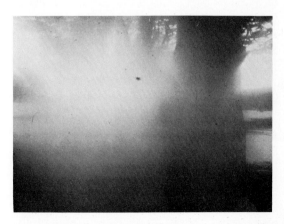

Figure 9–5. Senile cataract. In the photo at right the scene shown at left is reproduced as if seen by a person with a moderately advanced senile cataract (opacity denser centrally). (Courtesy of E Goodner.)

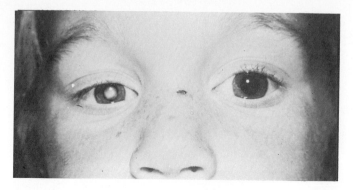

Figure 9–6. Congenital cataract.

cataracts involves lens extraction through a 3-mm lim-bal incision utilizing a mechanical irrigation-aspiration handpiece. Phacoemulsification is rarely required. In contrast to adult lens extraction, the posterior capsule and anterior vitreous are removed by most surgeons using a mechanical vitreous suction-cutting instrument. This prevents formation of secondary capsular opacification, or after-cataract. Primary removal of the posterior capsule therefore avoids the necessity for secondary surgery and enhances early optical correction.

Using today's sophisticated surgical techniques, operative and postoperative complications are similar to those reported with adult cataract procedures. With experience, the childhood cataract surgeon can expect good technical results in well over 90% of cases.

Optical correction can consist of spectacles in older bilaterally aphakic children, but most childhood cataract operations should be followed by contact lens correction. This is crucial in infants and requires much time and effort by the surgeon and the parents.

Prognosis

The visual prognosis for childhood cataract patients requiring surgery is not as good as that for patients with senile cataract. The associated amblyopia and occasional anomalies of the optic nerve or retina limit the degree of useful vision that can be achieved in this group of patients. The prognosis for improvement of visual acuity is worst following surgery for unilateral congenital cataracts and best for incomplete bilateral congenital cataracts that are slowly progressive.

TRAUMATIC CATARACT

Traumatic cataract (Figs 9–8 to 9–10) is most commonly due to a foreign body injury to the lens or blunt trauma to the eyeball. BB shot is a frequent cause; less frequent causes include arrows, rocks, contusions, overexposure to heat ("glassblower's cataract"), x-rays, and radioactive materials. Most

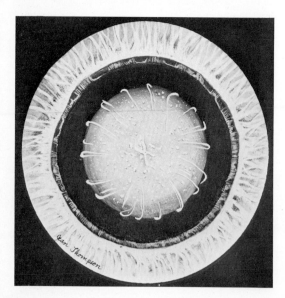

Figure 9–7. Congenital cataract, zonular type. One zone of lens involved. The cortex is relatively clear.

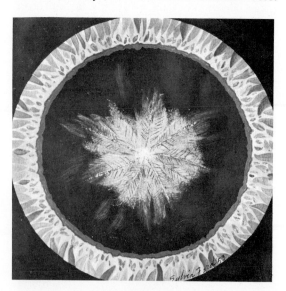

Figure 9–8. Traumatic "star-shaped" cataract in the posterior lens. This is usually due to ocular contusion and is only detectable through a well-dilated pupil.

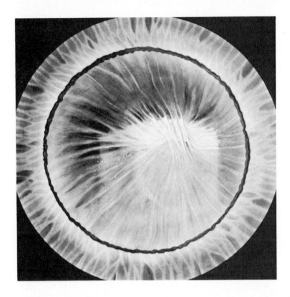

Figure 9–9. Traumatic cataract with wrinkled anterior capsule.

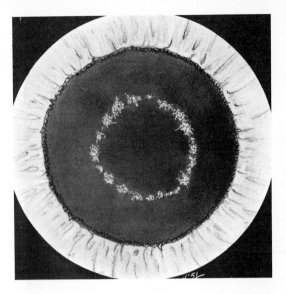

Figure 9–10. "Vossius' ring." Traumatic cataract caused by the imprint of the iris pigment on the anterior surface of the lens. The remainder of the lens is clear, and vision is not impaired.

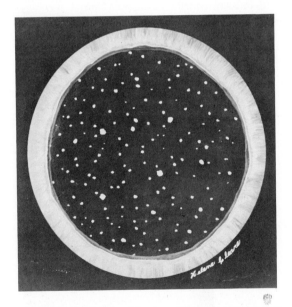

Figure 9–11. Punctate dot cataract. This type of cataract is sometimes seen as an ocular complication of diabetes mellitus. It may also be congenital.

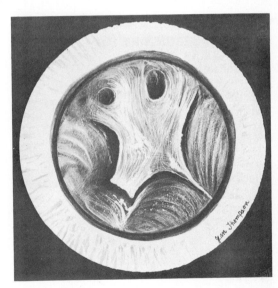

Figure 9–12. After-cataract.

[Figs 9–7 to 9–12 are reproduced, with permission, from Cordes FC: *Cataract Types,* 3rd ed. American Academy of Ophthalmology and Otolaryngology, 1954.]

traumatic cataracts are preventable. In industry, the best safety measure is a good pair of safety goggles.

The lens becomes white soon after the entry of the foreign body since the interruption of the lens capsule allows aqueous and sometimes vitreous to penetrate into the lens structure. The patient is often an industrial worker who gives a history of striking steel upon steel. A minute fragment of a steel hammer, for example, may pass through the cornea and lens at a tremendous rate of speed and lodge in the vitreous, where it can usually be seen with the ophthalmoscope.

The patient complains immediately of blurred vision. The eye becomes red, the lens opaque, and there may be an intraocular hemorrhage. If aqueous or vitreous escapes from the eye, the eye becomes extremely soft. Complications include infection, uveitis, retinal detachment, and glaucoma.

A magnetic intraocular foreign body should be removed without delay.

Systemic and topical antibiotics and topical corticosteroids should be given over a period of several days to minimize the chance of infection and uveitis. Atropine sulfate, 1%, 1 drop 3 times daily, is recommended to keep the pupil dilated and to prevent the formation of posterior synechiae.

The cataract can be removed at the same time the foreign body is removed or after the inflammation subsides. If glaucoma occurs during the waiting period, cataract surgery should not be delayed even though inflammation is still present. Some time after cataract surgery, a thin opaque membrane may occur, in which case discission with the neodymium-YAG laser (see After-Cataract) or a knife may be necessary to improve vision. The same techniques utilized for removal of congenital cataracts are generally used for the removal of traumatic cataracts, especially in patients under 30 years of age.

CATARACT SECONDARY TO INTRAOCULAR DISEASE ("Complicated Cataract")

Cataract may develop as a direct effect of intraocular disease upon the physiology of the lens (eg, severe recurrent uveitis). The cataract usually begins in the posterior subcapsular area and eventually involves the entire lens structure. Intraocular diseases commonly associated with the development of cataracts are chronic or recurrent uveitis, glaucoma, retinitis pigmentosa, and retinal detachment.

These cataracts are usually unilateral. The visual prognosis is not as good as in ordinary senile cataract.

CATARACT ASSOCIATED WITH SYSTEMIC DISEASE

Bilateral cataracts may occur in association with the following systemic disorders: diabetes mellitus (Fig 9–11), hypoparathyroidism, myotonic dystrophy, atopic dermatitis, galactosemia, and Lowe's, Werner's, and Down's syndromes.

TOXIC CATARACT

Toxic cataract is uncommon. Many cases appeared in the 1930s as a result of ingestion of dinitrophenol, a drug taken to suppress appetite. Other offenders are triparanol (MER/29) and corticosteroids administered over a long period of time. It has been suggested that echothiophate iodide, a strong miotic used in the treatment of glaucoma, may cause cataracts.

AFTER-CATARACT (Secondary Membrane)

After-cataract (Fig 9–12) denotes opacification of the posterior capsule due to partially absorbed traumatic cataract or following extracapsular cataract extraction.

Persistent subcapsular lens epithelium may attempt regeneration of lens fibers, giving the posterior capsule a "fish egg" appearance (Elschnig's pearls). The proliferating epithelium may produce multiple layers, leading to frank opacification. These cells may also undergo myofibroblastic differentiation. Their contraction produces numerous tiny wrinkles in the posterior capsule, resulting in visual distortion. All of these factors may lead to reduced visual acuity following extracapsular cataract extraction.

After-cataract has become a significant problem in that almost all pediatric patients and approximately half of adult patients develop an opaque secondary membrane after extracapsular cataract extraction. Before the neodymium-YAG laser came into use, this condition was treated by performing a small capsulotomy with a needle knife or barbed 27-gauge needle, either at the time of the original operation or as a secondary procedure.

In recent years, the neodymium-YAG laser has gained popularity as a noninvasive method for discission of the posterior capsule. Pulses of laser energy cause small "explosions" in target tissue, creating a small hole in the posterior capsule in the pupillary axis. Complications of this technique include a transient rise in intraocular pressure, damage to the intraocular lens, and rupture of the anterior hyaloid face with forward displacement of vitreous into the anterior chamber. The rise in intraocular pressure is usually detectable within 3 hours posttreatment and resolves within a few days with treatment. Rarely, the pressure may not return to normal for several weeks. One group has found that the rise in intraocular pressure is significantly greater in aphakic eyes than in pseudophakic eyes. Small pits or cracks may occur on the intraocular lens, but they usually have no effect on visual acuity. In the aphakic eye, rupture of the vitreous face with anterior displacement of vitreous may predispose to development of rhegmatogenous retinal detachment or cystoid macular edema. Current studies indicate that no significant damage is done to corneal endothelium with the neodymium-YAG laser.

CATARACT SURGERY

Cataract surgery has changed dramatically over the past 20 years, principally as a result of introduction of the operating microscope, better instrumentation, improved suture material, and refinement of the intraocular lens. In cataract surgery, the lens is removed from the eye (lens extraction) by an intracapsular or extracapsular procedure.

Intracapsular extraction, which is performed infrequently today, consists of removing the lens in toto, ie, within its capsule, through a 140- to 160-degree superior limbal incision. In **extracapsular extraction,** a superior limbal incision is also made; the anterior portion of the capsule is cut and removed; the nucleus is extracted; and the lens cortex is removed from the eye by irrigation with or without aspiration, leaving the posterior capsule behind. Some patients develop secondary opacity of the posterior capsule that requires discission using the neodymium-YAG laser (see After-Cataract, above).

Phacofragmentation and **phacoemulsification** with irrigation or aspiration (or both) are extracapsular techniques that utilize ultrasonic vibrations to remove the nucleus and cortex through a small limbal incision (2–5 mm), thus facilitating postoperative wound healing. These techniques are most useful in congenital, traumatic, and some senile cataracts. They are less effective with dense senile cataracts, and the advantage of a small limbal incision is somewhat negated if an intraocular lens is to be inserted, although flexible intraocular lenses that can be inserted through such small incisions are currently being developed.

Over the past 5 years, extracapsular operations have replaced intracapsular procedures by a large percentage as the most common type of cataract surgery. The principal reason is that an intact posterior capsule allows the surgeon to insert a posterior chamber intraocular lens. The incidence of postoperative complications, such as retinal detachment and cystoid macular edema, is less when the posterior capsule is intact.

Intraocular Lens

Over 90% of all cataract operations in the USA— or over 1 million per year—involve intraocular lens implantation. Refinements in surgical technique and improved lens implants have played major roles in this advance. However, the major stimulus has been the inherent disadvantages of aphakic spectacles, including image magnification, spherical aberrations, limited visual field, and no chance of binocular vision if the other eye is phakic.

About 90% of implants are in the posterior chamber and 10% in the anterior chamber. There are many styles of lenses, but all consist of 2 basic parts: a spherical optic, usually made of polymethylmethacrylate; and footplates or haptics to maintain the optic in position.

Posterior chamber lenses are generally used in extracapsular procedures. This combination is preferred over anterior chamber lenses because of a lower incidence of sight-threatening complications such as hyphema, secondary glaucoma, macular edema, and pupillary block. There is also a lower incidence of corneal endothelial damage and subsequent pseudophakic bullous keratopathy in patients with posterior chamber lenses. Anterior chamber lenses are used for patients undergoing intracapsular surgery or when the posterior capsule has been inadvertently ruptured in extracapsular surgery.

Contraindications to intraocular lens implantation include recurrent uveitis, proliferative diabetic retinopathy, rubeosis iridis, and neovascular glaucoma. Patients with open-angle glaucoma and ocular hypertension may receive an intraocular lens, but posterior chamber lenses are preferred. Age is considered by many to be a relative contraindication, but younger and younger patients are receiving intraocular lenses each year.

An alternative to the intraocular lens is the contact lens, but many elderly patients are unable to tolerate them or insert them easily. In rare situations where an intraocular lens or contact lens cannot be used, aphakic eyeglasses are prescribed.

Postoperative Care (Senile Cataract)

If a small-incision technique is used, the postoperative recovery period is usually shortened. The patient may be ambulatory on the day of surgery but is advised to move cautiously and avoid straining or heavy lifting for about a month. The eye can be bandaged for a few days, but if the eye is comfortable, the bandage can be removed and the eye protected by spectacles or by a shield during the day. Protection at night by a metal shield is required for several weeks. Temporary glasses can be used a few days after surgery, but usually the patient sees well enough through the intraocular lens to wait for permanent glasses (usually provided 6–8 weeks after surgery).

DISLOCATED LENS (Ectopia Lentis)

Partial or complete lens dislocation (Fig 9–13) may be hereditary or may result from trauma.

Hereditary Lens Dislocation

Hereditary lens dislocation is usually bilateral and may be associated with coloboma of the lens, homocystinuria, Marfan's syndrome, and Marchesani's syndrome. The vision is blurred, particularly if the lens is dislocated out of the line of vision. If dislocation is partial, the edge of the lens and the zonular fibers holding it in place can be seen in the pupil. If the lens is completely dislocated into the vitreous, it can be seen with the ophthalmoscope.

A partially dislocated lens is often complicated by cataract formation. If so, the cataract may have to be removed, but this should be delayed as long as possible

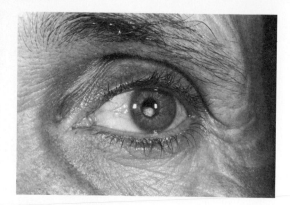

Figure 9–13. Dislocated lens.

If dislocation is partial and the lens is clear, the visual prognosis is good.

Traumatic Lens Dislocation

Partial or complete traumatic lens dislocation may occur following a contusion injury such as a blow to the eye with a fist. If the dislocation is partial, there may be no symptoms; but if the lens is floating in the vitreous, the patient has blurred vision and usually a red eye. **Iridodonesis,** a quivering of the iris when the patient moves the eye, is a common sign of lens dislocation and is due to the lack of lens support. This is present both in partially and completely dislocated lenses but is more marked in the latter.

Iritis, uveitis, and glaucoma are common complications of dislocated lens, particularly if dislocation is complete.

If there are no complications, dislocated lenses are best left untreated. If uveitis or uncontrollable glaucoma occurs, lens extraction must be done despite the poor results of this operation. The technique of choice is pars plana lensectomy using a motor-drive lens and vitreous cutter.

because vitreous loss, predisposing to subsequent retinal detachment, is prone to occur during surgery. If the lens is free in the vitreous, it may lead in later life to the development of glaucoma of a type that responds poorly to treatment.

REFERENCES

Birch EE, Stager DR: Prevalence of good visual acuity following surgery for congenital unilateral cataract. *Arch Ophthalmol* 1988;**106**:40.

Bradford JD, Wilkinson CP, Bradford RH Jr: Cystoid macular edema following extracapsular cataract extraction and posterior chamber intraocular lens implantation. *Retina* 1988;**3**:161.

Brown NAP, Hill AR: Cataract: The relation between myopia and cataract morphology. *Br J Ophthalmol* 1987;**71**:405.

Gross KA, Pearce JL: Modern cataract surgery in a highly myopic population. *Br J Ophthalmol* 1987;**71**:215.

Jacob TJ et al: Cytological factors relating to posterior capsule opacification following cataract surgery. *Br J Ophthalmol* 1987;**71**:659.

Jaffe NS, Clayman HM, Jaffe MS: Retinal detachment in myopic eyes after intracapsular and extracapsular cataract extraction. *Am J Ophthalmol* 1984;**97**:48.

Kraff MC, Sanders DR, Lieberman HL: Intraocular pressure and the corneal endothelium after noedymium-YAG laser posterior capsulotomy. *Arch Ophthalmol* 1985;**103**:511.

Leff SR, Welch JC, Tasman W: Rhegmatogenous retinal detachment after YAG laser posterior capsulotomy. *Ophthalmology* 1987;**94**:1222.

Lerman S: Ultraviolet radiation photodamage to the ocular lens: Diagnosis and treatment. *Ann Ophthalmol* 1982;**14**:411.

Lichter PR: Interpreting tests: Implications for cataract surgery. (Editorial.) *Ophthalmology* 1988;**95**:1.

Mammo RB, Allan D: Effect of age on visual acuity after cataract extraction. *Br J Ophthalmol* 1987;**71**:112.

McDonnell PJ, Krause W, Glaser BM: In vitro inhibition of lens epithelial cell proliferation and migration. *Ophthalmic Surg* 1988;**19**:25.

McDonnell PJ, Zarbin MA, Green WR: Posterior capsule opacification in pseudophakic eyes. *Ophthalmology* 1983;**90**:1548.

Mehra V, Minassian DC: A rapid method of grading cataract in epidemiological studies and eye surveys. *Br J Ophthalmol* 1988;**72**:801.

Percival SPD, Anand V, Das SK: Prevalence of aphakic retinal detachment. *Br J Ophthalmol* 1983;**67**:43.

Radius RL et al: Pseudophakia and intraocular pressure. *Am J Ophthalmol* 1984;**97**:738.

Rasooly R, BenEzra D: Congenital and traumatic cataract: The effect on ocular axial length. *Arch Ophthalmol* 1988;**106**:1066.

Rice NSC: Congenital cataract: A cause of preventable blindness in children. *Br Med J* 1982;**285**:581.

Schwab IR et al: Cataract extraction: Risk factors in a health maintenance organization population under 60 years of age. *Arch Ophthalmol* 1988;**106**:1062.

Shock JP: Phacofragmentation and irrigation. *Ann Ophthalmol* 1976;**8**:591.

Smiddy WE et al: Cataract extraction after vitrectomy. *Ophthalmology* 1987;**94**:483.

Taylor DM et al: Pseudophakic bullous keratopathy. *Ophthalmology* 1983;**90**:19.

Taylor HR et al: Effect of ultraviolet radiation on cataract formation. *N Engl J Med* 1988;**319**:1429.

Terry AC et al: Neodymium-YAG laser for posterior capsulotomy. *Am Ophthalmol* 1983;**96**:716.

Van Heyningen R, Harding JJ: A case-control study of cataract in Oxfordshire: Some risk factors. *Br J Ophthalmol* 1988;**72**:804.

West SK et al: Use of photographic techniques to grade nuclear cataracts. *Invest Ophthalmol Vis Sci* 1988;**29**:73.

Wilson J: Clearing the cataract backlog. *Br J Ophthalmol* 1987;**71**:158.

Vitreous

10

Conor O'Malley, MD

COMPOSITION & ANATOMY

The vitreous is about 99% water. The remaining 1% includes 2 components, collagen and hyaluronic acid, which give it its specific physical character.

The vitreous owes its gel-like form and consistency to a loose syncytium of long-chain collagen molecules capable of binding about 200 times their own weight in water.

The hyaluronic acid molecules are very large, loose skeins capable of binding about 60 times their weight in water. Combined with the collagen element, they account for the physical characteristics of normal vitreous.

The vitreous is a clear, avascular, gelatinous body that comprises two-thirds of the volume and weight of the eye. It fills the space bounded by the lens, retina, and optic disk (Fig. 10–1). Since it is quite inelastic and impervious to cells and debris, it plays an important role in maintaining the transparency and form of the eye. If the vitreous were removed, the eye would collapse. When the vitreous is replaced by saline, as in certain forms of vitreous surgery, cellular matter and particulate debris are free to migrate into the optical pathway.

The outer surface of the vitreous—the hyaloid membrane—is normally in contact with the following structures: the posterior lens capsule, the zonular fibers, the pars plana epithelium, the retina, and the optic nerve head. The base of the vitreous maintains a firm attachment throughout life to the pars plana epithelium and the retina immediately behind the ora serrata. The attachment to the lens capsule and the optic nerve head is firm in early life but soon disappears. This is

the principal reason that intracapsular cataract extraction without vitreous prolapse or ''loss'' is possible in adults and not in children. In addition, the vitreous is prone to vitreoretinal adhesions at the site of lattice degeneration of the retina, congenital retinal rosettes, meridional retinal folds, vitreoretinal scars, and new retinal blood vessels, as in diabetes and central retinal vein occlusion.

The hyaloid canal (Cloquet's canal), which in the fetus contains the hyaloid artery, passes anteroposteriorly from the lens to the optic nerve head. The hyaloid artery usually disappears soon after birth, but the hyaloid canal remains throughout life. It is not visible ophthalmoscopically. A rudimentary portion of the hyaloid artery occasionally remains and can be seen floating in the vitreous with its anterior portion attached to the posterior surface of the lens. This point of attachment can be seen as a black dot (Mittendorf's dot) with the ophthalmoscope.

EXAMINATION OF THE VITREOUS

Slit Lamp Examination

Normal vitreous is not visible by either direct or indirect ophthalmoscopy. The numerous ophthalmoscopically visible features are anomalies attributable either to structural changes, such as the floaters of syneresis and the ringlike form associated with posterior vitreous detachment (Fig 10–2), or to invasive elements, such as blood, white blood cell masses, or fibrovascular proliferations from adjacent tissues. Normal vitreous in situ and many important anomalies (eg, the retraction, condensation, and shrinkage of vitreous characteristic of diabetes or injury) can be viewed only with a slit lamp. **Slit lamps** are microscopes with specialized illuminating systems that make transparent and near-transparent ocular fluids and tissues visible. Although slit lamp examination of the vitreous is quite easy to learn and plays an important role in the management of vitreous disease, too few ophthalmologists make optimal use of this instrument.

Contact Lenses as Aid in Vitreous Examination

The anterior central vitreous is the only part of the inner eye (behind the lens) that can be seen with the slit lamp alone. In order to view other areas, special

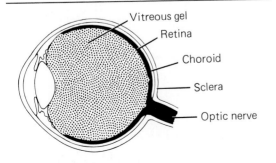

Figure 10–1. Normal: vitreous gel fills inner eye.

153

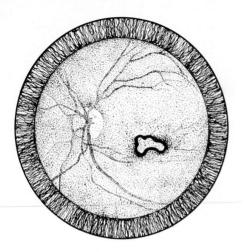

Figure 10–2. Vitreous detachment as seen with the +8 lens of the ophthalmoscope.

contact lenses must be placed in the patient's eye (1) to modify the light-focusing power of the aqueous lens and the lens lens and (2) to expand the limited range through which the illumination beam of the slit lamp can be angulated with respect to the visual axis of the eyeball.

A relatively thin contact lens with a flat front surface will neutralize the light-bending property of the eye, so that tissues *on and near the visual axis of the eye*—the optic disk, the posterior retina and choroid, and the axial vitreous—can be illuminated in 3-dimensional detail. Much thicker contact lenses with built-

in mirrors and a flat front surface can be used to displace the illumination and viewing pathways of the slit lamp with respect to the visual axis of the eyeball, so that much of the nonaxial retina and vitreous can be seen.

These special contact lenses are also used in therapeutic procedures. Fundus contact lenses with built-in mirrors are widely used in laser surgery for panretinal photocoagulation of the peripheral retina. This prevents vitreous hemorrhage that may result from the retinal neovascularizations of diabetic retinopathy, retinal vein occlusions, and (rarer) sickle cell anemia. The thinner contact lenses are sometimes used in ablation of macular lesions associated with age-related macular degeneration and histoplasmosis.

Use of special contact lenses, whether for diagnostic or therapeutic procedures, requires maximum dilation of the pupil with a combination of mydriatic and cycloplegic solutions; use of a topical anesthetic to make the patient more comfortable; and use of a clear viscous solution of methylcellulose to prevent air from entering the lens-cornea interface.

B-Scan Ultrasonography

B-scan ultrasonography is an important diagnostic and prognostic tool used in many posterior segment problems associated with gross vitreous opacification (Fig 10–3). Where light-dependent ophthalmoscopes and slit lamps are of limited value, skillful use of B-scan ultrasonography can provide much information about the vitreous and adjacent structures. For example, it is possible to identify and locate vitreous membranes (Fig 10–4), vitreoretinal relationships and retinal detachments greater than 1 mm in depth (Figs

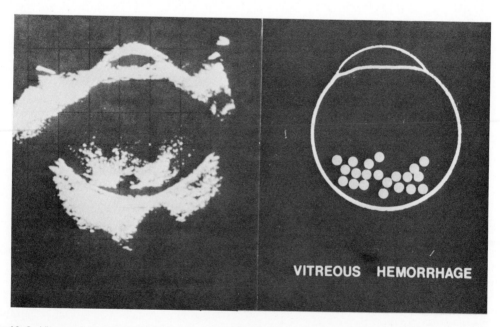

Figure 10–3. Vitreous hemorrhage limited to posterior vitreous region in aphakic eye. (Reproduced, with permission, from Coleman DJ: Ultrasound in vitreous surgery. *Trans Am Acad Ophthalmol Otolaryngol* 1972;**76**:469.)

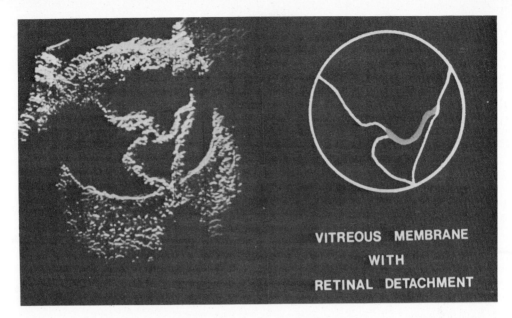

Figure 10–4. Total retinal detachment viewed horizontally below iris plane. A vitreous membrane connecting 2 leaves of retina is clearly demonstrated. (Reproduced, with permission, from Coleman DJ: Ultrasound in vitreous surgery. *Trans Am Acad Ophthalmol Otolaryngol* 1972;**76**:474.)

10–4 to 10–6), scleral ruptures, and intraocular foreign bodies (even nonlucent plastic and glass).

DISORDERS OF THE VITREOUS

"FLASHING LIGHTS"

"Flashing lights" are a common symptom of an abnormal relationship between the retina and the vitreous. The patient is aware of a localized "light," "glow," "streak of light," or "flashing" (as of a neon tube) in the field of vision in the absence of a corresponding light source in the environment. The patient can usually point to the area of the disturbance and often describes an arc-shaped flicker in the periphery of one or 2 quadrants. The light seldom persists for more than a fraction of a second. It frequently recurs at short intervals for a few minutes and then disappears for hours, days, or even weeks. It is most readily identified on moving the eye and when illumination is dim or absent. Bilateral episodes may occur simultaneously but more commonly are separated by an interval of days to many years.

The light represents a cerebral awareness of the initial physical traction on and excitation of the sensory retina by abnormal vitreous. It is most commonly associated with recent collapse and detachment of the vitreous due to syneresis with focal vitreous traction on vitreoretinal lesions such as lattice degeneration, meridional folds, congenital rosettes, and other visually subclinical vitreoretinal adhesions. A careful history will readily distinguish the light from the scintillating scotoma of migraine, which is characterized by a symmetric quivering scotoma usually in both eyes, of predictable configuration and progression, accompanied by variable nausea or headache.

The vitreoretinal traction may require no treatment. However, as it can induce retinal tears, retinal detachment (Fig 10–7), or vitreous hemorrhage, every new case requires a survey of the vitreoretinal relationship, especially in the periphery.

VITREOUS FLOATERS

Vitreous floaters are by far the most common symptom of abnormal vitreous. A given floater represents the patient's awareness of the shadow of a mobile vitreous opacity cast upon the retina. The mind projects the corresponding dark form onto the appropriate area of the visual field.

The term vitreous floaters denotes a common, potentially serious symptom that was formerly called *muscae volitantes*—Latin for flies that flit, flutter, or fly to and fro.

The onset may be either insidious or acute and unilateral or bilateral. The patient is aware of one or more (or even many) fine, dark forms in the field of vision. Their configuration is usually so pronounced that the patient spontaneously classifies them as "spots," "soot," "particles," "spiders," "cob-

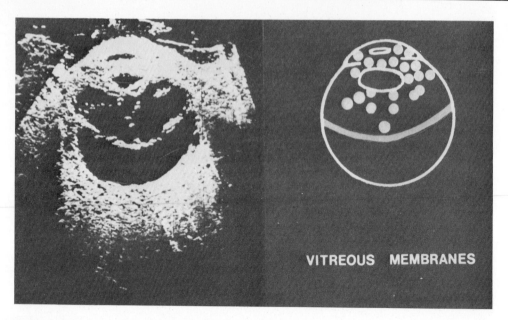

Figure 10–5. Vitreous membrane extending along posterior limiting membrane of vitreous from ora to ora. Retina is in place. (Reproduced, with permission, from Coleman DJ: Ultrasound in vitreous surgery. *Trans Am Acad Ophthalmol Otolaryngol* 1972;**76**:473.)

webs," "threads," "worms," "dark streaks," "a ring," etc. Combinations are often reported. The objects continue to migrate after the eye comes to rest—hence the name floaters.

Central, relatively immobile floaters are visually annoying and may even be disabling. Peripheral ones are readily overlooked, as they are intermittent and require large eye motion or special positions merely to be seen. Unlike "flashing lights," they are most readily seen against bright lights or a uniform light background. They are extremely common in myopes and people with syneresis.

Floaters are commonly caused by small hemorrhages into the vitreous due to retinal tears or hemorrhagic diseases such as diabetic retinopathy, hypertension, leukemia, old retinal branch vein

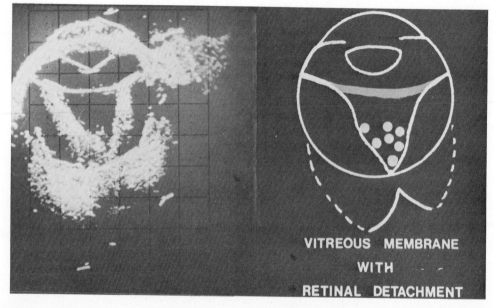

Figure 10–6. Vitreous membrane connecting 2 leaves of detached retina. Lens is normal. (Reproduced, with permission, from Coleman DJ: Ultrasound in vitreous surgery. *Trans Am Acad Ophthalmol Otolaryngol* 1972;**76**:474.)

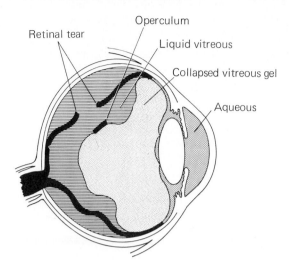

Figure 10–7. Schematic representation of vitreous collapse causing the retina to tear and detach.

occlusions, Eales's disease, Coats's disease, and subacute bacterial endocarditis. Individual red cells are seen as small round black spots. Recent hemorrhages are often seen as black streaks or cobwebs that later break up into small round spots.

White cell invasion of the vitreous gel associated with pars planitis may also cause "spots before the eyes."

Vitreous floaters due to pigment are usually a consequence of long-standing tear-induced detachment of the retina that has not yet reached the macula.

Vitreous floaters should never be dismissed as harmless or imaginary. A careful survey of the vitreous and retina is always indicated in order to identify the nature and origin of floaters and to decide on management. Failure to make such an examination not infrequently leads to missed diagnosis. In the absence of a serious causative pathologic process, the patient may be reassured that the condition is harmless.

ASTEROID HYALOSIS

Asteroid hyalosis is an uncommon condition that occurs in otherwise healthy eyes in elderly people. Unilateral cases are 3 times as common as bilateral cases. Hundreds of small yellow spheres consisting of calcium soaps are seen in the vitreous. These move when the eyes move but always return to their original positions because they are attached to interlacing fibers. There are no related ocular or systemic diseases. The opacities have little or no effect upon vision but reflect the examiner's light very strongly. If there are enough asteroid bodies, the fundus is not viewable by ophthalmoscopy.

ACUTE VITREOUS COLLAPSE

The vitreous cavity is bounded by the retina, optic disk, pars plana, zonule, and crystalline lens. Normal vitreous fills this cavity (Fig 10–1) and remains firmly attached to the retina and pars plana near the ora serrata.

All types of gels, whether vitreous or gelatin, become increasingly prone with the passage of time to a degenerative process known as **syneresis,** involving drawing together of particles of the dispersed medium, separation of the medium, and shrinkage of the gel. Syneresis affects at least 65% of persons over 60 years of age. Myopes are especially susceptible, even in childhood.

With age, the center of the vitreous may undergo syneresis and become filled with liquid breakdown products of the degenerated gel (Fig 10–8). The liquid contents of the cavity can migrate into the preretinal space. The more solid, heavier vitreous gel collapses downward and forward to create a posterior vitreous detachment (Fig 10–9). The dynamic forces that accompany this collapse can rupture the last vestiges of the adhesions that once connected the vitreous to the disk, blood vessels, and sensory retina in childhood.

The patient and examiner can often see portions of the adhesions that remain attached to the collapsed vitreous as opacities. If they arise from the disk margin, the patient and examiner may note a ring-shaped opacity on the back of the vitreous.

Since the front of the vitreous is attached to the globe and the back of the vitreous is collapsed in on itself, abrupt motions of the eye transmit a whiplike force to the back of the vitreous. The vitreous tends to fill out toward its normal configuration; liquid vitreous is drawn into the syneretic cavity, and the posterior separation tends to disappear (Fig 10–10).

The whiplike motions of the vitreous can give rise to **photopsia** (an appearance of sparks or flashes) by causing stimulation of the vitreoretinal juncture and may cause a characteristic floating motion of posterior vitreous opacities, or floaters. The floaters move with the eye and float to a resting position after the eye comes to rest.

Since acute vitreous collapse can also cause asymp-

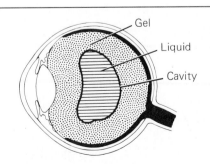

Figure 10–8. Large intravitreal cavity filled with liquid breakdown products of syneresis.

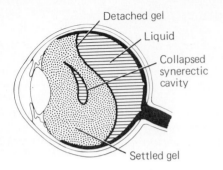

Figure 10–9. Posterior vitreous detachment.

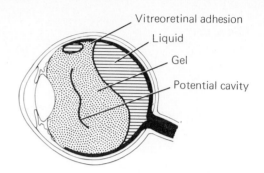

Figure 10–11. Local vitreoretinal adhesion.

tomatic retinal tears or detachment, *it should be assumed that patients with new floaters or photopsia have retinal tears or detachment until proved otherwise by thorough examination of the peripheral retina with an indirect ophthalmoscope.*

RETINAL TEARS
(See also Chapter 11.)

While retinal tears can be caused by trauma, vitreous shrinkage, or proliferative vitreoretinopathy, most are caused by acute vitreous collapse. Tears following acute vitreous collapse are the result of a dynamic interaction between a focal vitreoretinal adhesion, collapsed mobile vitreous, and normal eye movement (Fig 10–11).

Since the gel and liquid components of the collapsed vitreous are structurally relatively independent of the retina, they do not move synchronously with the retina. When the eye (and hence the retina) moves, the gel and liquid tend to lag behind the retina, and when the eye stops moving, the gel and liquid tend to continue in motion. The vitreous gel and liquid are said to exhibit inertial lag with respect to the retina. Inertial

lag of the gel can cause the vitreous to tear the friable sensory retina at the point where they adhere to each other (Fig 10–12). With the ophthalmoscope, the torn retina is seen to be pulled inward as a flap or a detached operculum (Fig 10–13). If retinal vessels are broken, they bleed briefly. A variable amount of blood accumulates in the vitreous cavity.

Some patients are not aware of the onset of retinal tears but often complain of photopsia and floaters. Some present with gross vitreous hemorrhage. Many retinal tears never lead to retinal detachment, but recent symptomatic tears, especially those with symptomatic vitreous hemorrhage, have a strong tendency to cause retinal detachment days to years later. Patients with symptoms of acute vitreous collapse or vitreous hemorrhage should therefore undergo careful examination of the retina from the optic disk to the ora serrata to rule out one or more tears. Management of tears by prophylactic laser therapy or cryopexy is relatively simple and very effective compared to the performance of silicone buckling once retinal detachment has occurred.

Retinal tears are usually located anterior to the equator and are more often in the upper quadrants (Fig 10–13 left).

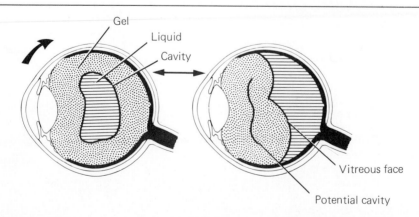

Figure 10–10. Liquid vitreous tends to be drawn into intravitreal cavity on abrupt eye motion *(left)* and expelled at rest *(right)*.

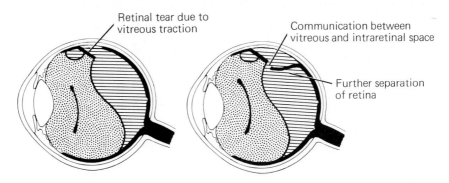

Figure 10-12. *Left:* Retinal tear. *Right:* Retinal detachment.

VITREOUS HEMORRHAGE

Vitreous hemorrhage can occur whenever the sensory retina is torn. Retinitis proliferans, central vein occlusion, branch vein occlusion, and hypertension are also frequent causes of vitreous hemorrhage. Acute collapse of the vitreous with posterior vitreous detachment will sometimes cause bleeding without tear formation. The patient often complains of floaters that suggest red blood cells, a sudden shower of small black dots, or even tiny ringlike forms with clear centers. Visual loss ranges from imperceptible to gross.

The appearance of the retina and its visibility vary with the cause and amount of bleeding in the vitreous cavity (see Chapter 11). Fresh blood is red and tends to be located behind the vitreous gel or within a syneretic cavity (Fig 10-14). Within weeks to months, the blood tends to break down, becomes a pale color, and migrates into the gel (Fig 10-15).

Vitrectomy may be indicated to facilitate surgical reattachment of the retina. For example, vitreous hemorrhage following recent retinal detachment (diagnosed possibly by ultrasonography) may be extensive enough to hamper retinal surgery, which may need to be performed promptly to prevent irreversible macular atrophy.

Vitrectomy is not indicated for 3-6 months if treatment of the underlying cause can wait, as the vitreous may clear adequately without surgery.

RETINAL DETACHMENT
(See also Chapter 11.)

In the normal eye, the intact sensory retina is kept opposed to the pigment epithelium by the suction the latter exerts on the watertight space between them. If a retinal tear is present, rapid eye motions and sudden rotation of the globe can readily generate enough inertial force to initiate retinal detachment (Fig 10-16). The space between the 2 layers of the retina fills with liquid vitreous, and eddy currents develop in this space, further accelerating the detachment process (Fig 10-17). Almost invariably, detachment continues until it is total.

Surgery with cryopexy and silicone buckling is required (1) to close the hole in the retina, reestablishing a watertight intraretinal space; (2) to restrict the inertial lag of the liquid and gel with respect to the retina; and (3) to approximate and seal together the 2 layers of the retina around the tear to counter the effects of eddy currents in the vitreous cavity. (See also Chapter 11.)

TRACTION RETINAL DETACHMENT

Traction retinal detachment is detachment of the sensory retina without retinal tears. The most common cause is long-standing diabetes. The detachment is typically found posterior to the equator and is due to

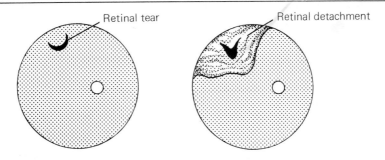

Figure 10-13. *Left:* Ophthalmoscopic view of retinal tear. *Right:* Ophthalmoscopic view of retinal detachment.

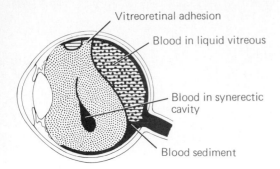

Figure 10–14. Acute vitreous hemorrhage: a retinal vessel ruptures due to vitreous traction.

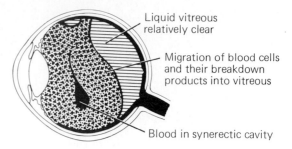

Figure 10–15. Chronic vitreous hemorrhage.

vitreous traction on an area of retinitis proliferans (Fig 10–18).

Reattachment by vitrectomy is indicated only if there is clear-cut recent extension of the detachment into the macula.

PROLIFERATIVE VITREORETINOPATHY

A considerable number of abnormal conditions of the vitreous and retina are characterized by contractile membranes arising metaplastically from abnormally located retinal pigment epithelial cells and retinal glial cells. The membranes can occur on either the inner or outer surface of the sensory retina or on several vitreous surfaces. The membranes may be weak and subtle or strong, easily seen, and capable of causing great distortion of the host tissues.

The causal retinal pigment epithelial cells and retinal glial cells are pluripotential cells, with great metaplastic potential. They may proliferate at remote sites and take on the characteristics of myofibroblasts. These myofibroblastlike cells readily form contractile membranes that may deform the inner and outer surfaces of the retina and the posterior vitreous surfaces (Fig 10–19).

The basic process, or its outcome, is known as massive vitreous retraction, preretinal traction, preretinal vitreous membrane (see Chapter 11), subretinal fibrosis, macular pucker, or surface wrinkling retinopathy.

Proliferative vitreoretinopathy requires no treatment unless it causes surface wrinkling retinopathy of the macula (also known as macular pucker) or unduly complicates therapy for retinal detachment. While research holds some promise for an antiproliferative pharmaceutical agent, current treatment involves a special surgical procedure that employs distention, severing, or removal of vitreous tissue (see below).

INJURY TO THE VITREOUS

Contusion

Because the vitreous is inelastic compared with the adjacent tissues, contusions that abruptly though briefly alter the shape of the eye are apt to cause injuries where the vitreous is adherent.

Disinsertion of the vitreous base is not uncommon. It is frequently associated with tearing of the pars plana or retina, vitreous hemorrhage, or detachment of the retina—as long as 20 years later.

Less commonly, "flashing lights," vitreous floaters, and even vitreous hemorrhage or detachment of

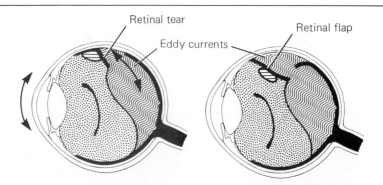

Figure 10–16. Abrupt rotation of globe generates eddy currents in liquid vitreous, a result of inertial lag *(left),* that tends to lift the retinal flap and surrounding sensory retina *(right).*

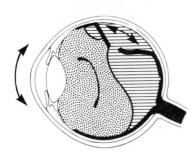

Figure 10–17. Enlargement of retinal detachment due to inertial lag of liquid vitreous within the retina.

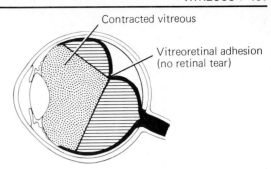

Figure 10–18. Traction detachment of retina.

the retina may result from stress behind the vitreous base. The affected sites may be previously subclinical anomalous vitreoretinal adhesions (eg, lattice degeneration) or areas of frank vitreoretinal disease such as diabetic retinopathy.

Rupture of the Globe

Rupture of the globe is always a serious injury that may result in early or late blindness or even loss of the eyeball. Prolapse of the vitreous through the wound is a severe complication often associated with acute secondary tearing or detachment of the retina. A seemingly uncomplicated prolapse may be followed by late retinal detachment with or without tears due to fibrous ingrowth from the orbit and subsequent contraction. The latter may be visible as membranes or bands in the vitreous. Various forms of vitreous surgery are used to prevent or treat such complications.

Penetration of the Globe

An almost endless variety of material may accidentally penetrate the globe. Common examples are needles, BB shot, and small particles of metal, stone, or plastic that fly into the eye at high velocity.

Prolapse of the vitreous may occur at the site of entry or exit or both. The part traversed by the foreign body is permanently damaged and is often marked by visible condensation, shrinkage, or fibrous elements. Vitreous surgery is increasingly used to prevent or treat complications such as retinal detachment with or without tears.

Vitreous Loss

Vitreous loss is an iatrogenic complication. The vitreous gel prolapses through a surgical wound, usually at (but not limited to) the corneal limbus during the course of operating on the lens, iris, or cornea.

Fibrous tissue invasion and contraction are frequent sequels that are prone to cause traction complications involving the retina. Corneal edema and iris displacement (eg, "updrawn pupil") may also occur. An acute prolapse can be effectively excised. An old prolapse may require surgery for release of vitreous traction.

VITREOUS INFLAMMATION

Vitreous inflammation includes a wide spectrum of disorders ranging from a few scattered white cells to abscess formation. Most commonly, one or more focal inflammatory lesions in the choroid or retina—as in chorioretinitis or retinitis—are responsible for a secondary cellular invasion of the liquid vitreous or relatively resistant gel. There may be a mild localized blurring of the fundus landmarks and lesions that pro-

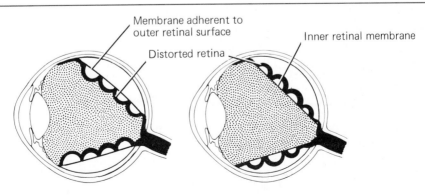

Figure 10–19. Proliferative vitreoretinopathy. **Left:** Contracture of membrane adherent to outer retinal surface. **Right:** Contracture of inner retinal membrane.

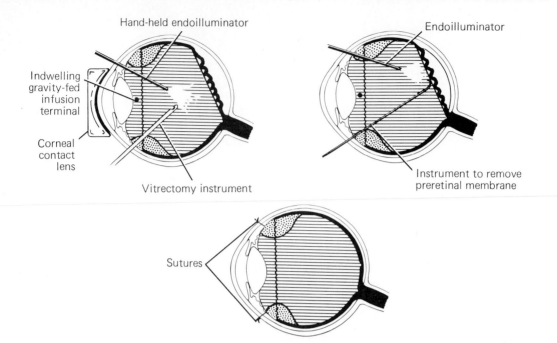

Figure 10–20. Vitreous surgery. *Top left:* Position of corneal contact lens and intraocular devices. *Top right:* Removal of preretinal membrane. *Bottom:* Placement of sutures at completion of procedure.

voke little or no visual complaint except for a possible vitreous floater effect. With greater infiltration, vision is decreased and the fundus is invisible or almost so. The condition may be so marked that the red reflection is lost and the vitreous appears opaque and white. Since these conditions spare the anterior segment, there is no pain and the external eye appears normal. The prognosis and treatment depend upon the underlying condition. The vitreous usually clears when the primary defect is quiescent. Vitreous surgery is used to remove gross residual opacities that show no sign of clearing spontaneously.

Vitreous Abscess (Endophthalmitis)*

Vitreous abscess may occur following penetrating ocular trauma. The vitreous is an excellent culture medium; following bacterial invasion, it undergoes liquefaction and abscess formation.

The diagnosis of vitreous abscess is confirmed by aspirating 0.5–1 mL of vitreous under local anesthesia through a pars plana sclerotomy using a 20- to 23-gauge needle. The aspirate should be examined with Gram's, Giemsa's, and Gomori's methenamine silver stains and inoculated into blood agar, chocolate agar, thioglycolate, and Sabouraud's agar.

---

* If all 3 coats of the eye as well as the vitreous are involved by an inflammatory process, the condition is known as panophthalmitis. The line of demarcation between endophthalmitis and panophthalmitis is usually obscure.

Once the organism is identified, the patient is hospitalized and given maximum medical treatment as outlined in Table 26–1. Subconjunctival and intravenous antibiotics are standard therapy; intravitreal injection is optional.

In some cases, vitrectomy is indicated to drain the abscess and allow better visualization of the fundus.

Even in the best hands, vitreous abscess carries a grave prognosis.

VITREOUS SURGERY

Vitreous surgery is useful for a broad spectrum of intraocular disorders. Airtight and watertight incisions measuring 1–4 mm are made in the pars plana and sclera (Fig 10–20). One incision is used for an indwelling gravity-fed infusion terminal, which maintains the desired tension and configuration of the globe. Surgical gases and medications are also instilled through this terminal. Another incision is used for a hand-held endoilluminator, which illuminates the contents and all of the walls of the vitreous cavity. The illuminated structures are viewed microscopically through the pupil with the aid of a corneal contact lens that neutralizes the light-focusing power of the

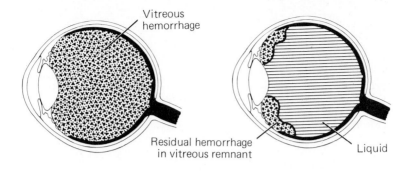

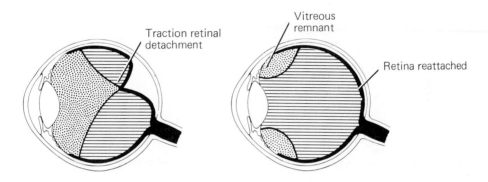

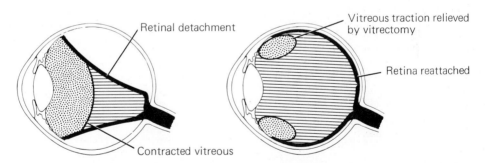

Figure 10–21. Scope of vitreous surgery. **Top:** Removal of vitreous hemorrhage. Residual hemorrhage will clear in time from vitreous remnants. **Middle:** Reattachment of traction retinal detachment following vitrectomy. **Bottom:** Vitreous contracture complicating retinal detachment. Removal of vitreous and repair of retinal detachment.

eye. The remaining incision is used to allow for instrumentation (severing or removal of tissue), diathermy, and laser photocoagulation (Fig 10–20).

Vitreous surgery provides access to virtually all of the intraocular tissues between the endothelium of the cornea and the retinal pigment epithelium. Surgery is most commonly done (1) to remove vitreous opacified by blood (Fig 10–21 top), (2) to remove shrunken vitreous causing traction retinal detachment (Fig 10–21 middle), (3) to treat vitreous contracture compli-

cating retinal detachment (Fig 10–21 bottom) (see preretinal membranes), (4) to remove metaplastic membranes that deform or detach the sensory retina (Figs 10–19 and 10–20), (5) to create an optical opening in recalcitrant pupillary membranes, and (6) to remove infected vitreous in endophthalmitis (so as to dilute the organismal toxins and reduce the population of causal organisms and to instill therapeutic solutions). Vitreous surgery is frequently combined with scleral buckling for retinal detachment.

REFERENCES

Charles S: *Vitreous Microsurgery*. Williams & Wilkins, 1981.

Machemer R, Aaberg TM: *Vitrectomy,* 2nd ed. Grune & Stratton, 1979.

O'Malley C et al: Closed eye intraocular microsurgery. Pages 39–216 in: *Highlights of Ophthalmology*. Vol 1. Boyd B (editor). Highlights of Ophthalmology Press, 1981.

Smiddy WE et al: Vitrectomy for macular traction caused by incomplete vitreous separation. *Arch Ophthalmol* 1988;**106:**624.

Williams GA et al: Treatment of postvitrectomy fibrin formation with intraocular tissue plasminogen activator. *Arch Ophthalmol* 1988;**106:**1055.

Retina & Intraocular Tumors 11

Patrick O'Malley, MD

I. RETINA

ANATOMY

The retina covers the inner aspect of the posterior two-thirds of the wall of the globe. A fundus photo of the posterior pole of a normal retina is shown in Fig 11–1. The principal landmarks of the retina are illustrated and labeled in Fig 2–14.

The retina is a multilayered sheet of neural tissue closely applied to a single layer of pigmented epithelial cells, which in turn is attached to Bruch's membrane (Fig 1–11). The anterior extremity of the retina is firmly bound to the pigment epithelium. Posteriorly, the optic nerve fixes the retina to the wall of the globe. Elsewhere, the retina and the pigment epithelium are easily separated. In adults, the ora serrata—the partly serrated anterior end of the retina—is about 6.5 mm behind Schwalbe's line on the temporal side of the eye and 5.7 mm behind it nasally.

The retina is 0.1 mm thick at the ora serrata and 0.23 mm thick at the posterior pole. It is thinnest at

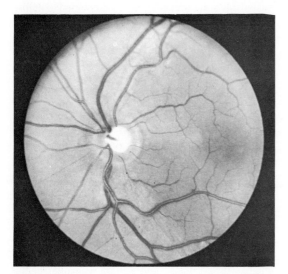

Figure 11–1. Ophthalmoscopic view of a normal retina. Note deep physiologic cup. (Courtesy of S Mettier, Jr.)

the fovea centralis, the center of the macula. The retina is normally transparent, and some of the incident light is reflected at the vitreoretinal interface. The resulting sheen is especially noticeable when young, heavily pigmented patients are examined with an indirect ophthalmoscope. On examination with the direct ophthalmoscope, the concave foveal surface produces a clearly visible inverted image of the lamp. Absence of this foveal reflection may indicate disease, but the reflection may be absent in blond or elderly patients even though the retina is normal.

The fovea centralis, which lies about 3.5 mm lateral to the optic disk, is specialized for fine visual discrimination. In the fovea, the receptors are all cones; the outer nuclear layer is thinned; the other parenchymal layers are displaced centrifugally; and the internal limiting membrane is thin. Throughout most of the retina, the axons of the receptor cells pass directly to the inner side of the outer plexiform layer, where they connect with dendrites of horizontal and bipolar cells, which extend outward from the inner nuclear layer. In the macula, however, the receptor cell axons follow an oblique course and are called the Henle fiber layer. The normally empty extracellular space of the retina is potentially greatest at the macula, and diseases that lead to accumulation of extracellular material cause considerable thickening of this area.

The axons of the bipolar cells are connected with amacrine and ganglion cells in the densely woven inner plexiform layer. The long axons of the ganglion cells pass in the nerve fiber layer to the optic nerve.

The retina receives its blood supply from 2 sources. The choriocapillaris is a single layer of closely spaced capillaries intimately attached to the outer surface of Bruch's membrane. The choriocapillaris supplies the outer third of the retina, including the outer plexiform and outer nuclear layers, the photoreceptors, and the pigment epithelium. The inner two-thirds of the retina receive branches of the central retinal artery. As the choriocapillaris is the only blood supply to the fovea centralis, this, the most important part of the retina, is susceptible to irreparable damage when the retina is detached.

PHYSIOLOGY

The optical system of the eye focuses a miniature image of the world upon the outer segments of the rods and cones, where the light starts a complex chain of chemical reactions beginning with a light-sensitive pigment composed of a small molecule, retinal (vitamin A aldehyde), bound to a large protein, opsin. The retinal is the same in both rods and cones, but the opsin differs. Light isomerizes the retinal from the 11-*cis* to an all-*trans* shape, so that it no longer remains adherent to the opsin. The liberated all-*trans* retinal may be metabolized to the 11-*cis* form and reattached to opsin, or it may be stored as vitamin A to be used later as the need arises.

The chemical sequence following the isomerization of retinal produces a transient excitation of the receptor that is propagated along its axon. A complex system of interconnections between the receptor axon and the cell processes of the horizontal and bipolar cells begins the process of analyzing the raw data from the receptors. The bipolar cells transmit this refined information to the inner plexiform layer, where it is once more modified through connections between amacrine, bipolar, and ganglion cells. The ganglion cells pass this reanalyzed information to the brain.

The cones are used for detailed vision (eg, reading) and color perception (Fig 11–2). They predominate at the macula, the center of visual attention; and they alone are present at the fovea, the site of best visual acuity. The rods, which predominate elsewhere, function best in reduced illumination. The principal roles of the extramacular retina are night vision and visual orientation. Examples of the latter are the ability to walk without tripping over objects or to fix one's gaze on a moving object.

Physiology of Symptoms

The function of the retina is to receive visual images, to partly analyze them, and to dispatch this modified information to the brain. In the absence of refractive errors or opacities of the media, the images are seen in sharp focus. If the macular area of the retina is diseased, the patient's central visual acuity is affected, causing difficulty in reading and in discerning small objects in the distance (eg, street signs). If the peripheral portion of the retina is diseased, side vision is impaired but the patient continues to read well. With extreme contraction of peripheral visual field, the patient can read the finest print but bumps into large objects such as chairs and desks.

The retina has no pain nerve fibers, so that diseases of the retina are painless. In addition, they do not cause the eye to become red. The clinical evaluation of patients with retinal disease includes history, visual acuity, refraction, biomicroscopy, ophthalmoscopy, visual fields, color vision tests, and fluorescein angioscopy. Other helpful diagnostic tests in the study of retinal disorders include fluorescein angiography, electroretinography (ERG), electro-oculography (EOG), dark adaptation, and ultrasonography. (See Chapter 2.)

DISEASES OF THE RETINA

RETINAL ARTERY OCCLUSION

Blockage of the central retinal artery or one of its branches is an uncommon unilateral disorder of older patients. The obstruction may be due to an embolus or may be caused by intimal atherosclerosis. When the central retinal artery is affected, the result is sudden complete or almost complete loss of vision. Ophthalmoscopic examination within 2 hours of the occlusion shows segmentation of the blood column. Later, the vessel may appear normal, but emboli are often visible at its bifurcations. The posterior retina is pale and opaque because of changes in the axons of the nerve fiber layer (Fig 11–3). Lacking the inner retinal layers, the fovea remains transparent with the choroid showing through as a cherry-red spot. The direct pupillary response is absent. The consensual light reaction is normal.

One should attempt to restore the blood flow if the patient is seen within 2 hours of the onset of symptoms. The suggested treatment is massaging the globe and anterior chamber paracentesis. The globe is massaged by pressing firmly through the closed lids for several seconds and then abruptly releasing the pressure. This maneuver is repeated several times.

Anterior chamber paracentesis is performed after anesthesia is achieved by instillation of drops and by local infiltration of the conjunctiva. The conjunctiva is held with a forceps, and a short 30-gauge needle, which is not attached to a syringe, is passed obliquely through the limbus at 4:30 or 7:30 o'clock. The needle

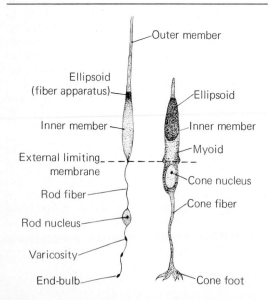

Figure 11–2. Rod *(left)* and cone *(right).* (Redrawn and reproduced, with permission, from Wolff E: *Anatomy of the Eye and Orbit,* 4th ed. Blakiston-McGraw, 1954.)

Labels: Outer member; Ellipsoid (fiber apparatus); Ellipsoid; Inner member; Inner member; Myoid; External limiting membrane; Cone nucleus; Rod fiber; Cone fiber; Rod nucleus; Varicosity; End-bulb; Cone foot

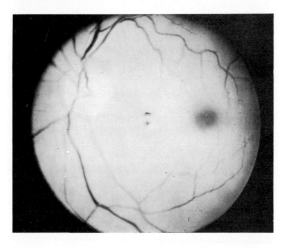

Figure 11–3. Twenty-four hours after left central retinal artery occlusion. Ischemic changes have made the nerve fiber layer pale and opaque. Because the fovea lacks this layer, the choroid can be seen as a cherry-red spot.

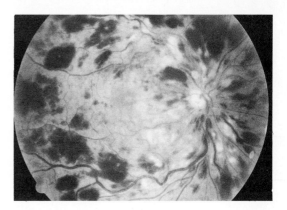

Figure 11–4. Central retinal vein occlusion. (Courtesy of University of California, San Francisco.)

is aimed at the 6 o'clock chamber angle so as to avoid the lens. One or 2 drops of aqueous are expressed through the needle by pressing on the globe, and the needle is removed. The rationale of the procedure is that the sudden lowering of the intraocular pressure might allow the blood in the central retinal artery to dislodge the embolus to a more peripheral branch of the vessel.

There is experimental evidence that 100% oxygen at atmospheric pressure may prolong retinal survival. However, if complete loss of vision persists for more than 2 hours, the value of therapy is questionable.

RETINAL VEIN OCCLUSION

1. CENTRAL RETINAL VEIN OCCLUSION (Fig 11–4)

Central retinal vein occlusion is an uncommon, usually monocular condition in which the retina and disk are swollen, the retinal veins are dilated and tortuous, and there are many retinal hemorrhages with a variable number of cotton wool patches. These findings, which are due to blockage of the central retinal vein at the level of the lamina cribrosa or behind it, are most prominent in the posterior pole and are less intense in the peripheral retina. The choriocapillaris protects the retina from ischemic death.

The patient generally presents with a slow, painless loss of vision. Predisposing systemic diseases are hypertension, diabetes, and conditions that slow venous blood flow. Many patients have elevated intraocular tension in both eyes.

One may divide the patients into 2 fairly distinct subgroups. In the less severely affected group, the

retinal bleeding is mild and there are few, if any, cotton wool patches. The visual acuity is generally no worse than 20/80 and the peripheral visual field is relatively normal. A few of the patients in this group may get worse, so that they will be included in the more severely affected group, but most dry out spontaneously when, in the course of weeks or months, the shunt vessels enlarge. Many regain normal vision, although some, in whom the fovea is permanently damaged by the edema, have a persistent central scotoma.

The usually older patients in the more severely affected subgroup are felt to have a deficient retinal arterial supply compounding the venous obstruction. In these patients, whose condition is sometimes labeled hemorrhagic retinopathy—as opposed to the name, venous stasis retinopathy, applied to the less severely affected group—the congestion and bleeding of the disk and retina are more pronounced and there may be many cotton wool exudates. These hemorrhagic retinopathy patients have a reduced peripheral visual field. Their visual acuity is 20/200 or worse. Fluorescein demonstrates absence of blood flow through the greater part of the retinal capillary bed, and histologically there is no viable retinal vascular endothelium. The protracted course of hemorrhagic retinopathy leads to the following states: cystoid degeneration and irreversible loss of foveal function; alterations of all parts of the retinal parenchyma; degeneration of the pigment epithelium; and liquefaction of the vitreous. When the vitreous is severely liquefied and thus no longer serves as a diffusion barrier to angiogenesis stimuli coming from the retina, new vessels often develop on the surface of the iris and the anterior chamber angle, causing peripheral anterior synechiae and intractable glaucoma.

Treatment

Many of the patients with venous stasis retinopathy recover spontaneously and require no treatment. Failing this, steroids may be considered.

Some practitioners advocate photocoagulation for

those with hemorrhagic retinopathy. Anticoagulants, if they do anything, make matters worse.

In the hope of preventing neovascular glaucoma, the iris surface should be periodically checked for new vessels. Fluorescein angiography helps visualize these vessels, which first appear at the pupillary margin. If they occur, panretinal photocoagulation—a polka-dot distribution of coagulations covering areas of the retina other than the macula—usually arrests the process. If the media are too opaque for photocoagulation, the equivalent—transcleral cryotherapy—may help.

The possibilities of systemic vascular occlusive disease or blood sludging problems should be considered.

2. RETINAL BRANCH VEIN OCCLUSION (Fig 11–5)

Retinal branch vein occlusion is more common than central retinal vein occlusion. The obstruction occurs at the site of an arteriovenous crossing. Distal to the obstruction, the vein is engorged and tortuous, the retina is edematous, and there are hemorrhages, microaneurysms, and sometimes cotton wool exudates. Fluorescein angioscopy emphasizes the venous dilation and demonstrates segmental dilation and leakiness of the retinal capillary bed.

The superior temporal vein is most often affected. When the macular area is involved, the vision is reduced. If one-quarter or less of the macula is edematous, the prognosis for spontaneous recovery is good. If more, the prognosis is poor.

A significant number of patients with occlusion of a branch of the retinal vein will subsequently develop new vessels. These proliferate from the surrounding, relatively normal retinal or disk vessels. If the vitreous still is against the retina, they fan out on its back surface and may bleed both behind the vitreous and into its substance, when eventually the vitreous detaches. Rarely, traction by the vitreous may tear the retina at the site of origin of the neovascular frond.

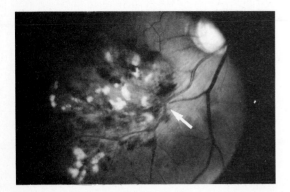

Figure 11–5. Inferotemporal branch vein occlusion in right eye. Hemorrhages and cotton wool spots are located distal to the point of obstruction at an arteriovenous crossing (arrow). (Courtesy of E Ai.)

In the presence of preexisting vitreous detachment, the new vessels present as minute protrusions at the inner retinal surface. Such vessels also may bleed, apparently because the mobile vitreous brushes against them.

Three-fourths of patients with branch vein occlusion have high blood pressure. Diabetes, sickle cell disease, polycythemia vera, lymphoma, leukemia, macroglobulinemia, and multiple myeloma are less common causes.

Treatment

Patients with retinal branch vein occlusion should be evaluated by an internist. If visually significant macular edema does not clear spontaneously, the area of capillary leakage identified by angiography can be treated with argon laser photocoagulation in a grid pattern that spares the fovea. If neovascularization is present, photocoagulation of the involved ischemic retinal sector may cause regression of the new vessels. Vitrectomy may become necessary if vitreous hemorrhage does not clear and obscures the retina.

DIABETIC RETINOPATHY

Diabetic retinopathy continues to be one of the leading causes of blindness in the Western world. Its frequency increases with the duration of the underlying disease. Several studies have suggested a strong correlation between poor antecedent blood glucose control and increased incidence and severity of retinopathy. However, it is unknown if there is a causal relationship or if these are separate manifestations of a more severe form of disease.

In terms of both prognosis and treatment, it is useful to divide diabetic retinopathy into nonproliferative and proliferative forms. The former can be further classified as background diabetic retinopathy or preproliferative retinopathy.

1. NONPROLIFERATIVE DIABETIC RETINOPATHY

Diabetic retinopathy is a progressive microangiopathy characterized by small vessel damage and occlusion. The earliest pathologic changes are thickening of the capillary endothelial basement membrane and reduction in the number of pericytes. **Background diabetic retinopathy** (Fig 11–6A) is a clinical reflection of the hyperpermeability and incompetence of these vascular walls. The capillaries develop tiny dotlike outpouchings called microaneurysms, while the retinal veins become dilated and tortuous.

Multiple hemorrhages may appear throughout different levels of the retina. Flame hemorrhages are so shaped because of their location within the horizontally oriented nerve fiber layer, while dot and blot hemorrhages are in the deeper retina, where cells and axons are vertically oriented.

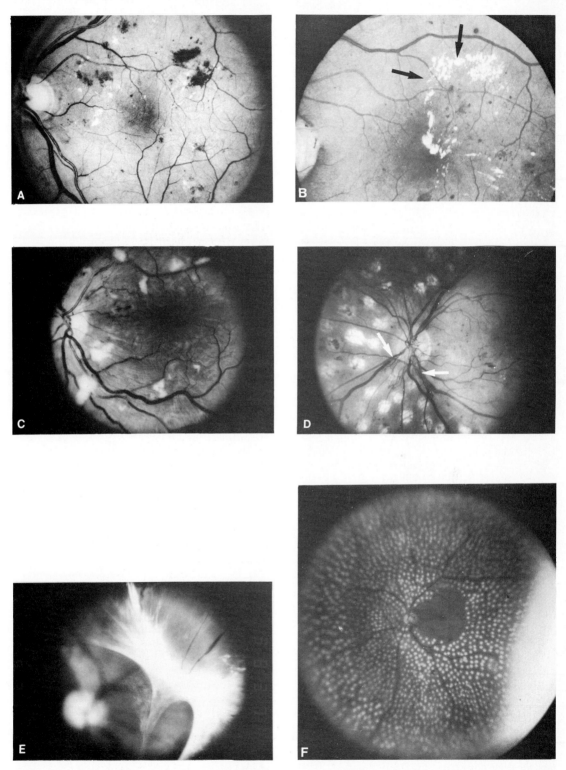

Figure 11–6. A: Background diabetic retinopathy. **B:** Background diabetic retinopathy with hard exudate (arrows). (Courtesy of P O'Malley.) **C:** Preproliferative retinopathy with multiple cotton wool spots (incorrectly named "soft exudates"). (Courtesy of E Ai.) **D:** Proliferative diabetic retinopathy with neovascularization of left disk (arrow) and panretinal photocoagulation scars sparing the macula. (Courtesy of E Ai.) **E:** Diabetic traction retinal detachment. (Courtesy of E Ai.) **F:** Wide-angle view of panretinal photocoagulation in left eye. (Reproduced, with permission, from Duane TD [editor]: Diabetic retinopathy. Chap 30, p 17, in: *Clinical Ophthalmology,* Vol 3. Lippincott. Series of 6 vols, 1978–1983.)

Leaking capillaries produce retinal edema with a predilection for the macula, giving the retina a thickened, cloudy appearance. In areas where serous fluid is resorbed, a yellowish lipid precipitate may remain in the form of "hard" exudate (Fig 11–6B). Central vision is variably impaired if the fovea becomes edematous or ischemic or contains deposits of hard exudate. Many diabetics will not progress beyond this stage.

With progressive microvascular occlusion, signs of increasing ischemia may be superimposed on the above background picture, producing so-called **preproliferative diabetic retinopathy.** The most typical change would be the appearance of multiple cotton wool spots (incorrectly termed "soft exudates"), which are microinfarcts of the nerve fiber layer (Fig 11–6C).

Other signs include gross venous abnormalities, such as loops, boxcarlike segmentation, and intraretinal microvascular abnormalities, which consist of irregularly dilated capillary beds and intraretinal shunts. Fluorescein angiography, which best demonstrates the extent of ischemia, shows "capillary nonperfusion," or large filling defects of capillary dropout usually most pronounced in the midperipheral retina.

Treatment

In background diabetic retinopathy, attention is focused on optimizing control of blood glucose and any associated hypertension. Macular edema may spontaneously improve, but if there is a significant loss of vision, laser photocoagulation may be considered if a focal source of leakage can be targeted by the angiogram. Randomly scattered laser therapy for diffuse macular leakage is controversial.

Preproliferative retinopathy is associated with increased risk for development of neovascularization, and these patients require close monitoring, even if they are asymptomatic. The effect of early laser panretinal photocoagulation during this stage and the benefit of laser treatment for macular edema are being evaluated in a national trial.

2. PROLIFERATIVE DIABETIC RETINOPATHY

The most severe complications of diabetic retinopathy are associated with the proliferative phase. Progressive retinal ischemia eventually stimulates the formation of delicate new vessels that leak serum and proteins (and fluorescein) profusely. Neovascularization is frequently located on the surface of the disk and at the posterior edge of peripheral zones of "nonperfusion" (Figs 11–6D and 11–7). Iris neovascularization, or rubeosis, can also result.

The fragile new vessels proliferate onto the posterior face of the vitreous and become elevated once the vitreous starts to contract away from the retina. If the vessels bleed, massive vitreous hemorrhage may cause sudden visual loss. As these elevated neovascular fronds undergo fibrous change, they form taut fibrovascular bands that tug on the retina with continued vitreous contraction (Fig 11–6E). This can cause either a progressive traction retinal detachment (without a hole) or a rhegmatogenous detachment if a tear is produced. A detachment may be concealed by vitreous hemorrhage.

Treatment

Argon laser panretinal photocoagulation is usually indicated in proliferative diabetic retinopathy. Patients at greatest risk are those with preretinal or vitreous hemorrhage or neovascularization of the disk. Panretinal photocoagulation can significantly reduce the chance of massive vitreous hemorrhage and retinal detachment in these patients by causing the regression, and in some cases, the disappearance of new vessels.

The technique involves scattering up to several thousand regularly spaced laser burns throughout the retina, sparing the central region bordered by the disk and the major temporal vascular arcades. (Fig 11–6F). Although the mechanism is not precisely understood, panretinal photocoagulation presumably works by reducing the angiogenic stimulus from ischemic retina.

If a significant vision-impairing vitreous hemorrhage has not spontaneously cleared by 6 months, vitrectomy may be performed. Operation should be performed immediately if progressive retinal detachment is suspected clinically or on ultrasound examination. Traction retinal detachments that involve or threaten the macula are treated by vitrectomy to release the traction and by scleral buckling to help reattach the retina.

The presence of retinal neovascularization alone will not affect vision. In the absence of macular pathology, such patients may be asymptomatic. Because many resulting severe complications can be presented by prompt laser treatment, the importance of early detection and regular monitoring cannot be overemphasized.

EDEMA OF THE RETINA

Between the retinal cells there is a potential space that fills with fluid when the retinal capillaries leak. The accumulation is greatest in the outer part of the outer plexiform layer, less in the outer and inner nuclear layers, and negligible in the remaining tightly woven layers. Because of the oblique course of the receptor cell axons in the Henle fiber layer, the macula swells more than the rest of the retina and the fluid is often visibly loculated in varicose tunnels radiating from the fovea, which itself becomes a single cystlike cavity.

Chronic edema is often accompanied by minute yellow deposits, mainly in the outer plexiform layer or beneath the retina. In the Henle fiber layer, the aggregates have a striking stellate distribution. Elsewhere, a nidus of edema is surrounded by a circular belt of these deposits. If the circinate figure is close

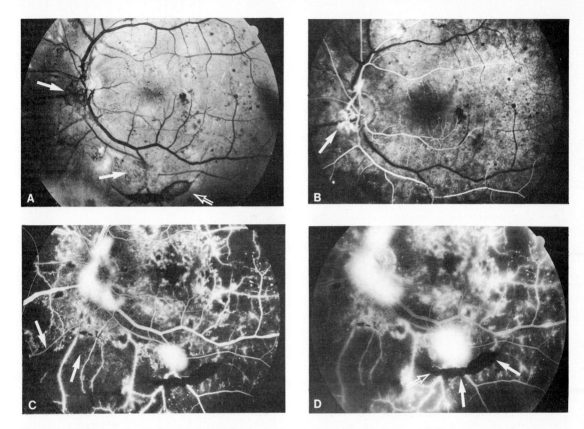

Figure 11–7. Proliferative diabetic retinopathy. **A:** Fundus photography of left eye, showing neovascularization of the disk and along the inferotemporal arcade (arrows). The latter area has bled, producing a preretinal hemorrhage (open arrow). **B:** Fluorescein angiogram (early phase) of the same eye, showing dye filling the area of neovascularization on the disk (arrows). **C:** Mid-phase angiogram, showing dye leakage from the 2 areas of neovascularization. In addition to the irregular venous caliber, extensive ischemic areas of capillary dropout can be seen (arrow). **D:** Late-phase angiogram, showing profuse leakage of fluorescein from the same areas. The retinal vessels are obscured by the preretinal hemorrhage (arrows). (Courtesy of University of California, San Francisco.)

to the macula, it spreads along the spaces of the Henle fiber layer, forming one arm of a star figure. Beneath the retina, the fatty material is irregularly clumped like the aggregates sometimes seen when new vessels grow through Bruch's membrane.

The causes of retinal edema include diabetes, retinal vein obstruction, hypertension, retinal angiomas or telangiectases, traction by the vitreous or preretinal membranes, macroaneurysms, and inflammations involving the vitreous or retina. A special case of retinal edema is the **Irvine-Gass syndrome,** which consists of rapid, usually temporary loss of visual acuity in aphakic patients. It occurs more commonly after intracapsular extraction, which allows the vitreous to adhere to the iris. It is probably due to chemicals in the anterior segment having free access to the retina through the liquefied vitreous core.

Clinical Findings

Blurred vision occurs only when the macula is edematous. Visual acuity may be only slightly affected or may be as low as finger counting. The elevation

and ground glass appearance of the macular area can be quite striking, and one may discern a cystoid accumulation of fluid. When retinal edema is widespread, with relative sparing of the macula—as can be the case in diabetic patients—the ophthalmoscopic diagnosis is difficult. The only clues are retinal pallor and difficulty in distinguishing details of the pigment epithelium and choroid.

Intravenous fluorescein confirms the diagnosis of retinal edema, because the dye leaks from the normally impermeable vessels and stains the extracellular fluid and because cystoid collections at the macula (which cannot be discerned with the ophthalmoscope) will become easily visible. Later, if there is frank cystoid degeneration, the cavity contents no longer stain. Fluorescein does not stain the waxy yellow deposits observed in chronic edema.

Treatment

If macular edema is due to inflammation, corticosteroids may help when given systemically or by parabulbar injection.

Most patients with the Irvine-Gass syndrome need only explanation and encouragement, since they will improve without treatment. Prophylactic therapy with indomethacin reduces the incidence of this complication. If the vitreous is detached from the retina and is extensively adherent to the iris and the cataract incision, the macular edema often persists until the fovea is irreversibly damaged. Patients with these developments are sometimes helped by vitrectomy.

Focal edema due to vasculopathies—including diabetic retinopathy—may respond to photocoagulation.

Prognosis

Persistent macular edema may eventually become transformed into cystoid generation, with irreversible loss of central vision. In some cases, this is compounded by development of an atrophic hole at the fovea.

RETINAL MACROANEURYSMS

Sometimes, patients with hypertension or other systemic vascular diseases develop focal aneurysmal dilation of a retinal arteriole.

The aneurysm may bleed, but this usually clears spontaneously.

Surrounding the aneurysm is a ring of retinal edema. If this is away from the macula, nothing need be done, for it will clear on its own. If the exudate encroaches on the macula, however, it reduces the visual acuity and usually causes irreversible cystoid degeneration before resorbing. Photocoagulation helps if done before the macula is irreparably damaged.

RETINOPATHY OF PREMATURITY

Retinopathy of prematurity is a retinal vascular disease of premature infants who have been treated with supplemental oxygen. In addition to the severity of prematurity, it is associated with multiple risk factors: oxygen concentration, apnea, patent ductus arteriosus, septicemia, blood transfusion, and intraventricular hemorrhage. The incidence of retinopathy of prematurity is estimated to be as high as 65% in infant survivors of birth weight less than 1500 g and to approach 77% in infants weighing less than 1000 g. About 500 new cases of infant blindness resulting from retinopathy of prematurity are reported yearly in the United States.

Retinopathy of prematurity results from an alteration in normal maturation of the retinal vascular system. At 4 months' gestation, vascularization of the inner retina begins at the optic nerve and proceeds anteriorly, normally reaching the nasal ora serrata at 8 months and the temporal ora serrata at 9 months. Consequently, the preterm infant lacks blood vessels in a part of the peripheral retina that is proportionate to the level of immaturity.

In the initial phase of the disease, the retinal vessels constrict. They then dilate and become tortuous ("plus disease"). The band of primitive vascular channels and mesenchymal cells separating vascularized from nonvascularized retina becomes clearly visible (stage I). This zone thickens to form a distinct ridge (stage II). Subsequently, blood vessels and fibrous tissue proliferate at the vitreoretinal interface in this area (stage III). Contraction of this scar tissue results in vitreous hemorrhage or retinal detachment (or both). Depending on the severity of contraction and how much of the circumference of the eye is involved, the detachment may be subtotal (stage IV) or may extend for 360 degrees, forming a funnel with its apex at the disk (stage V).

Eighty to 90 percent of cases of retinopathy of prematurity undergo spontaneous regression with no significant clinical consequences. This may occur at any stage, though the advanced stages are prone to cicatricial sequelae ranging from minor peripheral retinal pigment epithelial migration and scar formation to distortion and traction of the retina (Fig 11–8), sometimes pulling the macula eccentrically (usually temporally). In later years, rhegmatogenous retinal detachment may develop.

The retinas of infants delivered at 32 weeks of gestational age should be examined and clinical findings described utilizing a classification that includes localization of pathologic features according to zone, number of clock hours involved, and stage of disease (Table 11–1). Affected and suspect eyes should be followed. Those that show evidence of progression to stage III should be treated with external panretinal cryotherapy to the peripheral avascular zone if 4 or more clock hours are involved. Stages IV and V require invasive surgery.

RETINITIS PIGMENTOSA

Retinitis pigmentosa is a group of hereditary dystrophies of the retinal receptors transmitted as autosomal recessive, autosomal dominant, or X-linked traits. The rods slowly degenerate, with secondary atrophy of the remainder of the retina and the pigment epithelium. Cells filled with epithelial pigment aggregate along the retinal vessels to give the typical bone corpuscular appearance (Fig 11–9). These changes begin in the mid periphery, sparing the macular and peripheral regions until later. The retinal problems are often associated with deafness, mental retardation, and other systemic findings, making several distinct syndromes. The most common of these is Laurence-Moon-Biedl syndrome, which combines retinitis pigmentosa, obesity, mental retardation, polydactyly, and hypogenitalism.

Night blindness—the first symptom of retinitis pigmentosa—usually occurs in early youth. Thereafter, the visual fields gradually constrict ("gun barrel vision") to become disabling in the fifth or sixth decade, at which time macular vision may also be lost. The

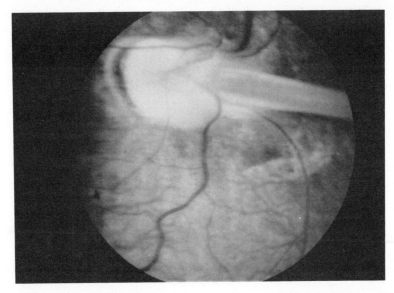

Figure 11–8. Retinopathy of prematurity (stage III). Note extraretinal fibrovascular proliferation with ridge formation. (Courtesy of R Stevens.)

fundi may appear normal at first. Later, most patients have the typical scattered black pigmentary disturbance. The retinal arterioles become attenuated, and the disk becomes pale and waxy. In rare instances, the disease may affect only one eye or just one sector of an eye.

The electroretinogram is reduced or absent, and the electro-oculogram gives a flat curve. Commonly associated eye findings are myopia, posterior polar cataract, and glaucoma.

In rare instances where retinitis pigmentosa is due to abetalipoproteinemia (Bassen-Kornzweig syndrome: steatorrhea, ataxia, and retinitis pigmentosa), its progress may be arrested in the early stages by massive doses of vitamin A. There is no specific therapy for the other causes of retinitis pigmentosa. Genetic counseling should be offered in an attempt to prevent propagation of the disease.

PERIPHERAL CYSTOID DEGENERATION

Cystoid degeneration of the retina consists of the permanent accumulation between the neural elements of a clear material that compresses the glial tissue into columns separating cystlike spaces. Some degree of cystoid degeneration is present in the peripheral retina of many infants and of everybody over age 8. It in-

Table 11–1. Stages of retinopathy of prematurity.

I. Demarcation line
II. Intraretinal ridge
III. Ridge with extraretinal fibrovascular proliferation
IV. Retinal detachment

variably begins at the ora serrata and progresses backward as a maze of contiguous varicose tunnels. It can extend behind the equator in later life, but not to the point where it causes symptoms or encroaches significantly on the peripheral field of vision.

Close to the ora serrata, the cystoid cavities are large and often cause the retina to have a moth-eaten appearance. Otherwise, the low magnification of the indirect ophthalmoscope does not normally allow the examiner to see this essentially innocuous condition.

SENILE RETINOSCHISIS

Peripheral cystoid degeneration may lead to splitting of the retina into 2 layers. Such "senile" retinoschisis occurs in about 3% of the population, increasing in frequency from the second decade onward.

The bulging internal wall of the cavity is thin and immobile and often has a "beaten metal" appearance. The thick external wall is hard to see in its usual position against the pigment epithelium, but there are often defects in it—in contrast to the inner layer, which usually is intact. Further diagnostic features include a band of prominent cystoid degeneration separating the cavity from the ora serrata and the presence of other areas of retinoschisis in the temporal half of the same eye or of the fellow eye.

If the contents of the cavity leak through a hole in the outer wall, a self-limited, usually harmless retinal detachment results. Rhegmatogenous detachment may develop when there is a hole in both walls. This rare complication is the only serious consequence of senile retinoschisis.

The bulging internal wall must not be mistaken for a retinal detachment and treated as such. Only when

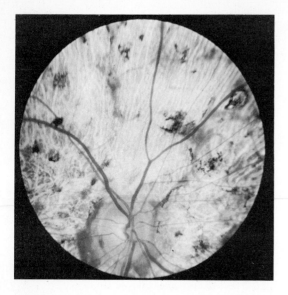 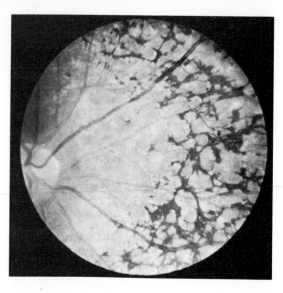

Figure 11–9. Retinitis pigmentosa. **Left:** Typical "bone spicule" arrangement of pigmentary changes. **Right:** Clumped, scattered pigment, attenuated arteries, and choroidal sclerosis. (Photos by L Arlinghaus.)

rhegmatogenous detachment has occurred or is imminent is it warranted to intervene with light coagulation, cryothermy, diathermy, or scleral buckling. In extremely rare instances, the retinal splitting threatens the macula and should be treated.

PAVING STONE DEGENERATION OF THE RETINA

Paving stone degeneration is a striking but harmless condition of the peripheral retina in which the pigment epithelium and outer retinal layers are damaged or absent. The intact inner retina is adherent to the exposed Bruch's membrane and also to the pigment epithelium at the edge of the lesion. The vitreous and the outer choroidal structures are normal.

The sharply outlined, rounded lesions are pale yellow, often with a partial rim of increased pigmentation. They range in size up to 1 disk diameter and may occur singly or in clusters. Several lesions may coalesce to form a circumferential band with a scalloped margin.

The process occurs mainly in the lower quadrants, though it is found in any part of the peripheral fundus. It is fairly common in young adults, and its incidence and the frequency of bilateral occurrence increase with age. It is quite innocuous, and the patient is unaware of its presence.

LATTICE DEGENERATION OF THE RETINA

Lattice degeneration (Fig 11–10) of the retina is characterized by elongated, excavated troughs in the peripheral retina. The lesions are surrounded by a distinct narrow rim, which projects above the level of the normal adjacent retina. The vitreous is firmly adherent to the rim and forms a canopy, which envelops a pocket of fluid lying in the trough. Close to their insertion, the vitreous fibrils are condensed and may be visible as a white frill.

Glistening white spots are common on the retinal surface, giving a snail-track appearance to some lattice

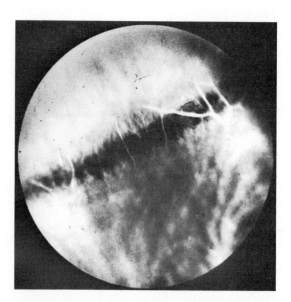

Figure 11–10. Lattice degeneration. (Reproduced, with permission, from O'Malley C, O'Malley P: *The Peripheral Fundus of the Eye.* Medcom, 1973.)

areas. Although the pigment epithelium beneath the lesions may appear normal, it is often disturbed and may vary from subtle disarray to gross disorganization. The walls of the retinal vessels are thickened where they cross the abnormal retina in over 10% of lesions. These sclerosed vessels form a white latticework that inspired the name.

The above features are often not visible on routine inspection, and areas of lattice might be missed were it not for the edge-on view afforded by scleral depression. With this aid to examination, the sharp rim and roughened, depressed surface of the trough are readily seen.

The individual lesions are about one-third disk diameter in width and one-half disk diameter to 1 quadrant long. They generally lie parallel to the ora serrata, are confined to the equatorial and oral zones, and are concentrated toward the vertical meridian. There may be as many as 20 lesions in one eye forming 2 or more parallel rows. Both eyes are affected in about a third of cases.

About 8% of the population have lattice degeneration, and the incidence is constant in each age group after 10. Surprisingly, teenagers may have heavily pigmented lesions with extreme thinning of the retina, whereas septuagenarians will often have rather superficial nonpigmented lesions. Atrophic round holes are common in all age groups.

Lattice degeneration is an etiologic factor in about one-third of all cases of rhegmatogenous retinal detachment. One of 2 distinct mechanisms is responsible for the detachment. In one group of patients, the leakage is through an atrophic hole. This may result in tiny localized areas of detachment that rarely spread and require no treatment other than periodic observation. In younger patients, such a detachment sometimes spreads slowly, with multiple demarcation lines, and surgery is required.

The more common mechanism by which lattice degeneration leads to retinal detachment derives from the fact that owing to their posterior location, about two-thirds of the lesions have established a firm vitreoretinal adhesion behind the vitreous base. If the vitreous detaches posteriorly, the stress at the ends and the posterior border of the lattice may be enough to produce a tear. The break is in the relatively normal retina beneath the rim and not through the thinned retina. Small lesions far back may be completely avulsed. Much more often, the tear is J-shaped and located at one end of the lattice. As the vitreous continues to tug on the retina, these tears usually cause extensive retinal detachment.

The threat of retinal detachment has given lattice degeneration notoriety in excess of what it deserves. Most people with this condition enjoy a normal asymptomatic existence. They should, however, be checked periodically, and they must be seen immediately if they report symptoms suggestive of vitreous detachment. If it is obvious that retinal detachment is likely—because of retinal detachment in the fellow eye, a family history of retinal detachment, or local find-ings—then one should perform prophylactic cryothermy or photocoagulation.

RETINAL HOLES

Retinal holes are either tears, which have an operculum (lid) of retinal tissue, or atrophic holes, which do not. The fovea and the peripheral retina are the sites of predilection for retinal holes. In both places, the internal limiting membrane and retinal parenchyma are thin. Extramacular tears and holes are described here. (For macular holes, see p 182.)

1. RETINAL TEARS
(Fig 11–11)

The retina is torn by mechanical force, usually vitreous traction (see also Chapter 10). The distinctive feature of a retinal tear is an operculum of avulsed tissue. The size of the tear may vary tremendously.

When the retina is torn, metaplastic pigment epithelial cells may enter the vitreous. If these tobacco-dustlike cells are found, a retinal tear is almost certainly present and must be sought.

Retinal tears may be due to constant or intermittent vitreous traction.

Tears due to constant vitreous traction. Proliferative diabetic retinopathy, penetrating injuries, and a variety of other disorders cause scarring of the vitreous. Contraction of the scarred vitreous may tear the retina at its point of attachment. Only a small percentage of retinal tears occurs by this mechanism,

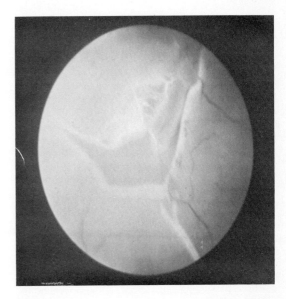

Figure 11–11. Retinal tear at an area of lattice degeneration. Operculum still attached to retina. (Reproduced, with permission, from O'Malley C, O'Malley P: *The Peripheral Fundus of the Eye.* Medcom, 1973.)

but it is important to recognize and treat them promptly for they may lead to extensive retinal detachment.

Tears due to intermittent vitreous traction. When the vitreous is partly liquefied and detached from the retina, acceleration or deceleration of the globe—either as a result of normal eye movements or trauma—will cause whiplike motions of the gel that may exert sufficient stress to tear the retina at normal and abnormal points of vitreoretinal attachments. The latter may be due to a number of anatomic anomalies and pathologic processes that may not be recognizable before the tear appears.

The greater the space inside the eye, the greater the force that can be exerted to tear the retina. This may explain why aphakia, the large globe commonly associated with myopia, forward displacement of the lens by miotics, and localized scleral ectasia predispose to retinal tears.

The operculum of most tears retains a partial attachment at the anterior margin of the break, so that the vitreous continues to tug on the retina. Even so, such retinal tears should be watched and not treated unless (1) the vitreous cavity is unduly large; (2) the holes are multiple, large, or far behind the ora serrata; (3) there is a history of retinal detachment in the fellow eye or a family history of retinal detachment; or (4) there are recent symptoms of vitreous detachment. In these situations, the danger of retinal detachment outweighs the small risk of complications from prophylactic therapy.

Retinal tissue may be torn completely free if the area of vitreoretinal adhesion is small. Such tears are generally round or oval and rarely exceed the diameter of the disk. They are much less likely to lead to retinal detachment than if the operculum is still adherent to the retina.

Relationship of Blood Vessels to Retinal Tears

At the time the retina is torn, capillaries are often ruptured and the patient reports a shower of black spots that represent shadows on the macula caused by red blood cells in the retrovitreal space. If a larger vessel is broken, the subvitreal bleeding may be so severe that the retina is obscured. A few hours of bed rest with bilateral eye patches and elevation of the head will generally allow the blood to settle enough to permit visualization of the retina.

As a rule, the larger vessels do not break, so that the retina either continues to tear beyond the vessel and a segment of the vessel is elevated off the retina or the vessel arrests the shearing force.

In younger patients, the acquired posterior extension of the vitreous base is narrow, so that tears may occur close to the ora serrata. Since the mechanical reinforcement of the retinal vessels is lacking here, the rip can extend a considerable distance around the circumference of the globe.

Causes of Retinal Tears

Vitreous traction, either intermittent or constant, accounts for the vast majority of retinal tears. This usually happens spontaneously, but indirect trauma occasionally precipitates a retinal tear in a predisposed individual.

Direct trauma deforms the globe transiently and can cause conventional tears, giant tears at the posterior margin of the vitreous base, or tears in the nonpigmented epithelium of the pars plana at the anterior margin of the vitreous base (see p 183).

Anomalous zonular attachments to the retina are also believed to cause tears. The detaching retina (for whatever reason) may also tear at the site of chorioretinal adhesions resulting from previous therapy, paving stone degeneration, or chorioretinitis, but this is rare. In these latter cases, the torn fragment remains adherent to the external structure—not in its usual location at or central to the detached retina.

2. ATROPHIC RETINAL HOLES

In addition to the atrophic holes associated with lattice degeneration and retinoschisis, about 1% of people have small, round, nonoperculated holes of unknown cause in the peripheral retina. These are usually close to the ora serrata and rarely cause significant retinal detachment, though a tiny self-limiting detachment is often present.

Most atrophic retinal holes are asymptomatic. Some are accompanied by symptoms of vitreous detachment (see Chapter 10).

Treatment

The greatest problem in treating retinal holes is deciding whether or not treatment is necessary. Unfortunately, the decision must be made with an inadequate knowledge of the natural history of most types of holes and almost total ignorance of the qualitative and quantitative parameters of vitreous traction. However, careful observation does give some clues, for with the passage of time the lips of a retinal hole become white and rounded because of gliosis; opercula slowly shrink; the subjacent pigment epithelium is often altered; and a ring of pigment epithelial reaction may appear at the edge of the narrow halo of retinal detachment, which often accompanies even innocuous holes. In the absence of frank retinal detachment, these findings tell the examiner that the potentially dangerous lesion has been present for some time without causing trouble; thus, a conservative attitude toward prophylactic therapy is required.

The objective of prophylactic treatment is to establish a firm chorioretinal bond around the retinal break. The scar should be broader on the side nearest the ora serrata, since this is usually the site of greatest vitreous pull. Indeed, it is often safest to treat forward to the vitreous base to forestall future vitreous traction.

There are 3 ways to seal a retinal hole: freezing, burning by light, or burning by electricity. The mechanism in each case is to cause an inflammatory response of the retina and choroid that subsequently binds them together.

A. Cryothermy: A supercooled metal probe is placed on the conjunctiva in an area corresponding to the borders of the retinal hole. The instrument must have an adequate heat sink to propagate a dome of ice through the wall of the eye. The surgeon ophthalmoscopically controls the freezing, which selectively destroys cells but leaves the fibrous structures intact.

B. Photocoagulation: A bright light focused on the pigment epithelium will coagulate it and the overlying retina. One may use a xenon arc or argon laser as the light source. This form of therapy is excellent for posterior lesions but is awkward to administer anterior to the equator.

C. Diathermy: The energy of a high-frequency current, when applied to the sclera, is transformed to heat, which coagulates choroid and retina.

RETINAL DETACHMENT

Because the retina is only loosely adherent to the pigment epithelium, the 2 may separate, allowing fluid to accumulate between them. The fluid usually comes from the vitreous, having passed through a hole in the retina. Less often, it leaks from blood vessels, as happens with central serous retinopathy, choroidal tumors, some inflammatory conditions, malignant hypertension, or when vitreous traction creates a subretinal space without perforating the retina. (See also Chapter 10.)

Mechanism of Rhegmatogenous Retinal Detachment

Rhegmatogenous (tear-induced) retinal detachment is dependent upon 3 factors: (1) a retinal hole, (2) liquid in the vitreous compartment with free access to the hole, and (3) a force sufficient to break the bond between the retina and the pigment epithelium and transfer fluid from in front of to behind the retina. The vitreous supplies this force in essentially the same way as it causes retinal tears (see p 176).

Until one or more of these factors is nullified, the detachment will continue to spread. Most of the retina may become detached in a few hours, or it may take years for this to happen.

Clinical Findings

The common sequence is for the symptoms of vitreous detachment (see Chapter 10) to be followed minutes to years later by a "shadow" or "curtain" spreading across the field of vision. When the detachment spreads very slowly, the patient may be unaware of any problem until the macula is affected.

On ophthalmoscopic examination, the detached retina bulges inward and is gently ripped or thrown into folds (Figs 11–12 to 11–16). It is translucent, obscuring the details of the pigment epithelium and choroid, and trembles with each movement of the eye. A careful search will almost always reveal one or

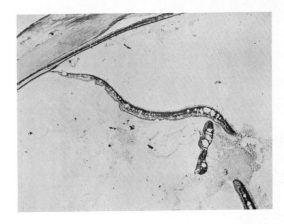

Figure 11–12. Tear in retina causing retinal detachment (microscopic section). Also shows cystoid degeneration of retina.

Figs 11–12 to 11–16 are reproduced, with permission, from Arruga H: *Detachment of the Retina.* Salvat, 1936.

more holes. If the detachment is of long standing, the retina will usually be more transparent and a characteristic demarcation line of pigment epithelial disturbance separates detached from normal retina.

The other eye must be examined, since it often has retinal holes or vitreoretinal adhesions that might lead to tears. These should be mapped carefully and treated prophylactically.

Differential Diagnosis

One must consider senile retinoschisis, choroidal detachment, and malignant melanoma of the choroid. The retinoschisis cavity has a thin, immobile inner wall. The honeycomb appearance and large breaks of the outer wall are pathognomonic but are not always

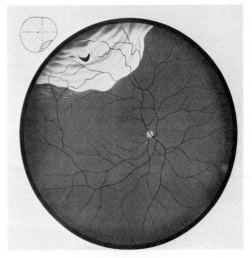

Figure 11–13. Retinal detachment 3 days after onset with crescent-shaped retinal tear.

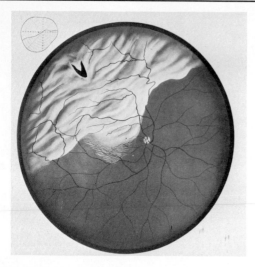

Figure 11–14. Retinal detachment and retinal tear 6 days after onset.

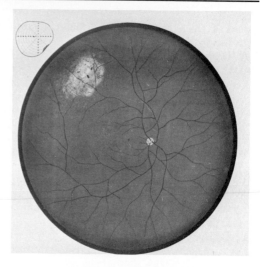

Figure 11–16. Operative cure of retinal detachment. Appearance of retina 2 months after surgical repair.

present. There may be other areas of retinoschisis on the temporal side of the same or fellow eye.

A detached choroid is not limited by the ora serrata but is prevented from spreading where the vortex vessels enter the sclera. The pigment epithelium is still visible, but the choroidal structures are not.

In malignant melanoma of the choroid, the subretinal fluid shifts on changing the patient's position. The tumor usually does not transilluminate, and its position disregards both ora serrata and vortex vessels.

Treatment

Surgical repair is mandatory in the treatment of rhegmatogenous retinal detachment, since spontaneous reattachment is extremely rare. The first step is ophthalmoscopic examination of the entire retina and

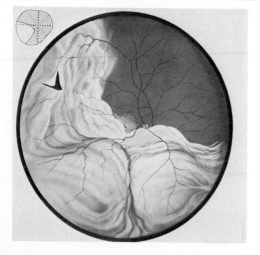

Figure 11–15. Appearance of retinal detachment 40 days after onset.

construction of a detailed map showing each hole and each area of vitreoretinal traction. The goal is to seal the holes and prevent further holes from developing. By reducing the volume of the vitreous compartment and distorting it in various ways, vitreous traction is relieved. The retina is thus placed in contact with choroid, and the tissues are stimulated by diathermy, cryothermy, or photocoagulation to establish a permanent chorioretinal bond around the hole.

Course & Prognosis

With care, 90% of retinal detachments can be repaired by one operation. Subsequent procedures salvage another 6%. If the retina is still in place after 6 months, it is unlikely to become detached again.

The fovea may suffer irreparable damage in a brief period of separation from its only blood supply, the choriocapillaris. By contrast, on reattaching the retina, extrafoveal function may recover to a remarkable degree even after several months of detachment.

PRERETINAL MEMBRANES

These thin sheets of contractile tissue on the inner retinal surface are produced by glia or by pigment epithelium that has undergone metaplasia. They arise in association with a variety of conditions, including spontaneous vitreous detachment, retinal tears with or without retinal detachment, diabetic retinopathy, occlusion of retinal veins, and penetrating injuries. The associated condition apparently provides a vitreous-free retinal surface in combination with a break in the inner limiting lamina, or a full-thickness retinal hole through which the offending cells migrate.

In the beginning, the membrane, which covers part or all of the retina behind the vitreous base, is composed of elongated cells and delicate supportive tissue;

later it contracts, exerting traction through scattered focal retinal attachments. This causes retinal folds if the retina is detached and mobile or if it causes the lips of a retinal tear to roll inward. If a large area of detached retina is involved, the condition is called **massive preretinal retraction.** In contrast, there is very little puckering when the retina is attached— whence the name **surface wrinkling retinopathy.** (See also Chapter 10.)

Clinical Findings

Vision is rapidly lost when a contracting preretinal membrane in the presence of a retinal hole causes retinal detachment. At the opposite end of the spectrum, if the retina is attached and a membrane is some distance from the macula, the patient is asymptomatic. If the macula is wrinkled, however, visual acuity may be reduced to less than 20/200.

It is usually impossible to detect an early preretinal membrane with the ophthalmoscope, since it is virtually transparent. When the membrane contracts, it may become visible, especially with the aid of redfree light. The membrane is slightly opaque, with an irregular, ill-defined outline. It bridges the apexes of the retinal folds when the retina is detached and is at the focus of the retinal wrinkles and has a shiny surface when the retina is attached.

Treatment

Treatment is usually not necessary for surface wrinkling retinopathy. However, if severe visual loss occurs, one may attempt the hazardous task of surgically cutting the membrane on the surface of the retina. If retinal detachment is present, scleral buckling and sometimes vitrectomy are indicated.

THE MACULA

CENTRAL SEROUS CHORIORETINOPATHY (Fig 11–17)

This disorder occurs at any age past the early teens and affects males more often than females. Although it is usually monocular, both eyes may be affected either concurrently or sequentially. One or more small defects appear in the pigment epithelial layer of an otherwise normal-appearing fundus, and fluid leaks from the choriocapillaris to the subretinal space. This transudate is either clear or partly opaque. The resulting smooth retinal detachment may extend up to 6 disk diameters in circumference.

The main symptom is blurred vision, and—as with most macular problems—exposure to bright light makes this worse. Visual acuity is reduced to a variable degree, and there is a slight shift toward hyperopia. Ophthalmoscopic and slit lamp examinations reveal a shallow retinal detachment with loss of the foveal reflection. Intravenous fluorescein demonstrates the site of leakage. Because the fresh fluorescein-stained fluid is warm, it rises by convection in the cooler preexisting fluid. The new fluid eventually becomes mixed with the old, and detectable fluorescence persists for about 30 minutes.

In most cases the leak closes spontaneously, and the subretinal fluid is resorbed within 3 months of the onset of the disease. Most of these patients recover good vision. Sometimes the detachment persists

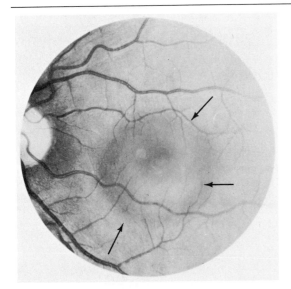 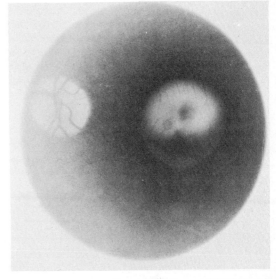

Figure 11–17. Central serous chorioretinopathy. **Left:** Fundus photo of a 34-year-old man with serous detachment of the macula (arrows). **Right:** Fluorescein angiogram showing leakage of fluid into the subretinal space. (Reproduced, with permission, from Gass J: *Stereoscopic Atlas of Macular Diseases.* Mosby, 1970.)

longer, increasing the likelihood of secondary cystoid degeneration of the macula. Permanent damage to the retina is also more likely if there are repeated episodes of central serous detachment.

If the pigment epithelial leakage persists longer than 3 months and if it is not directly beneath the fovea, photocoagulation is indicated. This seals the leakage site and the subretinal fluid is resorbed, with improvement in vision.

Although central serous chorioretinopathy appears to be a distinct entity, it must be stressed that any condition damaging Bruch's membrane and the pigment epithelium may cause leakage of serous fluid beneath the central retina. The differential diagnosis thus includes age-related macular degeneration, angioid streaks, tumors such as choroidal angioma, nevus, and malignant melanoma, familial drusen, high myopia, and trauma.

Very rarely, a pit of the optic nerve may be associated with detachment in the posterior polar retina. In these cases, there is no demonstrable leak in the pigment epithelium, and it is thought that the fluid may originate from the vitreous.

AGE-RELATED MACULAR DEGENERATION (Involutional or Senile Macular Degeneration)

Age-related macular degeneration is the leading cause of permanent blindness in the elderly. The exact cause is unknown, but the incidence increases with each decade over the age of 50. Other associations besides age include race (usually Caucasian), sex (slight female predominance), family history, and a history of cigarette smoking. Age-related macular degeneration includes a broad spectrum of clinical and pathologic findings, which can be classified into 2 groups: nonexudative ("dry") and exudative ("wet"). Although both types are progressive and usually bilateral, they differ in terms of their manifestations, prognosis, and management. The more severe exudative form accounts for approximately 90% of all cases of legal blindness due to age-related macular degeneration.

1. NONEXUDATIVE AGE-RELATED MACULAR DEGENERATION

Nonexudative age-related macular degeneration is characterized by variable degrees of atrophy and degeneration of the outer retina, retinal pigment epithelium, Bruch's membrane, and choriocapillaris (Fig 1–11). Of the ophthalmoscopically visible changes in the retinal pigment epithelium and Bruch's membrane, **drusen** are the most typical. These appear as variably sized, yellowish round spots that are located deep to the retina and scattered throughout the macula and posterior pole. With time, they may enlarge, coalesce, calcify, and increase in number (Fig 11–18).

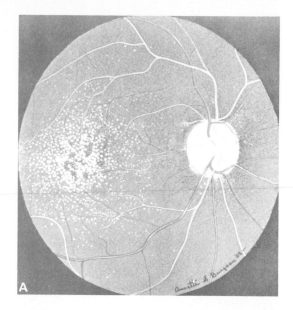

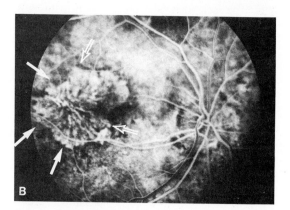

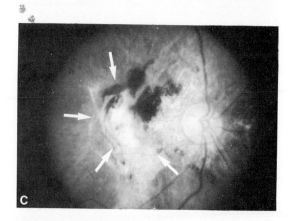

Figure 11–18. A: Nonexudative age-related macular degeneration, showing multiple drusen in the macula. (Reproduced, with permission, from Wilmer L: *Atlas Fundus Oculi.* Macmillan, 1934.) **B:** Fluorescein angiogram, showing dye filling a subretinal neovascular membrane beneath the macula (arrows). (Courtesy of E Ai.) **C:** Cicatricial stage, showing subretinal hemorrhage and a disciform macular scar (arrows). (Courtesy of E Ai.)

Microscopically, drusen are small mounds of amorphous material deposited within Bruch's membrane by retinal pigment epithelial cells. Other types of drusen can occur in younger patients and in dominantly inherited patterns, but these differ ultrastructurally from the age-related type. In addition to drusen, clumps of pigment irregularly interspersed with depigmented areas of atrophy may progressively appear throughout the macula. The level of associated visual impairment is variable and may be minimal. Fluorescein angiography demonstrates the irregular patterns of retinal pigment epithelial hyperplasia and thinning. Drusen hyperfluoresce owing to overlying retinal pigment epithelial attenuation.

Treatment

There is no known means of treatment or prevention for this stage of the disease. Fortunately, progression of the atrophic changes is slow and may stabilize. However, the exudative stage may suddenly develop at any time, and in addition to regular ophthalmic examinations, patients are given an Amsler grid (see Chapter 2) to help monitor themselves for any symptomatic changes.

2. EXUDATIVE AGE-RELATED MACULAR DEGENERATION

The impairment of Bruch's membrane as a barrier between the retinal pigment epithelium and the choriocapillaris gives rise to the complications of "wet" age-related macular degeneration. Serous fluid or blood from the choroid can leak through small defects in the collagenous membrane, causing a focal dome-shaped elevation of the pigment epithelium, or so-called retinal pigment epithelial detachment (Fig 11–19). Additional fluid may lead to further separation of the overlying sensory retina, and vision usually decreases if the fovea becomes detached. Retinal pigment epithelial detachments may spontaneously flatten, with variable visual results, and may leave a geographic area of depigmentation at the involved site.

The prognosis is much worse if a subretinal neovascular membrane is present. Degenerative breaks in Bruch's membrane provide a pathway through which choroidal neovascularization can proliferate beneath the retinal pigment epithelium. The stimulus for the growth of the vessels is unknown. They may behave in a variety of patterns, remaining unnoticed in a dormant "subclinical" state or actively leaking or bleeding while exhibiting amazingly rapid growth. Although fluorescein angiography may fail to detect occult neovascularization, this technique usually identifies these membranes, which are typically lacy, delicate vascular networks that leak dye profusely. (Figs 11–18 and 11–19.)

A leaking macular subretinal neovascular membrane may produce **metamorphopsia** (wavy distortion of vision), a blurred scotoma, or decreased central acuity. Any of these symptoms may develop suddenly. Funduscopic signs of subretinal neovascularization include subretinal hemorrhage, sub- and intraretinal hard exudate, overlying detachments of the retinal pigment epithelium and sensory retina, and the appearance of a "dirty gray" subretinal membrane, occasionally surrounded by a pigmentary ring.

Although some neovascular membranes may occasionally regress, the natural course of age-related macular degeneration associated with subretinal neovascularization is usually one of progressive, severe worsening. The time span is variable, but a rapid decline can occur within days. The sensory retina may be damaged by long-standing edema, detachment, or subretinal hemorrhage. Furthermore, a hemorrhagic detachment of the retina may undergo fibrous meta-

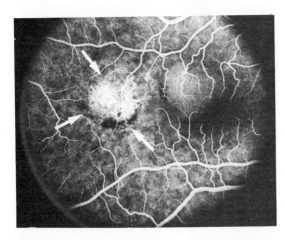 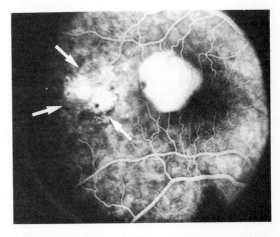

Figure 11–19. Early-phase *(left)* and late-phase *(right)* angiograms of the same eye, show a serous retinal pigment epithelial detachment on the right, adjacent to a subretinal neovascular membrane on the left (arrows). Note the irregular pattern of fluorescence of the neovascular membrane in contrast to the homogeneous pattern of the serous detachment. A subretinal hemorrhage is seen at the inferior edge of the membrane. (Courtesy of E Ai.)

plasia and organization, resulting in an elevated sub-retinal mass called a **disciform scar.** This fixed, but variably sized, fibrovascular mound represents the cic-atricial stage of exudative age-related macular degen-eration. If centrally located, it results in permanent loss of central vision (Fig 11–18).

Treatment

In the absence of subretinal neovascularization, la-ser treatment of serous retinal pigment epithelial de-tachments is of no proved benefit. However, if a sub-retinal neovascular membrane is present and has not yet involved the fovea, laser photocoagulation offers hope for stabilization or improvement.

An angiogram is used to define the precise location and borders of the neovascular membrane, which is then completely ablated by heavy confluent laser burns. Photocoagulation destroys the overlying retina as well but is worthwhile if the subretinal membrane can be halted short of the fovea. The opportunity for treatment is lost once the fovea is involved; this un-derscores the importance of prompt detection and eval-uation.

The argon blue-green laser was the first to be proved successful in the treatment of subretinal neovascular membranes located at least 200 μm away from the center of the fovea. Because of the particular absorp-tion characteristics of this technique, it is not as safe for treatment closer to the fovea. For the photoco-agulation of juxtafoveal membranes, 3 other laser wavelengths—red and yellow krypton and argon green—appear safer and are being clinically evalu-ated. Treatment is not indicated for subfoveal neo-vascularization.

Even when successfully treated, subretinal neo-vascular membranes can recur, either adjacent to the initial area or at new sites within the same or fellow eye. The incidence of membranes occurring in the fellow eye may be as high as 12–15% per year. Thus, careful monitoring with Amsler grids, ophthalmos-copy, and angiography is essential. Once both foveas have been damaged, the only helpful measures are low-vision aids and magnifiers.

ANGIOID STREAKS
(Fig 11–20)

Linear breaks in the fibroelastic layer of Bruch's membrane may ophthalmoscopically resemble blood vessels, for which reason they are called angioid streaks. They are brown, irregular bands radiating from the disk. Associated findings are pseudoxan-thoma elasticum (Groenblad-Strandberg syndrome), sickle cell disease, and Paget's disease (osteitis de-formans). From a practical point of view, the lacquer breaks of high myopia and traumatic ruptures of Bruch's membrane can be grouped with angioid streaks. The pigment epithelium overlying all of these lesions slowly degenerates, and new vessels some-times grow through the defect in Bruch's membrane

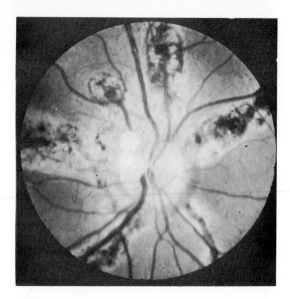

Figure 11–20. Retinal photograph showing angioid streaks in retina. (Courtesy of M Hogan and S Aiken.)

to cause a disciform lesion in a manner similar to that which occurs in age-related macular degeneration.

In the absence of neovascularization, angioid streaks are usually asymptomatic. If new vessels are present, photocoagulation occasionally helps.

PRESUMED HISTOPLASMOSIS SYNDROME

A considerable number of patients from the eastern half of the USA have combinations of the following findings: positive skin test for histoplasmosis, miliary opacities of the lungs, tiny choroidal scars, peripap-illary disruption of the choroid, and exudation or bleeding from subretinal neovascular lesions at or near the macula. Except for the macular complications, the condition is asymptomatic and benign. Once disciform changes commence, the prognosis is very poor. Pho-tocoagulation usually arrests the course of active le-sions that are eccentric to the fovea.

MACULAR HOLE

As in the retinal periphery, the parenchyma and internal limiting membrane at the avascular fovea are thin and prone to hole formation (Fig 11–21). These atrophic macular holes are fairly common and can be caused by prolonged macular edema or traction by a preretinal membrane. In older patients, they may de-velop spontaneously.

The loss of vision is proportionate to the size of the hole and the associated findings. If the retina is flat, it is often difficult to tell if the macula is really perforated. However, one can be reasonably confident

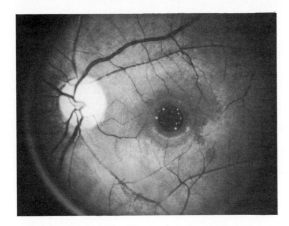

Figure 11–21. Macular hole. (Courtesy of E Ai.)

of the diagnosis if the view of the underlying pigment epithelium is sharp, the hole margin is rounded and more opaque than the contiguous retina, and the background choroidal fluorescence shows through clearly.

There is no effective treatment for macular atrophic holes. They very rarely lead to retinal detachment and should merely be watched.

HEREDITARY DISEASES OF THE MACULA

The hereditary diseases of the macula—all of which are untreatable—can be loosely divided into those that involve primarily the choriocapillaris and those that initially affect the pigment epithelium.

Central areolar choroidal sclerosis is an example of the former group. This autosomal dominant or recessive disease leads to slow loss of central vision in middle life. Abnormalities of the choriocapillaris and pigment epithelium are apparent early. By the time symptoms occur, there may be complete atrophy of the central pigment epithelium.

Stargardt-Behr disease and Best's disease are examples of macular diseases primarily affecting the pigment epithelium. Stargardt-Behr disease is usually transmitted in an autosomal recessive manner. Commencing at different ages, the macular pigment epithelium slowly degenerates. The intensity of the pigment epithelial changes and the degree of visual loss vary from family to family.

In Best's vitelliform macular degeneration, there is a diffuse abnormality of the pigment epithelium, but the visible changes are confined to the macula. Initially in this autosomal dominant disease—though the vision is good—there are deposits in the pigment epithelium, giving the appearance of a poached egg "sunny side up." Later, when the yolk of the egg appears scrambled, macular vision is seriously reduced.

TRAUMA

Though the eye as a whole must be considered when dealing with an injury (see Chapter 20), some details particular to the retina are described here.

BLUNT TRAUMA

A nonpenetrating injury to the globe may tear the retina or produce commotio retinae, or it may indirectly damage the retina as a result of fracturing Bruch's membrane.

Traumatic Retinal Tears

The severe, almost instantaneous distortion of the globe caused by blunt trauma can tear the retina, primarily because of the different rates at which the vitreous and the eye wall change shape. The nonuniform structure of the vitreous and the attachments of the vitreous to the retina dictate where the tears will occur. Thus, the vitreous base, the ribbon of very firm vitreoretinal adhesion extending 1–2 mm in front of and behind the ora, may be disinserted, or the tears may be confined to the retina at the posterior margin of the vitreous base or the nonpigmented epithelium of the pars plana at its anterior margin. Such tears can lead to retinal detachment and usually require treatment.

Trauma may prematurely cause a posterior vitreous detachment, such as normally happens as an aging phenomenon to most people. On detaching, the vitreous may tear the retina at focal vitreoretinal adhesions situated behind the vitreous base. These tears and the associated bleeding into the vitreous are handled the same way as those that occur spontaneously.

Commotio Retinae (Berlin's "Edema")

A blow to the front of the eye can sometimes avulse the outer segments of the retinal receptor cells in a discrete area at the back of the eye. In the following weeks, this debris is phagocytosed by the pigment epithelium. At first, the white subretinal material is easily visible. Eventually, little ophthalmoscopic evidence of it remains other than a localized mild disturbance of the underlying pigment epithelium. There is a permanent scotoma in the affected area. When it includes the macula, the symptoms are distressing. Otherwise, the loss of visual field may go unnoticed.

With involvement of the peripheral retina or the fovea, where the retina and its internal limiting membrane are thinnest, an atrophic retinal hole may later develop at the site of the contrecoup injury (Fig 20–3). Such holes rarely cause a significant retinal detachment.

Fracture of Bruch's Membrane

Blunt trauma will sometimes cause one or more easily visible linear fractures of Bruch's membrane, which are usually accompanied by subretinal bleeding. The break may occur anywhere. Those in the posterior pole are curved and are concentric with the optic nerve head. In the course of time, the subretinal blood resorbs, but the pigment epithelium bordering the fracture atrophies over the areas of choriocapillaris supplied by the affected ciliary arterioles. Later still, new vessels may grow into the subretinal space through the breaks in Bruch's membrane (see Exudative Age-Related Macular Degeneration, p 181).

If they are some distance from the macula, fractures of Bruch's membrane and possible complications are of little consequence to the patient. However, a fracture beneath the fovea usually causes permanent loss of function, though vision sometimes improves when the subretinal blood is resorbed. Late involvement of the macula by a disciform lesion usually causes permanent loss of macular vision. These disciform cases are occasionally helped by photocoagulation. (See Fig 20–4.)

PENETRATING INJURY

At the time of a penetrating injury, the retina may be directly damaged by the penetrating object or indirectly damaged through traction on the vitreous. The findings are protean and are handled surgically according to the anatomic situation.

Quite often, an injury involving the vitreous will cause late traction on the retina owing either to contraction of fibrous tissue, which grows along the penetration tract, or to the delayed detachment of the vitreous, which was initiated by the injury. In either case, the retina may be distorted or detached and may require surgical intervention.

INJURY DUE TO EXPOSURE TO ELECTROMAGNETIC ENERGY

Orson W. White, MD

Damage to retinal elements caused by exposure to excessive electromagnetic energy, including light, has occurred with increasing frequency in recent years. Causes include increased retinal exposure during operations with the operating microscope, prolonged and repeated retinal examinations, repeated retinal photographs, and therapeutic and accidental exposure to lasers.

The energy from light and other forms of radiomagnetic energy can be calculated with the following equation:

Energy = Planck's constant × Number of photons × Frequency

A deer struck by an automobile and one struck by a bullet from a high-powered rifle delivering the same amount of energy on impact would suffer different injuries. In similar fashion, the effect on the molecule or atom varies with the frequency (wavelength) of the energy absorbed. With a transition from the relatively longer wavelengths of radio waves, microwaves, and infrared rays, through the visible spectrum and ultraviolet light, to the shorter wavelength x-rays and gamma rays, there are qualitative differences in the damage caused.

It is important to be aware that excessive electromagnetic energy, including light energy, can result in permanent visual damage.

COLOR VISION & COLOR BLINDNESS

Light may be defined as that portion of the electromagnetic spectrum (400–700 nm) that readily stimulates human retinal receptors. To other species, "light" may encompass a different set of wavelengths.

The cones mediate color vision. In order to be stimulated, they require a greater intensity of light than the rods. Thus, one cannot detect color in moonlight. Each cone has one of 3 distinct spectral sensitivity patterns. These curves are overlapping, with maxima at red, green, or blue. A given light elicits different degrees of response in each type of cone. This generates data which the neural computer interprets as a specific color.

Color is dependent upon hue, saturation, and brightness. Objects appear to have a particular **hue** primarily because they reflect, irradiate, or transmit light of certain wavelengths. The addition of black to a given hue produces the various **shades.**

Saturation is an index of purity of a hue. For example, scarlet is more saturated than pink because pink is made up of red and white mixed together.

Brightness is that aspect of perception most closely related to light intensity.

Color blindness is a misleading term, since most color-blind people have normal visual acuity. According to Marriott, 8% of men and 0.4% of women interpret colors differently than the rest of humanity. They are classified as follows:

(1) Cone monochromats: These individuals have only one type of cone. The incidence is about 1:1,000,000.

(2) Dichromats: Persons having 2 rather than 3 types of cones. They are divided into 3 groups: Protanopes, or red-blind subjects, are insensitive to deep red light. Deuteranopes confuse shades of red, green, and yellow. Tritanopes are blue-blind subjects who confuse blue and green shades and, generally, orange and pink shades.

(3) Anomalous trichromats: This is by far the largest group. Protans have similar but milder defects than occur in protanopia; deutans have similar but milder defects than occur in deuteranopia; and tritans have similar but milder defects than occur in tritanopia.

(4) Rod monochromats: Rod monochromatism is a very rare disorder in which there is complete lack of cone function. It is always associated with photophobia, nystagmus, and poor visual acuity.

The common types of color blindness are inherited as X-linked characteristics. Acquired causes of color blindness include retinal disease and poisoning. In the acquired cases, the patient may be color-blind in only one area of the visual field.

The detection of color blindness is described in Chapter 2. Because of the relationship to choice of occupation, color vision testing should be done early in life (eg, age 8–12). However, the physician must be wary of attributing too much importance to a hereditary anomaly that in its more common milder forms is little more than an occasional social inconvenience.

Treatment is of no value.

II. TUMORS INVOLVING THE RETINA

J. Brooks Crawford, MD

PRIMARY BENIGN INTRAOCULAR TUMORS

Several important tumors that may be first identified during ophthalmoscopic examination are discussed below.

Nevus

Nevi (Figs 11–22 and 11–23) are usually flat pigmented lesions lying in the stroma of the tissue. On the anterior surface of the iris they may be noted as iris "freckles." Posteriorly in the choroid one may see flat pigmented areas. Large choroidal nevi are difficult to differentiate from malignant melanomas. Their unchanging slate-gray color and flat appearance and the lack of extension are important in the differential diagnosis from malignant melanoma.

Because of the difficulties in differentiation from malignant melanomas, fundus photographs or careful line drawings should be made of all suspicious lesions. Observations should be made periodically for changes.

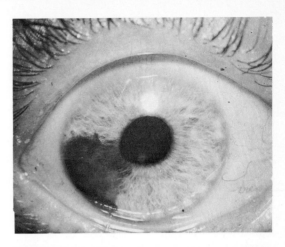

Figure 11–22. Nevus of the iris. (Courtesy of A Rosenberg.)

Retinal Angioma[*]

Angioma of the retina is a rare congenital disorder. Blurring of vision may result if bleeding occurs or if the retina is secondarily detached. Occasionally, angioma is associated with angioma in the cerebral cortex (Lindau's disease) (Fig 11–24). It is globular in outline and may be located near one of the pairs of enlarged retinal vessels. Angiomas may enlarge. Photocoagulation therapy (xenon or argon laser) and cryotherapy are currently utilized to eradicate these lesions.

Tuberous Sclerosis (Bourneville's Disease) (Fig 11–25)

The rare intraocular tumor (glial hamartoma) associated with tuberous sclerosis in about half of cases varies in size and color but is most often a yellow or white nodular swelling, frequently mulberry in appearance, located in any portion of the posterior fundus but with a predilection for the area near the optic nerve. Other manifestations of tuberous sclerosis include skin changes (adenoma sebaceum), intracranial changes causing epilepsy and mental retardation, and other neurologic symptoms (see p 186).

Hemangioma of the Choroid

Choroid hemangioma occurs in most cases of Sturge-Weber syndrome associated with unilateral infantile glaucoma (see p 186). Cases occurring with no other signs of Sturge-Weber syndrome are frequently mistaken for malignant melanoma of the choroid (see below), and the mistaken diagnosis has often led to unnecessary removal of the affected eye. The tumor involves the posterior pole, usually near the optic disk and sometimes extending out to the equator, most often on the temporal side. It may produce a solid elevation or a serous detachment of the retina.

---

[*] See also Angiomatosis Retinae in Chapter 15.

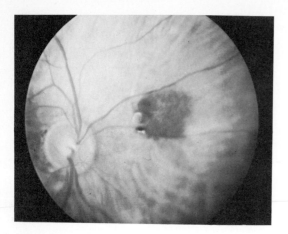

Figure 11–23. Nevus of the choroid. (Photo by Diane Beeston.)

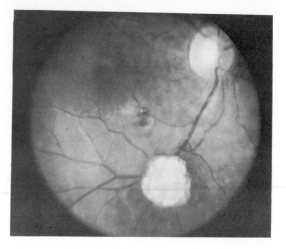

Figure 11–25. Tuberous sclerosis.

The borders are irregular, and the tumor is never pigmented. Hemangiomas can produce arcuate field defects or localized scotomas.

Histologically, the tumor consists of endothelium-lined spaces engorged with blood separated by sparse connective tissue. Retinal degeneration over the tumor is common.

Secondary glaucoma, usually severe and refractory to any treatment, is associated with larger choroidal hemangiomas.

The differentiation from malignant melanoma is most important and frequently difficult.

Occasionally, choroidal hemangiomas can be treated with photocoagulation to limit the extent and degree of associated serous detachment of the retina.

Enucleation may be necessary for those tumors associated with intractable, painful glaucoma.

PRIMARY MALIGNANT TUMORS OF THE INTRAOCULAR STRUCTURES

Malignant Melanoma

It has been estimated that intraocular malignant melanoma occurs in 0.02–0.06% of the total eye patient population in the USA. It is seen only in the uveal tract and is the most common intraocular malignant tumor in the white population. The average age of patients with this disorder is 50 years. It is almost always unilateral. Eighty-five percent appear in the choroid, 9% in the ciliary body, and 6% in the iris.

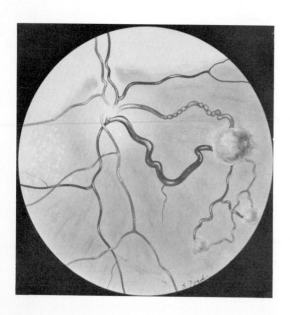

Figure 11–24. Angiomatosis retinae of Von Hippel-Lindau disease (drawing). (Courtesy of F Cordes.)

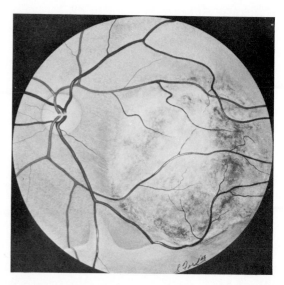

Figure 11–26. Malignant melanoma of the choroid, macular area, left eye (drawing). (Courtesy of F Cordes.)

Most of the choroidal tumors are in the posterior portion of the eye, especially on the temporal side. In the iris, the lower half is most often affected. Intraocular malignant melanoma is rare in blacks, although uveal nevi are common (Fig 11–24).

This tumor may be seen in its early stages only accidentally during routine ophthalmoscopic examination or because of blurring due to macular invasion. Blood-borne metastases may occur at any time, and death may occur before local spread or ocular symptoms appear. Glaucoma may be a late manifestation.

Histologically, these tumors are composed of spindle-shaped cells, with or without prominent nucleoli, and large epithelioid tumor cells. Tumors composed of the former have a good prognosis; tumors with the latter, a poor prognosis.

Intraocular malignant melanomas may spread directly through the sclera, by local invasion of intraocular structures, or by metastasis.

Clinical manifestations are usually absent unless the macula is involved. In the later stages, growth of the tumor may lead to retinal detachment with loss of a large amount of visual field. A tumor located in the iris may be large enough to change the color of the iris or deform the pupil. Pain does not occur in the absence of glaucoma.

The first step in diagnosis is to suspect the lesion. Most intraocular malignant melanomas can be seen ophthalmoscopically. Transillumination is of some value in differentiation from serous retinal detachment.

A high incidence of intraocular tumors has been found in the study of blind, painful, phthisic (atropic) eyes, one writer reporting that 10% of such eyes contained previously unsuspected malignant melanomas.

Enucleation of an eye with a choroidal melanoma has been the traditional treatment. Recently, other forms of therapy, particularly radiotherapy with charged particles such as helium ions and protons or with plaques of radioactive isotopes sutured to the sclera, have been used for eyes with small tumors and useful vision. Very small melanomas (< 10 mm in diameter) have an excellent prognosis and are often impossible to differentiate from benign nevi; therefore, many authorities advocate not treating these tumors until unequivocal growth can be documented

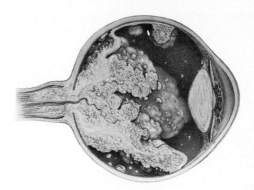

Figure 11–28. Retinoblastoma with multiple seedings and optic nerve invasion. (Courtesy of B Crawford and W Spencer.)

(usually with serial photographs or ultrasound measurements).

Small melanomas of the iris that have not invaded the iris root can be safely observed until growth is documented; then they can be removed by iridectomy. Lesions that invade the iris root and ciliary body can sometimes be treated with iridocyclectomy. Iris melanomas have an excellent prognosis; the mortality rate is less than 1%. Many pigmented iris tumors are actually large nevi rather than malignant melanomas.

Retinoblastoma
(Fig 11–25)

Retinoblastoma is a rare but life-endangering tumor of childhood. Two-thirds of cases appear before the end of the third year; rare cases have been reported at almost every age. The tumor is bilateral in about 30% of cases. Retinoblastoma was formerly thought to result from mutation of an autosomal dominant gene, but it is now thought that an allele at a single locus within chromosomal band 13q14 controls both the heritable and nonheritable forms of the tumor. (See Chapter 19 for further discussion of genetic aspects of ocular disease.) About 94% of retinoblastomas arise by mutation; therefore, only about 6% are familial. When the inheritance is familial or the mutation involves germinal tissue, a retinoblastoma survivor has approximately a 50% chance of producing an affected child.

Retinoblastomas usually arise from the posterior retina. Growth tends to be nodular, with numerous satellite or seeding nodules that may produce multiple secondary tumors (Fig 11–26). They gradually fill the eye and extend through the optic nerve to the brain and along the emissary vessels and nerves in the sclera to the orbital tissues. Microscopically, most retinoblastomas are composed of small, closely packed, round or polygonal cells with large, darkly staining nuclei and scanty cytoplasm. They sometimes form characteristic Flexner-Wintersteiner rosettes, which are indicative of photoreceptor differentiation. Degenerative changes are frequent, with necrosis and

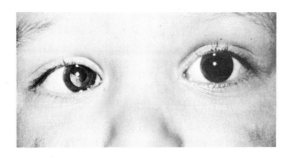

Figure 11–27. Retinoblastoma visible through pupil.

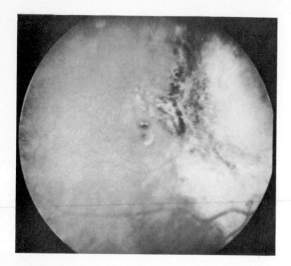

Figure 11–29. Retinoblastoma after x-ray radiation.

calcification. A few spontaneous cures have been reported.

Retinoblastoma usually remains unnoticed until it has advanced far enough to produce a white pupil—unless strabismus has occurred, leading to earlier diagnosis. Otherwise, the tumor is usually seen in the early stages only when sought for, as in children having a hereditary background or where the other eye has been affected. In the early stages small, yellowish-white nodular masses may be seen protruding into the vitreous from the retina. Infants and children with esotropia should be examined to rule out retinoblastoma, since blind eyes of children will often turn inward.

Retrolental fibroplasia, persistence of the primary vitreous, retinal dysplasia, Coats' disease, and nematode endophthalmitis may simulate retinoblastoma.

In general, the earlier the discovery and treatment of the tumor, the better the chance to prevent spread through the optic nerve and orbital tissues.

Enucleation is the treatment of choice for large retinoblastomas; smaller ones in eyes with potentially useful vision can be effectively treated with radiotherapy, sometimes augmented by chemotherapy, cryotherapy, or photocoagulation (Fig 11–27).

Medulloepitheliomas ("Diktyoma") of the Ciliary Body

Benign and malignant medulloepitheliomas are rare tumors that may arise from the ciliary body epithelium. Those with one or more heteroplastic elements, such as hyaline cartilage, brain tissue, or rhabdomyoblasts, are called teratoid medulloepitheliomas. Those that arise soon after birth may infiltrate the area around the lens and produce a white pupillary reflex similar to that seen in eyes with retinoblastoma.

REFERENCES

Retina & Retinal Disorders

Blankenship GW: A clinical comparison of central and peripheral argon laser panretinal photocoagulation for proliferative diabetic retinopathy. *Ophthalmology* 1988;**95:**170.

Bradford JD, Wilkinson CP, Bradford RH Jr: Cystoid macular edema following extracapsular cataract extraction and posterior chamber intraocular lens implantation. *Retina* 1988;**3:**161.

The Branch Vein Occlusion Study Group: Argon laser photocoagulation for macular edema in branch vein occlusion. *Am J Ophthalmol* 1984;**98:**271.

Byer NE: The natural history of asymptomatic retinal breaks. *Ophthalmology* 1982;**89:**1033.

Committee for Classification of Retinopathy of Prematurity: An international classification of retinopathy of prematurity. *Arch Ophthalmol* 1984;**102:**1130.

de Juan E, Machemer R: Vitreous surgery for hemorrhagic and fibrous complications of age-related macular degeneration. *Am J Ophthalmol* 1988;**105:**25.

Doft BH et al: The association between long-term diabetic control and early retinopathy. *Ophthalmology* 1984;**91:**763.

Foos RY: Vitreoretinal junction: Topographical variations. *Invest Ophthalmol* 1972;**11:**801.

Gass JDM: *Stereoscopic Atlas of Macular Diseases,* 2nd ed. Mosby, 1977.

Gass JDM, Weleber RG, Johnson DR: Non-Hodgkin's lymphoma causing fundus picture simulating fundus flavimaculatus. *Retina* 1987;**7:**209.

Hayreh SS: Classification of central retinal vein occlusion. *Ophthalmology* 1983;**90:**458.

Jaffe NS, Clayman HM, Jaffe MS: Cystoid macular edema after intracapsular and extracapsular cataract extraction with and without an intraocular lens. *J Am Acad Ophthalmol* 1982;**89:**25.

Kalina RE, Karr DJ: Retrolental fibroplasia: Experience over two decades in one institution. *J Am Acad Ophthalmol* 1982;**89:**91.

Kearns TP: Differential diagnosis of central retinal vein obstruction. *Ophthalmology* 1983;**90:**475.

Lucke KH, Foerster MH, Laqua H: Long-term results of vitrectomy and silicone oil in 500 cases of complicated retinal detachments. *Am J Ophthalmol* 1987;**104:**624.

Machemer R: The importance of fluid absorption, traction, intraocular currents, and chorioretinal scars in the therapy of rhegmatogenous retinal detachments: The 41st Edward Jackson Memorial Lecture. *Am J Ophthalmol* 1984;**98:**681.

Macular Photocoagulation Study Group: Argon laser photocoagulation for senile macular degeneration. *Arch Ophthalmol* 1982;**100:**912.

McDonald JM, Newsome DA, Rintelmann WF: Sensorineural hearing loss in patients with typical retinitis pigmentosa. *Am J Ophthal* 1988;**105:125.**

Meyers SM, Zachary AA: Monozygotic twins with age-related macular degeneration. *Arch Ophthalmol* 1988;**106:**651.

Michels RG, Rice TA, Rice EF: Vitrectomy of diabetic

traction detachment involving the macula. *Am J Ophthalmol* 1983;**95**:22.

Michels RG, Rice TA, Rice EF: Vitrectomy for diabetic vitreous hemorrhage. *Am J Ophthalmol* 1983;**95**:12.

Newsome DA et al: Oral zinc in macular degeneration. *Arch Ophthalmol* 1988;**106**:192.

O'Malley P et al: Paving-stone degeneration of the retina. *Arch Ophthalmol* 1965;**73**:169.

Palmer EA: Multicenter trial of cryotherapy for retinopathy of prematurity. *Arch Ophthalmol* 1988;**106**:471.

Patz A: Clinical and experimental studies on retinal neovascularization: The 29th Edward Jackson Memorial Lecture. *Am J Ophthalmol* 1982;**94**:715.

Patz A: Observations on the retinopathy of prematurity. *Am J Ophthalmol* 1985;**100**:164.

Patz A et al: Diseases of the macula: Diagnosis and management of choroidal neovascularization. *Trans Am Acad Ophthalmol Otolaryngol* 1977;**83**:468.

Rosenlund EF et al: Transient proliferative diabetic retinopathy during intensified insulin treatment. *Am J Ophthalmol* 1988;**105**:618.

Sherwin RS: Diabetic retinopathy after two years of intensified insulin treatment. *JAMA* 1988;**260**:37.

Sira IB, Nissenkorn I, Kremer I: Retinopathy of prematurity. (Major review.) *Surv Ophthalmol* 1988;**33**:1.

Soong HK et al: In situ actin distribution in excised retrolental membranes in retinopathy of prematurity. *Arch Ophthalmol* 1985;**103**:1553.

Spencer WH (editor): *Ophthalmic Pathology: An Atlas and Textbook.* Vol 2. *Vitreous and Retina.* Saunders, 1985.

Trese MT: Surgical results of stage V retrolental fibroplasia and timing of surgical repair. *Ophthalmology* 1984;**91**:461.

Virdi PS, Hayreh SS: Ocular neovascularization with retinal vascular occlusion. *Arch Ophthalmol* 1982;**100**:331.

Walsh JB: Hypertensive retinopathy: Description, classification, and prognosis. *Ophthalmology* 1982;**89**:1127.

Wilson CA et al: Optic disk neovascularization and retinal vessel diameter in diabetic retinopathy. *Am J Ophthalmol* 1988;**106**:131.

Tumors Involving the Retina

Abramson DH et al: The management of unilateral retinoblastoma without primary enucleation. *Arch Ophthalmol* 1982;**100**:1249.

Bedford MA, Bedotto C, Macfaul PA: Retinoblastoma: A study of 139 cases. *Br J Ophthalmol* 1971;**55**:19.

Blodi FC: Ocular melanocytosis and melanoma. *Am J Ophthalmol* 1975;**80**:389.

Char DH: The management of small choroidal melanomas. *Surv Ophthalmol* 1978;**22**:377.

Char DH: Therapeutic options in uveal melanoma. (Editorial.) *Am J Ophthalmol* 1984;**98**:796.

Davidorf FH et al: Conservative management of malignant melanoma. 2. Transscleral diathermy as a method of treatment for malignant melanomas of the choroid. *Arch Ophthalmol* 1970;**83**:273.

Davidorf FH, Lang JR: The natural history of malignant melanoma of the choroid: Small vs large tumors. *Trans Am Acad Ophthalmol Otolaryngol* 1975;**79**:op310.

Gallie BL, Phillips RA: Retinoblastoma: A model of oncogenesis. *Ophthalmology* 1984;**91**:666.

Gass JD: Problems in the differential diagnosis of choroidal nevi and malignant melanoma. *Trans Am Acad Ophthalmol Otolaryngol* 1977;**83**:19.

Geisse LJ, Robertson DM: Iris melanomas. *Am J Ophthalmol* 1985;**99**:638.

Halloran SL et al: Accuracy of detection of the retinoblastoma gene by esterase D linkage. *Arch Ophthalmol* 1985;**103**:1329.

Jensen RD, Miller RW: Retinoblastoma: Epidemiologic characteristics. *N Engl J Med* 1971;**285**:307.

Kopf AW, Bart RS, Rodriguez-Sains RS: Malignant melanoma: A review. *J Dermatol Surg Oncol* 1977;**3**:41.

12

Glaucoma

Daniel Vaughan, MD

Glaucoma includes a complex of disease entities that have in common an increase in intraocular pressure sufficient to cause degeneration of the optic disk and defects in the visual field. An estimated 50,000 persons in the USA are blind as a result of glaucoma. The incidence of glaucoma in unselected persons over age 40 is about 1.5%. The disease is particularly common in black individuals. In black persons age 45–65, the prevalence is 15 times that of whites in the same age group.

The chief threat of chronic (open-angle) glaucoma is insidious visual impairment. The degree of interference with vision varies from slight blurring to complete blindness. The disease is bilateral and is genetically determined, probably by multifactorial or polygenic inheritance. Infantile glaucoma usually has an autosomal recessive mode of inheritance, whereas some specific glaucoma syndromes are transmitted as autosomal dominant diseases. Acute glaucoma (angle-closure glaucoma) comprises less than 5% of primary glaucoma cases.

In most cases, blindness can be prevented if treatment is instituted early. The objective of therapy is to facilitate the outflow of aqueous through existing drainage channels by the use of miotics and to inhibit the secretion of aqueous by the ciliary processes, using systemically and topically administered drugs. The most commonly used miotic is pilocarpine. The most commonly used secretory suppressants are beta-blockers and epinephrine, which are applied topically, and carbonic anhydrase inhibitors, which are given orally. Increase in outflow can also be accomplished by laser trabeculoplasty. Operative treatment is sometimes indicated in the later stages of glaucoma when medical management is no longer sufficient to control the intraocular pressure.

The management of glaucoma is best left to the ophthalmologist, but all physicians should participate in the diagnosis by making ophthalmoscopy and tonometry a part of the routine physical examination of all patients old enough to cooperate. This is especially important in patients with a family history of glaucoma. The physician should learn to recognize optic nerve changes associated with glaucoma as seen with the ophthalmoscope. Doubtful cases should be referred to an ophthalmologist for confirmation and management.

Classification

A generally accepted classification of glaucoma is as follows:

A. **Primary glaucoma**
   1. Open-angle glaucoma—Also called chronic open-angle glaucoma, simple glaucoma, chronic simple glaucoma. The most common form.
   2. Angle-closure glaucoma—Also called narrow-angle glaucoma, closed-angle glaucoma.
      a. Acute.
      b. Subacute or chronic.
      c. Plateau iris.

B. **Congenital glaucoma**
   1. Primary congenital glaucoma, primary infantile glaucoma, trabeculodysgenesis.
   2. Glaucoma associated with congenital anomalies–
      a. Aniridia.
      b. Axenfeld's syndrome.
      c. Sturge-Weber syndrome.
      d. Infantile glaucoma developing late.
      e. Marfan's syndrome.
      f. Neurofibromatosis.
      g. Lowe's syndrome.
      h. Microcornea and megalocornea.

C. **Secondary glaucoma**
   1. Pigmentary glaucoma–
   2. Exfoliative syndrome (pseudoexfoliation of lens capsule, glaucoma capsulare).
   3. Due to changes of the lens—
      a. Dislocation.
      b. Intumescence.
      c. Phacolytic.
   4. Due to changes of the uveal tract–
      a. Peripheral anterior synechiae (PAS) (angle closure without pupillary block).
      b. Iridocyclitis.
      c. Tumor.
      d. Iridocorneoendothelial (ICE) syndrome (essential iris atrophy, Chandler's syndrome, iris-nevus syndrome).
   5. Due to trauma–
      a. Massive hemorrhage into the anterior chamber.

b. Massive hemorrhage into the posterior chamber.

c. Corneal or limbal laceration with iris prolapse into the wound.

d. Retrodisplacement of iris root following contusion (angle recession).

6. Following surgical procedures–
   a. Epithelial ingrowth into the anterior chamber.
   b. Failure of prompt restoration of the anterior chamber following cataract extraction.

7. Associated with rubeosis (diabetes mellitus and central retinal vessel occlusion).

8. Associated with pulsating exophthalmos.

9. Associated with topical corticosteroids.

10. Other rare causes of secondary glaucoma.

D. Absolute glaucoma: The end result of any uncontrolled glaucoma is a hard, sightless, and often painful eye.

PHYSIOLOGY

Aqueous Humor

The intraocular pressure is determined by the rate of aqueous production by the ciliary body epithelium and the resistance to outflow of aqueous from the eye. Some knowledge of the physiology of aqueous is necessary to an understanding of glaucoma.

A. Composition of Aqueous: The aqueous is a clear liquid that fills the anterior and posterior chambers of the eye. Its volume is about 125 μL. The osmotic pressure of aqueous is slightly higher than that of plasma. The total protein content is 0.02%. The albumin-globulin ratio is the same as that of blood serum (2:1). In general, the same electrolytes and other components are found in the aqueous as in plasma, although the concentrations differ.

Intraocular inflammation and surgical or traumatic emptying of the anterior chamber cause the formation of plasmoid aqueous, which closely resembles blood serum and has a much higher protein concentration than normal aqueous.

B. Formation and Flow of Aqueous: A great deal is known about the dynamics of aqueous humor, but the exact mechanism of production and elimination of aqueous is not completely understood. Water, electrolytes, and nonelectrolytes enter and leave the eye at varying rates. Water enters both by diffusion from the ciliary body and by secretion from the epithelium of the ciliary processes. From the posterior chamber the fluid passes through the pupil into the anterior chamber (Fig 12–1). The flow in the anterior chamber is peripheral, toward the filtering trabecular meshwork and into Schlemm's canal. Efferent channels from Schlemm's canal (about 30 collector channels and about 12 aqueous veins) conduct the fluid into the venous system. There is also a constant exchange of nonelectrolytes as well as a major exchange of water in and out of the iris stroma. A small amount of aqueous leaves the eye through the uveal vessels and the sclera (uveoscleral flow) (Fig 12–2).

Pressure Dynamics*

Intraocular pressure is such an important feature of glaucoma that a review of pressure dynamics is desirable.

A. Pressure-Tension-Strain Relationships: The terms pressure, tension, and strain are frequently

---

* By Orson W. White, MD.

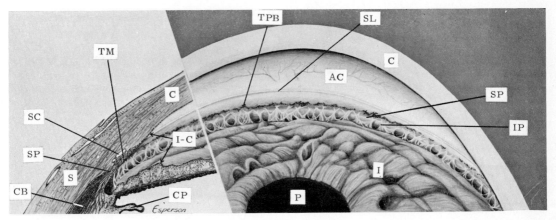

AC	= anterior chamber	I	= iris	S	= sclera	TM	= trabecular meshwork
C	= cornea	I-C	= iris-corneal angle	SC	= Schlemm's canal	TPB	= trabecular pigment band
CB	= ciliary body	IP	= iris processes	SL	= Schwalbe's line		
CP	= ciliary process	P	= pupil	SP	= scleral spur		

Figure 12–1. Composite illustration showing anatomic *(left)* and gonioscopic *(right)* view of normal anterior chamber angle. (Courtesy of R Shaffer.)

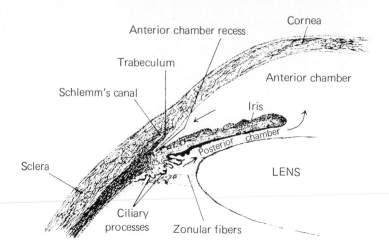

Figure 12–2. Anterior segment structures. Arrows indicate direction of flow of aqueous.

used interchangeably and are listed as synonyms in some dictionaries. However, the precise distinctions and interactions between these related but different terms must be appreciated before pressure dynamics in glaucoma can be understood.

1. Pressure–Hydrostatic pressure is the force per unit area exerted by a fluid (gas or liquid). With the eye, as with other pressure vessels, the pressure force is exerted normal to the structural wall (in the eye, this is the corneoscleral wall). Hydrostatic pressure per se causes no damage to the delicate neurons paralleling the scleral wall, even at high levels. A neuron in the eye may be compared to a diver resting on the ocean bottom; at a depth of 43 meters (1693 ft), the diver will experience no discomfort, even though at this depth, the total force being exerted on the body is about 9000 kg (10 tons). The concept that intraocular pressure damages neurons by pushing them against the sclera is false.

The unit of pressure in the International System of Units (SI) is the pascal (Pa), which is 1 newton per square meter (N/m^2). To convert millimeters of mercury to kilopascals (kPa), divide millimeters of mercury by 7.5. However, for calculation of pressure within the eye, it is helpful to convert millimeters of mercury to grams per square centimeter. Multiply millimeters of mercury by 1.36 to obtain grams per square centimeter, which is also the pressure in centimeters of water. One may thus determine the pressure effect in millimeters of mercury of an infusion bottle infusing the eye by measuring the height in centimeters from the eye to the top of the fluid in the bottle and dividing by 1.36. A satisfactory approximation is to double the height in inches; thus, a 12-inch-high infusion bottle creates an intraocular pressure of about 24 mm Hg.

2. Tension (tensile stress)–A jack supporting a car is subjected to compressive stress. A towline pulling a car is subjected to tensile stress, or tension. Stresses are assigned a magnitude of force per unit area. Tensile stress, or the tension force vector, acts parallel to the scleral wall (attempting to pull the sclera apart). In the same way, the pressure of the abdomen at right angles to a belt is almost analogous to intraocular pressure, while the tension along the belt acting to pull the belt apart is analogous to scleral tension.

Trampolines and drumheads are examples of pure tension without pressure. The pressure is the same on either side of the tensed membrane. Tension levels in the sclera, cornea, and lamina cribrosa are not equal. The tension equation for thin-walled spheres can be used to obtain a close approximation of tensions in various parts of the corneoscleral wall of the eye. Tension in the sclera is directly proportional to the intraocular pressure multiplied by the radius of curvature of the sclera and inversely proportional to twice the thickness of the sclera:

$$\text{Tension} = \frac{\text{Pressure} \times \text{Radius}}{2 \times \text{Thickness}}$$

An inflated surgical glove or balloon (Fig 12–3) illustrates this relationship. The palm of the glove has relatively high tension and the thumb has relatively low tension, though the pressure within the glove is equal at all locations. The thumb has low tension because the radius of curvature is small and the thickness large relative to the same factors at the palm. In the eye, tension is lower in the cornea or optic cup than in the sclera.

An eye under slowly increasing pressure usually ruptures beneath the lateral rectus, as the tension equation would suggest. The 43 meters' sea depth used in the example of harmless pressure was chosen because this same pressure within the eye residing at atmospheric pressure results, via tension and strain, in rupture of the eye. A precipitous pressure rise due to trauma (eg, a blow from a club) frequently ruptures the eye at the limbus owing to the anvil effect of the more viscous vitreous.

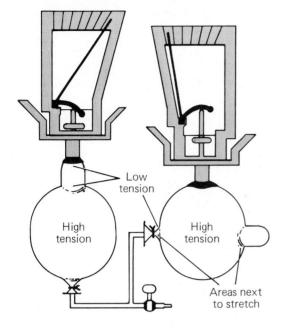

Figure 12–3. Equal-pressure balloons.

3. Strain–Strain is stretch or displacement per unit length. A strain gauge measures displacement. Strain can result in damage, and in the body can cause both pain and damage. Using the belt analogy, strain is the stretch per unit length of the belt resulting from the tension in the belt caused by the pressure of the abdomen.

To calculate the strain or stretch of a substance at a given pressure or tension, one of 3 moduli of elasticity is used. Each modulus is appropriate for a different type of structure. Thomas Young (1773–1829), an English physician, clarified these complex relationships as follows:

a. Young's modulus E–Young's modulus E is used for determining the elastic properties of structures such as cables, pressure vessels, submarines, *and eyes*. E is defined as the tension required to stretch a material of unit cross section to double its original length. This is represented by the following equation:

$$E = \frac{\text{Change in tension sclera}}{\text{Change in length of sclera per unit length}}$$

Thus, the stretch of the sclera per unit length (strain) is given by dividing the change in tension of the sclera by Young's modulus of the sclera E.

b. Shear modulus G–The shear modulus G is used for determining the elastic properties of structures such as drive shafts and bolts. G should not concern us in the discussion of elasticity of the eye. It is sometimes called the modulus of rigidity, and the unfortunate term "scleral rigidity" may have originated from inappropriate use of the shear modulus in ocular calculations.

c. Bulk modulus K–The bulk modulus K also should not concern us in our discussion of elasticity of the eye. The bulk modulus is the hydrostatic pressure (compressive stress) required to compress (strain) a solid material to half its original volume.

The empirical "scleral rigidity" equation found in some glaucoma literature resembles the bulk modulus equation. However, using the bulk modulus for the eye would be valid only if the eye were solid sclera and subjected to external hydrostatic pressure. However, the eye is a nearly spherical shell of elastic sclera filled with fluid under pressure and is therefore appropriately described only by Young's modulus, as are other thin-walled pressure vessels.

The belt analogy may now be used to illustrate the way in which neurons are damaged in glaucoma. Envision a very obese person wearing a large belt (sclera) with a delicate cloth liner (neurons). After fasting for several days, the obese subject feasts heavily, with the result that there is some ripping of the delicate cloth liner. The progression of the damage process is as follows: (1) The expanding abdomen (intraocular pressure) exerts gentle pressure at right angles to the belt, producing a summation tension parallel to the belt (sclera) tending to pull the belt apart. (2) The tension leads to stretching (strain) of the belt, following the rules of Young's modulus. (3) The stretching (strain) results in damage to the delicate cloth liner (neurons).

B. Devices for Measuring Ocular Tension and Pressure: The Goldmann applanation device is designed to measure intraocular pressure, with results recorded in millimeters of mercury. The Schiotz device is a true tonometer, primarily measuring tension. Recordings should be in tension units or scale units, as originally proposed by Schiotz, but they are commonly converted to millimeters of mercury (a pressure unit, not a tension unit).

C. Local Exceptions to the Mathematical Theory of Elasticity: The tension and strain exerted on areas of discontinuity, such as the optic disk and the limbal area, are not easy to calculate. These relationships can be studied by various methods of photoelasticity on models or actual eyes. Note in the balloon model (Fig 12–3) that the area next to stretch occurring when the pressure in the balloon is increased is analogous to the disk and limbal areas of the eye.

D. Biologic Exceptions to the Mathematical Theory of Elasticity: Living tissue reacts in the same way as nonliving material to brief changes in tension and strain. However, long-term tensions and strains have a unique effect on living tissue, causing changes in growth, shape, and strength. This is the basis of the "orthodontic shift" of teeth and the way in which deformities of the head, face, and foot have been created in some cultures over the course of history. The cupping of the disk may be a response to long-term tension and strain. *Nerve damage in glaucoma is not due directly to intraocular pressure on* *the neurons but may be due to deformation and stretching, caused by long-term tension-strain effects.*

SPECIAL DIAGNOSTIC TECHNIQUES
(See also Chapter 2.)

A number of special diagnostic tests have been developed to help detect, classify, and follow the course of glaucoma.

Tonometry

This is an important test in establishing the diagnosis of glaucoma. A single normal reading either with the Schiotz or applanation tonometer does not rule out glaucoma, however, as the intraocular pressures may vary within wide limits. A single "high normal" reading (24–32 mm Hg) is suggestive of glaucoma but always requires repeated testing before a definite diagnosis can be made.

Gonioscopy

Visualization of the anterior chamber angle differentiates angle-closure from open-angle glaucoma, demonstrates the extent of peripheral anterior synechiae, and offers the only means of detecting an impending angle closure before there is any rise in intraocular pressure. It is an essential part of any glaucoma evaluation and has replaced provocative tests for glaucoma.

Ophthalmoscopy

Direct visualization of the optic disk is the single most important test in diagnosing glaucoma and evaluating the response to treatment. A patient with elevated intraocular pressure (eg, 32 mm Hg) and normal-appearing optic disks may not require active treatment but only periodic examinations.

Visual Fields in Glaucoma

The visual field test is most important in detecting open-angle glaucoma and in following the course of visual deterioration caused by the disease. The tangent screen, the Goldmann perimeter, and various automated perimeters give important information. Small extentions of the blind spot or early nerve fiber bundle defects not necessarily connected to the blind spot are noted early in the disease. Ideally, the diagnosis is made before visual field loss occurs. Under these circumstances, medical control can usually prevent significant visual loss.

The nerve fibers are arranged in the retina as indicated in Fig 12–4. Increased intraocular pressure will gradually destroy the function of a bundle of these fibers, and the resulting visual field defect is spoken of as a "nerve fiber bundle defect." As the nerve fiber bundle defect enlarges, it takes an arcuate shape from the blind spot encircling the fixation area. It arches into either the superior or inferior field and ends at the horizontal meridian (Bjerrum scotoma).

A double arcuate scotoma (one in the superior and one in the inferior field) forms a full-ring scotoma around the central fixation area.

Loss of peripheral field occurs later in the course of the disease. The nasal and superior fields are usually lost first. The last remnant of the visual field is usually a temporal island.

The field of vision may slowly contract in some cases down to 5 degrees from fixation, leaving the patient with good central vision but no peripheral vision. Central visual acuity, therefore, is not a reliable index of the progress of the disease. There is no substitute for careful periodic study of the visual field, applanation tonometry, and, most importantly, ophthalmoscopic visualization of the optic disks.

PRIMARY GLAUCOMA

OPEN-ANGLE GLAUCOMA

At least 90% of cases of primary glaucoma are of the open-angle type. Open-angle glaucoma is bilateral, insidious in onset and slowly progressive. There are no symptoms until visual impairment occurs, often too late to salvage useful vision. It is threrefore the physician's responsibility to diagnose glaucoma before irreversible optic nerve damage has occurred. Early treatment prevents or delays visual deterioration.

Significant advances in the understanding of the course of open-angle glaucoma have been made in recent years, but unsolved problems remain and there are still differences of opinion among authorities on some issues. It now seems certain that increased intraocular pressure is caused by interference with aqueous outflow due to degenerative changes in the trabeculum, Schlemm's canal, and adjacent channels (see below). Increased pressure, whether caused by obstructed outflow or increased production of aqueous, affects primarily the retina and optic nerve, the functional elements of the eye.

Some authorities feel that in open-angle glaucoma, there is also a primary degenerative disorder of the optic nerve due to mechanical distortion of the lamina cribrosa, vascular insufficiency, or both. This view is supported by the observation that loss of function sometimes continues to progress even after the intraocular pressure has been normalized by medical therapy or surgery. Also, patients with systemic disease (eg, diabetes, arteriosclerosis) are more likely than others to suffer optic nerve damage as a result of ocular hypertension.

There are few detectable histologic changes in the early stages. Nonspecific changes common to all forms of primary glaucoma occur in later stages. Studies of early open-angle glaucoma reveal primary de-

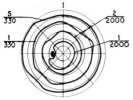

Baring of the blind spot. The earliest nerve fiber bundle defect.

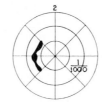

Incipient double nerve fiber bundle defect (Bjerrum scotoma).

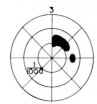

Bjerrum scotoma isolated from blind spot.

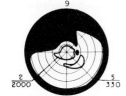

End stages in glaucoma field loss. Remnant of central field still shows nasal step.

Fully developed nerve fiber bundle defect with nasal step (arcuate scotoma).

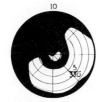

Peripheral depression with double nerve fiber bundle defect. Isolation of central field.

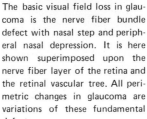

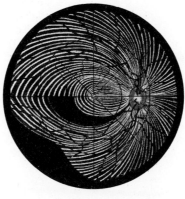

The basic visual field loss in glaucoma is the nerve fiber bundle defect with nasal step and peripheral nasal depression. It is here shown superimposed upon the nerve fiber layer of the retina and the retinal vascular tree. All perimetric changes in glaucoma are variations of these fundamental defects.

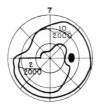

Double arcuate scotoma with peripheral breakthrough and nasal step.

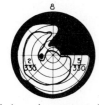

Nasal depression connected with arcuate scotoma. Nasal step of Rönne.

Peripheral breakthrough of large nerve fiber bundle defect with well developed nasal step.

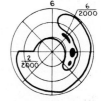

Seidel scotoma. Islands of greater visual loss within a nerve fiber bundle defect.

Figure 12–4. Visual field changes in glaucoma. (Reproduced, with permission, from Harrington DO: *The Visual Fields: A Textbook and Atlas of Clinical Perimetry,* 5th ed. Mosby, 1981.)

generation in the trabecular meshwork, degeneration of the collagen and elastic fibers of the trabeculum, a decrease in the number of trabecular cells, and an increased amount of electron-dense materials. The trabecular spaces tend to be obliterated. The collector channels also undergo degenerative changes.

If the pressure remains elevated, gross damage to the eye occurs. The optic nerve undergoes degener-

ation, often assuming a typical bean-pot cupping appearance (Figs 12–5 and 12–6). There is degeneration of ganglion cells and nerve fibers in the retina. The iris and ciliary body become atrophic, and the ciliary processes show hyaline degeneration.

Genetic aspects. Open-angle glaucoma is a familial, genetically determined disorder, probably multifactorial or polygenic in origin. In any case, family

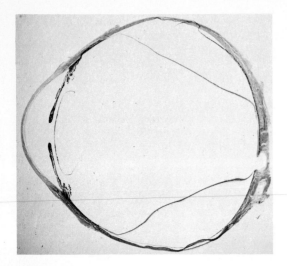

Figure 12–5. Cross section of an eye with open-angle glaucoma. Note open anterior chamber angle (peripheral iris is not in contact with the posterior corneal surface). Deep glaucomatous cupping ("bean-pot" appearance) shows the process to be well advanced. (Courtesy of R Carriker.)

history and routine systematic testing of relatives are most important in glaucoma detection.

Clinical Findings

Open-angle glaucoma causes no early symptoms. Subjective visual loss is nearly always a late finding. Although the disease is nearly always bilateral, one eye is frequently involved earlier and more severely than the other.

Optic disk changes are the most important early findings. The disk margin (neuroretinal rim) thins, especially superiorly and inferiorly (Fig 12–7), and the cup gradually becomes wider and deeper. The large vessels become displaced, and the affected area of the disk becomes atrophic (light gray or white rather than pink). The lamina cribrosa becomes more exposed.

The intraocular pressure is increased. The anterior chamber angle may be normal on gonioscopy. The loss of visual function from glaucoma can best be determined by repeated studies of the visual fields.

Treatment

A. Medical Treatment: Miotics facilitate aqueous outflow by increasing the efficiency of the outflow channels. The exact mechanism of their effect is not understood. The drug of choice is pilocarpine, 1–4%, instilled in each eye up to 5 times daily. Carbachol, 0.75–3%, may be effective when pilocarpine fails or in patients who are allergic to pilocarpine. These are cholinergic drugs.

Anticholinesterase drugs are the longest-acting miotics available. These include demecarium bromide (Humorsol), 0.06–0.25%, and echothiopate (Phospholine) iodide, 0.03–0.25%. These drugs are primarily useful in aphakic and pseudoaphakic glaucoma. *Caution:* These drugs should not be used in the presence of a narrow anterior chamber angle or in chronic angle-closure glaucomas since the extreme miosis increases relative pupillary block and can lead to angle closure. They also have cataractogenic properties and therefore should be avoided, if possible, in the phakic eye. They may cause iritis, bleeding, and excessive conjunctival scarring if used before surgery. Also, systemic effects have been noted in children who receive succinylcholine during anesthesia. Because of their high complication rate, their use is generally reserved for patients with open-angle glau-

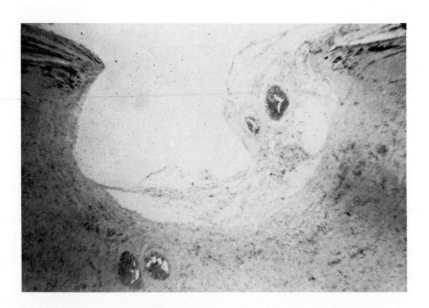

Figure 12–6. Glaucomatous ("bean-pot") cupping of the optic disk.

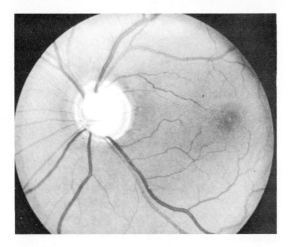

Figure 12–7. Typical glaucomatous cupping. Note the nasal displacement of the vessels and hollowed-out appearance of the optic disk except for a thin border. (Courtesy of S Mettier Jr.)

coma who are not good surgical candidates or who are aphakic.

Miotics frequently cause dimness of vision for 1–2 hours after instillation due to pupillary constriction, and younger glaucoma patients often have accommodative spasm with induced myopia.

Timolol maleate (Timoptic), a beta-adrenergic blocking agent, lowers intraocular pressure by decreasing aqueous production. It is available in 2 strengths, 0.25% and 0.5%, for use as eye drops instilled twice daily. Timolol can be used alone or in combination with other drugs. Although side effects of timolol are rare, they can be serious; the action of the beta blockade slows the heart rate and lowers the blood pressure. The drug is contraindicated in chronic obstructive lung diseases, particularly asthma. Depression, confusion, and fatigue may occur. Patients should be taught to occlude the tear ducts after instillation to reduce systemic absorption.

Betaxolol (Betoptic) and levobunolol (Betagan) are promising new alternatives to timolol in the treatment of glaucoma. They are also beta-adrenergic blocking agents with comparable effects on intraocular pressure but have the added advantage of β_1-receptor selectivity. Thus, systemic side effects are less likely to include bronchoconstriction, particularly the exacerbation of reactive airway disease, as demonstrated in a number of clinical trials. Cardiac or metabolic side effects may still occur.

Epinephrine, 0.5–2% instilled 1–2 times daily, decreases aqueous production and increases aqueous outflow. No miosis or myopia is induced, and it has a longer action than the miotics.

Epinephrine instilled once or twice daily dramatically reduces the intraocular pressure in selected cases of aphakic glaucoma. Watch for macular edema as a complication.

Dipivefrin (Propine) is a prodrug of epinephrine that is metabolized intraocularly to its active state. This decreases the side effects of the epinephrine.

Either timolol, betaxolol, or dipivefrin is commonly used as the primary drug in open-angle glaucoma. (Do not use dipivefrin or epinephrine in eyes with narrow anterior chamber angles.)

Carbonic anhydrase inhibitors such as acetazolamide (Diamox), 125–250 mg 4 times daily, or Diamox Sequels, 500 mg twice daily, are used in open-angle glaucoma if strong antiglaucoma solutions do not adequately control intraocular pressure. Dichlorphenamide (Daranide), methazolamide (Neptazane), and ethoxzolamide are similarly effective carbonic anhydrase inhibitors and, like acetazolamide, usually suppress aqueous production from 40 to 60%. Complications of long-term therapy with carbonic anhydrase inhibitors include renal calculi (see also p 198). Nevertheless, these drugs are indicated to avoid glaucoma surgery.

B. Laser Trabeculoplasty: Treatment of the trabecular meshwork by laser energy will reduce intraocular pressure by almost 25% in 80% of patients. It can be used as an adjunct to medical therapy before resorting to surgery. The initial gratifying decrease in pressure is often lost after a few months or years.

C. Surgical Treatment: (See p 204.) Surgery for open-angle glaucoma may be performed if the intraocular pressure is not maintained within normal limits by medical therapy and there is progressive visual field loss associated with optic nerve damage. There is no operation that can be called uniformly successful in the treatment of open-angle glaucoma. Standard filtration procedures such as trephine, sclerectomy, and thermal sclerostomy all have their advocates. Trabeculectomy and other forms of filtering procedures beneath a scleral flap have recently become popular. This is not because they are more effective but because they have a lower complication rate, since the anterior chamber remains formed following the procedure. The success rate without medication averages about 75%. Cataract formation does not occur as rapidly or as frequently following these latter procedures as it did with standard filtering operations.

If a cataract is present, it should be extracted and a posterior chamber implant introduced. This alone will help control the glaucoma in some cases. If the glaucoma is difficult to control or is uncontrolled prior to extraction, the cataract operation and trabeculectomy may be done simultaneously. The success rate of glaucoma surgery in the aphakic patient is approximately 60%. If medical therapy fails, however, subscleral filtration procedures may be used. Some authorities still use cyclodialysis.

In patients under 40 years of age, filtration surgery of any type has a low success rate. Standard filtering techniques are somewhat mutilating to the eye. The external trabeculotomy is somewhat more successful in these patients and is less mutilating. In general, surgery is recommended in open-angle glaucoma only when maximum medical therapy has failed to halt the progression of visual field and optic nerve deterioration.

Course & Prognosis

Without treatment, open-angle glaucoma may be insidiously progressive to complete blindness. If antiglaucoma drops control the intraocular pressure in an eye that has not suffered extensive glaucomatous damage, the prognosis is good (although visual field loss sometimes continues to progress in spite of normalized intraocular pressure). When the process is detected early, most glaucoma patients can be successfully managed medically.

LOW-PRESSURE GLAUCOMA

This term denotes a number of conditions in which there is evidence of intraocular glaucomatous damage (cupping of the optic disk, visual field defects, etc) with normal or low intraocular pressure. Most such cases can be classified in the following groups:

(1) Cases in which some type of glaucoma, usually secondary, has caused permanent changes and then regressed spontaneously. Tonography may reveal a diminished facility of outflow.

(2) Diurnal variation: The pressure is usually normal when taken but is elevated at other times. This may be due to diurnal variation, so that if the pressure is measured at the same time of day it seems normal. Diurnal pressure curves disclose the real diagnosis.

(3) Cases in which glaucomatous damage is evident despite no diurnal elevation. A weakness of the lamina cribrosa or vascular insufficiency of the optic nerve head may be contributing factors.

(4) A variety of miscellaneous cases of damage to the optic nerve and retina, including vascular, congenital, degenerative, and other diseases, or tumors involving the optic chiasm. Some of these are apparently due to reduced blood pressure and blood flow

to the optic nerve or perhaps to an easily distorted lamina cribrosa.

ANGLE-CLOSURE GLAUCOMA (Acute Glaucoma)

Angle-closure glaucoma occurs when there is a sudden increase in the intraocular pressure due to a block of the anterior chamber angle by the root of the iris, which cuts off all aqueous outflow, causing severe pain and sudden visual loss.

An acute attack of angle-closure glaucoma can develop only in an eye in which the anterior chamber angle is anatomically narrow. This situation can be easily assessed clinically by estimation of the depth of the anterior chamber, using oblique illumination from a penlight (Fig 12–8). The following factors may cause further encroachment upon the anterior chamber angle, setting the stage for angle-closure glaucoma.

(1) Physiologic pupillary block: When the anterior chamber angle is narrow, the iris has a relatively large arc of contact with the anterior surface of the lens. This may obstruct the free passage of aqueous from the posterior to the anterior chamber. As pressure builds up in the posterior chamber, the peripheral iris is pushed forward (iris bombé). If the iris is pushed forward far enough so that it lies against the trabeculum, aqueous humor drainage is impeded, resulting in acute angle-closure glaucoma.

(2) Increased size of the lens: Normally, the lens continues to enlarge slightly with age. During the act of accommodation there may be a further increase in the forward displacement of the lens, increasing the relative pupillary block.

Precipitating Factors

The more miotic the pupil, the more tightly the iris is held against the lens, thus increasing pupillary

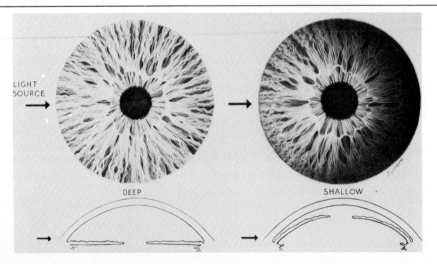

Figure 12–8. Estimation of depth of anterior chamber by oblique illumination (diagram). (Courtesy of R Shaffer.)

block. If a patient with a narrow angle is given pilocarpine, an acute attack of angle-closure glaucoma may be precipitated. Usually, however, the pull of the sphincter on the peripheral iris will tend to open the angle.

Dilating the pupil has the opposite effect, making it easier for the aqueous humor trapped behind the iris by the relative pupillary block to lift the peripheral iris against the trabecular meshwork. The most dangerous pupillary position in such an eye is mid-dilation. With further dilation, the arc of contact of iris to lens is reduced, lessening pupillary block. It is wise to perform gonioscopy of a shallow-chambered eye before the pupil is dilated or contracted, to avoid causing iatrogenic angle-closure glaucoma.

Plateau iris is a rare condition in which the central anterior chamber depth is normal but the angle is very narrow. Such an eye has little pupillary block, but dilation will cause "bunching up" of the peripheral iris, occluding the angle even if peripheral iridectomy has been performed. Miotics or laser iridoplasty can help open the angle.

A secondary cause of shallow anterior chamber and angle-closure glaucoma is a sudden increase in the volume of the posterior chamber. This can result from subchoroidal hemorrhage, a swollen lens, ciliary block (malignant) glaucoma or from therapeutic procedures such as panretinal photocoagulation or scleral buckling.

Pathology

The pathologic changes in acute glaucoma include peripheral anterior synechiae and edema and congestion of the ciliary processes and iris. These are secondary to the vascular strangulation that results from the high pressure. Late changes are the result of interference with circulation and the continued high pressure. The iris and ciliary body become atrophic, and the ciliary processes show hyaline degeneration. Chronic edema of the cornea results in loosening of the corneal epithelium and the formation of epithelial bullae (bullous keratopathy). The most important pathologic change is damage to the nerve elements: degeneration of nerve fibers and a loss of substance of the optic cup associated with a backward bowing of the cribriform plate. The ganglion cell layer and the nerve fiber layer of the retina undergo degeneration. Eventually the lens may show cataractous change.

Clinical Findings

Angle-closure (acute) glaucoma is characterized by a sudden onset of blurred vision followed by excruciating pain, and a rainbow-colored halo is seen around lights. Nausea and vomiting are often present. The pain is usually localized in and around the eye. Other findings include markedly increased intraocular pressure, a shallow anterior chamber, an edematous cornea, decreased visual acuity (at times limited to light perception only), a fixed, moderately dilated pupil, and ciliary injection.

Differential Diagnosis

Acute iritis and conjunctivitis must be considered with acute angle-closure glaucoma in the differential diagnosis of any acutely inflamed eye, although they seldom have shallow anterior chambers or increased tension. (1) Acute iritis causes more photophobia and less pain than acute glaucoma. Intraocular pressure may be normal, the pupil is constricted, and the cornea is not edematous. Marked flare and cells are present in the anterior chamber, and there is deep ciliary injection. (2) In acute conjunctivitis there is little or no pain and no visual loss. There is discharge from the eye and an intensely inflamed conjunctiva, but no ciliary injection. The pupillary responses are normal, the cornea is clear, and intraocular pressure is normal. (3) Iridocyclitis with secondary glaucoma occasionally presents a difficult problem of differentiation. Gonioscopy to define the type of angle is most helpful. If corneal or anterior chamber haze prevents good visibility, gonioscopy of the other eye will usually confirm the diagnosis.

Complications & Sequelae

A. Formation of Peripheral Anterior Synechiae: The peripheral iris adheres to the trabecular meshwork and blocks the outflow of aqueous.

B. Cataract Formation: The lens sometimes swells, and a cataract may develop. The enlarged lens pushes the iris even farther anteriorly; this increases the pupillary block, which in turn increases the degree of angle block.

C. Atrophy of the Retina and Optic Nerve: The nerve elements of the eye withstand the effects of increased intraocular pressure poorly. Glaucomatous cupping of the optic disk and retinal atrophy, particularly of the ganglion cell layer, occur.

D. Absolute Glaucoma: The end result of uncontrolled angle-closure glaucoma is absolute glaucoma. The eye is stony hard, sightless, and often quite painful, in which case enucleation or retrobulbar alcohol injection is necessary.

Prevention

Although miotics can usually widen a narrow angle and break an attack of angle-closure glaucoma, prevention is best accomplished by laser iridectomy that bypasses the pupillary block permanently.

Treatment

Angle-closure glaucoma is an ophthalmic surgical emergency.

A. Medical Treatment: Before surgery, every effort must be made to reduce the intraocular pressure by medical means. Osmotic agents, miotics, beta-blockers, and acetazolamide are usually required. The immediate administration of oral glycerin (glycerol), 1 mL/kg of body weight in a cold 50% solution mixed with chilled lemon juice, nearly always interrupts the acute attack by making the blood hypertonic and drawing fluid from the eye. Pilocarpine 2%, 2 drops every 15 minutes for several hours, will usually constrict the pupil and pull the iris away from the trabeculum, allowing aqueous outflow to be reestablished (unless permanent adhesions have formed).

If treatment with glycerin is not successful or if the patient is nauseated, intravenous hypertonic mannitol (20%) may be effective in total doses of 1.5–3 g/kg. Acetazolamide, 500 mg given intramuscularly if the patient is nauseated, will further reduce intraocular pressure by decreasing aqueous production.

Meperidine, 100 mg intramuscularly, or other systemic analgesic should be given as necessary to relieve pain.

B. Surgical Treatment: (See p 204.) Although surgical intervention can be delayed for several hours to permit clearing of the cornea, surgery is indicated whether or not pressure has been reduced. The safest method of breaking the pupillary block is laser iridectomy.

SUBACUTE OR CHRONIC ANGLE-CLOSURE GLAUCOMA

Chronic angle-closure glaucoma is caused by the same etiologic factors as acute angle-closure glaucoma. The difference is that there is no sudden complete block to aqueous outflow by the iris being pushed against the trabeculum. The iris extends its arc of contact with the trabeculum gradually until an adequate area of angle is no longer available for aqueous outflow. The pressure rises and glaucoma results that may be clinically similar to open-angle glaucoma.

Clinical Findings

Symptoms are minimal or absent. Occasional mild attacks of increased intraocular pressure cause transient blurring of vision, halos around lights, and possibly slight pain in or about the eyes. On examination, one finds a shallow anterior chamber, high intraocular pressure (25–50 mm Hg), and a partially closed chamber angle as seen on gonioscopic examination. The iris is in apposition to the trabeculum except in an area covering one-fifth or less of the chamber angle.

Treatment

Treatment is the same as for acute angle-closure glaucoma. After breaking of the pupillary block by iridectomy, residual glaucoma should be treated in the same way as open-angle glaucoma.

CILIARY BLOCK GLAUCOMA (Malignant Glaucoma)

Surgery upon an eye with markedly increased intraocular pressure and a closed angle can lead to ciliary block glaucoma. Immediately after surgery, the intraocular pressure increases markedly and the lens-iris diaphragm is pushed forward as a result of the collection of aqueous in and behind the vitreous body.

Treatment

Treatment consists of cycloplegics, mydriatics, aqueous suppressants, and hyperosmotic agents. Atropine, 2–4%, should be used topically every 2 hours for the first day and may need to be continued indefinitely on a daily basis thereafter. Phenylephrine, 10%, is used 4 times a day. Hyperosmotic agents are used to shrink the vitreous body and let the lens-iris diaphragm fall posteriorly.

Posterior sclerotomy, vitrectomy, and even lens extraction may be needed.

PRIMARY CONGENITAL OR INFANTILE GLAUCOMA (Trabeculodysgenesis)

Primary infantile glaucoma is a form of developmental glaucoma with onset in the first year of life. One-fourth of cases are present at birth. A few are diagnosed after the second year of life. The pathologic picture is produced by an arrest in development of the angle structures at about the seventh month of fetal life. The iris is hypoplastic and inserts onto the trabecular surface in front of a poorly developed scleral spur (Fig 12–9).

Clinical Findings

The earliest and most constant symptom is epiphora. Photophobia may be present. Increased intraocular pressure is the cardinal sign. Glaucomatous cupping of the optic disk is a relatively early and most important change. Later findings include increased corneal diameter (above 11.5 mm is considered significant), epithelial edema, tears of Descemet's membrane, and increased depth of the anterior chamber (associated with general enlargement of the anterior segment of the eye), as well as edema and opacity of the corneal stroma. The iris inserts anteriorly onto the trabeculum instead of into the ciliary body.

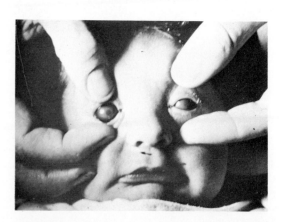

Figure 12–9. Infantile glaucoma (buphthalmos.)

Differential Diagnosis

Megalocornea, secondary glaucoma, and traumatic corneal haze should be ruled out. Measurement of intraocular pressure, gonioscopy, and evaluation of the optic disk are important in making the differential diagnosis.

Treatment

Unlike open-angle glaucoma, in which the best treatment is often nonsurgical, primary infantile glaucoma must be treated surgically to obtain lasting results. Medical treatment with miotics is at best a preoperative adjunctive measure.

Goniotomy is the treatment of choice. If repeated goniotomies fail or are not possible due to corneal haze, external trabeculotomy is often effective. Subscleral filtration (trabeculectomy) may be tried if these measures fail. The long-term visual prognosis is then much less favorable.

Course & Prognosis

In untreated cases, blindness occurs early. The eye undergoes marked stretching and may even rupture with minor trauma. Typical glaucomatous cupping occurs relatively soon, emphasizing the necessity of early effective treatment.

The earlier the disease becomes manifest, the less favorable the prognosis, since the early appearance of symptoms implies a more severe defect of aqueous drainage. Over 80% of cases are evident by age 3 months. Goniotomy controls the pressure permanently in 70–80% of cases. The long-term visual prognosis in such cases is good.

DEVELOPMENTAL GLAUCOMA ASSOCIATED WITH OTHER CONGENITAL ANOMALIES*

A number of syndromes characterized by increased intraocular pressure in persons under 40 have been grouped under this broad heading, which includes late-developing infantile glaucoma.

Aniridia

The distinguishing feature of aniridia, as the name implies, is the vestigial iris. Often, little more than the root of the iris or a thin iris margin is present. Other deformities of the eye may be present, such as congenital cataracts, corneal dystrophy, and foveal hypoplasia. Vision is usually poor. Glaucoma frequently develops before adolescence and is usually refractory to medical or surgical management.

This rare syndrome is genetically determined. Numerous examples of both autosomal dominant and recessive inheritance have appeared in the literature.

If medical therapy is ineffective, goniotomy or trabeculotomy may occasionally normalize the intraoc-

ular pressure. Often, filtering operations are necessary, but the long-term visual prognosis is poor.

Iridocorneal Trabeculodysgenesis (Axenfeld's Syndrome, Peters' Anomaly, Rieger's Syndrome)

These rare diseases represent a spectrum of improper development of the mesodermal structures of the anterior segment. The result is an abnormally developed angle, iris, and cornea. Occasionally, lens changes are present. Usually there is some hypoplasia of the anterior stroma of the iris, with bridging filaments connecting the iris stroma to the cornea. If these bridging filaments occur peripherally and connect to a prominent, axially displaced Schwalbe's line (posterior embryotoxon), the disease is known as **Axenfeld's syndrome.** If adhesions are between the central iris and central posterior surface of the cornea, the disease is known as **Peters' anomaly.** If there are broader iridocorneal adhesions associated with the disruption of the iris with polycoria and, in addition, skeletal and dental anomalies, the disorder is called **Rieger's syndrome.**

These diseases are usually dominantly inherited, although sporadic cases have been reported. Glaucoma occurs in approximately 50% of such eyes. Since no highly effective surgical procedure is available for these syndromes, they are treated as open-angle glaucomas. Filtering surgery or trabeculotomy may be used if medical therapy fails. The prognosis is guarded for long-term retention of good visual function.

SECONDARY GLAUCOMA

Increased intraocular pressure occurring as one manifestation of some other intraocular disease is called secondary glaucoma. These diseases are difficult to classify satisfactorily.

In addition to treatment of the underlying disease, several drugs are of value in control of secondary glaucoma. With moderate elevation of intraocular pressure, reduction of aqueous production with epinephrine or timolol with or without acetazolamide is adequate management. With extreme elevations, osmotic agents are indicated. These ocular antihypertensive drugs may prevent permanent damage due to increased intraocular pressure until the underlying cause of secondary glaucoma can be controlled.

PIGMENTARY GLAUCOMA

This syndrome seems to be primarily a degeneration of the pigmented epithelium of the iris and ciliary body. The pigment granules flake off the iris as a result of friction against the underlying packets of

*Formerly classified as juvenile glaucoma.

zonular fibers, resulting in iris transillumination. The pigment is deposited on the posterior corneal surface (Krukenberg's spindle) and becomes lodged in the trabecular meshwork, impeding the normal outflow of aqueous. The syndrome occurs most often in myopic males between the ages of 25 and 40 who have a deep anterior chamber with a wide anterior chamber angle.

A number of pedigrees of autosomal dominant inheritance of pigmentary glaucoma have been reported. The pigmentary changes may be present without glaucoma, but such persons must be considered "glaucoma suspects."

This type of glaucoma responds to timolol and to epinephrine. Miotics can seldom be used in these young patients because of induced myopia. The prognosis is not favorable if the process is severe enough to require a filtering operation. Laser trabeculoplasty may improve the prognosis.

EXFOLIATIVE SYNDROME (Pseudoexfoliation of the Lens Capsule, Glaucoma Capsulare)

In exfoliative syndrome, flakelike deposits of epithelial cell origin are seen on the lens surface, ciliary processes, zonule, posterior iris surface, loose in the anterior chamber, and in the trabecular meshwork. The disease is usually found in patients over the age of 65. Glaucoma and sometimes cataract may eventually develop. Lens extraction has no effect on the glaucoma. Miotics, timolol, and epinephrine are moderately effective, but laser trabeculoplasty or a filtering operation may be necessary.

GLAUCOMA SECONDARY TO CHANGES IN THE LENS

Lens Dislocation (Traumatic)

The lens may dislocate anteriorly, pressing the iris against the posterior cornea and blocking aqueous outflow, or it may dislocate posteriorly. Secondary glaucoma is a frequent complication of posterior dislocation of the lens and is not easy to explain. Often it may be due to angle recession or trabecular damage that occurred at the time of the trauma. In other cases pupillary block occurs when a wedge of vitreous curls around the dislocated lens and plugs the pupillary opening. Surgery may be necessary if the intraocular pressure cannot be controlled medically.

Intumescence of the Lens

The lens may take up considerable fluid during cataractous change, increasing its size markedly. It may then encroach upon the anterior chamber and produce a pupillary block, resulting in angle-closure glaucoma. Treatment consists of lens extraction.

Phacolytic Glaucoma

As cataract formation proceeds, the lens cortex elements may undergo liquefaction and seep out through the lens capsule. Lens protein products may cause an inflammatory reaction within the eye. In this case, uveitis occurs, and the protein and cellular debris lodge in the outflow system to obstruct the free passage of aqueous. Edema of the trabeculum itself is probably associated, further decreasing the facility of aqueous outflow. Lens extraction is indicated.

GLAUCOMA SECONDARY TO CHANGES IN THE UVEAL TRACT

Uveitis

Often the intraocular pressure is below normal early in uveitis. This is because the inflamed ciliary body is functioning poorly and does not secrete the elements that produce the difference in osmotic pressure between aqueous and plasma. There is edema of the trabeculum as well as the ciliary body and iris, and this may result in a decreased facility of aqueous outflow. As long as there is no osmotic difference between blood and aqueous there will be no rise in pressure, but when the ciliary body begins secreting there will be an abrupt rise of pressure unless there has been a simultaneous improvement in the patency of the outflow channels. Long-standing or repeated attacks of iridocyclitis cause permanent anterior synechiae. In these cases, after the inflammatory reaction has subsided, miotics or even filtering procedures may be needed to control the intraocular pressure.

Tumor

Rapidly growing melanomas originating in the uveal tract can cause increased intraocular pressure by volume replacement, by encroachment on the filtration angle, or by blocking of a vortex vein. Enucleation is indicated.

Iridocorneoendothelial (ICE) Syndrome (Essential Iris Atrophy, Iris Nevus Syndrome, Chandler's Syndrome, Cogan-Reese Syndrome)

Slowly progressive atrophy of iris tissue is a rare disorder of unknown cause that is almost always associated with glaucoma. Anterior synechiae form and the degenerated iris elements block the trabecular meshwork, creating a glaucoma that is very difficult to control either medically or surgically. Endothelial degeneration occurs with edema of the cornea at relatively low intraocular pressures. The condition is nearly always unilateral.

GLAUCOMA SECONDARY TO TRAUMA

Massive Hemorrhage Into the Anterior Chamber

Contusion or penetrating injuries of the globe can cause tears in the iris or ciliary body and thus massive hemorrhage into the anterior chamber. The intraocular pressure may be elevated, and blood breakdown products or organized clots lodge in the outflow mechanism. One serious complication is blood staining of the cornea. Once well established, the staining may require several years to absorb. If the intraocular pressure cannot be controlled with systemic hypotensive drugs, the anterior chamber should be lavaged through a limbal incision. Patients with sickle cell trait or disease are at greater risk of developing glaucoma following anterior chamber hemorrhage.

Corneal or Limbal Laceration
With Prolapse of Iris
Into the Wound

Lacerations of the anterior eye or contusions causing anterior rupture of the eye precipitate a loss of the anterior chamber and the rapid closure of the chamber angle by the adherence of the iris to the cornea. Occasionally, a prolapse of uveal tissue into the wound will seal the defect and maintain the anterior chamber. The primary objective of the treatment is the reformation of the anterior chamber to prevent permanent anterior peripheral synechiae. Excision of prolapsed uvea, tight closure of the wound. and injection of saline into the anterior chamber are of paramount importance.

Contusion Causing
Retrodisplacement of the Iris
Root & Deepening of the Anterior
Chamber Angle
(Angle Recession Glaucoma)

A number of clinicians have called attention to this type of trauma-induced unilateral secondary glaucoma. Following a contusion injury, the anterior chamber may be significantly deeper than in the uninjured eye. Gonioscopically, one sees a recession of the angle and a torn ciliary body. Glaucoma occurs if there is sufficient associated damage to the trabecular meshwork to interfere with aqueous outflow. The condition often responds to standard open-angle glaucoma therapy, although occasionally a filtering operation is necessary.

GLAUCOMA FOLLOWING SURGERY

Epithelial Ingrowth
Into the Anterior Chamber

Following cataract surgery with resultant poor healing of the wound edges, epithelium may grow into the anterior chamber and eventually line the anterior chamber angle structures, preventing normal outflow of aqueous. This is a difficult complication to treat once it is well established. An effort can be made to scrape the newly deposited epithelium off the angle structures. Corneal transplant may be beneficial. The problem is primarily one of prevention.

Flat Anterior Chamber Following
Cataract Surgery

Following caratact surgery, aqueous may escape through an imperfectly closed wound resulting in a flat (absent) anterior chamber. If the chamber fails to re-form within 1–3 days, repair of the wound is required to avoid anterior synechiae and endothelial damage.

GLAUCOMA SECONDARY
TO RUBEOSIS IRIDIS

Rubeosis often follows central retinal vein occlusion and occurs frequently in advanced diabetes mellitus. Small vessels grow on the anterior surface of the iris and into the anterior chamber angle, interfering with normal aqueous outflow. Miotics are of little value. Early panretinal photocoagulation can arrest the blood vessel proliferation. Filtering surgery can then be successful in some cases. Ciliary body destructive procedures are often necessary.

GLAUCOMA SECONDARY
TO ARTERIOVENOUS FISTULAS

Pulsating exophthalmos from arteriovenous fistula is usually accompanied by a slightly elevated intraocular pressure due to increased venous pressure. Treatment is directed at the underlying condition.

GLAUCOMA SECONDARY
TO THE USE OF TOPICAL
CORTICOSTEROIDS

Much interest has been aroused by the observation that topically administered corticosteroids may produce a type of glaucoma that simulates open-angle glaucoma. Most persons do not develop significant intraocular pressure elevations while on such treatment. In those who do, withdrawal of the medication eliminates the glaucoma; but permanent damage can occur if the condition goes unrecognized too long. If topical steroid therapy is absolutely necessary, miotics or other open-angle glaucoma therapy usually will control the glaucoma. It is imperative that patients receiving long-term topical steroid therapy have periodic tonometry and ophthalmoscopy. It is equally important to beware of topical administration of corticosteroids in the eyes of patients known to have glaucoma or a family history of glaucoma. Less commonly, glaucoma can occur in patients being given long-term systemic corticosteroids over prolonged periods. Injections of corticosteroids under the conjunctiva and under Tenon's capsule may cause elevated intraocular pressure for several months. Surgical excision of the residual steroid deposit may allow the pressure to return to normal.

OCULAR HYPERTENSION

Ocular hypertension is the term coined to denote an elevated intraocular pressure (above the statistically normal level of 10–21 mm Hg) without evidence of anatomic or functional damage to the eye. The diagnosis changes to glaucoma if there is asymmetry of the disk cups (cup in one eye larger than the cup in the other) or increase of the size of the disk cup over a period of time. Obviously, functional loss represents visual field defects specific for glaucoma.

The patient with ocular hypertension should be considered a glaucoma suspect. Although no evidence of damage from the elevated intraocular pressure may be apparent, there is as yet no sure means of predicting which patient will subsequently develop damage. Frequent observation (1–3 times yearly) of the optic disk, tonometry, and visual field testing are indicated in order to make certain that proper treatment is initiated immediately if the optic nerve appears threatened.

SURGICAL PROCEDURES USED IN THE TREATMENT OF THE GLAUCOMAS

PERIPHERAL IRIDECTOMY

In acute or chronic angle-closure glaucoma when extensive peripheral anterior synechiae have not formed, peripheral iridectomy is the operation of choice. It offers the one hope of a permanent cure by reestablishing ready communication between the posterior and anterior chambers. This relieves pupillary block and allows the iris root to drop away from the filtration angle, thus reestablishing the outflow of aqueous by normal channels.

In recent years, laser iridectomy has become the procedure of choice.

LASER TRABECULOPLASTY

When maximal medical therapy fails to control the pressure of open-angle glaucoma, laser trabeculoplasty is usually indicated before filtration surgery is considered. Laser energy is focused through a goniolens onto the trabecular meshwork. Intraocular pressure is reduced by improved aqueous outflow in about 80% of cases. Medications must usually be continued. The effect of the laser decreases with time. The procedure may be repeated but with much less effectiveness.

FILTRATION SURGERY

When pressures cannot be maintained at a safe level in open-angle glaucoma despite the use of medications and laser therapy, filtration surgery is indicated. The variety of procedures available indicates that none is perfect. In "full-thickness" operations (trephine, thermal sclerostomy, posterior lip sclerectomy), a channel is created from the anterior chamber into the subconjunctival space. There, the aqueous is absorbed by the lymphatics and blood vessels and via transudation through the conjunctiva. In about 25% of cases, postoperative scarring closes the opening, and reoperation becomes necessary.

In recent years, a protected filtration operation, trabeculectomy, has achieved universal popularity. A half-thickness scleral flap is sutured over the limbal opening in addition to closure of the conjunctival flap. Complications are reduced, but pressure reduction is somewhat less than with the unprotected methods.

GONIOTOMY

Primary infantile glaucoma is best treated by goniotomy. This procedure was introduced for treatment of infantile glaucoma by Otto Barkan in 1938 and changed the prognosis of the disease from very bad to good (70–80% cure). The operation aims to establish normal aqueous outflow through physiologic channels.

CILIARY BODY DESTRUCTIVE PROCEDURES

Cyclocryotherapy has generally replaced cyclodiathermy in the treatment of glaucomas where filtering surgery has failed. It has the advantage of destroying the ciliary body without causing damage to the sclera. No cutting is required. The highly vascular reaction in the ciliary body leads to fibrosis, decreased ciliary body function, and consequent decreased aqueous production.

Therapeutic ultrasound is a new noninvasive treatment of all types of glaucoma was introduced by Dr. Jackson Coleman of the Cornell Medical Center. To date, it has been used only in advanced cases, with a success rate of more than 50%. High-frequency sound waves are focused on the ciliary body and targeted through the sclera near the limbus. The damaged ciliary body produces less aqueous, and the weakened sclera allows seepage of aqueous.

Neodymium:YAG laser cyclodiathermy offers an alternative method for decreasing aqueous production. The treatment is applied transsclerally using the thermal mode to damage the ciliary body.

The neodymium:YAG laser and therapeutic ultrasound are promising techniques that may provide an advance over cyclocryotherapy in the treatment of difficult glaucomas.

REFERENCES

Abraham RK, Miller GL: Argon laser iridectomy for angle-closure glaucoma. (Letter.) *Ann Ophthalmol* 1973;**5:**613.

Airaksinen PJ et al: A double-masked study of timolol and pilocarpine combined. *Am J Ophthalmol* 1987;**104:**587.

Cartwright MJ, Anderson DR: Correlation of asymmetric damage with asymmetric intraocular pressure in normal-tension glaucoma (low-tension glaucoma). *Arch Ophthalmol* 1988;**106:**898.

Chandler PA et al: *Glaucoma,* 2nd ed. Lea & Febiger, 1980.

Coleman DJ et al: Therapeutic ultrasound in the treatment of glaucoma. 1. Experimental model. 2. Clinical applications. *Ophthalmology* 1985;**92:**339, 347.

Cowan CL et al: Glaucoma in blacks. *Arch Ophthalmol* 1988;**106:**739.

Del Priore LV, Robin AL, Pollack IP: Long-term follow-up of neodymium:YAG laser angle surgery for open-angle glaucoma. *Ophthalmology* 1988;**95:**277.

Devenyi RG et al: Neodymium:YAG transscleral cyclocoagulation in human eyes. *Ophthalmology* 1987;**94:**1519.

Dickens C, Hoskins HD Jr: *Developmental Glaucoma in the Eye in Infancy.* Yaer Book, 1988. Drance SM et al: Diffuse visual field loss in chronic open-angle and low-tension glaucoma. *Am J Ophthalmol* 1987;**104:**577.

Edwards RS: Behaviour of the fellow eye in acute angle-closure glaucoma. *Br J Ophthalmol* 1982;**66:**576.

Glaucoma: 1984 Annual Meeting of the American Academy of Ophthalmology, Atlanta, November 11–15. *Ophthalmology* 1984;**91:**307, 1005. [Entire issues.]

Glaucoma: 1985 Annual Meeting of the American Academy of Ophthalmology, San Francisco, September 29–October 3. *Ophthalmology* 1985;**92:**853. [Entire issue.]

Harrington DO: *The Visual Fields: A Textbook and Atlas of Clinical Perimetry,* 5th ed. Mosby, 1981.

Heuer DK: Glaucoma update. *Ophthalmology* 1988; **95:**282.

Hoskins HD Jr, Gelber EC: Optic disk topography and visual field defects in patients with increased intraocular pressure. *Am J Ophthalmol* 1975;**80:**284.

Hoyt WF: Ophthalmoscopy of the retinal nerve fibre layer in neuro-ophthalmologic diagnosis. *Aust J Ophthalmol* 1976;**4:**14.

Jay JL, Murray SB: Early trabeculectomy versus conventional management in primary open angle glaucoma. *Brit J Ophthalmol* 1988;**72:**881.

Jocson VL, Sears ML: Channels of aqueous outflow and related blood vessels. 1. *Macaca mulatta* (rhesus). 2. *Cercopithecus ethiops. Arch Ophthalmol* 1968;**80:**104 and 1969;**81:**244.

Kitazawa Y, Horie T: Diurnal variation of intraocular pressure in primary open-angle glaucoma. *Am J Ophthalmol* 1975;**79:**577.

Kolker AE, Hetherington J: *Becker-Shaffer's Diagnosis and Therapy of the Glaucomas,* 5th ed. Mosby, 1983.

McDonnell PJ et al: Molteno implant for control of glaucoma in eyes after penetrating keratoplasty. *Ophthalmology* 1988;**95:**364.

Newsome DA et al: Oral zinc in macular degeneration. *Arch Ophthalmol* 1988;**106:**192.

Quigley HA: Early detection of glaucomatous damage. 2. Changes in the appearance of the optic disk. *Surv Ophthalmol* 1985;**30:**111.

Quigley HA, Dunkelberger GR, Green WR: Chronic human glaucoma causing selectively greater loss of large optic nerve fibers. *Ophthalmology* 1988;**95:**357.

Schwartz L, Moster M: Neodymium-YAG laser cyclodiathermy. *Ophthalmic Laser Ther* 1986;**1:**135.

Shaffer RN et al: The use of diagrams to record changes in glaucomatous discs. *Am J Ophthalmol* 1975;**80:**460.

Shingleton BJ et al: Long-term efficacy of argon laser trabeculoplasty. *Ophthalmology* 1987;**94:**1513.

Tuulonen A, Niva A-K, Alanko HI: A controlled five-year follow-up study of laser trabeculoplasty as primary therapy for open-angle glaucoma. *Am J Ophthalmol* 1987;**104:**334.

Van Buskirk EM: *Clinical Atlas of Glaucoma.* Saunders, 1986.

Van Meter WS et al: Laser trabeculoplasty for glaucoma in aphakic and pseudophakic eyes after penetrating keratoplasty. *Arch Ophthalmol* 1988;**106:**185.

Van Buskirk EM, Fraunfelder FT: Ocular beta-blockers and systemic effects. (Editorial.) *Am J Ophthalmol* 1984;**98:**623.

Williams MT: Community screening for glaucoma and diabetes. *Sight Sav Rev* 1974;**44:**79.

Wise JB: Long-term control of adult open-angle glaucoma by argon laser treatment. *Ophthalmology* 1981;**88:**197.

Wise JB: Ten year results of laser trabeculoplasty: Does the laser avoid glaucoma surgery or merely defer it? *Eye* 1987;**1:**45.

Wise JB, Munnerlyn CR, Erickson PJ: A high-efficiency laser iridotomy-sphincterotomy lens. *Am J Ophthalmol* 1986;**101:**546.

Zimmerman TJ: Medication versus surgery: Are we doing it wrong? (Editorial.) *Ann Ophthalmol* 1981;**13:**783.

13

Strabismus

Taylor Asbury, MD, and Howard M. Eggers, MD

Under normal binocular viewing conditions, the image of the object of regard falls simultaneously on the fovea of each eye (bifoveal fixation), and the vertical retinal meridians are both upright. Either eye can be misaligned, so that only one eye at a time views the object of regard. Deviation from perfect alignment (strabismus) may be in any direction—inward, outward, up, down, or in a rotary direction about the line of sight. The amount of deviation is the angle by which the deviating eye is misaligned. Strabismus present under binocular viewing conditions is called manifest strabismus, heterotropia, or tropia. Deviation present only after binocular vision has been interrupted (ie, deviation controlled by binocular vision) is called latent strabismus, heterophoria, or phoria.

Strabismus is present in about 2% of children. Treatment should begin as soon as the diagnosis is made in order to ensure the best possible visual acuity and binocular visual function. It is extremely rare for true strabismus to be outgrown.

ANATOMY

Muscles

Six extraocular muscles control the movement of each eye; 4 rectus and 2 oblique muscles.

A. Rectus Muscles: The 4 rectus muscles originate at a common ring tendon (annulus of Zinn) surrounding the optic nerve at the posterior apex of the orbit. They are named according to their insertion into the sclera on the medial, lateral, inferior, and superior surfaces of the eye. The muscles are about 40 mm long, becoming tendinous 4–6 mm from insertion, and are about 10 mm wide at the point of insertion. The approximate distances of insertion from the corneal limbus are as follows: medial rectus, 5 mm; inferior rectus, 6 mm; lateral rectus, 7 mm; and superior rectus, 8 mm (Fig 13–1). With the eye in primary position, the vertical rectus muscle makes an angle of 23 degrees with the optic axis.

B. Oblique Muscles: The 2 oblique muscles control primarily torsional movement and, to a lesser

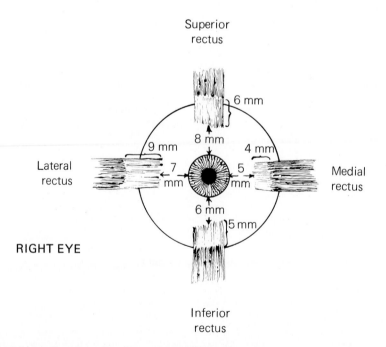

Figure 13–1. Approximate distances of the rectus muscles from the limbus, and the approximate lengths of tendons.

extent, upward and downward movement. The inferior oblique muscle arises from the nasal orbital wall several millimeters behind the orbital rim; it passes under the inferior rectus and curves around the eyeball, making a large arc of scleral contact, and inserts in the posterior lateral quadrant of the eye just lateral to the fovea. The main muscle body of the superior oblique muscle originates from the annulus of Zinn just above the origin of the superior rectus muscle and passes to the cartilaginous pulley (trochlea) attached to the nasal side of the superior orbital rim. At the pulley it is reflected downward, outward, and posteriorly, passing under the tendon of the superior rectus muscle to insert into the sclera. In the primary position, the muscle plane of the superior and inferior oblique muscles forms an angle of 51–54 degrees with the optic axis.

Innervation

The abducens nerve innervates the lateral rectus muscle; the trochlear nerve innervates the superior oblique muscle; and the oculomotor nerve innervates the other 3 rectus muscles and the inferior oblique muscle.

Fascia

The rectus and oblique muscles are ensheathed by fascia. Near the points of insertion of these muscles the fascia is continuous with Tenon's capsule, which is between the sclera and conjunctiva. Fascial condensations to adjacent orbital bony structures serve as check ligaments for the extraocular muscles and limit ocular rotation (Figs 13–2 and 13–3).

DEFINITIONS

Angle kappa: The angle between the visual axis and the central pupillary line. When the eye is fixing a light, if the corneal reflection is centered on the pupil, the visual axis and the central pupillary line coincide and the angle kappa is zero. Ordinarily, the light reflex is 2–4 degrees nasal to the pupillary center, giving the appearance of slight exotropia (positive angle kappa). A negative angle kappa gives the false impression of esotropia.

Conjugate: Movement of the eyes in the same direction at the same time.

Ductions: (Fig 13–4.) Monocular rotations with no consideration of the position of the other eye.

Adduction: Inward rotation.

Abduction: Outward rotation.

Sursumduction (elevation): Upward rotation.

Infraduction (depression): Downward rotation.

Fusion: Formation of one image from the 2 images seen simultaneously by the 2 eyes. Fusion has 2 aspects:

Motor fusion: Adjustments made by the brain in innervation of extraocular muscles in order to bring both eyes into bifoveal and torsional alignment.

Sensory fusion: Integration in the visual sensory areas of the brain of images seen with the 2 eyes into one sensory percept.

Heterophoria (phoria): Latent deviation of the eyes held in check by binocular vision.

Esophoria: Tendency for one eye to turn inward.

Exophoria: Tendency for one eye to turn outward.

Hyperphoria: Tendency for one eye to deviate upward.

Hypophoria: Tendency for one eye to deviate downward.

Heterotropia (tropia):

Strabismus: Manifest deviation of the eyes uncontrolled by binocular vision.

Estropia: Convergent manifest deviation ("crossed eyes").

Exotropia: Divergent manifest deviation ("wall-eyes").

Hypertropia: Manifest deviation of one eye upward.

Hypotropia: Manifest deviation of one eye downward. By convention, in the absence of specific pathologic disease to explain the low visual direction of one eye, vertical deviations are named according to the high eye.

Incyclotropia: Rotation of one eye about the line of sight to produce a convergence of the 12 o'clock meridians of the 2 eyes.

Excyclotropia: Rotation of one eye about the line of sight to produce a convergence of the 6 o'clock meridians of the 2 eyes.

Orthophoria: The absence of any tendency of either eye to deviate when fusion is suspended. This state is rarely seen clinically. A small degree of phoria is normal.

Primary deviation: The deviation measured with the normal eye fixing and the eye with the paretic muscle deviating.

Prism diopter (Δ): A unit of angular measurement used to characterize ocular deviations. One centimeter subtends 1 prism diopter at 1 meter. This is along a tangent scale, so that with larger angles, each incremental prism diopter is progressively smaller. A 1-diopter prism deflects a ray of light toward the base of the prism by 1 centimeter at 1 meter. One degree of arc equals approximately 1.7 Δ. (For technique of measurement, see p 206.)

Secondary deviation: (Fig 13–5.) The deviation measured with the paretic eye fixing and the normal eye deviating.

Torsion: Rotation of the eye about its anteroposterior axis.

Intorsion (incycloduction): Rotation of the 12 o'clock meridian of the eye toward the midline of the head.

Extorsion (excycloduction): Rotation of the 12 o'clock meridian of the eye away from the midline of the head.

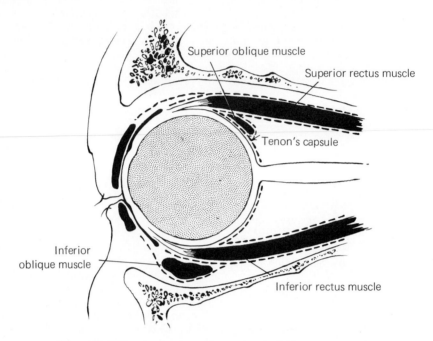

Figure 13–2. Fascia about muscles and eyeball (Tenon's capsule).

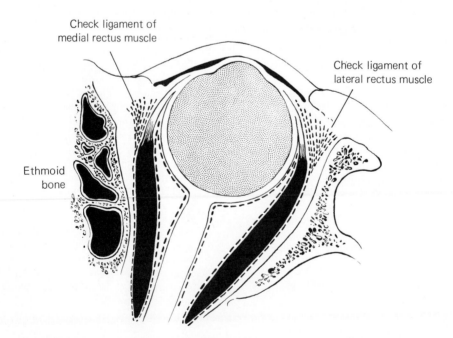

Figure 13–3. Check ligaments of medial and lateral rectus muscles, right eye (diagrammatic).

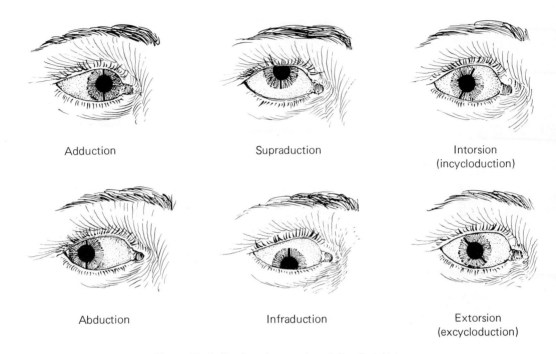

Adduction   Supraduction   Intorsion (incycloduction)

Abduction   Infraduction   Extorsion (excycloduction)

Figure 13–4. Ductions (monocular rotations), right eye.

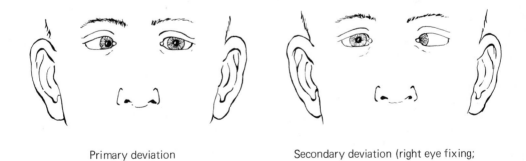

Primary deviation (left eye fixing)

Secondary deviation (right eye fixing; "inshoot" of sound left eye)

Figure 13–5. Paresis of horizontal muscle (right lateral rectus). Secondary deviation is greater than primary deviation because of Hering's law. With the left eye fixing, the right eye is deviated inward because of the paretic right lateral rectus. For the right eye to fix, the paretic right lateral rectus muscle must receive excessive stimulation. The yoke muscle, the left medial rectus, also receives the same excessive stimulation (Hering's law), which causes "inshoot" shown above.

Vergences (disjunctive movements): Movement of the 2 eyes in opposite directions.
Convergence: The eyes turn inward.
Divergence: The eyes turn outward.
Versions: Binocular rotations of the eyes in qualitatively the same direction.
Dextroversion (levoversion): Movement of the eyes to the right (or left).
Supraversion (infraversion): Movement of the eyes up (or down).
Dextrocycloversion: Torsional movement of both eyes to the right (clockwise).
Levocycloversion: Torsional movement of both eyes to the left (counterclockwise).

PHYSIOLOGY

1. MOTOR ASPECTS

Individual Muscle Functions (Table 13–1)

Each of the 6 extraocular muscles plays a role in positioning the eye about 3 possible axes of rotation. The primary action of a muscle is the principal effect it has on eye rotation. Lesser effects are called secondary or tertiary actions. The exact action of any muscle depends on the direction of the eye in space.

The medial and lateral rectus muscles adduct and abduct the eye, respectively, with little effect on elevation or torsion. The vertical rectus and oblique muscles have vertical rotation and torsion as their chief functions. In general terms, the vertical recti are the main elevators and depressors of the eye, and the obliques are mostly involved with torsional positioning. The vertical effect of the superior and inferior recti is greater in abduction than in adduction. The vertical effect of the obliques is greater in adduction than in abduction.

Field of Action

The position of the eye is determined by the equilibrium position achieved by the pull of all 6 extraocular muscles. In any direction of gaze, the agonist muscles contract to pull the eye into that direction and the antagonist muscles relax. When the eye is at rest in any direction of fixation, the pull exerted by the agonist muscles is exactly equal to that of the antag-

onist muscles plus the load of deflecting the eye from primary position. The field of action of a muscle is the direction of gaze in which that muscle has its greatest contraction as agonist, eg, the lateral rectus undergoes the greatest contraction in abducting the eye. The fields of action of the vertical rectus and oblique muscles overlap to some extent.

Donder's Law

The orientation of the eye about the fixation axis is determined by the direction of gaze (Donder's law). The eye has 3 degrees of rotational freedom in space; one degree is constrained by the innervation pattern of the 6 extraocular muscles, and 2 degrees are independent rotational coordinates.

Synergistic & Antagonistic Muscles (Sherrington's Law)

Synergistic muscles are those having the same field of action. Thus for vertical gaze, the superior rectus and inferior oblique muscles are synergists. Muscles synergistic for one function may be antagonistic for another. The superior rectus and inferior oblique muscles are antagonists for torsion, the superior rectus causing intorsion and the inferior oblique extorsion. The extraocular muscles, like skeletal muscles, show reciprocal innervation of antagonistic muscles (Sherrington's law). Thus, in dextroversion (right gaze), the right medial and left lateral rectus muscles are inhibited in proportion to the gaze effort.

Yoke Muscles (Hering's Law)

For movements of both eyes in the same direction, the corresponding agonist muscles receive approximately similar innervation (Hering's law). The pair of agonist muscles with the same primary action is called a yoke pair. The right lateral rectus and the left medial rectus muscles are a yoke pair for right gaze. The right inferior rectus and the left superior oblique muscles are a yoke pair for gaze down to the right. Table 13–2 lists the yoke muscle combinations.

Development of Binocular Movement

Eye movements in the infant are strongly dependent on the amount of illumination. In bright light, the eyes are fully or partially closed much of the time and there

Table 13–1. Functions of the ocular muscles.

Muscle	Primary Action	Secondary Action
Lateral rectus	Abduction	None
Medial rectus	Adduction	None
Superior rectus	Elevation	Adduction, intorsion
Inferior rectus	Depression	Adduction, extorsion
Superior oblique	Depression	Intorsion, abduction
Inferior oblique	Elevation	Extorsion, abduction

Table 13–2. Yoke muscle combinations.

Cardinal Direction of Gaze	Yoke Muscles
Eyes up, right	Right superior rectus and left inferior oblique
Eyes right	Right lateral rectus and left medial rectus
Eyes down, right	Right inferior rectus and left superior oblique
Eyes down, left	Right superior oblique and left inferior rectus
Eyes left	Right medial rectus and left lateral rectus
Eyes up, left	Right inferior oblique and left superior oblique

is more nystagmus on lateral gaze. In dim illumination, the eyes are opened and the infant scans the environment. The eyes linger over areas rich in visual contours, such as a face. Eye control is better in dim illumination. The eye movements of the infant are generally conjugate, although the control of convergence is inexact until 3–4 months of age. Transient exodeviations may be seen and are of no great import, since they tend to disappear with maturation. Esodeviations are more significant and tend to be permanent. An infant can be productively examined at any age and should be brought to an ophthalmologist as soon as any abnormality is suspected.

2. SENSORY ASPECTS

Binocular Vision

In each eye, whatever is imaged on the fovea is seen subjectively as being straight ahead. Thus, if 2 dissimilar objects were imaged on the 2 foveas, the 2 objects would be seen superimposed, but the dissimilarities would prevent fusion into a single impression. Because of the different vantage point in space of each eye, the image in each eye is actually slightly different from that in the other. Sensory fusion and stereopsis are the 2 different physiologic processes that are responsible for binocular vision.

A. Sensory Fusion: Sensory fusion is the process whereby dissimilarities between the 2 images are not appreciated. On the peripheral retina of each eye, there are **corresponding points** that in the absence of fusion localize stimuli in the same direction in space. In the process of fusion, the direction values of these points can be modified. Thus, each point of the retina in each eye is capable of fusing stimuli that strike sufficiently close to the corresponding point in the other eye. This region of fusible points is called **Panum's area.**

B. Stereopsis: While fusion is possible because subtle differences between the 2 images are ignored, stereopsis, or binocular depth perception, is possible because of recognition of these very same differences. When disparate retinal points are stimulated at the same time, fusion of the different images results in perception of an object in 3 dimensions.

Sensory Changes in Strabismus

Up to age 7 or 8 the brain may develop several responses to abnormal binocular vision that cannot occur later in life.

A. Diplopia: If strabismus is present, each fovea receives a different image. The objects imaged on the 2 foveas are seen in the same direction in space. This process of localization of spatially separate objects to the same location is called **visual confusion.** The object viewed by one of the foveas is imaged on a peripheral retinal area in the other eye. The foveal image is localized straight ahead, while the peripheral image of the same object in the other eye is localized

in some other direction. Thus, the same object is seen in 2 places (diplopia).

B. Suppression: Under binocular viewing conditions, the images seen by one eye become predominant and those seen by the other eye are not perceived (suppression). Suppression takes the form of a **scotoma** (an area of depressed vision within the visual field, surrounded by an area of less depressed or normal vision) in the deviating eye only under binocular viewing conditions. Suppression scotomas in esotropia are usually approximately elliptical in shape, extending on the retina from just temporal to the fovea to the point in the peripheral retina where the object of regard for the other eye is imaged. In exotropia, the suppression area tends to be larger and extends from the fovea to usually the entire temporal half of the retina. When fixation shifts to the other eye, the suppression scotoma also switches to the newly deviating eye. In the absence of strabismus, a blurred image in one eye may also lead to suppression. The lack of simultaneous perception in the central retina prevents fine stereopsis, although crude stereopsis from the peripheral retina may still be present.

C. Amblyopia: Prolonged abnormal visual experience may also lead to amblyopia (reduction in visual acuity in the absence of detectable organic disease). The 2 clinical contexts in which amblyopia occurs are strabismus and disorders producing degradation of retinal image quality in one eye, such as **anisometropia.** Anisometropic amblyopia is the amblyopia produced by anisometropia, ie, unequal refractive error in the 2 eyes. The eye with the greater refractive error (the more ametropic eye) is at risk for developing amblyopia. Accommodation provides clear vision through the eye with the lesser refractive error, and the more ametropic eye never has a clear image since accommodation is always equal binocularly.

In strabismus, the eye used habitually for fixation retains normal acuity and the nonpreferred eye becomes amblyopic. If spontaneous alternation of fixation is present, there is usually no amblyopia. Suppression and amblyopia are different processes. While amblyopia usually occurs in the presence of suppression, suppression may occur without amblyopia (eg, in strabismic patients with alternating fixation).

Anomalous Retinal Correspondence

In strabismus under binocular viewing conditions, the peripheral retinal areas outside the suppression scotoma may take on new direction values shifted in space by the amount of deviation. There is thus an anomalous correspondence of direction values between the retinal points in the 2 eyes. The direction values in the deviating eye are remapped just enough to avoid diplopia. Stereopsis is not possible under these conditions, and the new direction values may be labile, readjusting themselves from moment to moment as the exact deviation changes with direction of gaze. Should fixation shift to the opposite eye, the anomalous direction values also shift eyes. On monocular testing, the direction values are normal.

Eccentric Fixation

In eyes with sufficiently severe amblyopia, an extrafoveal retinal area may be used for fixation under monocular viewing conditions. It is only a sign of severe amblyopia and does not depend on anomalous retinal correspondence. The area used instead of the fovea may be the area of best remaining visual acuity. The eccentric fixation point is usually but not necessarily displaced in a direction appropriate to the direction of strabismus (eg, the nasal retina in esotropia). Gross eccentric fixation can be readily identified clinically by occluding the dominant eye and directing the patient's attention to a light source held directly in front. An eye with gross eccentric fixation will not point toward the light source but will appear to be looking in a different direction. More subtle degrees of eccentric fixation may be detected by an ophthalmoscope that projects a small fixation target onto the retina. The area of the retina used for fixation may then be directly observed.

EXAMINATION

History

A careful history is of great aid in the diagnosis, prognosis, and treatment of strabismus.

A. Family History: Strabismus is frequently present; autosomal dominant inheritance is common.

B. Age at Onset: This is the single most important factor in prognosis. The earlier the onset, the worse the prognosis for fusion.

C. Type of Onset: The onset may be gradual, sudden, intermittent, or associated with systemic disease.

D. Type of Deviation: Under what conditions does the patient notice strabismus? When viewing near objects? When tired? Is the amount of deviation constant? Does the patient shut one eye in the sunlight? It is most important to know if the eyes are straight at any time.

E. Fixation: Is it always the same eye that deviates? Is there alternating strabismus?

Visual Acuity

Visual acuity must be evaluated, even if only a rough approximation or comparison of the 2 eyes is possible. Each eye must be evaluated by itself, as binocular testing will not reveal poor vision in one eye. For the very youngest children, sometimes all that can be established is that the eye can fixate or follow a target. The target should be made as small as is compatible with the child's age, interest, and level of alertness. If occlusion of one eye produces resistance but occlusion of the other eye does not, poor vision may be present in the eye that can be occluded without provoking a response. A dot test, in which the child puts its finger on a dot of calibrated size, is the earliest quantitative test done routinely

(starting at 2–2½ years). At 2½–3 years, it is possible to perform recognition testing of small pictures (Allen card). At age 3, many children will play the "E" game: a conventional Snellen chart with "E's" pointing in various directions is used, and the child points a hand in the direction of the "E."

Visual acuity and other visual capabilities of infants can be determined by preferential looking methods, which rely on the infant's habit of looking at a patterned field in preference to a uniform field. (See also Chapters 2 and 18.) The baby is seated on its mother's lap facing a blank screen with porthole-sized apertures on either side in which are presented either (1) a stripe pattern of the desired width and the same average mean luminance as the surrounding screen, or (2) a uniform blank screen also of the same average mean luminance as the background. For each presentation trial, an independent observer—or the mother through a TV system—to whom the location of the pattern is not visible is asked to decide, by observing the baby's reactions, on which side the stripe presentation was made. The baby will look toward visible stripes and will gaze randomly around when the stripes are not visible. A rigorous psychophysical staircase statistical method is used to select the next stimulus and to determine when the observations unequivocally indicate that the child saw the stripes.

The disadvantages of this method are the number of trials required, the number of people required to run the test, the expense of the equipment, and the need for dependence on the cooperation of the baby.

Determination of Refractive Error

It is very important to determine the cycloplegic refractive error by retinoscopy (see Chapter 27). The standard of comparison for producing complete cycloplegia is atropine. This may be given as a drop or ointment, 0.5 or 1%, several times a day for several days to produce complete cycloplegia. It is much less desirable to use atropine in older children, since the prolonged cycloplegia, lasting up to 2 weeks, can interfere with schoolwork. At all ages, homatropine, 5%, or cyclopentolate, 1 or 2%, may also be used successfully.

Inspection

Inspection alone may show whether the strabismus is constant or intermittent, alternating or nonalternating, and variable or constant. Associated ptosis and abnormal position of the head may also be noted. The quality of fixation of each eye separately and both eyes together is important. Nystagmoid movements indicate poor fixation and reduced visual acuity.

Prominent epicanthal folds commonly confuse laymen as well as some physicians. The folds obscure a portion of the nasal sclera and may give the child the appearance of esotropia ("pseudoesotropia"). This pitfall can be avoided if the positions of the corneal reflections are noted. When the child is observing a light source, the corneal reflection of this light should be centered in the 2 pupillary areas. Prominent epicanthal folds usually disappear by 4 or 5 years of age.

Determination of Angle of Strabismus (Angle of Deviation)

A. Prism and Cover Tests: (Fig 13–6.) Cover tests consist of 3 parts: (1) the cover test, (2) the uncover test, and (3) the alternate cover test. In all 3 tests the patient looks intently at a target, which may be in any direction of gaze, distance or near.

1. Cover test–As the examiner observes one eye, a cover is placed in front of the other eye so as to block its view of the target. If the observed eye moves to take up fixation, it clearly is not also fixating the target, and manifest deviation (strabismus) is present. The direction of movement reveals the direction of deviation (eg, the eye moves laterally if there is esotropia).

2. Uncover test–As the cover is removed from the eye following the cover test, the eye emerging from under cover is observed. If the position of the eye changes, interruption of binocular vision has allowed it to deviate, and heterophoria is present. The directions of corrective movement shows the type of heterophoria.

3. Alternate cover test–The cover is alternately placed in front of one eye and then the other. This tends to break up the control of heterophoria that may last through a single cover-uncover cycle. This test shows the total deviation of heterotropia plus heterophoria.

4. Prism plus cover testing–To quantitatively measure the deviation, prisms are placed in front of one or both eyes so as to slightly reverse the direction of the refixation movements produced by the cover. For example, to measure the full esodeviation, the cover is alternated, and prisms of increasing base-out strength are placed in front of one or both eyes until the lateralward refixation movement of the deviated eye is reversed to a just observable movement in a medial direction. The threshold for naked eye observation of eye movements is generally considered to be about 2 prism diopters, so 2 prism diopters are then subtracted from the prism strength to obtain the final deviation. Prism measurements are done either as simultaneous prism and cover measurements, using the cover test, to determine the manifest deviation; or as prism and alternate cover measurements, to record the total deviation in the fusion-free position.

B. Maddox Rod Test: (Fig 13–7.) This test is an accurate method of measuring a deviation if normal retinal correspondence is present. It is particularly useful for measurement of heterophoria but can also be used in heterotropia. A Maddox rod consists of a series of thin red glass cylinders placed side by side,

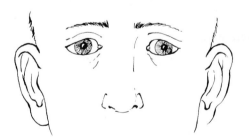

Eyes straight (maintained in position by fusion).

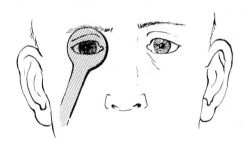

Position of eye under cover in orthophoria (fusion-free position). The right eye under cover has not moved.

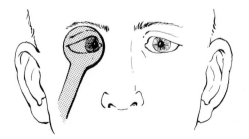

Position of eye under cover in esophoria (fusion-free position). Under cover, the right eye has deviated inward. Upon removal of cover, the right eye will immediately resume its straight-ahead position.

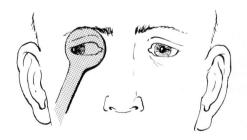

Position of eye under cover in exophoria (fusion-free position). Under cover, the right eye has deviated outward. Upon removal of the cover, the right eye will immediately resume its straight-ahead position.

Figure 13–6. Cover testing. The patient is directed to look at a target at eye level 6 m (20 ft) away. *Note:* In the presence of heterotropia, the deviation will remain when the cover is removed.

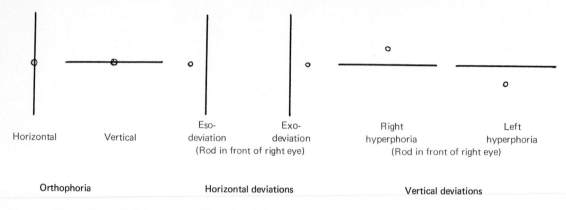

Horizontal	Vertical	Eso- deviation	Exo- deviation	Right hyperphoria	Left hyperphoria

Eso-deviation / Exo-deviation (Rod in front of right eye)

Right hyperphoria / Left hyperphoria (Rod in front of right eye)

Orthophoria   Horizontal deviations   Vertical deviations

Figure 13–7. Maddox rod test. Normal and abnormal responses. (Subjective view of the patient.)

usually mounted in a circular holder that can be held before the eye. When a target light is seen through the Maddox rod, its image is a red focal line perpendicular to the axes of the cylinders. Thus, one eye sees the light directly while the other views its image through the Maddox rod. In orthophoria the red line appears to run through the light. When the Maddox rod is held so that the cylinders are horizontal, a vertical red line is seen that in cases of horizontal deviation is displaced laterally. A prism can be held in front of one eye so that the red line appears to "run through the light." The strength of such a prism measures the angle of deviation. By rotating the Maddox rod 90 degrees, a horizontal line is produced (cylinders of the rod are vertical). Its displacement can also be measured by prisms as described for horizontal deviations.

C. Objective Tests: Prism and cover measurements are objective in the sense that no report of sensory observations is required from the patient. However, cooperation and some degree of vision are required. The Maddox rod test is more subjective because the end point of the measurement is based on a report of sensory observations by the patient. Confused, obtunded, or immature patients may be unable or unwilling to cooperate sufficiently. Clinical determinations of eye position that require no sensory observation by the patient (objective tests) are considerably less accurate, although still useful at times. Two methods commonly used depend on observing the position of the corneal reflection of a light. Results by both methods or any objective method must be modified by allowing for the angle kappa.

1. Hirschberg method–The patient fixes a light at a distance of about 33 cm (13 inches). The decentering of the light reflection is noted in the deviating eye. By allowing 15 diopters for each millimeter of decentration, an estimate of the angle of deviation can be made.

The ratio of accommodative convergence to accommodation (AC/A ratio) is a way of quantitating the relationship of convergence to accommodation. Accommodative convergence is convergence elicited by viewing an accommodative target, ie, one that has resolvable contours or letters that stimulate accommodation. The result is commonly expressed as prism diopters of convergence per diopter of accommodation. The AC/A ratio is useful as a research tool to further investigate and clarify this relationship and has contributed significantly to our understanding and therefore to the treatment of accommodative esotropia—particularly in prescribing bifocals, as described later in this chapter.

2. Prism reflex method (modified Krimsky test)–The patient fixes a light at any distance. A prism is placed before the fixing eye, and the strength of the prism required to center the corneal reflection of the deviating eye measures the angle of deviation.

Ductions (Monocular Rotations)

With one eye covered, the other eye follows a moving light in all directions of gaze, so that any weakness of rotation can be noted. Such a weakness can be due to muscle paralysis or to a mechanical anatomic anomaly.

Versions (Conjugate Ocular Movements)

According to Hering's law, yoke muscles receive equal stimulation during any conjugate ocular movement. The versions are tested by having the eyes follow a light at 33 cm in the 9 diagnostic positions: primary—straight ahead; secondary—right, left, up, and down; and tertiary—up and right, down and right, up and left, and down and left. Apparent rotation of one eye relative to the other is noted as overaction or underaction. By convention, in the tertiary positions, the oblique muscles are said to be overacting or underacting with respect to the yoke rectus muscle. Fixation in the field of action of a paretic muscle results in overaction of the yoke muscle, since greater innervation is required for contraction (Figs 13–8 and 13–9). Conversely, fixation by the normal eye will lead to underaction of the paretic muscle.

Disjunctive Movements

A. Convergence: (Fig 13–10.) As the eyes fol-

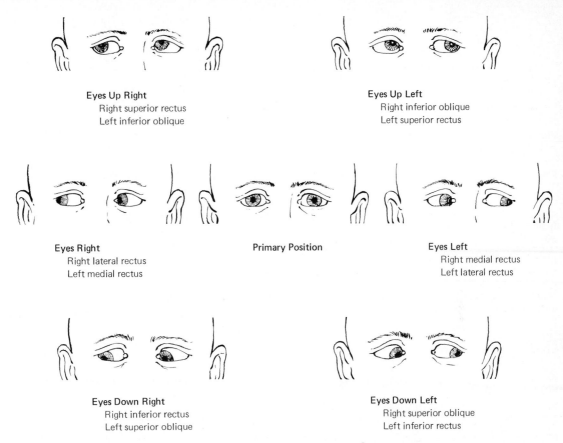

Figure 13–8. Normal version movement (binocular rotations). Pairs of yoke muscles concerned with ocular movement in various directions are shown.

low an approaching object, they must turn inward in order to maintain alignment of the visual axes with the object of regard. The medial rectus muscles are contracting and the lateral rectus muscles are relaxing under the influence of neural stimulation and inhibition. (Neural pathways of supranuclear control are discussed in Chapter 15.)

Convergence is an active process with a strong voluntary as well as involuntary component. An important consideration in evaluating the extraocular muscles in strabismus is convergence.

To test convergence, a small object or light source is slowly brought toward the bridge of the nose. The patient's attention is directed to the object by saying, "Keep the light from going double as long as possible." Convergence can normally be maintained until the object is nearly to the bridge of the nose. An actual numerical value is placed on convergence by measuring the distance from the bridge of the nose (in millimeters) at which the eyes "break" (ie, when the nondominant eye swings laterally so that convergence is no longer maintained). This point is termed the

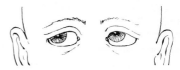

Eyes Up Right (Right Eye Fixing). Shows upshoot of left eye, indicating overaction of left inferior oblique. The fixating eye determines the innervation level to the yoke pair of right superior rectus and left inferior oblique. The left eye overacts because the paretic superior oblique does not load or resist the inferior oblique, which then rotates the left eye further than it ordinarily would.

Eyes Up Right (Left Eye Fixing). Shows relative underaction of right superior rectus. The fixating left eye determines the innervation level. Since the superior oblique is paretic, the inferior oblique rotates further at any innervation level than it otherwise would. Since the innervation level is less than normally required, the right superior rectus rotates less than normally. On duction testing, it will rotate fully.

Figure 13–9. Testing versions. Example of paretic left superior oblique.

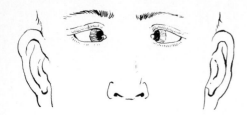

Figure 13-10. Convergence. The normal position of the eyes at the near point of convergence (NPC) is shown above. The break point is within 50 mm of the bridge of the nose.

near point of convergence, and a value of up to 50 mm (2 inches) is considered within normal limits.

B. Divergence: Electromyography has established that divergence is an active process, not merely a relaxation of convergence as previously believed by some authorities. Clinically, this function is seldom tested except in considering the amplitude of fusion (see below).

Sensory Examination

Many tests of the status of binocular vision have been devised, only a few of which can be mentioned here. The chief tests are for stereopsis, suppression, and anomalous retinal correspondence. They all require the simultaneous presentation of 2 targets separately to the 2 eyes.

A. Stereopsis Testing: Most stereopsis testing is done with polaroid glasses and targets to separate the stimuli. The monocularly observed targets have nearly imperceptible clues to depth. **Random dot stereograms** have no monocular depth clues. A field of random dots is seen by each eye, but the dot-to-corresponding-dot correlation between the 2 targets is such that if stereopsis is present, a form is seen standing out from the background.

B. Suppression Testing: The presence of suppression is readily demonstrated with the **Worth 4-dot test.** Glasses containing a red lens over one eye and a green lens over the other are placed on the patient. A flashlight containing red, green, and white spots is viewed. The color spots are markers for perception through each eye, and the white dot, potentially visible to each eye, can indicate the presence of diplopia. The separation of the spots and the distance at which the light is held determine the size of the retinal area tested. Foveal and peripheral areas may be tested at distance and near.

C. Anomalous Retinal Correspondence Testing: Anomalous retinal correspondence may be demonstrated in 2 ways: (1) by showing that one of the foveas does not have straight-ahead localization or (2) by showing that a peripheral retinal point in one eye shares a common visual direction with the fovea of the other eye.

1. After-image test–The first method is used in the after-image test and various projection methods.

A bright line with a centered fixation gap is used to produce a vertical after-image in one eye and a horizontal after-image in the other eye. The gaps superimpose in the after-images if the 2 foveas have the same visual direction.

2. Bagolini striated glass test–The Bagolini striated glass test uses the second testing method. Clear glasses containing fine striations in a different direction for each eye are placed in front of the eyes. The test conditions are as close as possible to natural vision. A point source of light is viewed, and streaks of light perpendicular to the direction of striation are seen with each eye. If peripheral retinal elements in the deviated eye localize the streak through the light, anomalous retinal correspondence is present.

OBJECTIVES & PRINCIPLES OF THERAPY OF STRABISMUS

The main objectives of strabismus treatment in children are (1) reversal of the deleterious sensory effects of strabismus (amblyopia, suppression, and loss of stereopsis) and (2) maintenance of improvement through medical or surgical straightening of the eyes. In adults with acquired strabismus, the aims are to alleviate diplopia and restore a range of binocular single vision.

Timing of Treatment in Children

A child can be productively examined at any age, and treatment for amblyopia or strabismus should be instituted as soon as the diagnosis is made. Neurophysiologic studies in animals have shown that the infant brain is very responsive to sensory experience, and the quality of function possible later in life is determined by the quality of early life experiences. It is generally believed that a better long-term result is obtained if the eyes are made as straight as possible by age 2 years. This is not a magic cutoff age by any means, and good results can be obtained later; however, improvements in brain function and modifications in synaptic connections become more difficult as time passes. By age 8 in most children, no permanent changes can be established. Treatment of amblyopia must be started as soon as possible; after age 8, efforts are usually futile.

Goals of Treatment

The 2 goals of eliminating suppression and restoring stereopsis are achieved by restoring alignment of the 2 eyes. Prisms can be useful in diagnosis or treatment (usually as a temporary measure) of deviation. Treatment of anomalous retinal correspondence by itself is not necessary. It disappears with improvement in eye position, and in cases with unimproved position, it is protective against diplopia.

Medical Treatment

Nonsurgical treatment of strabismus is achieved through treatment of amblyopia and the use of optical devices (prisms and glasses), pharmacologic agents, and various eye exercises.

A. Treatment of Amblyopia: The elimination of amblyopia is crucial in the treatment of strabismus and is always one of the first goals. Occasionally, strabismus will disappear entirely once amblyopia is cured. The deviation to be operated on can change considerably following treatment of amblyopia, and surgical results tend to be better.

1. Occlusion therapy–The mainstay of amblyopia treatment and the standard of comparison for all other treatments is occlusion therapy. In its simplest form, the sound eye is covered with a patch, and all seeing must be done with the amblyopic eye. Partial occlusions may also be created with plastic membranes, tape, blurring lenses, or alternate patching in various patterns. Sometimes an eye is blurred only for distance or only for near. All amblyopia treatment assumes that any refractive error has been determined with cycloplegic refraction and correction has been made, usually with spectacles if the refractive error is sufficient. Of particular importance is refractive asymmetry between the eyes. A very small refractive difference can produce amblyopia.

Two stages in amblyopia treatment can be distinguished: initial improvement and maintenance treatment.

a. Initial stage–Full-time occlusion is the standard initial treatment. Sometimes only partial occlusion is used at the beginning if the amblyopia does not seem to be too severe. As a rule of thumb, full-time occlusion may be done for as many weeks as the child's age in years without damaging the vision in the sound eye. If vision in the sound eye drops more than a line or so, a brief vacation from patching may be given or a less vigorous patching regimen selected. Occlusion treatment is continued in some form as long as vision continues to improve (sometimes for 2 or more years). Six months of full-time occlusion with no improvement at all is a treatment failure, and in such cases, it is usual to look again for any detectable organic lesion to explain the lack of response. Amblyopia is functional by definition (ie, there is no identifiable lesion). In most cases, if treatment is begun soon enough, substantial improvement or complete normalization of visual acuity can be achieved. Occasionally, there is no improvement and no reason can be found. Poor compliance with treatment (peeking around or through a patch by the child or inadequate enforcement of patching by the parents) must always be ruled out in these cases.

b. Maintenance stage–Maintenance treatment consists of intermittent patching continued after the improvement phase, with the goal of preserving improvement to beyond an age when amblyopia can be reacquired (about age 8 years). Whenever treatment is discontinued, there may be some loss of acuity. Later in life, acuity can be recovered to the best level achieved with occlusive treatment.

2. Other therapies–Other forms of amblyopia therapy mostly require periods of attentive vision, with variable patching regimens. With brief periods of intense visual effort, acuity can sometimes be improved with only minimal occlusion. Devices that have been employed are video games, rotating gratings (Cam stimulator), red filters, and games with small drawings. No method has been shown to be more effective than patching, and most are frequently less effective.

B. Optical Devices:

1. Spectacles–The most important optical device in the treatment of strabismus is accurate spectacles. The clarification of the retinal image produced by glasses allows the natural fusion mechanisms to operate to the fullest. Small refractive errors need not be corrected. If there is significant hyperopia and esotropia, the esotropia probably is at least partially due to the hyperopia (accommodative esotropia). The prescription should take into account the full cycloplegic findings. If a bifocal lens permits sufficient relaxation of the near synkinesis to allow fusion at near, it may also be prescribed.

2. Prisms–Prisms produce an optical redirection of the line of sight. Corresponding retinal elements are brought into line, and binocular diplopia is alleviated if the prism strength is correct. Correct sensory alignment of the eyes is also a form of antisuppression treatment. Used preoperatively, prisms can simulate the sensory effect of surgery and predict whether symptoms will be improved. In patients with horizontal deviation, prisms will show the patient's ability to fuse a simultaneous small vertical deviation, thereby indicating whether surgery also needs to be done for the vertical deviation. In children with esotropia, prisms can be used preoperatively to predict a post-operative shift in position that might nullify the surgical result, and the planned surgery can be modified accordingly (prism adaptation test).

Prisms can be implemented in several ways. A particularly convenient form is the plastic Fresnel press-on prism. These inexpensive plastic membranes can be placed on the glasses without the help of an optician and are very useful for diagnostic and temporary therapeutic purposes. For permanent wear, prisms are best ground into the spectacle prescription.

C. Pharmacologic Agents: The conventional pharmacologic agents used to treat strabismus are of 2 types: cycloplegic agents and miotics. A recently introduced pharmacologic substitute for surgical muscle-weakening procedures is the injection of botulinum toxin into the extraocular muscle.

1. Cycloplegic agents–Cycloplegic agents paralyze the ciliary muscle through a competitive inhibition of acetylcholine at the neuromuscular junction and thus prevent accommodation. They are most useful in the treatment of amblyopia, to allow clearer vision with the glasses on than is provided by peeking over the lenses. Another use is to provide blurred vision at near in the sound eye, so that all near vision must be performed with the amblyopic eye. The long-acting cycloplegic agent used for these purposes is atropine solution or ointment, usually 0.5 or 1% concentration. Weak short-acting cycloplegic agents have been used to stimulate accommodation in exotropia in an attempt to reduce the deviation.

2. Miotics–Miotics are used to reduce excess convergence at near in esotropia, referred to as a high accommodative convergence to accommodation ratio, or AC/A ratio. The agents usually used are echothiophate iodide (Phospholine Iodide) or isoflurophate (Floropryl), both of which irreversibly inactivate acetylcholinesterase at the neuromuscular junction and thus potentiate the effect of every nerve impulse. Accommodation should therefore be more effective with respect to convergence than before treatment. Since accommodation drives the near synkinesis (the triad of accommodation, convergence, and miosis), less convergence will be invoked with accommodation at near. Treatment with miotics is useful only if esodeviation is substantially reduced. Miotic treatment can be continued for years.

3. Botulinum toxin–The injection of botulinum A toxin into an extraocular muscle produces a dose-dependent depth and duration of paralysis of that muscle. The injection is given under electromyographic position control of the needle, and the toxin is tightly bound to the muscle tissue. The doses used are so small that systemic toxicity does not occur. Paralysis typically lasts for several months. The eye shifts into the field of action of the antagonist muscle and then starts to return to its original position as the injected muscle recovers its strength. During the time the eye is deviated, the tissues about the eye become adapted to the new position and apply a force opposing the returning muscle force. Frequently, multiple sequential injections must be given to obtain a lasting effect. The end result is a small net shift in position.

The method is useful for single-muscle weakening. If a muscle needs to be strengthened, the direction of action of a muscle shifted, adhesions lysed, or the strength of several muscles modified, surgery must be done instead. Botulinum toxin is useful in treating symptomatic heterophorias, shifting blind eyes (because it can be so readily repeated), or fine-tuning the results of surgery and whenever a small correction in position achieved by muscle weakening is needed to correct the deviation. Occasionally, botulinum toxin is used to correct larger deviations, but the results are not consistent. As with surgery, the best results are obtained in patients with good binocular function.

D. Eye Exercises: Various sensory exercises are sometimes used. These are best done by the patient at home. Exercises requiring fine vision can be used in treating amblyopia. Antisuppression exercises may also be done at home. These are most useful in intermittent exotropia to try to eliminate the facile suppression that prevents the patient from being aware that the eye has drifted out and correcting it voluntarily. The amplitudes of fusional vergence may be increased by exercising with prisms. Progressively larger prisms are place in front of one or both eyes and the separated images re-fused. Poor convergence can also be exercised. This can be combined with antisuppression treatment, ie, a card having large colored spots on each side is placed in the midline sagittal plane in front of the nose. The task is to see the dots singly while being aware of the color rivalry. So-called pencil push-ups, in which an approaching rod is kept single, can also be of some help. It is important that accommodation be controlled during convergence exercises.

Exercises for intermittent exotropia are rarely curative—only delaying—and patients who have been taught to inappropriately converge their eyes have a much higher incidence of postoperative overcorrection when they finally do come to surgery. Finally, the richness and variety of naturally occurring stimuli provide a rather complete repertoire of tasks for the visual system. The most effective exercises are those that can be performed naturally during daily oculomotor behavior or done at home. Exercise sessions in the physician's office are costly and rarely have any lasting effect.

Surgical Treatment
(Figs 13–11 and 13–12)

A. Surgical Procedures: A variety of changes in the rotational effect of an extraocular muscle can be achieved with surgery.

1. Resection and recession–Conceptually, the simplest procedures are strengthening and weakening. A muscle is strengthened by a procedure called resection. The muscle is detached from the eye, stretched out longer by a measured amount, and then resewn to the eye, usually at the original insertion site. The small amount of extra length is trimmed off. Recession is the standard weakening procedure. The muscle is detached from the eye, freed from fascial attachments, and allowed to retract. It is resewn to the eye a measured distance behind its original insertion.

The superior oblique is strengthened by tucking its tendon. This can be done by a graded amount. Superior oblique weakening is limited to the all-or-none procedure of cutting through its tendon (tenotomy). Attempts at measured recessions of the superior oblique tendon have been made. There is no effective strengthening procedure on the inferior oblique. The inferior oblique can be weakened by recession, myectomy, or disinsertion, with generally equivalent results.

2. Shifting of point of muscle attachment–In addition to simple strengthening or weakening, the point of attachment of the muscle can be shifted; this may give the muscle a rotational action it did not have before. For example, a vertical shift of both horizontal rectus muscles affects the vertical position of the eye. Shifts of the horizontal recti in opposite vertical directions affect the horizontal position in upgaze and downgaze. This is done for "A" or "V" patterns, in which the horizontal deviation is more of an esodeviation in upgaze or downgaze, respectively. The torsional effect of a muscle can also be changed. Tightening of the anterior fibers of the superior oblique tendon gives that muscle enhanced torsional action.

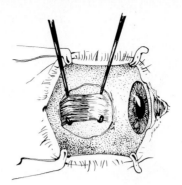

Exposure of lateral rectus

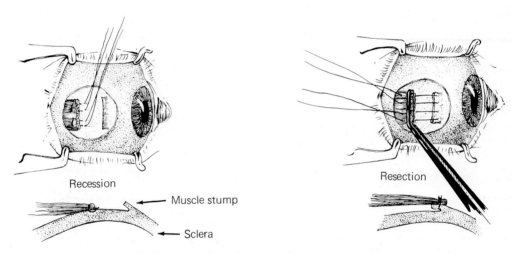

Recession

Resection

Muscle stump

Sclera

Figure 13–11. Surgical correction of strabismus (right eye).

3. Faden procedure–A special procedure for muscle weakening is called the Faden procedure (Fig 13–12) after the German word for "thread." In this operation, a new insertion for the muscle is created far in the back of the eye by suturing the muscle to the sclera, so that it cannot unwrap as the eye rotates into its field of action. This weakens the muscle only in its field of action and not in primary position. When combined with a muscle recession operation, the Faden operation can have a profound weakening effect on a muscle. This procedure is used in dissociated vertical divergence, nystagmus, high AC/A ratio, and miscellaneous other disorders.

B. Choice of Muscles to Be Corrected: Deciding which muscles to correct and how much correction to make is a technical decision based on measurements of the deviation in various directions of gaze. The usual positions measured are distance and near in primary position, secondary gaze directions at distance, and tertiary gaze directions at near, as well as lateral gaze to either side at near. Frequently, the near deviation is also measured with the patient looking down while wearing bifocals. In choosing which muscles to correct, both the primary and secondary actions of the muscles must be taken into account. Lateral or vertical incomitances must be planned for. To avoid a deviation in gaze away from primary position, the gaze effort required by the 2 eyes must be matched. For this, the strength of the 2 muscles in a yoke pair is balanced. With regard to near or distance positions, the medial recti have more effect at near and the lateral recti more effect at distance. For esotropia greater at near, both medial rectus muscles would be weakened. For exotropia greater at distance, both lateral recti would be weakened. For deviation the same at distance and near, both the medial and lateral recti of one eye may be corrected. Both eyes may be corrected if the deviation is large or if there is lateral incomitance requiring treatment of a pair of yoke muscles.

The same operation performed on 2 different people will give somewhat different results because of the varying mechanical properties of the muscles and surrounding soft tissues. Prior to operation, it is not known exactly how much of a deviation is due to abnormal muscle force and how much to abnormal surrounding tissues, such as adhesions or fibrous bands, or to abnormal points of muscle insertion. Consequently, several operations are frequently required to obtain a satisfactory position.

C. Adjustable Sutures: (Fig 13–13.) The de-

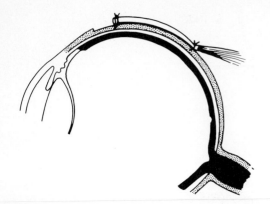

Figure 13–12. Faden procedure. The rectus muscle is tacked to the sclera far posterior to its insertion. This prevents unwrapping of the muscle as the eye turns into the muscle's field of action. The muscle is progressively weakened in its field of action. If this procedure is combined with recession, the alignment in primary position is also affected.

velopment of adjustable sutures has been a great boon in muscle surgery and the greatest advance in the field in the past decade. During operation, the muscles are reattached with a bow knot placed so that it is accessible to the surgeon. The next day, a topical anesthetic drop is placed in the eye, and the sutures can be tightened or loosened to change the eye position as necessary, under the guidance of prism and cover measurements.

The operation can be done effectively a second time, as long as approximately the correct procedure was done the first time. Adjustable sutures can be used on any rectus muscle for either recession or resection and on the superior oblique muscle for correction of torsion. Any patient willing to cooperate is suitable. With care in selection, even 5-year-old children can undergo suture adjustment without any special anesthetic measures, although the method is commonly not used for children age 12 or under.

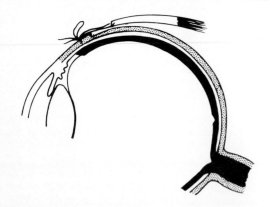

Figure 13–13. Adjustable suture. The suture is placed on the sclera at any point that will be accessible to the surgeon the next day. The bow is untied and the position of the muscle changed as desired.

CLASSIFICATION OF STRABISMUS

Classification of strabismus is based on the forms that are found to occur most commonly in practice.

A. Esotropia
  1. Nonparetic
     a. Nonaccommodative
     b. Accommodative
     c. Partially accommodative
  2. Paretic
B. Exotropia
  1. Intermittent
  2. Constant
C. "A" and "V" syndromes
D. Hypertropia
  1. Nonparetic
  2. Paretic

ESOTROPIA (Convergent Strabismus, "Crossed Eyes")

Esotropia is the most common type of strabismus. Most cases acquired in adulthood are paretic, caused by lateral rectus weakness following injury to the sixth cranial nerve. Esotropia in childhood is usually, but not always, nonparetic. The most common forms of childhood esotropia are infantile esotropia, accommodative esotropia, and partially accommodative esotropia.

I. NONPARETIC ESOTROPIA

NONACCOMMODATIVE ESOTROPIA

1. INFANTILE ESOTROPIA

The most common form of nonparetic, nonaccommodative esotropia is infantile esotropia. By convention, the onset must be before 6 months of age to qualify under the definition. The cause is not established.

Clinical Findings
The deviation is usually large ($\geq$ 50 degrees) and usually comitant. Abduction may be somewhat limited but can be demonstrated. Vertical deviations are frequently observed (commonly, dissociated vertical divergence; sometimes, overaction of the inferior oblique muscle). Either of these deviations may produce an upshoot in adduction. Nystagmus, manifest or latent, is frequently present. The commonest refractive error is low-to-moderate hyperopia (< 3 di-

opters). Amblyopia may occur, especially if there is anisometropia.

The eye that appears to be straight is the eye used for fixation. Almost without exception, it is the eye with better vision or lower refractive error, or both. If there is anisometropia, there will probably be some amblyopia as well. If at various times either eye is used for fixation, the patient is said to show spontaneous alternation of fixation; in this case, vision will be nearly equal in both eyes. Sometimes, the eye preference is determined by the direction of gaze. For example, with large-angle esotropia, there is a tendency for the right eye to be used in left gaze and the left eye to be used in right gaze (cross fixation).

Treatment

Congenital esotropia almost invariably requires surgical correction. Nonsurgical treatment is aimed at correcting refractive errors and treating amblyopia. It is essential that amblyopia be fully treated prior to surgery. Hyperopic refractive errors greater than 2 diopters are worth treating. A miotic agent can substitute for a trial of glasses in an uncooperative infant.

Surgery is indicated after medical therapy and treatment of amblyopia have been tried and there remains a significant deviation. Examination must be performed, and reproducible measurements of deviation must be obtained. There is nothing to be gained by waiting beyond this point, and there is evidence that sensory results are better the sooner surgery is undertaken. Many procedures have been recommended, but the 2 most popular procedures are (1) weakening of both medial rectus muscles and (2) recession of the medial rectus and resection of the lateral rectus on the same eye.

2. ACQUIRED NONACCOMMODATIVE ESOTROPIA

Several types of strabismus are included under this heading, with onset after the age of 6 months.

Basic Esotropia

The onset is in childhood, but there is no accommodative factor. The angle of strabismus is originally much smaller than in congenital esotropia but may increase with time. Treatment is correction of any refractive error and treatment of amblyopia, followed by surgical correction.

Esotropia of Myopia

This typically begins in young adults as diplopia at distance gradually extending to near. It must be distinguished from divergence insufficency or lateral rectus paresis associated with elevated intracranial pressure. A severe form of esotropia may also be associated with high myopia, in which the medial recti become extremely tight. Prisms for distance vision may help the former type of esotropia for a time. Surgery is otherwise indicated in both conditions.

ACCOMMODATIVE ESOTROPIA

Accommodative esotropia occurs when there is a normal physiologic mechanism of accommodation but insufficient relative fusional divergence to hold the eyes straight. There are 2 pathophysiologic mechanisms at work: (1) sufficiently high hyperopia requiring so much accommodation to clarify the image that esotropia results and (2) a high AC/A ratio, which may be accompanied by refractive error. The 2 mechanisms may be present in the same patient.

Accommodative Esotropia Due to Hyperopia

Accommodative esotropia due to hyperopia typically begins at age 2–3 but may occur in infancy or later in life. Deviation is variable prior to treatment. Treatment is full cycloplegic refraction.

Accommodative Esotropia Due to High AC/A Ratio

In accommodative esotropia due to a high AC/A ratio, a deviation is greater at near than at distance. The refractive error is hyperopic. Treatment is full cycloplegic refraction, amblyopia therapy, and bifocals or miotics, or both, to relieve excess deviation at near.

PARTIALLY ACCOMMODATIVE ESOTROPIA

An accommodative element frequently occurs superimposed into infantile or basic esotropia. Antiaccommodative therapy is of partial benefit. Surgery is reserved for the nonaccommodative component of the deviation that remains after antiaccommodative therapy and treatment for amblyopia.

II. PARETIC (INCOMITANT) ESOTROPIA (Abducens Palsy) (Fig 13–14)

In incomitant strabismus there are always one or more paretic extraocular muscles. In the case of incomitant esotropia, the paresis is always one of the lateral rectus muscles, usually as a result of palsy of the abducens nerve. These bases are most often seen in adults who have had cerebrovascular accidents or diabetes, but abducens palsy may occasionally be the first sign of a tumor or of inflammatory disease involving the central nervous system. Head trauma is a frequent cause of abducens palsy.

Incomitant esotropia is also seen in infants and children, but much less commonly than comitant esotro-

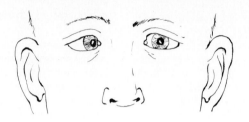

Primary position: right esotropia

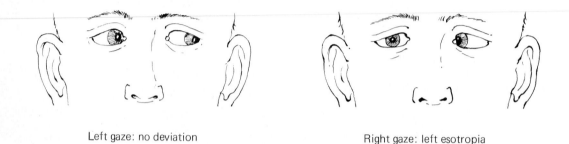

Left gaze: no deviation   Right gaze: left esotropia

Figure 13–14. Incomitant strabismus (paralytic). Paralysis of right lateral rectus muscle, with left eye fixing.

pia. These cases result from birth injuries affecting the muscle directly, from injury to the nerve, or, less commonly, from a congenital anomaly of the lateral rectus muscle or its fascial attachments.

Clinical Findings

If the lateral rectus muscle is totally paralyzed, the eye will not abduct past the midline. Esotropia is characteristically greater at distance than at near and greater to one side. Paresis of the right lateral rectus causes esotropia that becomes greater to the right and, if paresis is sufficiently mild, no deviation in far left gaze.

Treatment

A prism may be helpful in milder cases. Any spontaneous improvement should be allowed to develop as far as possible. If there is no improvement by 6 months, it is unlikely that any will occur, and surgery is indicated. Botulinum toxin injections may be helpful or curative in mild cases. More severe cases require surgery in proportion to the amount of deviation. Resection of the paretic muscle along with recession of some or all of the remaining horizontal recti (depending on the measurements) is required. For complete paralysis, the insertions of the superior and inferior rectus muscles may be transferred to the lateral rectus and the other horizontal recti may be recessed. Adjustable sutures allow the titration of surgery to each of the muscles, so that frequently, single vision may be obtained in many fields of gaze. Abduction of the paretic muscle will always be limited. Completely successful results are possible only with mild paresis.

EXOTROPIA
(Divergent Strabismus)

Exotropia is less common than esotropia, particularly in infancy and childhood. Its incidence increases gradually with age. Not infrequently, a tendency to divergent strabismus beginning as exophoria progresses to intermittent exotropia and finally to constant exotropia if no treatment is given. Other cases begin as constant or intermittent exotropia and remain stationary. As in esotropia, there may be a hereditary element in some cases. Exophoria and exotropia (considered as a single entity of divergent deviation) are frequently passed on as autosomal dominant traits, so that one or both parents of an exotropic child may demonstrate exotropia or a high degree of exophoria.

Alternative Classification of Exotropia

Constant or intermittent exotropia can also be classified on a descriptive basis, according to whether there is apparent excess of divergence or insufficiency of convergence. These terms should not be understood to imply the cause.

A. Basic Exotropia: Distance and near deviations are approximately equal.

B. Divergence Excess: Distance deviation is significantly larger than near deviation.

C. Convergence Insufficiency: Near deviation is significantly larger than distance deviation.

D. Pseudodivergence Excess: Distance devi-

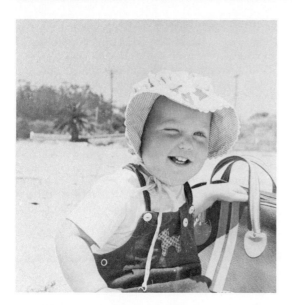

Figure 13–15. Child with intermittent exotropia squinting in sunlight.

ation is significantly larger than near deviation: however, use of a 3-diopter lens for near measurement will cause the near deviation to become approximately equal to the distance deviation.

INTERMITTENT EXOTROPIA

Clinical Findings

Intermittent exotropia (Fig 13–15) comprises well over half of cases of exotropia. The onset of the deviation may be in the first year, and practically all have shown up by age 5. The history reveals that the condition has become progressively worse. A characteristic sign is closing one eye in bright sunlight, as this avoids diplopia. There is usually a manifest exotropia for distance. The patient can fuse for near visions, overcoming moderate- to large-angle exophoria. Convergence is frequently excellent. There is no correlation with a specific refractive error.

Since the child fuses at least part of the time, there is usually no gross sensory abnormality. For distance, with one eye deviated, there is suppression but normal retinal correspondence and no amblyopia.

Treatment

A. Medical Treatment: Nonsurgical treatment is largely confined to refractive correction and amblyopia therapy. If the AC/A ratio is high, the use of minus lenses may delay surgery for a while. Occasionally, antisuppression or convergence exercises may be of some, albeit usually temporary, benefit.

B. Surgical Treatment: Surgery should be considered in adult patients with sufficiently severe symptoms or in children with signs of progression of the deviation (eg, increasing frequency of exotropia (implying loss of fusional control), larger deviation, de-

velopment of convergence insufficiency or lateral incomitance, or development of suppression [lack of diplopia during the manifest phase of deviation]). The goal of surgery is restoration of normal binocular function.

The choice of procedure depends on the measurements of the deviation. The 2 lateral rectus muscles alone may be corrected in cases in which deviation is mostly at distance. If there is much deviation at near, it is best to perform resection of a medial rectus as well as weakening of a lateral rectus. Both eyes may need to be corrected for larger deviations. Because all exodeviations tend to recur, it is best to produce slight overcorrection at the time of surgery. The use of botulinum toxin injections may help to prevent recurrences.

CONSTANT EXOTROPIA
(Fig 13–16)

Constant exotropia is less common than intermittent exotropia. It may be present at birth or may occur when intermittent exotropia progresses to constant exotropia. Some cases have their onset later in life, particularly following loss of vision in one eye. Except for cases due to loss of vision, the fundamental cause is usually not known.

Clinical Findings

Constant exotropia may be of any degree. With chronicity or poor vision in one eye, the deviation can be quite large. Adduction may be limited; hypertropia may occur along with exotropia; and stereopsis is lost. There is usually extensive suppression if the deviation was acquired by age 6–8; otherwise, diplopia is present. If exotropia is due to very poor vision, there may be no diplopia, although poor vision per se is not protective against diplopia. Anomalous retinal correspondence is unusual in the presence of extensive suppression. Amblyopia is uncommon in the absence of anisometropia, and spontaneous alternation of the fixating eye is frequently observed.

Treatment

The best treatment is surgery. Overcorrection is attempted because exotropia frequently recurs. The prognosis for maintenance of the improved position is particularly poor if one eye is blind. Botulinum toxin injections can be useful as primary treatment if the deviation is small or as a backup to surgery if exotropia begins to recur.

"A" & "V" SYNDROMES

A horizontal deviation may be vertically incomitant, ie, the deviation is different in upgaze versus primary position versus downgaze ("A" or "V" pat-

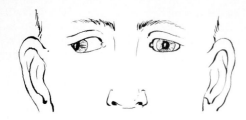

Figure 13–16. Right exotropia.

tern). An "A" pattern shows more esodeviation or less exodeviation in upgaze compared to downgaze. A "V" pattern shows less esodeviation or more exodeviation in upgaze compared to downgaze. An "A" pattern is diagnostically significant when greater than 10 Δ and a "V" pattern when greater than 15 Δ. Whether the pattern is clinically significant must be determined from the other findings. When the patient comes to surgery, the procedure is frequently modified to allow for "A" or "V" patterns.

HYPERTROPIA
(Fig 13–17)

Vertical deviations are customarily named according to the high eye, regardless of which eye has the better vision and is used for fixation. Hypertropias are less common than horizontal deviations and are usually acquired after childhood.

There are many causes of hypertropia. Congenital anatomic anomalies may result in muscle attachments in abnormal locations. Occasionally, there are anomalous fibrous bands that attach to the eye. Closed head trauma frequently produces paresis of the superior oblique muscle. Orbital tumors, brain stem lesions, and systemic diseases such as myasthenia gravis, multiple sclerosis, and Graves' disease can all produce hypertropias. Many of these specific entities are discussed in Chapter 15, Neuro-ophthalmology.

Clinical Findings

The clinical findings may vary, depending on the cause. The history is particularly important in diagnosis of hypertropias. Prism and cover measurements are the mainstay of clinical evaluation and may be diagnostic. Observation of ocular rotations for limitations can also be of great value.

Prism and cover measurements must be made in primary position at distance and near, at distance in secondary position, at near in tertiary position, and to the right, left, and down in reading position.

Diplopia is almost invariably present if strabismus develops past age 6–8. As in other forms of strabismus, sensory adaptation occurs if the onset is before this age range. Suppression and anomalous retinal correspondence may be present in gaze directions where there is strabismus. In gaze directions without strabismus, there may be no suppression and normal stereopsis.

There may be head tilt, turn, or abnormal posture of the head. The deviation may be of any magnitude and usually changes with the direction of gaze. Most hypertropias are incomitant. The deviation tends to be greatest in the field of action of one of the 4 vertically acting muscles. There may be associated **cyclotropia,** especially with oblique dysfunction. To measure cyclotropia, a Maddox rod in a trial frame may be rotated in front of each eye in turn, until the observed line is parallel to the subjective horizontal with the head erect. The angle of tilt is then read from the angular scale on the trial frame.

The superior oblique is the most commonly paretic vertical muscle. The vertical rectus muscles are commonly involved in trauma, as with entrapment of the inferior rectus in an orbital floor fracture, and in thyroid eye disease, in which the inferior rectus becomes hypertrophied, inelastic, and fibrotic and pulls the eye downward.

Paresis of the superior oblique may present in several patterns. It is not understood why different patients show different patterns. The simplest pattern is maximum deviation in the field of action of the muscle (ie, the lower field of gaze to the contralateral side). Another pattern is maximum deviation in the field of action of the ipsilateral antagonist, the inferior oblique. Deviation is then maximum in the upper field of gaze to the contralateral side. Deviation in the lower field need not be entirely lateralized and may have spread across to the other side as well. Deviation may also be to one side only without being much greater up or down, or it may be up and down the side and across the bottom as well. Most cases show some degree of excyclotorsion.

The Bielschowsky head tilt test (Fig 13–18) is useful to confirm the diagnosis of superior oblique paresis. The test exploits the differing effects of each vertical muscle on torsion and elevation. Thus, with a paretic right superior oblique when the head is tilted to the right, both muscles that attach to the top of the eye contract to intort the eye and maintain the position of the retinal vertical meridian as much as possible. The superior rectus elevates the eye, and the superior oblique depresses the eye. Because of weakness of the superior oblique muscle, the vertical forces do not cancel out as they normally would, and right hyper-

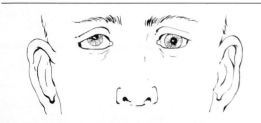

Figure 13–17. Right hypertropia.

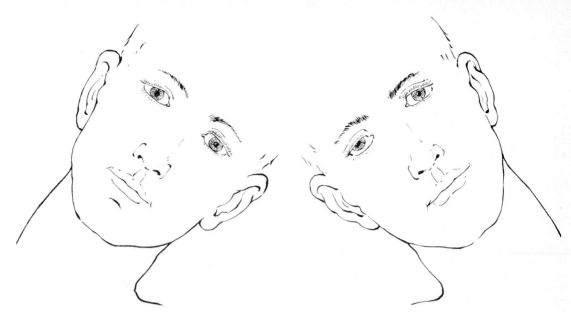

Figure 13–18. Head tilt test (Bielschowsky test). Paresis of right superior oblique. ***Left:*** Hypertropia is minimized on tilting the head to the sound side. The right eye may then extort and the intorting superior oblique and superior rectus relax. ***Right:*** When the head is tilted to the paretic side, the intorting muscles contract together, but their vertical actions do not cancel out as usual, because of superior oblique paresis. Hypertropia is worse with head tilt to the paretic side.

tropia becomes worse. In head tilt to the left, the intorting muscles for the right eye relax and the inferior oblique and inferior rectus both contract to extort the eye. Both the paretic superior oblique and superior rectus relax, and hypertropia is minimized. Hypertropia should be quantified with prism and cover measurements with the head tilted to either side.

Treatment

A. Medical Treatment: For smaller and less incomitant deviations, a prism may be all that is required. As with any form of strabismus, one eye may be occluded if the patient can function adequately without binocular vision. Many patients find occlusion of an eye with good vision to be unpleasant, if not intolerable. If there is systemic disease, it must be fully treated. Botulinum toxin injections may be of help in some cases, if muscle strengthening is not required.

B. Surgical Treatment: Surgery is the remaining possibility for cases that have not improved with the preceding methods (see p 218). The choice of procedure depends on the cause and the quantitative measurements. The use of adjustable sutures (Fig 13–13) is nearly indispensable in vertical muscle surgery, because the precision of the required result is greater than in horizontal rectus surgery.

DUANE'S RETRACTION SYNDROME

Duane's retraction syndrome is typically characterized by marked limitation of abduction, mild limitation of adduction, retraction of the globe and narrowing of the palpebral fissure on attempted adduc-

tion, and, frequently, upshoot or downshoot of the eye in adduction. Usually, only the left eye is affected. Most cases are sporadic, although some families with dominant inheritance have been described. A variety of other anomalies may be associated, such as dysplasia of the iris stroma, heterochromia, cataract, choroidal coloboma, microphthalmos, Goldenhar's syndrome, Klippel-Feil syndrome, cleft palate, and anomalies of the face, ear, or extremities. The causes of the motility defects are varied, and some anomalies of the muscles have been found. Most cases can be explained by an inappropriate innervation pattern to the lateral rectus and sometimes other muscles as well. Sherrington's law of reciprocal innervation is not obeyed, because nerve fibers to the medial rectus also go to the lateral rectus. Cases with proved absence of the abducens nucleus and nerve have been found.

Treatment

Treatment for the abnormal motility pattern is surgical. Traditionally, for a typical case, only recession of the medial rectus on the affected side has been done if esotropia is present in primary position. Care must be taken to preserve good binocular function if it exists. For more complicated cases, the technique must be adjusted for each individual.

SPECIAL FORMS OF VERTICAL STRABISMUS

1. DISSOCIATED VERTICAL DIVERGENCE

Dissociated vertical divergence is frequently associated with congenital and rarely with otherwise normal muscle balance. The exact cause is not known, although it can be said to be supranuclear.

Clinical Findings

Each eye drifts upward under cover, frequently with extorsion and small exotropic shift, and then returns close to its resting binocular position when the cover is removed. Sometimes the eye rests in a hypotropic position and comes up to assume fixation when the other eye is covered. Most cases are bilateral, although asymmetry of involvement is usual. There are usually no symptoms in children, but later in life there are occasionally strange, indescribable, sometimes annoying sensations produced when one eye is dissociated upward. Rarely, there is diplopia.

Treatment

Treatment is indicated if the problem is symptomatic or disfiguring. Nonsurgical treatment is limited to refractive correction to maximize the potential of motor fusion and therapy for amblyopia. Surgical results have traditionally been variable and somewhat disappointing. Currently, the most popular and successful procedures are very large recession of the superior rectus or recession of the superior rectus combined with the Faden procedure (see p 219).

2. BROWN'S SUPERIOR OBLIQUE TENDON SHEATH SYNDROME

Brown's syndrome is due to fibrous adhesions in the superonasal quadrant of the eye, which mechanically limit elevation of the eye when in an adducted position. Differential diagnosis is concerned mainly with paresis of the inferior oblique muscle. When inferior oblique paresis is present, a forced duction test will show free rotation of the eye into elevation in adduction; this will not be seen with Brown's syndrome. There is hypertropia of the other eye on gaze to the uninvolved side, which increases on upgaze and may extend to primary position. The condition may be idiopathic or may be due to trauma or systemic inflammatory disorders.

After appropriate therapy for any systemic illness, the only remaining treatment is surgery. The general strategy is to free the mechanical adhesion. Restoration of full mobility is seldom achieved.

HETEROPHORIA

Heterophoria is deviation of the eyes that is held in check by binocular vision. Almost all individuals have some degree of heterophoria, and small amounts are considered normal. Larger amounts may or may not cause symptoms, depending on the level of effort required by the individual to control latent muscle imbalance.

Clinical Findings

The symptoms of heterophoria may be clear-cut (intermittent diplopia) or vague ("eyestrain" or asthenopia). Diplopia may come on only with fatigue or with poor lighting conditions, as in night driving. Usage requirements for the eyes and personality type are additional variable factors. Thus, there is no degree of heterophoria that is clearly abnormal, although larger amounts are more likely to be symptomatic. Except for hyperopia, high AC/A ratios, and mild cases of muscle paresis not resulting in frank heterotropia, the fundamental causes of heterophorias are unknown.

Asthenopia is sometimes caused by uncorrected refractive errors as well as by muscle imbalance. One possible mechanism is aniseikonia, in which an image seen by one eye is a different size and shape from that seen by the other eye. Because it is difficult to prove that aniseikonia is a cause and because of the variability of patient responses in treating symptomatic disease, the diagnosis of aniseikonia has been made infrequently in recent years. Spectacles with unequal lens power in the 2 eyes can cause asthenopia by creating prismatic displacement of the image in one eye for gaze away from the optic axis that is too large to control (induced prism). Another mechanism that may produce symptoms is a change in space perception due to the curvature of the lenses or astigmatic corrections.

The symptoms encountered in asthenopia take a wide variety of forms. There may be a feeling of heaviness, tiredness, or discomfort of the eyes, varying from a dull ache to deep pain located in or behind the eyes. Headaches of all types occur. Easy fatigability, blurring of vision, and diplopia, especially after prolonged use of the eyes, also occur. Symptoms are more common for near visual work than for distance. Frequently, an aversion to reading develops. Symptoms can be brought on by fatigue or illness or following the ingestion of medications or alcohol.

Diagnosis

The diagnosis of heterophoria is based on prism and cover measurements. Heterophoria or intermittent heterotropia must be present before a diagnosis of asthenopia can be justified. The relative fusional vergence amplitudes should be measured. While the patient views an accommodative target (ie, a target that calls for a performance that tests visual acuity and thus controls the level of accommodation) at distance or reading position, prisms of increasing strength are placed in front of one eye to displace the image. The fusional vergence amplitude is then the amount of prism the patient is able to overcome and still maintain single vision. This measurement is done both at distance and at near with base-out and base-in prisms. The prisms may also be placed vertically to measure positive vertical vergence with the right eye directed upward and negative vergence with the left eye directed upward. Absolute fusional vergence amplitudes measured on a light are more indicative of the maximum effort that can be put forth than what happens under normal physiologic conditions. The important feature is the size of the amplitudes in comparison to the angle of heterophoria. While one cannot give exact norms for normal relative fusional vergences, guidelines for typical normal findings are as follows: at distance, convergence is 14 Δ, divergence is 6 Δ, and vertical is 3 Δ; at near, convergence is 25 Δ, divergence is 15 Δ, and vertical is 3 Δ.

Treatment

Heterophoria requires treatment only if symptomatic. Untreated heterophoria or asthenopia does not cause any permanent damage to the eyes. Treatment methods are all aimed at reducing the effort required to achieve fusion or at changing muscle mechanics so that the muscle imbalance itself is reduced.

A. Medical Treatment:

1. Accurate refractive correction–Occasionally, poor visual acuity is found in the presence of symptomatic heterophoria. Spectacles providing clear vision are sometimes all that is needed to alleviate symptoms. The clearer image allows the patient's fusional capacity to function to its fullest.

2. Manipulation of accommodation–The general principle is that esophorias are treated with antiaccommodative therapy and exophorias by stimulating accommodation. Plus lenses for near work will reduce the accommodative load and the accompanying convergence. A high AC/A ratio may be treated with plus lenses or miotics.

In exophoria, minus lenses may be used to stimulate accommodation. This works only in young children; otherwise, presbyopia may be produced. A weak cycloplegic drop applied in the morning may also stimulate accommodation. This produces other undesirable symptoms in adults but may be helpful in children.

3. Prisms–The use of prisms requires the wearing of glasses; for some patients, this is unacceptable. A trial of plastic Fresnel press-on prisms should be made before expensive ground-in prisms are ordered. For optical reasons, larger amounts of prismatic correction produce distortions of the geometry of space. Furthermore, very thick lenses can result. The usual practice is to prescribe about one-third to one-half of the measured deviation. This should lessen the work load on the visual system while keeping the fusional amplitudes built up, minimizing the tendency for frank diplopia due to reduced fusional amplitudes when the glasses are not being worn. Prisms are useful for esophoria, exophoria, and vertical phorias, as well.

4. Botulinum toxin injection–(See above.) This treatment is well suited to producing small shifts in ocular alignment. It may be used as a substitute for small to moderate amounts of surgical weakening of one muscle. One disadvantage is that results may not be known for many months. In time, this method may prove to be quite useful in treating heterophorias.

B. Surgical Treatment: Surgery should be the last resort after medical methods have been tried. As in strabismus, muscles are chosen for correction according to the measured deviation at distance and near in various directions of gaze. Sometimes, only one muscle needs to be corrected, although a new incomitant deviation may then be created. Adjustable sutures are very helpful (Fig 13–13).

REFERENCES

Cross HE, Pfaffenbach DD: Duane's retraction syndrome and associated congenital malformations. *Am J Ophthalmol* 1972;**73**:442.

Duke-Elder S, Wybar K: *Ocular Motility and Strabismus.* Vol 6 of: *System of Ophthalmology.* Duke-Elder S (editor). Mosby, 1973.

Eggers HM: Functional anatomy of the extraocular muscles. Chapter 31 in: *Biomedical Foundations of Ophthalmology.* Duane TD (editor). Harper & Row, 1982.

Foster RS, Paul TO, Jampolsky A: Management of infantile esotropia, *Am J Ophthalmol* 1976;**82**:291.

Helveston EM: *Atlas of Strabismus Surgery,* 3rd ed. Mosby, 1984.

Huber A: Electrophysiology of the retraction syndrome. *Br J Ophthalmol* 1974;**58**:293.

Ing MR: Early surgical alignment for congenital esotropia. *Trans Am Ophthalmol Soc* 1981;**79**:625.

Ingram RM: Refraction as a basis for screening children for squint and amblyopia. *Br J Ophthalmol* 1977;**61**:8.

Knapp P: Diagnosis and surgical treatment of hypertropia. *Am Orthopt J* 1971;**21**:29.

Lennerstrand G, Bach-y-Rita P (editors): *Basic Mechanisms of Ocular Motility and Their Clinical Implications.* Pergamon, 1975.

New Orleans Academy of Ophthalmology: *Symposium on Strabismus.* Mosby, 1971, 1978.

Parks MM: The monofixation syndrome. *Trans Am Ophthalmol Soc* 1969;**67**:609.

Robinson DA: A quantitative analysis of extraocular muscle cooperation and squint. *Invest Ophthalmol* 1975; **14:** 801.

Romano PE, Robinson JA: General anesthesia morbidity and mortality in eye surgery at a children's hospital. *J Pediatr Ophthalmol Strabismus* 1981;**18**:17.

Scott AB: Botulinum toxin injection of eye muscles to correct strabismus. *Trans Am Ophthalmol Soc* 1981;**79**:734.

Scott AB: Ocular motility. Chapter 21 in: *Physiology of the Human Eye and Visual System.* Records R (editor). Harper & Row, 1979.

Stockbridge L., Moore S: Prisms to determine the importance of a vertical component associated with esotropia. Page 213 in: *Orthoptics: Past, Present, Future.* Moore S, Mein J, Stockbridge L (editors). Stratton, 1976.

von Noorden GK: *Burian-von Noorden's Binocular Vision and Ocular Motility,* 3rd ed. Mosby, 1985.

von Noorden GK: *von Noorden–Maumenee's Atlas of Strabismus,* 4th ed. Mosby, 1983.

14

Orbit

John H. Sullivan, MD

ANATOMY
(Figs 14–1 to 14–5; Fig 1–12)

The orbital cavity is schematically represented as a pyramid of 4 walls that converge posteriorly. The medial walls of the right and left orbit are parallel and are separated by the nose. In each orbit the lateral and medial walls form an angle of 45 degrees, which results in a right angle between the 2 lateral walls. The orbit is compared to the shape of a pear, with the optic nerve representing its stem. The anterior circumference is somewhat smaller in diameter than the region just within the rim, which makes a sturdy protective margin.

The orbits are related to the frontal sinus above, the maxillary sinus below, and the ethmoid and sphenoid sinuses medially. The thin orbital floor is easily damaged by direct trauma to the globe, resulting in a "blowout" fracture with herniation of orbital contents into the maxillary antrum. Infection within the sphenoid and ethmoid sinuses can erode the paper-thin medial wall (lamina papyracea) and involve the contents of the orbit. Erosion of the roof (eg, neurofibromatosis) may result in visible pulsations of the globe transmitted from the brain.

Orbital Walls

The roof of the orbit is composed principally of the orbital plate of the **frontal bone.** The lacrimal gland is located in the lacrimal fossa in the anterior lateral aspect of the roof. Posteriorly, the lesser wing of the **sphenoid bone** containing the optic canal completes the roof.

The lateral wall is separated from the roof by the superior orbital fissure, which divides the lesser from the greater wing of the **sphenoid bone.** The anterior portion of the lateral wall is formed by the orbital surface of the **zygomatic (malar) bone.** This is the strongest part of the bony orbit. Suspensory ligaments, the lateral palpebral tendon, and check ligaments have their connective tissue attachment to the lateral orbital tubercle.

The orbital floor is separated from the lateral wall

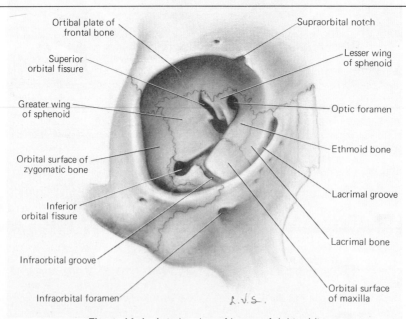

Ortibal plate of frontal bone

Superior orbital fissure

Greater wing of sphenoid

Orbital surface of zygomatic bone

Inferior orbital fissure

Infraorbital groove

Infraorbital foramen

Supraorbital notch

Lesser wing of sphenoid

Optic foramen

Ethmoid bone

Lacrimal groove

Lacrimal bone

Orbital surface of maxilla

Figure 14–1. Anterior view of bones of right orbit.

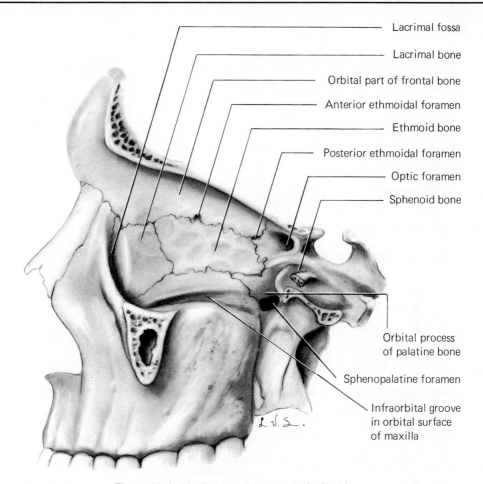

Lacrimal fossa

Lacrimal bone

Orbital part of frontal bone

Anterior ethmoidal foramen

Ethmoid bone

Posterior ethmoidal foramen

Optic foramen

Sphenoid bone

Orbital process of palatine bone

Sphenopalatine foramen

Infraorbital groove in orbital surface of maxilla

Figure 14–2. Medial view of bony wall of left orbit.

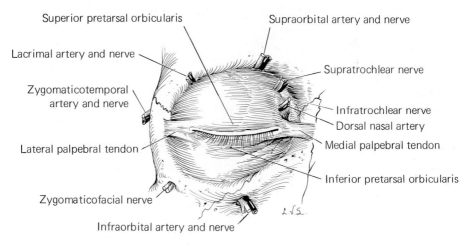

Superior pretarsal orbicularis

Supraorbital artery and nerve

Lacrimal artery and nerve

Supratrochlear nerve

Zygomaticotemporal artery and nerve

Infratrochlear nerve

Dorsal nasal artery

Lateral palpebral tendon

Medial palpebral tendon

Zygomaticofacial nerve

Inferior pretarsal orbicularis

Infraorbital artery and nerve

Figure 14–3. Vessels and nerves to extraocular structures.

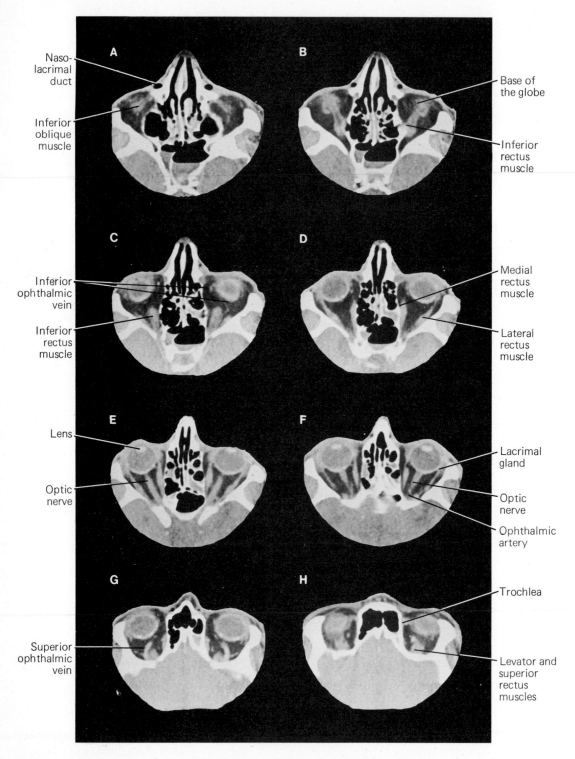

Figure 14–4. Normal CT scan showing the anatomy of the orbit. Axial CT sections, thickness 1.5 mm. *A,* lowest section; *H,* highest section. Note clear delineation of individual muscles, optic nerve, and major veins within the orbital fat.

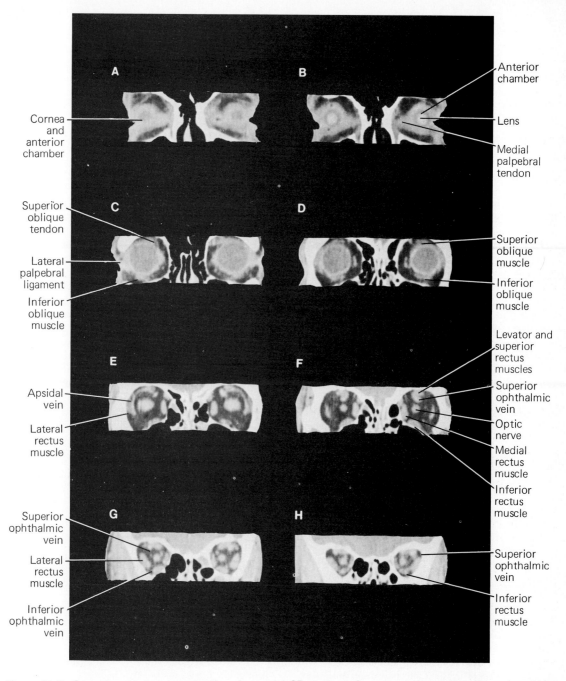

Figure 14–5. Coronal computer reconstructions from axial CT sections. **A,** most anterior section; **H,** most posterior section. Note detailed demonstration of ocular and orbital structures.

by the inferior orbital fissure. The orbital plate of the **maxilla** forms the large central area of the floor and is the region where blowout fractures most frequently occur. The frontal process of the **maxilla** medially and the **zygomatic bone** laterally complete the inferior orbital rim. The orbital process of the **palatine bone** forms a small triangular area in the posterior floor.

The boundaries of the medial wall are less distinct.

The **ethmoid** bone is paper-thin but thickens anteriorly as it meets the **lacrimal bone.** The body of the **sphenoid** forms the most posterior aspect of the medial wall, and the angular process of the **frontal bone** forms the upper part of the posterior lacrimal crest. The lower portion of the posterior lacrimal crest is made up of the **lacrimal bone.** The anterior lacrimal crest is easily palpated through the lid and is composed of the frontal process of the **maxilla.** The lacrimal groove lies between the 2 crests and contains the lacrimal sac.

Contents of the Orbit

The volume of the adult orbit is approximately 30 mL, and the eyeball occupies only about one-fifth of the space. Fat and muscle account for the bulk of the remainder.

The anterior limit of the orbital cavity is the **orbital septum.** It is a thin sheet of fascia extending from the orbital rim to the tarsus in the lower lid and to a point slightly above the border of the tarsus in the upper lid. The orbital septum acts as a barrier between the eyelids and the orbit. The extraocular muscles are described and discussed in Chapter 13.

The principal arterial supply of the orbit and its structures derives from the **ophthalmic artery,** the first major branch of the intracranial portion of the internal carotid artery. This branch passes beneath the optic nerve and accompanies it through the optic canal into the orbit. The first intraorbital branch is the central retinal artery, which enters the optic nerve about 8–15 mm behind the globe. The ophthalmic artery also sends branches to the lacrimal gland as well as to the intraocular structures via the short, long, and anterior ciliary arteries. The most anterior branches contribute to the formation of the arterial arcades of the eyelids, which make an anastomosis with the external carotid circulation via the facial artery.

The venous drainage of the orbit is primarily through the superior and inferior orbital veins. The superior orbital vein is important because it drains the skin of the periorbital region directly to the cavernous sinus. This forms the basis of the potentially lethal septic cavernous sinus thrombosis resulting from a superficial infection in this region.

The apex of the orbit is the entry portal for all nerves and vessels to the eye and the site of origin of all extraocular muscles except the inferior oblique. Expanding lesions of the apex result in a predictable neurologic deficit known as the orbital apex syndrome. The nerves enter the orbit through the **superior orbital fissure.** In its pathway to the cavernous sinus, the superior ophthalmic vein usually crosses at the highest point of the superior orbital fissure. Beneath the skin of the eyelid, this vein makes an anastomosis with the angular vein. The blood thus may drain posteriorly through the orbit or anteriorly to the facial vein.

The upper lateral aspect of the superior orbital fissure carries the **lacrimal nerve,** a branch of the first (ophthalmic) division of the trigeminal nerve. This small twig remains outside the area of origin of the rectus muscles (annulus of Zinn) and continues its lateral course in the orbit to terminate in the lacrimal gland, providing its sensory innervation. Slightly medial to the lacrimal nerve within the superior orbital fissure is the **frontal nerve,** which is the largest of the first division of branches of the trigeminal nerve. It also crosses over the annulus of Zinn and follows a course over the levator to the medial aspect of the

orbit, where it divides into the supraorbital and supratrochlear nerves. These provide sensation to the brow and forehead. The only other nerve to enter the orbit outside the annulus of Zinn is the **trochlear nerve.** Although the thinnest of the cranial nerves, the trochlear nerve has the longest intracranial course, and it is also the only nerve to originate on the dorsal surface of the brain stem. The fibers decussate before they emerge from the brain stem just before the inferior colliculi, where they are subject to injury from the tentorium. The nerve pierces the dura behind the sella turcica and travels within the lateral walls of the cavernous sinus to enter the superior orbital fissure medial to the frontal nerve. From this point it travels within the periorbita of the roof over the levator muscle to the upper surface of the superior oblique muscle.

The rectus muscles originate from a fibrous ring (the annulus of Zinn), which surrounds the remainder of the superior orbital fissure as well as the optic canal. The superior division of the **oculomotor nerve** is adjacent to the trochlear nerve but lies within the annulus of Zinn at its highest point. The oculomotor nerve originates from between the cerebral peduncles and passes near the posterior communicating artery of the circle of Willis. Lateral to the pituitary gland, it is closely approximated to the optic tract, and here it pierces the dura to course in the lateral wall of the cavernous sinus. As the nerve leaves the cavernous sinus, it divides into superior and inferior divisions. The superior division enters high within the annulus of Zinn and passes over the optic nerve to innervate the levator and superior rectus muscles. The inferior division enters the annulus of Zinn low and passes below the optic nerve to supply the medial and inferior rectus muscles. A large branch from the inferior division extends forward to supply the inferior oblique. A small twig from the proximal end of the nerve to the inferior oblique carries parasympathetic fibers to the ciliary ganglion.

Between the superior and inferior divisions of the oculomotor nerve within the annulus of Zinn lie the last 2 orbital nerves. On the lateral aspect is the **abducens nerve,** and medially the **nasociliary nerve.** The abducens originates between the pons and medulla and pursues an extended course up the clivus to the posterior clinoid, penetrates the dura, and passes within the cavernous sinus. (All other nerves course through the lateral wall of the cavernous sinus.) After passing through the superior orbital fissure within the annulus of Zinn, the nerve continues laterally to innervate the lateral rectus muscle.

The nasociliary nerve is the third branch of the first (ophthalmic) division of the trigeminal nerve and is the sensory nerve of the eye. The trigeminal nerve originates from the pons, and its sensory roots form the trigeminal ganglion. The first of the 3 divisions passes through the lateral wall of the cavernous sinus and divides into the lacrimal, frontal, and nasociliary nerve. The nasociliary nerve, after entering through the annulus of Zinn, lies between the superior rectus and the optic nerve. It sends a branch to the ciliary ganglion and other branches to supply the cornea (the posterior ciliary nerves), eventually terminating near the tip of the nose. Thus, the skin on the tip of the nose may be affected with vesicular lesions prior to the onset of herpes zoster ophthalmicus.

The second (maxillary) division of the trigeminal nerve passes through the foramen rotundum and enters the orbit through the inferior orbital fissure. It passes through the infraorbital canal and exits via the infraorbital foramen, supplying sensation to the lower lid and adjacent cheek. It is frequently damaged in fractures of the orbital floor.

PHYSIOLOGY OF SYMPTOMS

Owing to the rigid bony structure of the orbit, with only an anterior opening for expansion, any increase in the orbital contents taking place to the side of or behind the eyeball will displace that organ. Pressure behind the eyeball will push it forward (proptosis). Pressure on one side will displace the eyeball to the other side.

With the change in position of the eyeball, especially if it takes place rapidly, there may be enough interference with the movement of the eye to cause disssociation of ocular movements and diplopia (double vision). Pain is absent unless there is extreme swelling of the tissues or unless the eyelids are unable to protect the cornea adequately and there is irritation from exposure.

DIAGNOSTIC STUDIES

Imaging

Imaging by **computed tomography (CT scan)** has been a major advance in orbital diagnosis. Continued improvement in resolution quality—as well as 3-dimensional reconstructions—have made CT the single most important diagnostic study in the investigation of orbital disease. Contrast enhancement with CT during study of vascular lesions sometimes provides additional information.

Magnetic resonance imaging (MRI) has yet to achieve the same quality of image resolution as CT for most orbital problems. It is, however, capable of displaying subtle changes within soft tissue.

Ultrasonography

The use of ultrasonography in the diagnosis of orbital disease has largely been supplanted by CT. Although it is a noninvasive and cost-effective form of imaging, its usefulness in both A and B mode is limited to the anterior portion of the orbit. Its greatest value is reaped by the clinician-ultrasonographer capable of interpreting "real time" images.

Venography

Venography is occasionally useful in defining the extent of orbital venous disease. Although the diagnosis can usually be made by other means, contrast injection into the orbital veins via a scalp vein can sometimes reveal the presence of varices that have escaped detection by CT.

Angiography

Selective carotid angiography with bone subtraction is sometimes necessary to make the diagnosis of some orbital vascular disorders. In spontaneous, low-flow dural carotid artery-cavernous sinus fistula, angiography is required for management, since treatment by embolization is based on angiographic findings.

Radiography

Plain x-rays are often sufficient for diagnosis of some orbital disorders such as fractures. Soft tissue imaging, however, is usually valuable prior to surgery.

Dacryocystography and radionuclide scanning can be helpful in localizing the site of lacrimal obstructions, but these procedures are seldom used. The results are difficult to interpret, and treatment is rarely altered by the findings.

Positive contrast radiography and pneumo-orbitography are no longer used. Orbital thermography is a research procedure.

DISEASES & DISORDERS OF THE ORBIT

PROPTOSIS

Protrusion of the eyeball is the result of expansion of tissue within the orbital cavity and is the hallmark of orbital disease. Expansive lesions may be benign or malignant and may arise from bone, muscle, nerve, blood vessels, or connective tissue. A mass may be inflammatory, neoplastic, cystic, or vascular.

Protrusion is not in itself injurious unless the lids are unable to cover the cornea. The underlying cause, however, is usually serious and sometimes life-threatening.

Pseudoproptosis is apparent proptosis in the absence of orbital disease. Such confusion may arise with high myopia, buphthalmos, and lid retraction.

Etiology

History and examination provide many clues to the

cause of proptosis. The position of the eye is determined by the location of the mass. Expansion within the muscle cone displaces the eye straight ahead. A mass on one side will displace the eye to the other side. Bilateral involvement generally indicates systemic disease, such as Graves' disease. The term "exophthalmos" is often used when describing proptosis associated with Graves' disease. Pulsating proptosis reflects the pulse of an orbital vascular malformation or transmission of cerebral pulsations in the absence of the superior orbital roof, as in neurofibromatosis. Positional proptosis—which changes with Valsalva's maneuver—is a sign of orbital varices. Intermittent proptosis is likely to be from a sinus mucocele.

Clinical Findings

A. Symptoms and Signs: Diplopia may result from proptosis, especially if it occurs rapidly. Pain may occur as a result of rapid expansion, inflammation, or infiltration of sensory nerves. Vision is not usually affected early unless the lesion arises from the optic nerve. Pupillary signs and color vision testing may identify subtle optic nerve compression or involvement before acuity is reduced significantly.

The Hertel exophthalmometer (see Chapter 2) is the standard method of quantifying the magnitude of proptosis. Serial measurements are most accurate if performed by the same individual with the same instrument.

B. Imaging: Orbital imaging provides invaluable information, but biopsy or fine-needle aspiration is often necessary to make the diagnosis.

Treatment

Treatment of proptosis may involve surgery, corticosteroids, or radiation. A multidisciplinary approach is sometimes required for conditions involving adjacent structures.

ORBITAL INFECTIOUS & INFLAMMATORY DISORDERS

1. ORBITAL CELLULITIS (Fig 14–6)

Orbital cellulitis is the most common cause of proptosis in children. Immediate treatment is essential. Fortunately, the diagnosis usually is not difficult, because the clinical findings are characteristic. Although most cases occur in children, aged and immunocompromised individuals may also be affected.

Trauma may be responsible for introduction of contaminated material into the orbit through the skin or paranasal sinuses. In preantibiotic days, orbital cellulitis frequently led to blindness or death resulting from septic cavernous sinus thrombosis. Prompt treatment is critical.

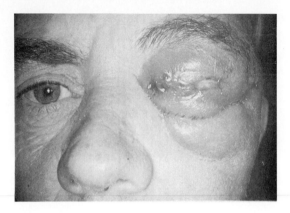

Figure 14–6. Orbital cellulitis. Abscess draining through upper eyelid.

The orbit is surrounded by the paranasal sinuses, and part of their venous drainage is through the orbit. Most cases of orbital cellulitis arise from extension of sinusitis through the thin ethmoid bones. The organisms usually responsible are those most frequently found in sinuses: *Haemophilus influenzae, Streptococcus pneumoniae,* streptococci, and staphylococci.

Clinical Findings

Preseptal cellulitis is the most common presentation. CT scan or MRI is helpful in distinguishing between pre- and postseptal involvement as well as identifying and localizing an orbital abscess or foreign body. Plain x-rays alone can only identify the presence of sinusitis.

It is important to distinguish between preseptal and orbital infections. Both present with edema, erythema, hyperemia, pain, and leukocytosis. Chemosis, proptosis, limitation of eye movement, and reduction of vision indicate deep orbital involvement. Extension to the cavernous sinus may cause bilateral involvement of cranial nerves II through VI, with severe edema and septic fever. Erosion of the orbital bones may cause brain abscess and meningitis.

In children, few orbital diseases develop as rapidly as cellulitis. Confusion may exist with rhabdomyosarcoma, pseudotumor, and Graves' ophthalmopathy.

Treatment

Treatment should be initiated before the causative organism is identified. As soon as nasal, conjunctival, and blood cultures are obtained, intravenous antibiotics should be administered. Beta-lactamase-resistant antibiotic should be given for staphylococcal infection and ampicillin for *H influenzae.* In the case of *H influenzae* resistant to ampicillin, one may give amoxicillin with clavulanic acid (Augmentin) or chloramphenicol. Posttraumatic cellulitis—especially following animal bites—must be covered for gram-negative and gram-positive bacilli. Hot compresses help localize the inflammatory reaction. Nasal decongestants and vasoconstrictors help drain the paranasal sinuses. Early surgical drainage is indicated in suppurative preseptal cellulitis. CT scan is useful in deciding when and where to drain an orbital abscess.

Most cases respond promptly to antibiotics. Those that do not may require drainage of the paranasal sinuses. Early consultation with an otolaryngologist may be helpful.

2. MUCORMYCOSIS

Diabetics and immunocompromised patients have a propensity to develop severe and often fatal fungal infections of the orbit. The organisms are of the Phycomycetes group, which have a tendency to invade vessels and create ischemic necrosis. Infection usually begins in the sinuses and erodes into the orbital cavity. A necrotizing reaction destroys muscle, bone, and soft tissue, frequently without causing signs of orbital cellulitis.

The patient is usually quite ill and presents with pain and proptosis. Examination of the nose usually reveals a necrotic area of mucosa, a smear of which shows broad branching hyphae.

Without treatment, the infection gradually erodes into the cranial cavity, resulting in meningitis, brain abscess, and death usually within days to weeks. Treatment is difficult and often inadequate and consists of correction of the underlying disease combined with surgical debridement and administration of amphotericin B intravenously. Recurrences are common.

3. GRAVES' OPHTHALMOPATHY

The most common cause of unilateral or bilateral proptosis in adults is Graves' disease.

The terminology of ocular involvement in thyroid disease is a bit confusing. Some degree of ophthalmopathy—usually mild—occurs in a high percentage of hyperthyroid patients. Severe infiltrative orbital myopathy with significant proptosis and restricted motility occurs in about 5% of cases of Graves' disease (Fig 14–7). This severe form, however, can also occur with hypothyroidism or with no detectable thyroid abnormality.

Thyroid ophthalmopathy is thought to be an autoimmune disease. It is often seen in autoimmune (Hashimoto's) thyroiditis. Antithyroglobulin, antimicrosomal, and other antibodies can usually be demonstrated, but their role in pathogenesis is in question.

Clinical Findings

The proptosis associated with thyroid disease is characterized by lid retraction, which serves to distinguish it from other causes of proptosis. Ocular myopathy usually begins with limitation of upgaze as a response to lymphocytic infiltration and edema of the

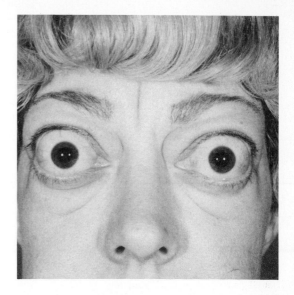

Figure 14–7. Graves' ophthalmopathy.

inferior rectus muscle. Permanent restriction eventually occurs because of fibrosis.

Diplopia usually begins in the upper field of gaze because of infiltrative myopathy of the inferior rectus muscle. All extraocular muscles may eventually be involved, and there may be no position of gaze free of diplopia. The eye may be tethered so tightly as to significantly raise the intraocular pressure when it is measured in the primary position.

The extraocular muscles may become massively enlarged and, in addition to restricting eye movement, may compress the optic nerve. Optic neuropathy is most common with enlargement of the posterior aspect of the muscles, but severe proptosis is often absent. Early signs include an afferent pupillary defect, impairment of color vision, and slight loss of visual acuity. Blindness is likely if compression is unrelieved. Lagophthalmos results from proptosis and lid retraction. Corneal exposure is a factor even in mild cases.

Treatment

The goal of treatment of Graves' ophthalmopathy is chiefly to maintain corneal hydration. Management of severe cases is difficult and multidisciplinary. An endocrinologist should monitor the metabolic activity, administer ^{131}I for ablation, or provide supplemental hormone therapy as indicated. Oral corticosteroids (prednisone, 60–100 mg/d) may be helpful in controlling the acute phase of infiltrative myopathy. Complications and side effects limit the use of corticosteroids in long-term maintenance.

Orbital radiation is most effective during the active phase of the disease. Soft tissue signs of swelling and chemosis are often relieved. Diplopia may be improved, as well as proptosis to some extent.

Early compression neuropathy may also be relieved

by radiation therapy, but compression neuropathy unresponsive to medical management is an indication for surgical decompression of the orbit. Several approaches have been devised to expand the orbital volume by fracture of the bony walls. The method of choice is fracture of the orbital floor into the maxillary sinus and the medial wall into the ethmoid sinus. Proptosis can be reduced by surgery, but there is a high risk of intractable diplopia and a lesser risk of orbital infection. For these reasons, decompression for cosmetic reasons alone is controversial.

Eyelid retraction is often more disturbing than proptosis—both functionally, because of exposure keratitis, and cosmetically. Decompression does not usually relieve lid retraction, but correction of the retraction camouflages proptosis to some extent. Lid retraction is corrected by surgery. The upper and lower lid retractors (aponeurosis and sympathetic muscles) can be lengthened by inserting a spacer such as eye bank sclera. Small amounts (2 mm) of lid retraction can be corrected by simply disinserting the retractors from the upper tarsal border.

Strabismus surgery should not be undertaken until the myopathy has stabilized. The adjustable suture technique is useful. Most patients can achieve at least a small area of single-image binocular vision in a useful position of gaze. Tortional diplopia, the result of oblique muscle involvement, complicates management.

Some patients have intractable diplopia despite all attempts at correction.

4. PSEUDOTUMOR

A frequent cause of proptosis in adults and children is inflammatory pseudotumor. This entity consists of a heterogeneous group of inflammatory diseases of unknown cause. The site of inflammation is usually diffuse and not amenable to excision. Onset is usually rapid, and pain is often present.

Pseudotumor is usually unilateral; when both orbits are involved, it is more often a manifestation of systemic lymphomas. In addition to lymphoma, the condition may be confused with Graves' ophthalmopathy, Wegener's granulomatosis, and systemic vasculitis.

Treatment with systemic corticosteroids or with radiation is usually effective. Surgery often exacerbates the inflammatory reaction.

CYSTIC LESIONS INVOLVING THE ORBIT

DERMOID

Dermoids are not true neoplasms but benign choristomas arising from embryonic tissue not usually found in the orbit. Orbital dermoids arise from surface ectoderm and often contain epithelial structures such as keratin, hair, and even teeth. Most are cystic and filled with an oily fluid that can incite a severe inflammatory reaction if liberated into the orbit. Most dermoids occur in the superior temporal quadrant of the orbit, but they can occur at any bony suture line.

X-rays show a sharp, round bony defect from the pressure of a slowly growing mass affixed to the periosteum.

Epidermoid cyst is a superficial keratin-filled mass, usually near the superior orbital rim. It may be congenital or posttraumatic. Excision is usually not difficult.

A **lipodermoid** is a solid mass of fatty material that occurs below the conjunctival surface. Hair growth on the overlying conjunctiva is not uncommon. Lipodermoids are often much larger than they appear to be, and excision may cause considerable damage to vital structures. If treatment is necessary, a limited excision is usually advised.

SINUS MUCOCELE

The proximity of the orbit to the paranasal sinuses may lead to invasion of the bony walls and extension of an obstructed sinus into the orbit. Plain x-ray will usually make the diagnosis, but CT scan may be required to differentiate sinus mucocele from dermoid cyst and to define the extent of the lesion (Fig 14–8).

Otolaryngologic and neurosurgical assistance may be necessary for surgical removal.

VASCULAR ABNORMALITIES INVOLVING THE ORBIT

ARTERIOVENOUS MALFORMATION

Arteriovenous malformations are an uncommon cause of proptosis. Varices produce intermittent prop-

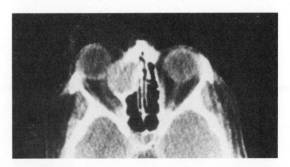

Figure 14–8. CT scan of orbital mucocele.

tosis sometimes associated with transient reduction of vision. Some degree of proptosis can be induced with Valsalva's maneuver or by placing the head in a dependent position. MRI or CT scan is helpful, and venography is diagnostic.

Surgery is the only method of treatment available and is fraught with hazard. Although there is usually pain and some disfigurement with intermittent proptosis, vision is usually spared. Surgical morbidity following eradication of the varix, however, may jeopardize visual function. Most varices are best left untreated unless vision is at risk.

CAROTID ARTERY-CAVERNOUS SINUS FISTULA

Carotid artery-cavernous sinus fistulas with high-flow shunts are easily diagnosed. Although sometimes occurring spontaneously, they usually follow trauma. Physical signs include severe congestion and chemosis, with pulsating proptosis and a loud bruit.

Low-flow shunts are usually spontaneous and often misdiagnosed. Mild congestion, venous engorgement and arterialization, elevated intraocular pressure, mild proptosis, and a faint bruit are the usual features. Diagnosis is by angiography, and treatment is by selective intra-arterial embolization.

PRIMARY ORBITAL TUMORS

CAPILLARY HEMANGIOMA

Capillary hemangioma—also called strawberry nevus—is common in neonates. In the orbital area, as elsewhere, the tumor is usually superficial and red, with a dimpled surface. Deep lesions appear as a bluish mass that often enlarges with crying (Fig 14–9). After an initial growth phase that typically lasts less than 1 year, most tumors regress slowly, and 70% resolve completely after 7 years. The tumors are not encapsulated and not easily excised.

Surgery is not recommended in young children unless amblyopia is threatened by occlusion of the lids or astigmatism from pressure on the globe. Tumors large enough to cause amblyopia can rarely be excised completely. The goal of surgery is to debulk the tumor sufficiently to prevent amblyopia without destroying vital structures. These tumors never become malignant, but large tumors frequently cause amblyopia and cosmetic disfigurement. Corticosteroids may cause prompt remission, but in infants their use is limited by the side effects. Intralesional injections may overcome these problems, but a significant number of children do not respond.

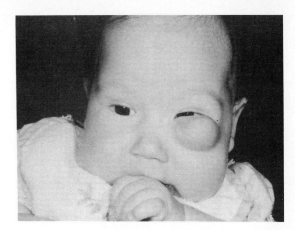

Figure 14–9. Capillary hemangioma.

Surgery for cosmetic improvement should be delayed until regression is completed, usually before age 10.

CAVERNOUS HEMANGIOMA

The most common orbital neoplasm of adults is cavernous hemangioma. The tumor grows slowly and usually becomes symptomatic in mid-life, typically in women. It often occurs within the muscle cone, producing axial proptosis, hyperopia, and in many cases choroidal folds on ophthalmoscopic examination. There is no relationship to capillary hemangioma. The tumor is encapsulated and contains large "cavernous" spaces lined with smooth muscle.

Surgical excision is usually successful, and recurrence is uncommon.

LYMPHANGIOMA

In its early stages, lymphangioma may be very similar to hemangioma—even histologically. Both usually begin in infancy, but lymphangioma may present later in life. Lymphangioma does not regress and is characterized by intermittent hemorrhage and gradual worsening. Large blood cysts may cause proptosis and diplopia and may require evacuation.

The tumor is often multifocal and frequently occurs in the soft palate and other areas of the face as well as the orbit. On histologic examination, it consists of large serum-filled channels and lymphoid follicles.

Local excision is almost always incomplete. Laser surgery and cryotherapy have limited usefulness.

RHABDOMYOSARCOMA
(Fig 14–10)

Rhabdomyosarcoma is the most common malignant tumor of the orbit in childhood. Presentation is before

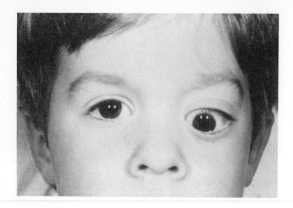

Figure 14–10. Rhabdomyosarcoma.

age 10, and rapid growth is characteristic. Tumors arising from the extraocular muscles—rather than de novo in the orbit—are least common but have the best prognosis. Manipulation of the tumor is thought to induce metastasis; consequently, it is advisable to be gentle during examination and biopsy.

Early treatment can be curative. Treatment in the past consisted of orbital exenteration, resulting in a 35% survival rate. In recent years, chemotherapy and x-ray without surgery have been employed with a 70% survival rate.

NEUROFIBROMA

Neurofibromatosis (Recklinghausen's disease) is inherited as an autosomal dominant trait. The diagnosis is made on the basis of cutaneous neurofibroma formation and café au lait spots. Plexiform neuroma of the upper lid produces a characteristic S-shaped blepharoptosis (Fig 14–11). Orbital involvement can produce massive disfigurement ("elephant man" disease). Erosion of the superior orbital roof permits transmission of pulsations from the brain to the prop-

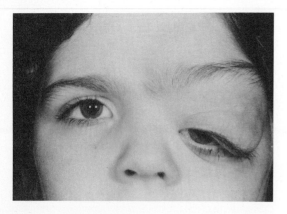

Figure 14–11. Neurofibromatosis.

totic globe. Meningioma, astrocytoma, and malignant schwannoma may also occur.

Surgery is generally palliative but can provide temporary relief from gross disfigurement.

OPTIC NERVE GLIOMA

Optic nerve glioma usually presents between the ages of 2 and 6 years as proptosis directed straight ahead. The tumor—usually a low-grade astrocytoma—originates from the optic nerve, resulting in early visual loss and enlarged optic canals on x-ray. Typical ophthalmoscopic findings are optic atrophy with opticociliary shunts (arteriovenous shunts adjacent to the disk).

Treatment is controversial, because there is no compelling statistics to indicate that either surgery or radiation is effective. Despite this, an attempt is usually made to excise the tumor from the nerve to prevent intracranial involvement. Once the chiasm has been invaded, radiation therapy is often recommended even though the tumor is generally not radiosensitive. Enucleation, however, is indicated for a blind proptotic eye.

LACRIMAL GLAND TUMORS

Fifty percent of masses presenting in the lacrimal gland are either inflammatory or secondary tumors. Signs of acute inflammation with pain characterize dacryoadenitis and pseudotumor. Lymphoma is usually painless and may be associated with a salmon-colored conjunctival patch. Primary tumors of the lacrimal gland are epithelial and similar to those of the parotid gland; half are benign and half are malignant. The most common epithelial tumor is "benign mixed"—by which is meant a mixture of epithelial and mesenchymal elements. These tumors should be excised—not biopsied—because of their propensity for recurrence and malignant transformation.

A malignant tumor of the lacrimal gland is suspected when the patient presents with pain and destructive bony changes are evident on x-ray. Biopsy should be performed through the eyelid to avoid tumor seeding in the orbit. Orbital exenteration with ostectomy is required if there is to be any chance of survival. Even with radical treatment, the prognosis is poor.

LYMPHOMA

Lymphomatous tumors of the orbit are divided into true malignant lymphomas and reactive lymphoid hyperplasia, or pseudolymphoma. A third category called "atyical lymphoid hyperplasia" is used when unequivocal attribution of malignancy cannot be made.

Classification is usually based on the histologic features of preexistent lymphoid architecture. The distinction is especially difficult in the orbit, which has no lymphoid system. Electron microscopy and immunocytochemical techniques are becoming more important for clinical management.

Patients with orbital lymphoid lesions are usually in the sixth or seventh decade of life. The lesions tend to occur in the superior orbit—the most frequent site of involvement being the lacrimal gland and conjunctiva. Lymphocytes are normally present in the substantia propria of the conjunctiva and scattered among the acini of the lacrimal gland.

Ninety percent of conjunctival lymphoid lesions are localized and not part of any systemic disease. They present as salmon patches and are mobile over the epibulbar surface. Of pseudolymphoma lesions that present in the orbit, 15–25% are presently or ultimately associated with concomitant systemic lymphoma. In over 60% of cases classified as malignant, systemic disease develops in 5 years; the remainder are believed to be of primary orbital provenance. Although 30% of cases of systemic lymphoma represent Hodgkin's disease, almost all orbital lymphomas are non-Hodgkin's tumors.

HISTIOCYTOSIS X

Histiocytosis X is a general term for a group of rare diseases that tend to occur in children and are usually manifested chiefly in bones. Hand-Schüller-Christian disease is characterized by typical punched-out skull defects along with proptosis and diabetes insipidus. Letterer-Siwe disease is an acute form in infants, often accompanied by systemic and visceral involvement, that progresses rapidly to death. The orbital lesions in both diseases are similar. Eosinophilic granuloma occurs in older patients and has a better prognosis, involving solitary granulomas of bone. Orbital lesions produce mild proptosis and are similar to fibrous dysplasia of bone.

Treatment is by surgical excision or radiation.

SECONDARY & METASTATIC TUMORS

NEUROBLASTOMA

Neuroblastoma is one of the most common malignant tumors of childhood. In late stages, it may metastasize to one or both orbits. Spontaneous periocular hemorrhage may occur as the rapidly growing tumor becomes necrotic. The prognosis is much better in children under age 2.

After chemotherapy or radiation, the survival rate of infants with orbital metastasis is 50%.

CUTANEOUS TUMORS

Basal cell, squamous cell, and meibomian gland carcinomas may spread locally into the anterior orbit. Nasopharyngeal carcinoma and meningioma invade the posterior orbit. Metastatic tumors reach the orbit by hematogenous spread, since the orbit is devoid of lymphatics. Metastasis is usually from the breast in women and from the lung in men. In children, the most common metastatic tumor is neuroblastoma. Metastatic tumors are much more common in the choroid than in the orbit, probably because of the nature of the blood supply.

Radiation therapy is effective in treatment of orbital metastasis. Life expectancy is short.

TRAUMA TO THE ORBIT

BLOW-OUT FRACTURE

Blunt trauma to the globe creates a sudden rise in pressure within the orbit and may result in fracture of the floor, the weakest area. Such an injury is called a blow-out fracture. Pure blow-out fractures are not as common as a combination of fractures involving the floor, the medial wall, and the orbital rim. Blow-out fractures are often associated with intraocular injury, and patients should be evaluated for hyphema, angle recession, retinal dialysis, and other sequelae of blunt trauma.

Floor fracture causes herniation of orbital contents into the maxillary sinus. Entrapment of the inferior rectus muscle or its adjacent fascia results in restricted upgaze and diplopia (Fig 14–12). Decompression of orbital volume leads to enophthalmos. Trauma to the infraorbital nerve as it crosses the floor of the orbit causes anesthesia of the upper lip and gum.

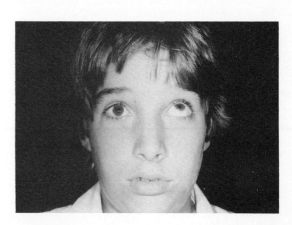

Figure 14–12. Right orbital blowout fracture in upgaze.

Not all blow-out fractures have to be repaired surgically. The presence of diplopia on upgaze and infraorbital anesthesia may be due to contusion, which will spontaneously improve. The presence of enophthalmos on initial examination, however, usually signifies a large fracture likely to require early operation. An unequivocally positive forced duction test, in which the globe cannot be passively elevated with forceps, is also an indication for surgery. If the patient is examined several hours after the injury, enophthalmos may be camouflaged by tissue swelling. CT demonstration of a large fracture with herniation—especially in the presence of restricted motility—is an indication for surgery. In doubtful cases, the patient may be observed for as long as 2 weeks before fibrosis makes the repair more difficult. Repair that has been delayed for several months is not likely to correct enophthalmos, because contracture of the rectus muscles will have occurred by that time.

The surgical approach may be through the maxillary sinus (Caldwell-Luc) or anteriorly through the skin. The latter approach is usually favored because it offers better visualization of the fracture and exposure to the medial wall or other fracture sites.

MAXILLARY FRACTURES

Trauma to the cheek bone may result in trimalar (tripod) fracture involving the inferior and lateral orbital rim and the zygomatic arch. The maxilla may be rotated or impacted into the sinus and may require reduction and fixation. Midfacial trauma may separate the maxilla from adjacent bones.

The Le Fort classification of maxillary fractures is useful even though most fractures are combinations of levels. Le Fort I involves the palate and upper jaw; Le Fort II separates the nose and upper teeth from the orbits; and Le Fort III separates the cranium from the face by a fracture across both orbits. Reduction and fixation of the fracture prevents gross facial deformity.

REFERENCES

Avery G, Tang RA, Close LG: Ophthalmic manifestations of mucoceles. *Ann Ophthalmol* 1983;**15**:734.

Beard C, Quickert MH: *Anatomy of the Orbit.* Aesculapius, 1969.

Char DH: *Thyroid Eye Disease.* Williams & Wilkins, 1985.

Clarke JR, Spalton DJ: Treatment of senile entropion with botulinum toxin. *Br J Ophthalmol* 1988;**72**:361.

Engstrom PF et al: Effectiveness of botulinum toxin therapy for essential blepharospasm. *Ophthalmology* 1987;**94**: 971.

Fells P: Orbital decompression for severe dysthyroid eye disease. *Br J Ophthalmol* 1987;**71**:107.

Ferry AP, Abedi S: Diagnosis and management of rhino-orbitocerebral mucormycosis (phycomycosis): A report of 16 personally observed cases. *Ophthalmology* 1983; **90**:1096.

Grove AS: Evaluation of exophthalmos. *N Engl J Med* 1975;**292**:1005.

Haik BG et al: Capillary hemangioma of the lids and orbit: An analysis of the clinical features and therapeutic results in 101 cases. *Ophthalmology* 1979; **86**:760.

Henderson JW: *Orbital Tumors,* 2nd ed. Decker, 1980.

Hoyt WF, Baghdassarian SA: Optic glioma of childhood: Natural history and rationale for conservative management. *Br J Ophthalmol* 1969;**53**:793.

Jacobson DM et al: Maternal orbital hematoma associated with labor. *Am J Ophthalmol* 1988;**105**:547.

Jakobiec FA, Bonanno PA, Sigelman J: Conjunctival adnexal cysts and dermoids. *Arch Ophthalmol* 1978; **96**:1404.

Jones IS, Jakobiec FA: *Diseases of the Orbit.* Harper & Row, 1979.

Keltner JL et al: Dural and carotid cavernous sinus fistulas: Diagnosis, management, and complications. *Ophthalmology* 1987;**94**:1585.

Kersten RC: Blowout fracture of the orbital floor with entrapment caused by isolated trauma to the orbital rim. *Am J Ophthalmol* 1987;**103**:215.

Leone CR Jr, Wissinger JP: Surgical approaches to diseases of the orbital apex. *Ophthalmology* 1988;**95**:391.

Macy JI, Mandelbaum SH, Minckler DS: Ocular pathology for clinicians. 8. Orbital cellulitis. Ophthalmology 1980; **87**:1309.

Rootman J, Nugent R: The classification and management of acute orbital pseudotumors. *Ophthalmology* 1982; **89**:1040.

Rootman J et al: Orbital-adnexal lymphangiomas: A spectrum of hemodynamically isolated vascular hamartomas. *Ophthalmology* 1986;**93**:1558.

Sergott RC, Glaser JS: Graves' ophthalmopathy: A clinical and immunologic review. *Surv Ophthalmol* 1981;**26**:1.

Shields CL et al: Orbital metastasis from a carcinoid tumor: Computed tomography, magnetic resonance imaging, and electron microscopic findings. *Arch Ophthalmol* 1987;**105**:968.

Shields JA, Shields CL, Eagle RC: Cavernous hemangioma of the orbit. *Arch Ophthalmol* 1987;**105**:853.

Warwick R: *Eugene Wolff's Anatomy of the Eye and Orbit,* 7th ed. Saunders, 1977.

Wharam M et al: Localized orbital rhabdomyosarcoma. *Ophthalmology* 1987;**94**:251.

Wilson WB et al: Magnetic resonance imaging of nonmetallic orbital foreign bodies. *Am J Ophthalmol* 1988; **105**:612.

Wojno TH: The incidence of extraocular muscle and cranial nerve palsy in orbital floor blow-out fractures. *Ophthalmology* 1987;**94**:682.

Neuro-ophthalmology

15

Pamela S. Chavis, MD, & William F. Hoyt, MD

The eyes are intimately related to the brain and frequently give up important diagnostic clues to central nervous system disorders. Indeed, the optic nerve is part of the central nervous system.

Intracranial disease frequently causes visual disturbances because of destruction of or pressure upon some portion of the optic pathways. Cranial nerves III, IV, and VI, which control ocular movements, may be involved; and nerves V and VII are also intimately associated with ocular function.

Fig 15–1 shows the normal brain as portrayed by the technique of magnetic resonance imaging (MRI).

THE SENSORY VISUAL PATHWAY

Topographic Overview (Fig 15–2)

Cranial nerve II subserves the special sense of vision. Light is detected by the rods and cones of the

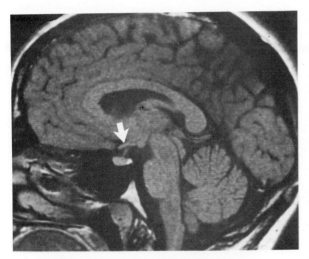

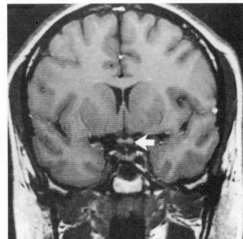

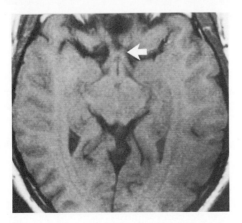

Figure 15–1. Magnetic resonance imaging (MRI) of normal brain in sagittal section *(upper left)*, coronal section *(upper right)*, and axial section *(lower left)*. The white arrows indicate the chiasm. The future impact of this technique on localization of lesions affecting the intracranial visual and ocular motor pathways will be profound.

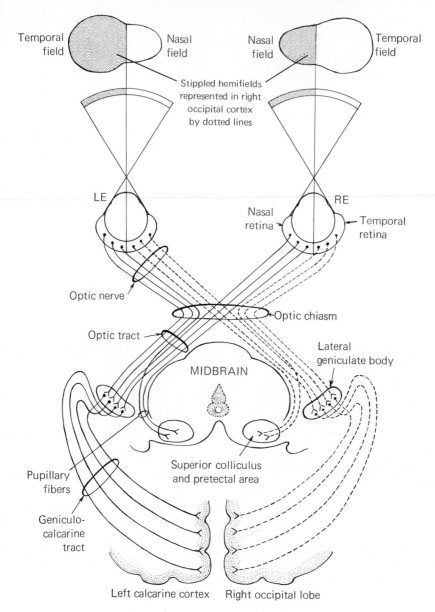

Temporal field

Nasal field

Nasal field

Temporal field

Stippled hemifields represented in right occipital cortex by dotted lines

LE

RE

Nasal retina

Temporal retina

Optic nerve

Optic chiasm

Optic tract

Lateral geniculate body

MIDBRAIN

Pupillary fibers

Superior colliculus and pretectal area

Geniculo-calcarine tract

Left calcarine cortex   Right occipital lobe

Figure 15–2. The optic pathway. The dotted lines represent nerve fibers from the retina to the occipital cortex that carry visual and pupillary afferent impulses from the left half of the visual field.

retina, which may be considered the special sensory end organ for vision. The cell bodies of these receptors send out processes that synapse with the bipolar cell, the second neuron in the visual pathway. The bipolar cells synapse, in turn, with the retinal ganglion cells. Ganglion cell axons comprise the nerve fiber layer of the retina and converge to form the optic nerve. The nerve emerges from the back of the globe and travels posteriorly within the muscle cone to enter the cranial cavity via the optic canal.

Intracranially, the 2 optic nerves join to form the optic chiasm. At the chiasm, more than half of the fibers (those from the nasal half of the retina) decussate

and join the uncrossed temporal fibers of the opposite nerve to form the optic tracts. The optic tract synapses in the lateral geniculate body. Each optic tract sweeps around the cerebral peduncle toward the lateral geniculate nucleus. All of the fibers receiving impulses from the right half of the visual field thus make up the left optic tract and project to the left cerebral hemisphere. Similarly, the left half of the visual field projects to the right cerebral hemisphere. Twenty percent of the fibers in the tract subserve pupillary function. These fibers leave the tract just anterior to the nucleus and pass via the brachium of the superior colliculus to the midbrain pretectal nucleus. The remaining fibers synapse in the lateral geniculate nucleus. The cell bodies of this structure give rise to the geniculocalcarine tract. This tract passes through the posterior limb of the internal capsule and then fans into the optic radiations that traverse parts of the temporal and parietal lobes en route to the occipital cortex (calcarine cortex).

Analysis of Visual Fields in Localizing Lesions in the Visual Pathways

In clinical practice, lesions in the visual pathways are localized by means of central and peripheral visual field examination. The technique (perimetry) is discussed in Chapter 2. Fig 15–3 shows the types of field defects caused by lesions in various locations of the pathway. Lesions anterior to the chiasm (of the retina or optic nerve) cause unilateral field defects; lesions anywhere in the visual pathway posterior to the chiasm cause contralateral homonymous defects. These may be congruent (ie, identical in size, shape, and location) or incongruent. Chiasmal lesions usually cause bitemporal defects.

Multiple isopters (field tests with several objects of different sizes) should be used in order to evaluate the defects thoroughly. A field defect shows evidence of actively spreading disease when there are areas of "relative scotoma" (ie, a larger field defect for a smaller test object). Such visual field defects are said to be "sloping." This is in contrast to vascular lesions with steep borders, (ie, the defect is the same size no matter what size test object is used). Such visual field defects are said to be "absolute."

Another important generalization is that the more congruous the homonymous field defects (ie, the more similar the 2 hemifields), the farther posterior the lesion is in the visual pathway. A lesion in the occipital region causes identical defects in each field, whereas optic tract lesions cause incongruous (dissimilar) homonymous field defects. Also, the more posterior the lesion, the more likely macular sparing and, therefore, maintenance of good visual acuity in both hemifields. Certainly, a complete homonymous hemianopia should have intact visual acuity in the sprayed visual field since that part of the visual system for macular and peripheral function is spared.

THE OPTIC NERVE

Anatomy (Fig 15–4)

The optic nerve is a trunk containing about 1.1 million axons arising from the ganglion cells of the retina. The nerve emerges from the back of the globe through a short circular opening (0.7 mm long, 1.5 mm in diameter) in the sclera situated 1 mm below and 3 mm nasal to the posterior pole of the eye. The orbital portion is 25–30 mm long and travels posteriorly within the muscle cone. The nerve than passes via the bony optic canal into the cranial cavity. This intracanalicular portion measures 4–9 mm. After a 10-mm intracranial course, the nerve joins the opposite optic nerve to form the optic chiasm.

The nerve fibers become myelinated upon leaving the eye; this increases the diameter from 1.5 mm (within the sclera) to 3 mm (within the orbit). Since the ganglion cells of the retina and their axons that make up the optic nerve are actually extensions of the central nervous system, they have no capacity to regenerate if severed.

Sheaths of the Optic Nerve (Fig 15–4)

The fibrous wrappings that ensheathe the optic nerve are continuous with the meninges. The pia mater is loosely attached about the nerve near the chiasm and only for a short distance within the cranium, but it is closely attached around most of the intracanalicular and all of the intraorbital portions. The pia consists of some fibrous tissue with numerous small blood vessels (Fig 15–5). It divides the nerve fibers into bundles by sending numerous septa into the nerve substance. The pia continues to the sclera, with a few fibers running into the choroid and lamina cribrosa.

The arachnoid comes in contact with the optic nerve at the intracranial end of the optic canal and accompanies the nerve to the globe, where it ends in the sclera and overlying dura. This sheath is a diaphanous connective tissue membrane with many septate connections with the pia mater, which it closely resembles. It is more intimately associated with pia than with dura.

The dura mater lining the inner surface of the cranial vault comes in contact with the optic nerve as it leaves the optic canal. As the nerve enters the orbit from the optic canal, the dura splits, one layer (the periorbita) lining the orbital cavity and the other forming the outer dural covering of the optic nerve. The dura becomes continuous with the outer two-thirds of the sclera. The dura consists of tough, fibrous, relatively avascular tissue lined by endothelium on the inner surface.

The subdural space is between the dura and the arachnoid; the subarachnoid space is between the pia and the arachnoid. Both are more potential than actual spaces under normal conditions but are direct continuations of their corresponding intracranial spaces. Subarachnoid or subdural fluid under sufficient pressure will fill these potential spaces about the optic nerve. The meningeal layers are adherent to each other and to the optic nerve and the surrounding bone within the optic foramen, making the optic nerve resistant to traction from either end.

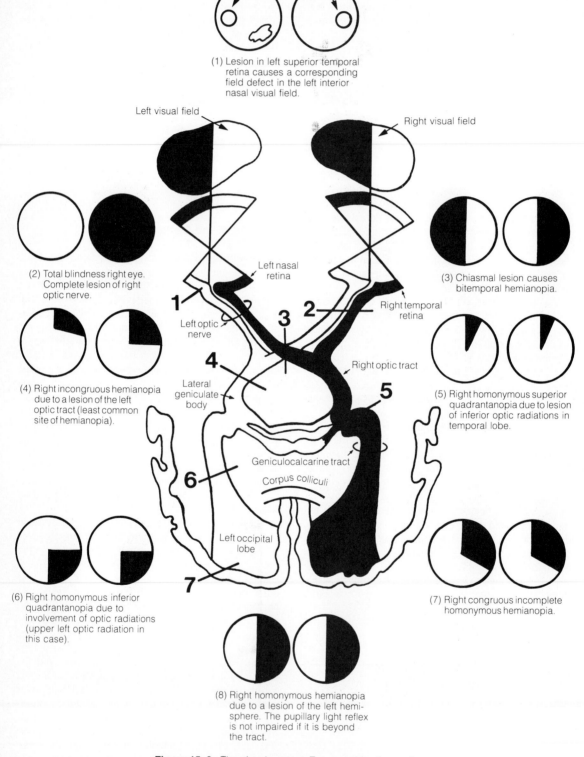

Normal blind spots

(1) Lesion in left superior temporal retina causes a corresponding field defect in the left interior nasal visual field.

Left visual field

Right visual field

(2) Total blindness right eye. Complete lesion of right optic nerve.

(3) Chiasmal lesion causes bitemporal hemianopia.

Left nasal retina

Right temporal retina

Left optic nerve

Right optic tract

(4) Right incongruous hemianopia due to a lesion of the left optic tract (least common site of hemianopia).

Lateral geniculate body

(5) Right homonymous superior quadrantanopia due to lesion of inferior optic radiations in temporal lobe.

Geniculocalcarine tract

Corpus colliculi

Left occipital lobe

(6) Right homonymous inferior quadrantanopia due to involvement of optic radiations (upper left optic radiation in this case).

(7) Right congruous incomplete homonymous hemianopia.

(8) Right homonymous hemianopia due to a lesion of the left hemisphere. The pupillary light reflex is not impaired if it is beyond the tract.

Figure 15–3. The visual system. Topographic diagnosis.

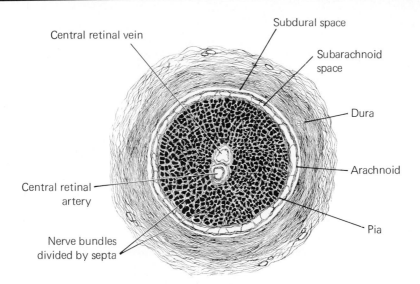

Figure 15–4. Cross section of the optic nerve. (Redrawn and reproduced, with permission, from Wolff E: *Anatomy of the Eye and Orbit*, 6th ed. Blakiston-McGraw, 1968.)

Etiologic Classification of Diseases of the Optic Nerve

A. Idiopathic optic neuritis
B. Demyelinating diseases
  1. Multiple sclerosis
  2. Other rare demyelinating syndromes—eg, neuromyelitis optica (Devic's disease)

C. Viral infections
  1. Postviral optic neuritis (measles, mumps, chickenpox, influenza)
  2. Postinfectious encephalomyelitis
  3. Polyradiculoneuronitis (Guillain-Barré syndrome)
  4. Infectious mononucleosis
  5. Herpes zoster

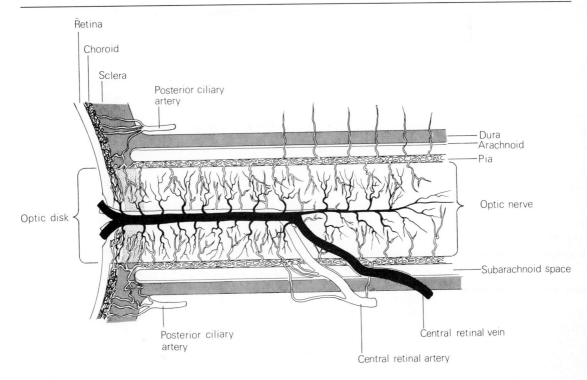

Figure 15–5. Blood supply of the optic nerve. (Redrawn and reproduced, with permission, from: Hayreh SS: *Trans Am Acad Ophthalmol Otolaryngol* 1974;**78**:240.)

D. Local extension of inflammatory disease
1. Sinusitis
2. Intracranial disease—meningitis, encephalitis
3. Orbital disease—cellulitis, vasculitis
4. Intraocular disease—chorioretinitis, endophthalmitis, iridocyclitis

E. Systemic infections and inflammation
1. Syphilis
2. Tuberculosis
3. Cryptococcosis
4. Coccidioidomycosis
5. Infective endocarditis
6. Sarcoidosis

F. Nutritional and metabolic
1. Diabetes mellitus
2. Vitamin deficiencies—beriberi, pellagra

G. Toxic
1. Tobacco—alcohol amblyopia
2. Heavy metal—arsenic, lead, thallium
3. Drugs—ethambutol, isoniazid, streptomycin, disulfiram, digitalis, chloramphenicol, chloroquine, chlorpropamide, halogenated hydroxyquinolines (eg, iodochlorhydroxyquin)
4. Methanol

H. Hereditary optic atrophy
1. Leber's disease
2. Dominant (juvenile) optic atrophy
3. Recessive (infantile) optic atrophy
4. Heredodegenerative diseases
5. Optic nerve anomalies

I. Vascular disease
1. Temporal arteritis
2. Arteriosclerosis (anterior ischemic optic neuropathy), diabetes mellitus, hypertension
3. Polyarteritis nodosa
4. Takayasu's disease

J. Neoplastic
1. Direct infiltration of optic nerve, leukemic or malignant
2. Compressive neuropathy (tumors, thyroid eye disease)
3. Paraneoplastic syndrome

K. Trauma

L. Radiation neuropathy

OPTIC NEURITIS
(Papillitis) (Fig 15–6)

Optic neuritis and papillitis are broad terms denoting inflammation, degeneration, or demyelinization of the optic nerve due to a wide variety of diseases. Loss of vision is the cardinal symptom and serves to differentiate papillitis from papilledema, which it may resemble on ophthalmoscopic examination.

Retrobulbar neuritis is optic neuritis that occurs far enough behind the optic disk so that early changes at the optic disk are not visible by means of the oph-

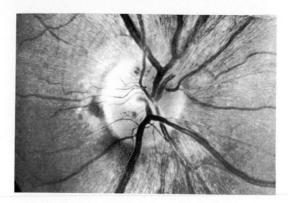

Figure 15–6. Mild disk swelling in papillitis.

thalmoscope. Visual acuity is markedly reduced. ("The patient sees nothing, and the doctor sees nothing.") Papillitis is disk swelling caused by local inflammation at the nerve head (intraocular optic nerve) (Fig 15–6).

The most frequent cause of retrobulbar neuritis is multiple sclerosis. A diagnosis of multiple sclerosis is eventually made in 25–60% of patients between 20 and 45 years of age who have an attack of retrobulbar neuritis. The percentage of progression to multiple sclerosis after an episode of optic neuritis tends to be higher with increased length of patient follow-up. Other causes are late neurosyphilis, toxic amblyopias, other demyelinating diseases, Leber's optic atrophy, diabetes mellitus, and vitamin deficiency. If the process is sufficiently destructive, retrograde optic atrophy results and nerve fiber bundle defects appear in the retinal nerve fiber layer (Fig 15–7). The disk loses its normal pink color and becomes pale. In very severe recurrent cases, a chalky-white disk with sharp outlines in a blind eye results.

Clinical Findings

There is usually a temporary but severe loss of vision. There may be pain in the region of the eye, especially upon movement of the globe. Vision characteristically improves dramatically within 2–6 weeks.

Central scotomas are the most common visual field defect. They are usually circular, varying widely in size and density. A central scotoma that has broken out to the periphery, however, should make the clinician suspect a compressive lesion, although it can happen in severe papillitis. Almost any unilateral field change is possible. The pupillary light reflex is sluggish, and if the optic nerves are asymmetrically involved, an afferent pupillary defect will be present.

Ophthalmoscopically, hyperemia of the optic disk and distention of large veins are early signs in papillitis. Blurred disk margins and filling of the physiologic cup are common. The process may advance to marked edema of the nerve head, but elevations of more than 3 diopters (1 mm) are unusual. Extensive

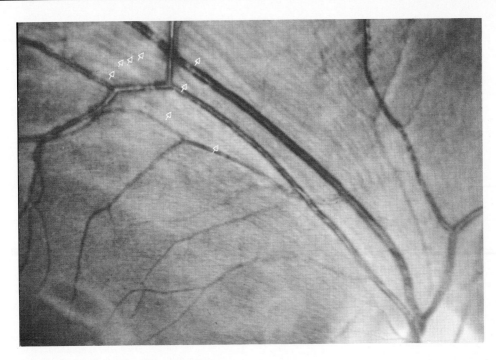

Figure 15–7. Retinal nerve fiber layer in demyelinative optic neuropathy of multiple sclerosis. The upper temporal nerve fiber bundles show multiple slitlike areas of thinning (arrows) representing retrograde axonal atrophy from subclinical disease in the optic nerve. Vision in the eye was 6/6 (20/20).

surrounding retinal edema may be present. Flame-shaped hemorrhages may occur in the nerve fiber layer near the optic disk.

Differential Diagnosis

Papilledema is the most common differential diagnostic problem (Fig 15–8). In papilledema, there is often greater elevation of the optic nerve head, nearly normal visual acuity, a normal pupillary response to light, associated increased intracranial pressure, and no visual field defect except an enlarged blind spot unless the visual pathway has been interrupted intracranially or there has been acute papilledema with vascular decompensation (ie, hemorrhage and cotton-wool spots) or chronic papilledema with secondary ischemia to the optic nerve. Nasal nerve fiber bundle defects and nasal quadrantanopias can then occur. Papilledema is usually bilateral, whereas papillitis is usually unilateral. Despite these obvious differences, differential diagnosis continues to be a problem because of the similarity of the ophthalmoscopic findings and because papilledema can be quite asymmetric and papillitis bilateral in some postviral events (eg, Devic's disease, or neuromyelitis optica).

Treatment

Ideally, treatment is directed toward the underlying cause. Systemic corticosteroids have not been proved to be helpful in retrobulbar neuritis by shortening the course of optic neuritis. However, in papillitis with minimal evidence of collagen vascular disease or other

signs of multiple sclerosis, intravenous pulses of methylprednisolone can be used over days to weeks, since visual loss can be more extensive.

Course & Prognosis

Loss of vision occurs within the first few hours after onset and is maximal within several days. Visual acuity usually begins to improve 2–3 weeks after onset and sometimes returns to normal in a few days. Improvement may continue slowly over a period of 6 weeks. The appearance of optic atrophy indicates some permanent destruction of nerve fibers with permanent loss of function. Optic neuritis associated with lupus erythematosus or other collagen vascular disease can be indistinguishable clinically from multiple sclerosis. Individual attacks of optic neuritis have a favorable prognosis without treatment, but over a period of years significant visual loss is the rule, since permanent damage results from recurrent attacks.

MULTIPLE SCLEROSIS
(Fig 15–7)

Multiple sclerosis is a chronic, relapsing demyelinating disorder of the central nervous system of unknown cause. Characteristically, the lesions occur at different times and in different noncontiguous locations in the nervous system. Onset is usually in young adult life—rarely before 15 years or after 55 years of age. There is a tendency to involve the optic

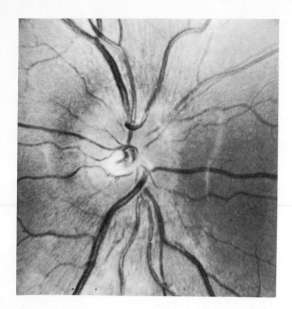

Figure 15–8. Early papilledema. The disk margins are blurred superiorly and inferiorly by the thickened layer of nerve fibers entering the disk.

nerves and chiasm, brain stem, cerebellar peduncles, and spinal cord, though no part of the central nervous system is protected. The peripheral nervous system is seldom involved.

Clinical Findings

A. Symptoms and Signs: Clinically, there are a variety of symptoms and signs that may vary in number and nature from time to time. In addition to ocular disturbances, there may be motor weakness with pyramidal signs, ataxia, urinary disturbances, paresthesias, dysarthria, intention tremors, and sensory disturbances. Sensory hyperesthesias and urinary incontinence are common early signs. The other problems can occur over months to years.

Patients may complain first of blurring of vision, as if a mist or film were covering the eye. This is due to optic neuritis (especially retrobulbar neuritis) and is characterized by acute unilateral loss of vision with a tendency toward recovery. Because of the transient nature of the visual defect and the absence of physical findings, the complaint is sometimes misdiagnosed as hysteria. The other eye is involved eventually. With each attack, there may be some residual permanent damage (eg, loss of visual acuity or defective color vision).

Because of the tendency toward selective involvement of the papillomacular bundle within the optic nerve, central scotoma is by far the most common visual field defect during the acute stage.

The pupil reacts sluggishly to light. If optic neuritis is severe, there may be atrophy of the optic disk that is ophthalmoscopically visible as temporal pallor.

Diplopia is a common early symptom of extraocular muscle involvement, due most frequently to internuclear ophthalmoplegia. This condition, caused by a lesion of the medial longitudinal fasciculus, is characterized by paresis of one or both medial rectus muscles on conjugate lateral gaze to the opposite side and symptoms in the opposite (abducting) eye; thus, diplopia can occur on lateral gaze, whereas medial rectus function can be normal for convergence. Ptosis may also occur; less commonly, weakness of the lateral rectus or other msucles, singly or together, occurs.

Nystagmus is a common early sign, and—unlike most manifestations of the disease (which tend toward remission)—it is often permanent (70%).

Peripheral retinal vessel vasculitis and low-grade uveitis are occasionally associated with multiple sclerosis. This can be either a granulomatous or lymphocytic retinal periphlebitis with venous sheathing and gray-white neovascular dots. Focal retinitis is less common.

B. Laboratory Findings: The cerebrospinal fluid gamma globulin concentration is frequently high, and oligoclonal bands in the cerebrospinal fluid can be elevated, representing either local production of IgG and IgA—which may signify a response to a viral infection—or an aberrant immune response to a viral antigen. Some patients with multiple sclerosis have no spinal fluid abnormalities, especially if the disease process is in a less acute or milder phase. Oligoclonal bands can be followed in the spinal fluid as a marker of disease activity in patients being treated with corticosteroids.

Pathologically, multiple areas of demyelination are present in the white matter. Early, there is degeneration of myelin sheaths and a relative sparing of the axons. Glial tissue overgrowth and complete nerve fiber destruction with some round cell infiltration are seen later. The disease affects the optic nerve and the chiasm more than the rest of the visual sensory system.

C. Special Examinations: Visual evoked response (VER) may help confirm involvement of the visual pathway. VER has been reported to be abnormal in 80% of definite, 43% of probable, and 22% of suspected cases of multiple sclerosis. A normal VER in patients with suspected multiple sclerosis makes the diagnosis questionable; but with positive oligoclonal bands or abnormal contrast sensitivity, the diagnosis can be made with greater confidence. CT scan and especially MRI can detect subclinical demyelinating lesions in white matter and can confirm that there are disseminated lesions.

Treatment, Course, & Prognosis

There is no specific therapy for multiple sclerosis, but corticosteroids are being used earlier to stop the central nervous system inflammatory process. Treatment is symptomatic and supportive. The course of the disease is unpredictable, and remissions and exacerbations may occur at other times and with new symptoms.

The prognosis for vision in retrobulbar neuritis is fairly good, but with successive attacks there may be an increased permanent defect. Complete blindness may occur when there is severe optic atrophy. Death may occur within a decade, but survival for 25–30 years is not uncommon.

NEUROMYELITIS OPTICA
(Devic's Disease)

This rare demyelinating disease of the central nervous system—considered by many to be a severe and acute form of multiple sclerosis—is characterized by bilateral optic neuritis and paraplegia. The cause is not known, but the disorder appears to be a postviral phenomenon. There is usually a subacute onset of blindness in one eye, followed soon by blindness in the other eye and paraplegia. Approximately 50% of patients progress to death within the first decade as a result of the paraplegia, but the remainder may have a prolonged remission and ultimately a better prognosis than those with chronic demyelinating disease or multiple sclerosis.

Treatment may be with a loading dose of intravenous methylprednisolone followed by oral steroids with monitoring of oligoclonal bands in cerebrospinal fluid.

ISCHEMIC OPTIC NEUROPATHY

Ischemic optic neuropathy is acute, pallid disk swelling, often associated with one or 2 splinter hemorrhages, and is associated with arteriosclerosis or vasculitis, thus occurring generally in the 60s or 70s and only occasionally at a younger age (Fig 15–9). It is due to occlusion of the posterior ciliary arteries in the retrolaminar cribrosa area (a few millimeters behind the optic nerve head), where the optic nerve capillaries are relatively less abundant, and for that reason, acute visual loss due to ischemic optic neuropathy should be associated with ophthalmoscopic evidence of disk edema within 24 hours after onset of visual symptoms.

These patients are commonly diabetic or hypertensive (or both) but any condition capable of producing intracranical stroke can affect the posterior ciliary arteries as well. Most important to the ophthalmologist is temporal arteritis, which can present with bilateral visual loss; this occurs most often in elderly people and is associated with a high sedimentation rate; painful, tender temporal arteries; pain on mastication; and general malaise, anorexia, weight loss, fever of unknown origin, and muscular aches and pains. It may represent an autoimmune response to internal elastic lamina which is bared to the systemic circulation by ulcerated arteriosclerotic plaques.

Impairment of visual acuity in ischemic optic atrophy may range from slight (with a corresponding decrease in color vision) to no light perception; visual field defects are commonly altitudinal (inferior defects more commonly than superior), quadrantanopias, and nerve fiber bundle defects. Occasionally, central scotomas are present. The initial visual loss tends to be more severe in arteritic than nonarteritic ischemic optic neuropathy, and subsequent visual recovery parallels this as well. As the acute process resolves, a pale disk with or without what may mistakenly appear to be "glaucomatous" cupping results (Fig 15–10).

PAPILLEDEMA
(Figs 15–8, 15–11, 15–12, and 15–13)

Papilledema (choked disk) is noninflammatory congestion of the optic disk associated with increased intracranial pressure. Papilledema will occur in any condition causing persistent increased intracranial pressure; the most common causes are cerebral tumors, abscesses, subdural hematoma, hydrocephalus, arteriovenous malformations, and malignant hypertension. It can also occur in spinal cord tumors and the mucopolysaccharidoses. In an ophthalmologic practice where patients walk in and are usually healthy except for visual complaints, it is often due to benign intracranial hypertension.

For papilledema to occur, the subarachnoid spaces around the optic nerve must be patent and connect the retrolaminar optic nerve through the bony optic canal to the intracranial subarachnoid space, thus allowing increased intracranial pressure to be transmitted to the retrolaminar optic nerve. Slow and fast axonal flow is blocked, and axonal distention occurs as the first sign of papilledema. Hyperemia of the disk, dilated surface capillary telangiectasias, blurring of the peripapillary disk margin, and loss of spontaneous venous pulsations occur later. Edema around the disk can cause decreased sensitivity to small isopters on visual field testing, but circumferential retinal folds and internal limiting membrane reflexes (Paton's lines) will eventually become evident as the retina is pushed away from the choked disk; when the retina is pushed away, the blind spot will be enlarged to large isopters on visual field testing as well. Fully developed papilledema is associated with peripapillary edema, choroidal folds, hemorrhages, and cotton-wool spots. Hemorrhages and cotton-wool spots herald vascular and axonal decompensation and then nerve fiber layer infarcts, and nasal quadrantanopias will occur. It takes 24–48 hours for early papilledema to occur and 1 week for it to develop fully.

Papilledema can occur if ocular hypotony is present, since in this situation intracranial pressure would appear falsely high relative to low pressure within the globe. Uveitis has also been associated with papilledema, either due to hypotony or to posterior vitreous changes at the optic nerve head. It takes 6–8 weeks for fully developed papilledema to resolve during adequate treatment. Papilledema can be associated with sudden visual loss after sudden intracranial decompression (ventriculography) or decreased systolic perfusion pressure. In chronic papilledema (Fig 15–13),

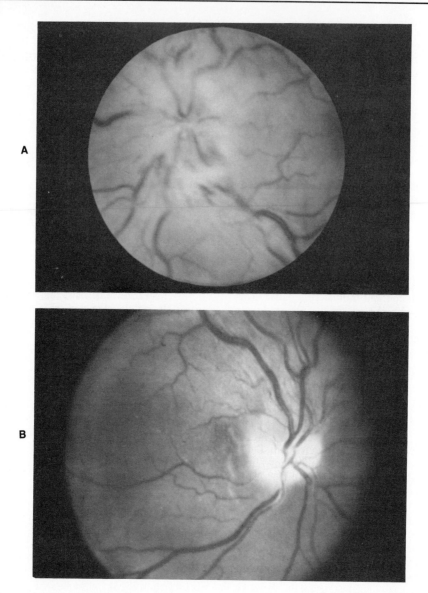

Figure 15–9. Acute ischemic optic atrophy. **A:** Diffuse ischemia. **B:** Old ischemia at bottom, new ischemia at top.

the hyperemic elevated disk becomes grayish-white due to astrocytic gliosis, and neural atrophy with constriction of retinal blood vessels occurs. There can be optociliary shunts and fine exudates or drusen (Fig 15–15). In this situation, there is loss of peripheral visual field, and transient visual obscurations occur.

Papilledema is often asymmetric and will be greater on the side of a supratentorial lesion. It can be strictly unilateral if there is an orbital lesion. Papilledema will occur late in glaucoma and will not occur at all if there is optic atrophy or if the optic nerve sheath on that side is not patent. Foster Kennedy syndrome is papilledema on one side with optic atrophy on the other (optic nerve and sheath compressed by neo-plasm) (Fig 15–15). This is commonly due to meningiomas of the sphenoid wing—classically, to meningiomas of the olfactory groove. However, this clinical presentation can be mimicked (pseudo-Foster Kennedy syndrome) by ischemic optic neuropathy when an old ischemic optic neuropathy with atrophy is associated with a new hyperemic ischemic optic neuropathy.

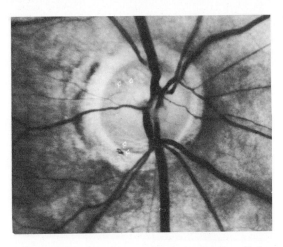

Figure 15–10. Chronic ischemic optic atrophy with loss of neuroglial tissue and exposure of the lamina cribrosa. The pale disk has a shallow cup without nasal displacement of the central retinal vessels. Multiple dark holes are present in the disk surface. The disk is ringed by a zone of choroidal atrophy. The retinal arterioles are narrowed irregularly.

OPTIC NERVE ATROPHY
(Figs 15–12 to 15–15)

Etiologic Classification

A. Vascular: Occlusion of the central retinal vein or artery; arteriosclerotic changes within the optic nerve itself, disturbing its vascular supply; or posthemorrhagic, due to sudden massive blood loss (eg, bleeding peptic ulcer).

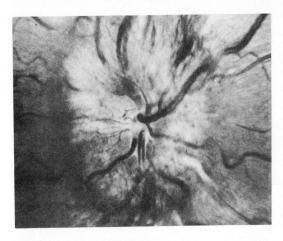

Figure 15–12. Fully developed papilledema. The disk tissue is swollen, elevated, and congested, and the retinal veins are markedly dilated.

B. Degenerative: Consecutive atrophy secondary to retinal disease, with destruction of ganglion cells (eg, retinitis); or as part of a systemic degenerative disease (eg, cerebromacular degeneration).

C. Secondary to papilledema: See p 249.

D. Secondary to optic neuritis (including retrobulbar neuritis): See p 246.

E. Pressure against the optic nerve: Aneurysm of the anterior circle of Willis; bony pressure at the optic foramen (eg, osteitis deformans);

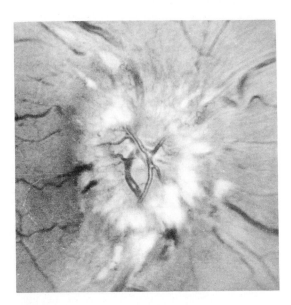

Figure 15–11. Papilledema with opaque (white) patches of swollen nerve fibers and hemorrhages.

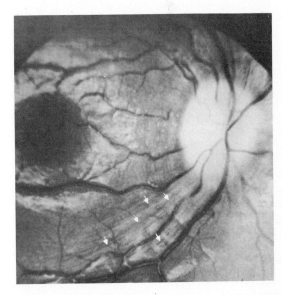

Figure 15–13. Chronic atrophic papilledema in a child with a cerebellar medulloblastoma. The disk is pale and slightly elevated and has blurred margins. The white areas surrounding the macula are reflected light from the vitreoretinal interface. The inferior temporal nerve fiber bundles are partially atrophic (arrows).

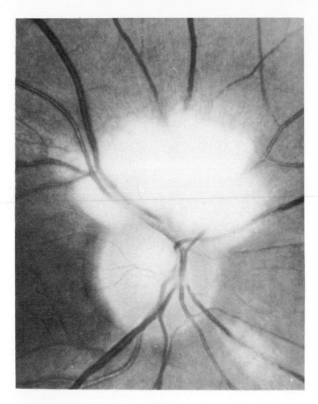

Figure 15–14. Large path of myelinated nerve fibers originating from superior edge of disk. Another smaller patch is present near inferior nasal border of disk. (Right eye.)

intracanalicular, parasellar, or orbital tumors, or even thyroid eye disease.

F. Toxic-nutritional: End result of toxic amblyopia (see below).

G. Metabolic: Eg, diabetes, ganglioside disease.

H. Traumatic: Direct injury to a nerve (ie, severing, avulsion, or contusion).

I. Glaucomatous: See Chapter 12.

Clinical Findings

Loss of vision is the only symptom. Pallor of the optic disk and loss of pupillary reaction are usually proportionate to visual loss except in compressive lesions. Compressive lesions can produce extensive central visual acuity changes and peripheral visual field changes long before there are fundus changes of relative severity, because axons can be dysfunctional long before they become atrophic.

Hereditary optic neuropathies produce bilateral temporal segmental disk pallor with special loss of papillomacular axons. Central retinal artery occlusion produces segmental retinal arteriolar narrowing and loss of the nerve fiber layer in the same distribution. Attenuated retinal blood vessels plus segmental or diffuse disk pallor with or without "glaucomatous" optic nerve cupping can signify a prior ischemic optic neuropathy. Peripapillary exudates are the hallmark of papillitis and occasionally papilledema. Peripapil-

lary atrophy, chorioretinal folds, and internal limiting membrane wrinkling can also be helpful signs of prior disk edema.

Treatment, Course, & Prognosis

Changes in visual function occur very slowly over weeks or months. It is difficult to assess prognosis on the basis of ophthalmoscopic findings alone. Even with experimental chiasmal section, it can take 2 months for axonal degeneration to extend from the chiasm to the retinal ganglion cell. Treatment is variable depending on the cause, as are the course and prognosis.

TOXIC-NUTRITIONAL AMBLYOPIA

1. TOBACCO-ALCOHOL AMBLYOPIA

Nutritional amblyopia is the preferred term for the entity sometimes referred to as tobacco-alcohol amblyopia. Persons with poor dietary habits—particularly if the diet is deficient in thiamine—may develop centrocecal scotomas that are usually of constant density. When density of the scotoma varies, the most dense portion usually lies between fixation and the blind spot in the papillomacular bundle.

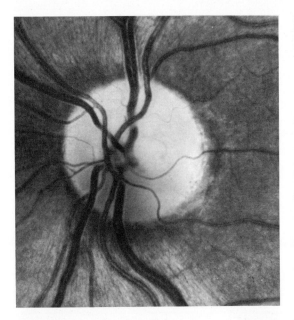
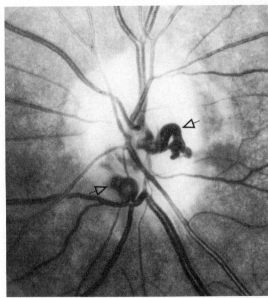
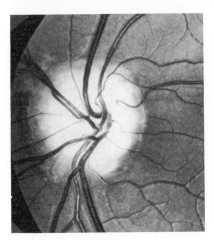
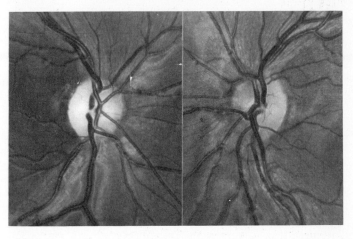

Figure 15–15. Examples of optic atrophy. ***Upper left:*** Primary optic atrophy due to nutritional amblyopia. ***Upper right:*** Secondary optic atrophy with optociliary shunts (arrows) due to optic nerve sheath meningioma. ***Lower left:*** Optic atrophy with optic disk drusen. ***Lower right:*** Pallor (atrophy) of right optic disk due to nerve compression by sphenoid meningioma. The left disk is normal.

Heavy drinking with or without heavy smoking is most often associated with a poor nutritional state. Bilateral loss of central vision is present in over 50% of patients, reducing visual acuity below 20/200. Most of the others have severe central loss in one eye with some deficit—often about 20/50 visual acuity—in the better eye. Central visual fields reveal scotomas that nearly always include both fixation and the blind spot (centrocecal scotoma) (Fig 15–16). Pallor of the optic disks may be present (Fig 15–15). Loss of the ganglion cells of the macula and destruction of myelinated fibers of the optic nerve—and sometimes of the chiasm as well—are the main histologic changes.

Much consideration has been given in the literature to other toxic causes such as cyanide intoxication from tobacco, producing low vitamin stores and low levels of sulfur-containing amino acids, but experimental studies with cyanide in primates have not confirmed this hypothesis. Rarely, multiple sclerosis, pernicious anemia, methanol poisoning, retrobulbar neuritis, or macular degeneration may cause diagnostic confusion.

Adequate diet plus thiamine, folic acid, and vitamin B_{12} is nearly always effective in completely curing the disease if it is recognized early. Withdrawal of tobacco and alcohol is advisable and may hasten the cure, but innumerable cases are known in which adequate nutrition alone effected the cure despite continued excessive intake of alcohol or tobacco. Improvement usually begins within 1–2 months,

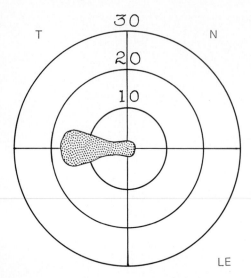

Figure 15–16. Nutritional amblyopia showing centrocecal scotoma. VA = 20/200.

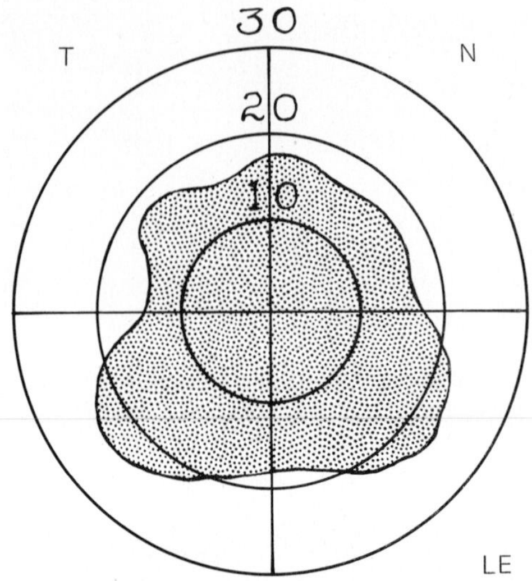

Figure 15–17. Methyl alcohol amblyopia showing very large centrocecal scotoma. VA = hand movements only.

although in occasional cases significant improvement may not occur for a year. Visual function may not return to normal; permanent optic atrophy or at least optic disk pallor can occur depending upon the stage of disease at the time treatment was started. If there has been neuronal degeneration, permanent dysfunction results.

2. AMBLYOPIA DUE TO DRUG TOXICITY

Ethambutol, isoniazid (INH), rifampin, and disulfiram can all produce a clinical picture similar to that of retrobulbar neuritis that will improve upon stopping the drug with or without nutritional supplements.

Chronic lead exposure can produce a toxic effect on the optic nerve. Thallium is present in many depilatory creams and can produce nutritional amblyopia.

Quinine can cause optic neuropathy with severely narrowed retinal arterioles as well.

3. AMBLYOPIA DUE TO METHANOL POISONING

Methanol is used widely in the chemical industry as antifreeze, solvent varnish, or paint remover; it is also present in fumes of some industrial solvents such as those used in old Xerox machines. Significant systemic absorption can occur from inhaled fumes in a room with inadequate ventilation and rarely through the skin.

Clinical Findings

The principal manifestations of methanol poisoning are visual disturbances and acidosis. The metabolites

of methanol are formic acid and formaldehyde, which produce acidosis and cause gastroenteritis, pulmonary edema, and retinal ganglion cell and diffuse retinal damage.

Visual impairment may be the first sign; it begins with mild blurring of vision and progresses to contraction of visual fields and sometimes to complete blindness. Visual disturbances range from "spots before the eyes" to complete blindness. The field defects are quite extensive and nearly always include the centrocecal area (Fig 15–17).

Hyperemia of the disk is the first ophthalmoscopic finding. Within the first 2 days, a whitish, striated edema of the disk margins and nearby retina appears. Disk edema may last up to 2 months and is followed by optic atrophy of mild to severe degree (Fig 15–18).

Decreased pupillary response to light occurs in proportion to the amount of visual loss. In severe cases, the pupils become dilated and fixed. Extraocular muscle palsies and ptosis may also occur.

Treatment

Treatment consists of correction of acidosis with intravenous sodium bicarbonate and oral or intravenous ethanol to compete with and prevent the slower metabolism of methanol into its by-products. Hemodialysis is indicated for blood methanol levels over 50 mg/dL.

GENETICALLY DETERMINED OPTIC ATROPHY

1. LEBER'S OPTIC NEUROPATHY

This rare disease, characterized by sequential, rapidly progressive optic neuropathy, occurs in young

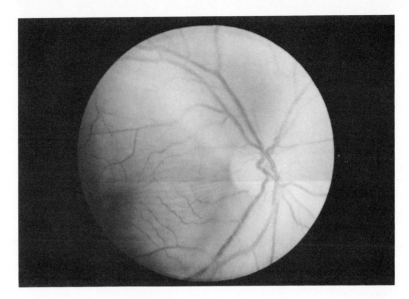

Figure 15–18. Methanol poisoning.

men aged 20–30 years (occasionally in women). It has classically been considered to be due to an X-linked recessive gene, but instead it may be an example of cytoplasmic inheritance. Blurred vision and a central scotoma appear in one eye, followed within days, weeks, or months by the other eye. The diagnosis of this familial disorder can only be confirmed during the acute episode by documenting a hyperemic edematous disk that does not leak during fluorescein injection despite the fact that it has many dilated capillary telangiectasias on its surface and on the immediate peripapillary retina. The nerve fiber layer around the disk can appear gray, due to the pseudo-edema of axonal congestion. Eventually, both optic nerves will become atrophic, and vision may be about 20/200 or better. Total loss of vision or recurrences of visual loss do not occur.

Leber's optic neuropathy can also be associated with the heredofamilial ataxias as well as cardiac and skeletal anomalies.

2. CONGENITAL OR INFANTILE HEREDITARY OPTIC ATROPHY

This disorder occurs in a severe autosomal recessive form and a milder autosomal dominant form. The recessive form is present at birth or appears within 2 years and is accompanied by nystagmus. The more common dominant form has an insidious onset in childhood, with little progression thereafter. There is characteristically a centrocecal scotoma with variable loss of central visual acuity.

The dominant form may be associated with congenital or progressive deafness and ataxia. The recessive form may be associated with progressive hear-

ing loss, spastic quadriplegia, and dementia, although an inborn error of metabolism must be first considered. There is also a recessive optic atrophy associated with juvenile diabetes mellitus, diabetes insipidus, and hearing loss.

3. OPTIC ATROPHY WITH NEURODEGENERATIVE DISEASES

Various neurodegenerative diseases can begin in childhood to early adult life and have steadily progressive neurologic and visual signs. Included among this group are the hereditary ataxias and Charcot-Marie-Tooth disease. Most of the sphingolipidoses late in their course are associated with optic atrophy. The leukodystrophies (Krabbe's dystrophy, metachromatic leukodystrophy, Pelizaeus-Merzbacher disease, Schilder's disease) are associated with optic atrophy earlier. Canavan's spongy degeneration and glioneuronal dystrophy (Alpers' disease) are associated with optic atrophy as well.

OPTIC NERVE ANOMALIES

Tilted disks, optic nerve hypoplasia, dysplasia, and coloboma are all congenital optic nerve anomalies. Closure of the fetal fissure, ocular melanogenesis, and disk development occur at the same time as development of the skull, face, and limbs. Accordingly, tilted disks, which occur in 3% of normal patients, may be seen with hypertelorism or the craniofacial dysostoses (Crouzon's disease, Apert's disease). They

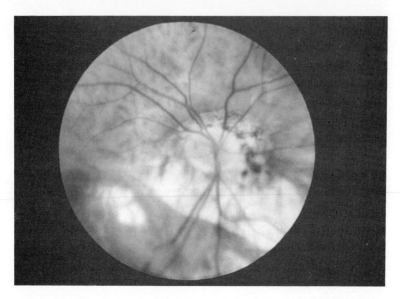

Figure 15–19. Tilted disk.

are oval disks with a usually inferior crescent and usually an associated area of fundus hypopigmentation (Fig 15–19).

Optic nerve hypoplasia, dysplasia, and coloboma have all been associated with basal encephaloceles as well as with varying intracranial anomalies ranging from Duane's refraction syndrome to agenesis of the corpus callosum. Hypoplastic optic nerves are small optic nerves with normal-sized retinal blood vessels (Fig 15–20). They are associated with a wide range of visual acuity losses, a peripapillary halo that may have a pigmented rim, and visual field defects. Dysplastic optic disks usually are associated with poor vision and show abnormal vasculature, retinal pigment epithelium, and glial tissue. They are often surrounded by a chorioretinal pigmentary disturbance. Colobomas of the optic nerve have been called "pseudoglaucoma" because of their resemblance to glaucomatous cupping.

THE OPTIC CHIASM

Anatomy

The optic chiasm is variably situated near the top of the diaphragm of the sella turcica (most often posteriorly, projecting 1 cm above it and at a 45-degree angle upward from the optic nerves as they emerge from the optic canals) (Fig 15–21). The lamina terminalis forms the anterior wall of the third ventricle. The internal carotid arteries lie just laterally, adjacent to the cavernous sinuses. The chiasm is made up of the junction of the 2 optic nerves and provides for crossing of the nasal fibers to the opposite optic tract and passage of temporal fibers to the ipsilateral optic tract. The macular fibers are arranged similarly to the rest of the fibers except that their decussation is farther posteriorly and superiorly. In general, lesions of the chiasm cause bitemporal hemianopic defects. Early, these defects are typically incomplete and often asymmetric. However, as compression progresses, the nasal field may then be involved and central visual acuity may be decreased. The chiasm receives many small blood vessels from the neighboring circle of Willis. Thus, most processes that affect it are neoplastic, with vascular or inflammatory processes only occasionally producing chiasmatic visual field loss.

PITUITARY TUMORS

The anterior lobe of the pituitary gland is the site of origin of pituitary tumors (Fig 15–22). Symptoms and signs include loss of vision, field changes, pituitary dysfunction, extraocular nerve palsies, and evidence on CT scan of seller and suprasellar tumors.

Combination therapy with radiation and surgery is now being challenged by medical treatment with bromocriptine, which has been effective classically in tumors associated with galactorrhea but also in some null cell (not endocrinologically active) tumors. Visual loss or endocrine dysfunction is an indication for treatment. Visual acuity and visual fields may improve dramatically after pressure has been removed from the chiasm. The appearance of the fundus does not predict the ultimate visual outcome.

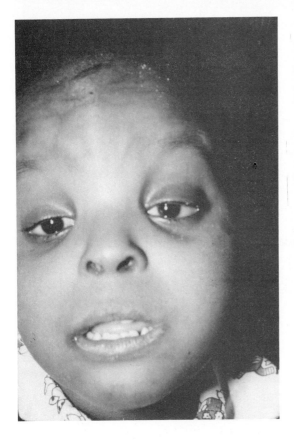

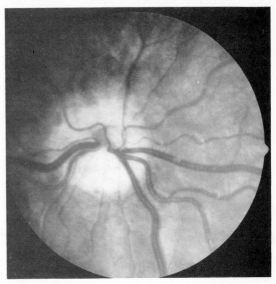

Figure 15–20. *At left:* Hypertelorism. ***Above:*** Optic nerve hypoplasia.

CRANIOPHARYNGIOMA

Craniopharyngiomas are an uncommon group of tumors arising from epithelial remnants of Rathke's pouch (80% of the population normally have such remnants) and characteristically become symptomatic between the ages of 10 and 25 years. They are usually suprasellar, occasionally intrasellar. The signs and symptoms vary tremendously with the age of the patient and the exact location of the tumor as well as its rate of growth. When a suprasellar tumor occurs, asymmetric chiasmal or tract field defects are prominent. Papilledema is more common than is the case in pituitary tumors. Optic nerve hypoplasia can be seen in tumors presenting in infancy. Pituitary deficiency may result, and involvement of the hypothalamus may cause stunted growth. Calcification of parts of the tumor contributes to a characteristic appearance on CT scan, especially in children.

Treatment consists of surgical removal—as complete as possible at the first procedure, since reoperation tends to involve the hypothalamus and the patients then do poorly.

SUPRASELLAR MENINGIOMAS

Suprasellar meningiomas arise from the meninges covering the tuberculum sellae and the planum sphenoidale. A high proportion of patients are female. The tumor is usually anterior and superior to the chiasm, and visual field changes are frequent. The optic nerves and chiasm are often involved early (but asymmetrically) in the slowly progressive damage to the visual pathway. CT scans with contrast enhancement easily demonstrate these tumors (Fig 15–23). Bony hyperostoses associated with bony erosion and a dense calcified tumor are the radiologic hallmarks of the meningioma. Treatment consists of surgical removal at this time.

GLIOMA OF THE OPTIC CHIASM & OPTIC NERVE

Optic nerve and chiasmal gliomas are rare, usually indolent disorders of childhood that sometimes occur as part of the clinical picture of neurofibromatosis.

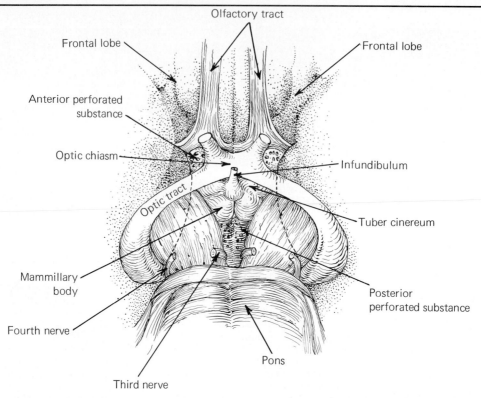

Figure 15–21. Relationship of optic chiasm from inferior aspect. (Redrawn and reproduced, with permission, from Duke-Elder WS: *System of Ophthalmology.* Vol 2. Mosby, 1961.)

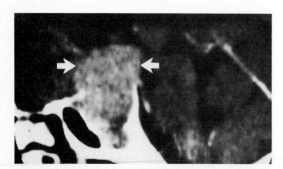

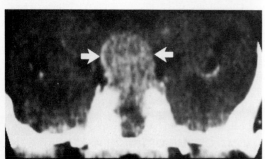

Figure 15–22. Pituitary adenoma with suprasellar extension (arrows) causing bitemporal hemianopia. CT scans with contrast enhancement. Sagittal re-formation *(top).* Coronal re-formation *(bottom).*

Onset may be sudden, with rapid loss of vision. Optic atrophy occurs, and visual field defects reveal an optic nerve or chiasmal syndrome. CT scans may reveal enlarged optic nerves and a mass in the region of the chiasm and hypothalamus. Treatment is variable depending on the location of the tumor and its clinical course. Irradiation can be given during a tumor growth spurt, and optic nerve resection is sometimes done when an optic nerve tumor starts to extend intracranially.

THE RETROCHIASMAL VISUAL PATHWAYS

Anatomy

Each optic tract begins at the posterolateral angle of the chiasm and sweeps around the upper part of the cerebral peduncle to end in the lateral geniculate nucleus. Afferent pupillary fibers leave the tract just anterior to the nucleus and pass via the brachium of the superior colliculus to the midbrain. (The pupillary pathway is diagrammed in Fig 15–24.) Afferent visual

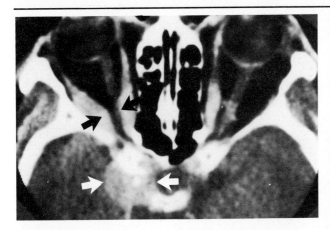
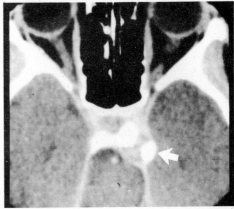
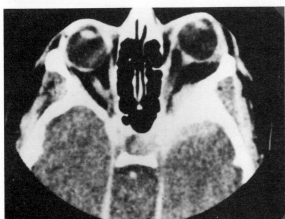
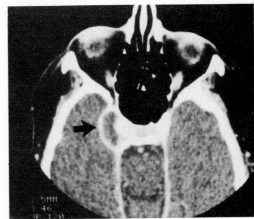

Figure 15–23. CT scans of 4 patients with eye signs of basal cranial tumors. ***Upper left:*** Optic nerve compression due to thyroid myopathy (black arrows) and meningioma (white arrows). ***Upper right:*** Sixth nerve palsy due to chordoma of petrous tip (arrow). ***Lower left:*** Proptosis due to sphenoid ridge meningioma. ***Lower right:*** Third nerve palsy due to intracavernous aneurysm (black arrow).

fibers terminate on cells in the lateral geniculate nucleus that give rise to the geniculocalcarine tract. This tract traverses the posterior limb of the internal capsule and then fans out into a broad bundle called the optic radiation. The fibers in this bundle curve backward around the anterior aspect of the temporal horn of the lateral ventricle and then medially to reach the calcarine cortex of the occipital lobe, where they terminate. The most inferior fibers, which carry projections from the superior aspect of the contralateral half of the visual field, course anteriorly into the temporal lobe in a configuration known as Meyer's loop. Lesions of the temporal lobe that extend 5 cm back from the anterior tip involve these fibers and can produce superior quadrantanopic field defects.

The primary visual cortex (area 17) occupies the upper and lower lips and the depths of the calcarine fissure on the medial aspect of the occipital lobe. Each lobe receives input from the 2 ipsilateral half-retinas, representing the contralateral half of the binocular visual field. Projection of the visual field onto the visual cortex occurs in a precise and orderly retinotopic pattern. The macula is represented at the medial posterior pole, and the peripheral parts of the retina project to the most anterior part of the calcarine cortex. Area 18 is a connection area to areas 17 and 19 through interhemispheric pathways. Area 19 is a visual association or integration area that really lies in the posterior parietal and posterior temporal lobe and is associated with pursuit or following eye movements.

LESIONS OF THE RETROCHIASMAL PATHWAYS

Cerebrovascular diseases and tumors are responsible for most lesions of the retrochiasmal visual pathways, although almost any intracranial disease process can involve these structures. Retrochiasmal visual field defects are homonymous. Partial lesions in the optic tract and lateral genicular nucleus produce incongruous (dissimilar) visual field defects due to a medial rotation of axons in each tract and to the fact that half of them have just decussated through the chiasm. Thus, there may be more involvement of a nasal hemifield than its corresponding temporal

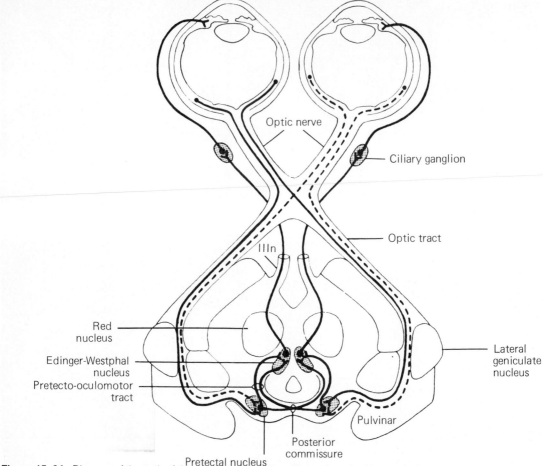

Figure 15–24. Diagram of the path of the pupillary light reflex. (Reproduced, with permission, from Walsh FB, Hoyt WF: *Clinical Neuro-ophthalmology*, 3rd ed. Vol 1. Williams & Wilkins, 1969.)

hemifield. Once the lesion becomes complete, however, incongruity cannot be assessed, and this sign loses its localizing ability. Retrochiasmal visual field defects should spare visual acuity, since the visual pathway from the other hemibrain is intact. The optic tracts and lateral geniculate nucleus are infrequently affected. After several weeks to months, the disks may appear pale, and the retinal nerve fiber layer is deficient. The optic tract and lateral geniculate have at least a dual blood supply, so that primary vascular lesions are uncommon. Most cases are due to trauma, tumors, arteriovenous malformations, abscesses, and demyelinating diseases.

Lesions involving the geniculocalcarine pathway to the occipital cortex produce homonymous field defects but do not result in optic atrophy (because of the synapse at the geniculate). Generally, the more posterior a lesion is located, the more congruous the homonymous visual field defect. The inferior geniculocalcarine pathway passes through the temporal lobe and the superior pathway through the parietal lobe, with macular function between them. Lesions of the inferior pathway project into superior visual

fields. Processes affecting the anterior and midtemporal lobe are commonly neoplastic; posterior temporal lobe and parietal processes can be either vascular or neoplastic. An insidious onset with mild and multiple neurologic deficits would be more typically neoplastic, whereas an acute cataclysmic neurologic event would be more typically vascular. Vascular lesions of the occipital lobe, on the other hand, are common and account for over 80% of cases of isolated homonymous visual field loss in patients over age 50 years. Optokinetic nystagmus is generated cortically by occipital association area 19, which anatomically lies in vascular territory of the middle cerebral artery and the posterior parietal area; it will be abnormal with parietal lesions but normal with occipital vascular lesions. This clinical sign will also suggest an occipital tumor if it is positive or asymmetric with an occipital visual field defect, thus suggesting a process not related to the vascular anatomy of the occipital lobe and extending into the parietal lobe, as tumors do. CT scans demonstrate vascular and neoplastic disease of the occipital lobe with remarkable clarity (Figs 15–25 and 15–26).

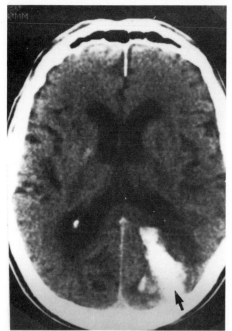

Figure 15–25. Occipital hematoma (arrow) resulting from a bleeding arteriovenous malformation. This lesion produced homonymous hemianopia and headache.

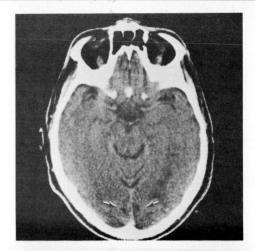

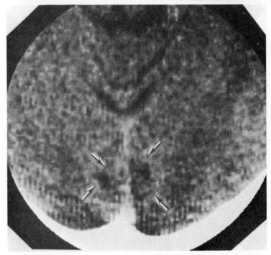

Figure 15–26. CT scans showing bilateral small infarctions of the visual cortex causing a ringlike scotoma in the middle field of vision. ***Top:*** Axial section. ***Bottom:*** Magnified view of the occipital cortex. The infarcted areas appear as zones of low density between the splenium and the occipital pole.

THE PUPIL

The size of the normal pupil varies at different ages and from person to person. The normal pupillary diameter is usually about 3–4 mm—smaller in infancy, tending to be larger in childhood, and again progressively smaller with advancing age. Many normal persons have a slight difference in pupil size—usually about 0.5 mm—in the 2 eyes (physiologic anisocoria). Mydriatic and cycloplegic drugs work more effectively on blue eyes than on brown eyes.

The function of the pupil is to control the amount of light entering the eye so as to give best visual function under varying degrees of light intensity. The pathways controlling this purely reflex function are described below and diagrammed in Fig 15–2.

Neuroanatomy of the Pupillary Pathways

Evaluation of pupillary reactions is important in localizing lesions involving the optic pathways. The examiner should be familiar with the neuroanatomy of the pathway for reaction of the pupil to light and the miosis associated with accommodation (Fig 15–24.

A. Light Reflex: The pathway for the light reflex is entirely subcortical. The afferent pupillary fibers are included within the optic nerve and pathway until they leave the optic tract just before the visual fibers synapse in the lateral geniculate body. They go to the pretectal area of the midbrain and synapse in the pretectal nucleus. Each pretectal nucleus then sends a neuron to the ipsilateral and contralateral Edinger-Westphal nucleus through the posterior commissure and periaqueductal gray matter. The efferent pathway is via the third nerve to the ciliary ganglion in the lateral orbit. The postganglionic fiber goes via the short ciliary nerves to innervate the sphincter muscle of the iris.

B. The Near Reflex: When the eyes look at a near object, 3 reactions occur—accommodation, convergence, and constriction of the pupil—bringing a sharp image into focus on corresponding retinal points. There is convincing evidence that the final common pathway is mediated through the oculomotor nerve with a synapse in the ciliary ganglion. The afferent pathway has not been worked out, but there is evidence that it enters the midbrain ventral to the Edinger-Westphal nucleus and sends fibers to both sides of the cortex. Although the 3 components are closely associated, the near reflex cannot be considered a pure reflex since each component can be neutralized while leaving the other 2 intact—ie, by prism (neutralizing convergence), by lenses (neutralizing accommodation), and by weak mydriatic drugs (neutralizing miosis).

ARGYLL ROBERTSON PUPIL

A typical Argyll Robertson pupil is strongly suggestive of central nervous system syphilis associated with tabes dorsalis or general paresis. The pupil is less than 3 mm in diameter (miotic), does not respond to light stimulation, and does constrict with accommodation. This finding is nearly always bilateral. The pupils are commonly irregular and eccentric and dilate poorly with mydriatics because of concomitant iris atrophy. Less commonly, the sign is incomplete (slow response to light) or unilateral. Some degree of Argyll Robertson pupil is present in over 50% of patients with central nervous system syphilis. A wide variety of other central nervous system diseases infrequently cause incomplete Argyll Robertson pupil. These include diabetes, chronic alcoholism, encephalitis, multiple sclerosis, central nervous system degenerative disease, and tumors of the midbrain. The periaqueductal gray matter of the midbrain is the usual site of the lesion and thus affects the light reflex. The near reflex pathway is more ventral and is spared.

TONIC PUPIL

Tonic pupil occurs because of an abnormal pupillary constrictor mechanism, in which the sphincter muscle contracts slowly (tonically) to near stimulation and little or not at all to direct light stimulation. It may be associated with loss of deep tendon reflexes (Adie's syndrome). It results from damage to the ciliary ganglion. A weak (0.1%) solution of pilocarpine instilled into the conjunctival sac causes a tonic pupil to constrict as a result of denervation hypersensitivity; normal pupils are not affected. The tonic pupil dilates slowly in the dark and reacts promptly to mydriatics.

HORNER'S SYNDROME

Horner's syndrome is caused by a lesion of the sympathetic pathway in the brain stem, upper spinal cord, or peripheral sympathetic chain, each representing a limb of a 3-neuronal loop. Unilateral miosis, ptosis, and absence of sweating on the ipsilateral face and neck make up the complete syndrome. Causes of Horner's syndrome include cervical vertebral fractures, tabes dorsalis, syringomyelia, cervical cord tumor, apical bronchogenic carcinoma, aneurysm of the carotid or subclavian artery, neck injuries, and injuries to the carotid artery high in the neck. Pharmacologic testing with topical cocaine in the conjunctival sac can differentiate Horner's syndrome from central anisocoria, and hydroxyamphetamine (Paredrine) can further localize the process to a postganglionic neuron. This helps in sorting through the many causes of Horner's syndrome that may be specific to each neuronal arc.

AFFERENT PUPILLARY DEFECT

Light entering the right eye decussates at the chiasm to the left tract as well as continuing into the right tract, and the same is true on the left side. As the pupillary light pathways enter the midbrain to the pretectal nucleus, they again decussate as each pretectal nucleus connects to the ipsilateral and contralateral Edinger-Westphal nucleus. For this reason, light shone into the right eye produces an immediate direct response in the right eye and an immediate indirect or consensual response in the left eye (Fig 15–27). The intensity of this response in each eye is proportionate to the light-carrying ability of the optic nerve stimulated directly.

One of the most important assessments to make in the patient complaining of decreased vision is whether it is due to a local ocular problem—eg, cataract—or to a more serious optic nerve problem. Even dense cataracts do not change the afferent light pathways to the brain, so that comparison is possible. If an optic nerve lesion is present, the direct light response in the involved eye is less intense than the consensual response (in the involved eye) evoked when the normal eye is stimulated. (If both optic nerves are equally affected, there is no relative difference in light-carrying ability.) This phenomenon is called an afferent pupillary defect, or Marcus Gunn pupil (Fig 15–28). Causes of unilateral decreased vision without an afferent pupillary defect include refractive error, cloudy media (cataract), amblyopia, hysteria or malingering, macular lesions, and chiasmal problems.

Amaurotic pupil is the term applied to an eye that does not even see light because of severe unilateral retinal or optic nerve disease. Obviously, a blind eye would not have a direct light response, nor could it induce a consensual response in the normal eye. However, a light shone directly into the normal eye would induce a direct response there and a consensual response in the blind eye (Fig 15–29).

EXTRAOCULAR MOVEMENTS

This section deals with the neural apparatus that controls the movements of the eyes and causes them

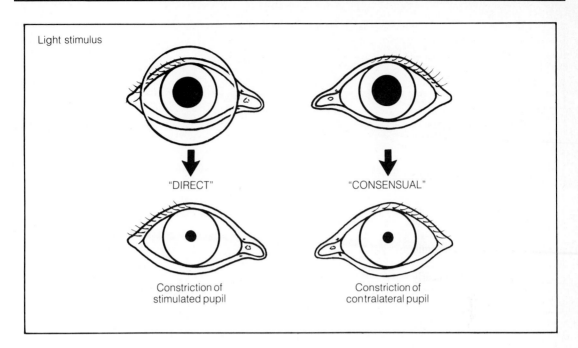

Figure 15–27. Normal pupillary light reactions test.

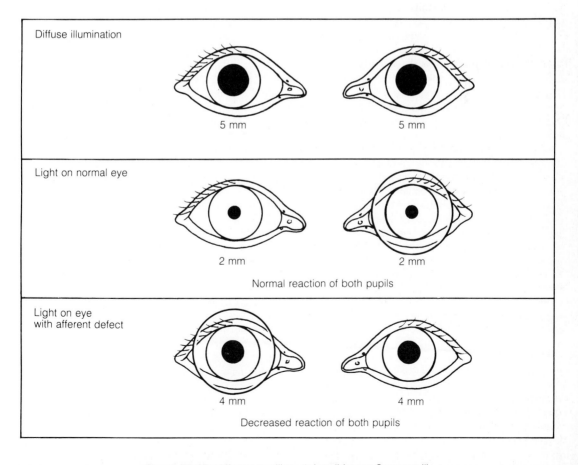

Figure 15–28. Afferent pupillary defect (Marcus Gunn pupil).

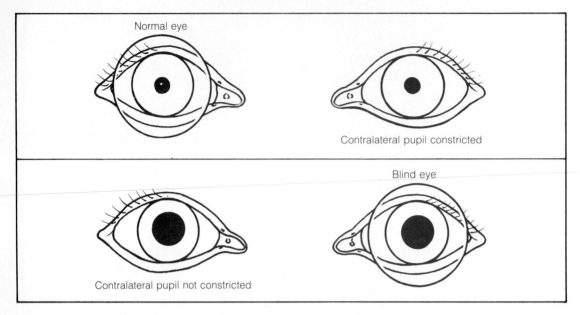

Figure 15–29. Amaurotic pupillary response.

to move simultaneously in tandem up or down and from side to side as well as in convergence or divergence.

THE SUPRANUCLEAR PATHWAYS

The supranuclear neural pathways of the extraocular muscles innervate conjugate lateral and vertical gaze as well as the disjunctive movements of convergence and divergence. They consist of central nervous system connections to the nuclei of cranial nerves III, IV, and VI located in the midbrain. The highest centers for these functions are located in the frontal lobe (fast or saccadic movement) and the occipital lobe (smooth or pursuit movement) (Fig 15–31).

Fast eye movements (saccades) are voluntary or involuntary refixation movements, the fast phase of vestibular nystagmus, optokinetic nystagmus, and microsaccades. This system is tested by command refixation movements and by the fast phase of vestibular nystagmus and optokinetic nystagmus.

Slow eye movements (pursuit) are involved in tracking a slowly moving target once the saccadic system places it on the fovea. This system is tested by asking a patient to follow a slowly and smoothly moving target and by the following or slow phase of optokinetic nystagmus.

Anatomy of Voluntary Conjugate Movements

A. Horizontal: The location of the cortical center that controls horizontal saccadic conjugate movements of the eyes is situated in the frontal lobe (frontal eye field area 8). The pathway descends through the basal ganglia and the anterior limb of the internal capsule into the brain stem and crosses to the opposite side of the pons into the paramedian pontine reticular formation. The ipsilateral lateral rectus and contralateral medial rectus muscles are stimulated to produce ipsilateral conjugate movement (Fig 15–30). This pathway then connects to the ipsilateral medial longitudinal fasciculus.

B. Vertical: The centers and pathways are probably the same as for horizontal movement, except that the subcortical pathway terminates in the pretectal area. The impulses then go to the medial longitudinal fasciculus and are distributed to the appropriate oculomotor nuclei to effect vertical gaze.

C. Vergence: It is probable that the supranuclear impulses for convergence travel much the same pathway as do those for conjugate horizontal and vertical gaze, arriving at a midbrain synapse near or in the oculomotor nucleus. From this synapse, stimulating impulses go to each medial rectus, and inhibitory impulses go to each lateral rectus via the medial longitudinal fasciculus. Supranuclear disease states and trauma can present as convergence insufficiency and bifocal failures. It is probable that the cerebellum integrates all of this oculomotor input and ultimately mediates gaze; defects in this neural integration probably result in nystagmus.

Electromyography has established divergence as an active process (not a relaxation of convergence, as was once thought). The supranuclear pathway is probably more or less the same as for convergence, arriving at a midbrain center and then proceeding to the sixth nerve nuclei.

D. Pursuit: Pursuit (following) eye movements originate in the occipital cortex in area 19 (Brodmann),

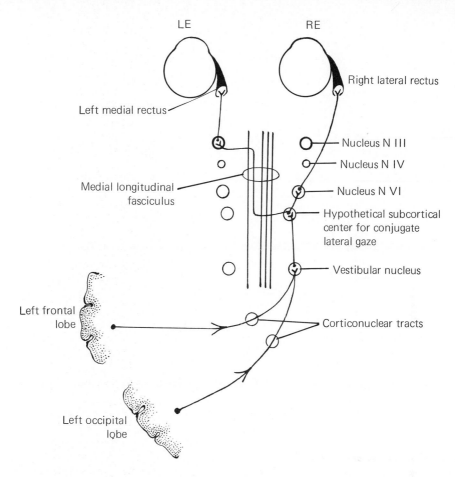

LE   RE

Right lateral rectus

Left medial rectus

Nucleus N III

Nucleus N IV

Medial longitudinal fasciculus

Nucleus N VI

Hypothetical subcortical center for conjugate lateral gaze

Vestibular nucleus

Left frontal lobe

Corticonuclear tracts

Left occipital lobe

Figure 15–30. Conjugate gaze. The impulses for voluntary conjugate movements in right lateral gaze are initiated in the left frontal lobe. Involuntary conjugate movements in right lateral gaze are initiated in the left occipital lobe or, according to recent reports, the ipsilateral occipital lobe. (After Spiegel and Sommer. Redrawn with modifications and reproduced, with permission, from Moses R: *Adler's Physiology of the Eye,* 5th ed. Mosby, 1970.)

descend through the posterior limb of the internal capsule through the midbrain and superior colliculus, and end in the ipsilateral paramedian pontine reticular formation (PPRF). The PPRF projects to the frontal eye fields for fast eye movements as well (this helps coordinate the optokinetic nystagmus response). The flocculus of the cerebellum and other cerebellar areas also project to the ipsilateral paramedian pontine reticular formation and help synthesize gaze to provide smooth tracking.

1. LESIONS OF THE SUPRANUCLEAR PATHWAYS

Frontal Lobe

A seizure focus in the frontal lobe may cause involuntary turning of the eyes to the opposite side. Destructive lesions cause transient deviation to the same side, and the eyes cannot be turned voluntarily to the opposite (saccadic) side. This is called frontal gaze palsy. Ocular pursuit to the opposite side is retained. There is no diplopia.

Occipital Lobe

Smooth ocular pursuit may be lost with posterior lesions of the hemispheres. The patient is unable to follow a slowly moving object in the direction of the gaze palsy. The command (fast) eye movement is not lost, and pursuit is saccadic.

A. Midbrain (Thalamus): Lesions of the posterior commissure cause impairment of conjugate upgaze. Lesions dorsal and medial to the red nuclei (trauma, infarcts) produce downgaze paresis.

B. Parinaud's Syndrome (Pretectal Syndrome): This syndrome is characterized by loss of voluntary upward gaze and convergence-retraction nystagmus and (frequently) loss of the pupillary light response with retention of miosis in response to the near reflex. Convergence-retraction movements of the globe on attempted upward gaze are due to cofiring of the rectus muscles as a result of loss of supranuclear

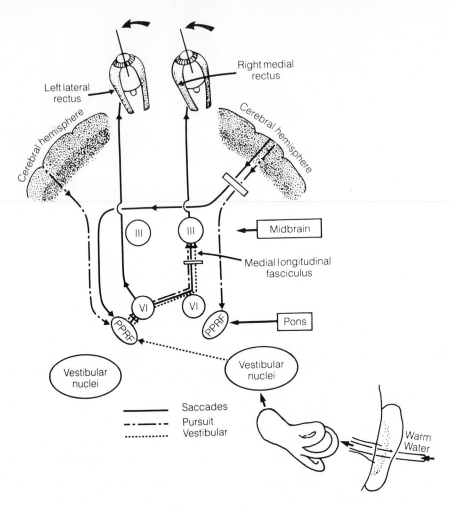

Figure 15–31. Nystagmus.

control. There may also be an apparent accommodative spasm, loss of conjugate voluntary downward gaze associated with loss of convergence and accommodation, ptosis or lid retraction, papilledema, or third nerve palsy. Surrounding structures may also be involved, depending upon the size and location of the lesion. Conjugate horizontal ocular movements are usually not affected. The syndrome results from tectal or pretectal lesions affecting the periaqueductal area. Pinealomas, infiltrating gliomas, vascular lesions, demyelinating disease, and trauma may produce this picture.

Pons

Lesions of the paramedian pontine reticular formation produce an ipsilateral saccadic and pursuit gaze palsy since the formation is the final resting place for both functions; PPRF lesions recover only slowly and incompletely, in contrast to supranuclear lesions. A patient so afflicted would have an asymmetric response on caloric testing.

Lesions of the brain stem are common causes of gaze palsies. The lesions most often encountered (in order of frequency) are vascular accidents, arteriovenous malformations, multiple sclerosis, tumors (pontine gliomas, cerebellopontine angle tumors), and encephalitis.

2. SUPRANUCLEAR SYNDROMES INVOLVING DISJUNCTIVE OCULAR MOVEMENTS

Spasm of the Near Reflex

The near reflex consists of 3 components: convergence, accommodation, and constriction of the pupil. Spasm of the near reflex is usually caused by hysteria, although encephalitis, tabes dorsalis, and meningitis may cause spasm by irritation of the supranuclear pathway. It is characterized by convergent strabismus with diplopia, miotic pupils, and spasm of accommodation.

If hysteria is the cause, atropine 1%, 2 drops in each eye twice daily, or minus (concave) lenses may give temporary relief. Psychiatric consultation is indicated for treatment of an underlying mental cause.

Convergence Paralysis

Convergence paralysis is characterized by a sudden onset of diplopia for near vision, with absence of any individual extraocular muscle palsy. It is caused by hysteria or destructive lesions of the supranuclear pathway for convergence. Multiple sclerosis, myasthenia gravis, head trauma, encephalitis, tabes dorsalis, tumors, aneurysms, minor cerebrovascular accidents, and Parkinson's disease are the most common organic causes.

3. NUCLEAR & INFRANUCLEAR CONNECTIONS

Peripheral & Intermediate Connections of the Nuclei of Cranial Nerves III, IV, & VI

A. Oculomotor (III): The motor fibers arise from a group of nuclei (Edinger-Westphal) in the central gray matter ventral to the cerebral aqueduct at the level of the superior colliculus. Mainly uncrossed fibers (superior rectus axons cross from the nucleus to the contralateral third nerve) course through the red nucleus and the inner side of the substantia nigra to emerge on the medial side of the cerebral peduncles. The nerve runs alongside the sella turcica, in the outer wall of the cavernous sinus, and through the superior orbital fissure to supply the medial, superior, and inferior rectus muscles and the inferior oblique and levator palpebrae muscles.

The parasympathetics arise from the Edinger-Westphal nucleus just rostral to the motor nucleus of the third nerve and pass via the inferior division of the third nerve to the ciliary ganglion. From there the short ciliary nerves are distributed to the sphincter muscle of the iris and to the ciliary muscle, which controls the shape of the lens during accommodation.

B. Trochlear (IV): Motor (entirely crossed) fibers arise from the trochlear nucleus just caudal to the third nerve at the level of the inferior colliculus, run posteriorly, decussate in the anterior medullary velum, and wind around the cerebral peduncles. The fourth nerve travels near the third nerve along the wall of the cavernous sinus to the orbit, where it supplies the superior oblique muscle.

C. Abducens (VI): Motor (entirely uncrossed) fibers arise from the nucleus in the floor of the fourth ventricle in the lower portion of the pons near the internal genu of the facial nerve. Piercing the pons, the fibers emerge anteriorly, the nerve running a long course over the tip of the petrous portion of the temporal bone into the cavernous sinus. It enters the orbit with the third and fourth nerves to supply the lateral rectus muscle.

Central Reflex Connections of the Nuclei of Cranial Nerves III, IV, & VI

The central reflex connections of these nuclei originate in 5 areas:

(1) From the pretectal region via the posterior commissure to the Edinger-Westphal nuclei for mediation of ipsilateral and consensual light reflexes. Interruption of this pathway may cause Argyll Robertson pupil.

(2) From the superior colliculi via the tectobulbar tract to the nuclei of cranial nerves III, IV, and VI for mediation of miosis associated with accommodation.

(3) From the inferior colliculi via the tectobulbar tract to the eye muscle nuclei for reflexes correlated with hearing.

(4) From the vestibular nuclei via the medial longitudinal fasciculus for reflex gaze movement correlated with equilibrium.

(6) From the cortex through the corticobulbar tract for mediation of voluntary and involuntary conjugate movements of the eye.

SUMMARY OF DISORDERS OF CRANIAL NERVES III, IV, & VI

Oculomotor Paralysis (Cranial Nerve III)

A. Complete Oculomotor Paralysis: Affected muscles innervated by the third nerve are the superior, medial, and inferior recti, the levator palpebrae superioris (lid), and the inferior oblique. The third nerve also carries the parasympathetics to the pupil. Ipsilateral lesions of the nucleus will affect these ipsilateral muscles except for the superior rectus nucleus, which decussates to the opposite third nerve; the patient will be unable to look up with the contralateral eye and will have intact elevation in the ipsilateral eye. From the fascicle of the nerve in the midbrain out to their eventual termination in the orbit, all other lesions produce purely ipsilateral results.

If the lesion involves the third nerve anywhere from the nucleus (midbrain) to the peripheral branches in the orbit, it causes divergent strabismus, since the eye is turned out by the intact lateral rectus muscle and slightly depressed by the intact superior oblique muscle. There can be a dilated fixed pupil, absent accommodation, and ptosis of the upper lid, often severe enough to cover the pupil. The eye can only be moved laterally. Trauma, carotid aneurysm, and diabetes are the most common causes. The latter 2 can be differentiated clinically since in diabetes the pupillary responses are usually spared, whereas in aneurysms the pupil is fixed and dilated.

B. Complete Internal Ophthalmoplegia: This consists of a dilated and fixed pupil and paralysis of accommodation. The lesion is nearly always peripheral in the ciliary ganglion and often results in tonic pupil.

C. Oculomotor Synkinesis (Aberrant Regeneration of the Third Nerve): This phenomenon is characterized by (1) lid dyskinesias on horizontal gaze (ie, the levator palpebrae superioris fires when the medial rectus fires); (2) adduction on attempted upgaze (ie, the medial rectus fires when the superior rectus fires); (3) retraction on attempted upgaze (ie, cofiring of recti, which are retractors); (4) pseudo-Argyll Robertson pupil (ie, no light response, no near response in the primary position but a "near" response on adduction or adduction-depression—pupillary innervation from medial or inferior rectus); (5) pseudo Von-Graefe's sign (ie, no lid lag on downgaze but lid retraction due to lid innervation from inferior rectus); and (6) a monocular vertical optokinetic nystagmus response (due to cofiring muscles). This oculomotor synkinesis occurs probably as a combination of misdirection of sprouting axons into the wrong sheaths and subsequent muscle cofiring but also to ephaptic transmission or cross-talk between axons without covering sheaths.

Oculomotor synkinesis can occur secondarily after a defined ictus of trauma or posterior communicator-internal carotid aneurysm compressing the third nerve, especially if compression lasts several weeks. It can also occur as a primary event without a clear-cut ictus in patients who have meningioma or internal carotid aneurysm in the cavernous sinus.

D. Marcus Gunn Phenomenon (Jaw Winking): This rare congenital condition consists of elevation of a ptotic eyelid upon movement of the jaw. Acquired cases occur after damage to the oculomotor nerve with subsequent innervation of the lid (levator palpebrae superioris) by a branch of the fifth cranial nerve.

E. Trochlear Paralysis (Cranial Nerve IV): Lesions of the fourth nerve are usually vascular or traumatic. However, cerebellar tumors can also present with a fourth nerve lesion as an early sign. The nerve is vulnerable to injury at the site of exit from the dorsal aspect of the posterior midbrain pons. Both nerves may be damaged as they decussate in the anterior medullary velum, resulting in bilateral superior oblique palsies. Superior oblique palsy results in upward deviation (hypertropia) of the eye. The hypertropia increases when the patient looks down and with adduction. In addition, there is excyclotropia, and one of the diplopic images will be tilted with respect to the other. Tilting the head toward the involved side increases the deviation. Tilting the head away from the side of the involved eye may relieve the diplopia, and patients frequently present with a head tilt.

F. Abducens Paralysis (Cranial Nerve VI): This is the most common isolated muscle palsy. Abduction of the eye is absent; esotropia is present in the primary position and increases upon gaze to the affected side. Movement of the eye to the opposite side is normal. Cerebrovascular accidents are a common cause; basilar artery disease, increased intracranial pressure, post-lumbar puncture, tumors at the base of the skull, meningitis, diabetes, and trauma are other frequent causes. A child with a sixth nerve palsy should be evaluated for a brain stem tumor or inflammation if trauma was not present or if trauma was minimal. Pseudo-sixth nerve palsies can occur in Duane's retraction syndrome, spasm of the near reflex, thyroid eye disease, myasthenia, and dorsal midbrain compression (Parinaud's syndrome).

G. Duane's Syndrome: This uncommon congenital, stationary, nearly always unilateral condition consists of deficient horizontal ocular motility, originally thought to be due to fibrous rectus muscle. Recent evidence based on pathologic studies has demonstrated that Duane's syndrome is a result of congenital absence of the sixth nerve. The lateral rectus is innervated by a branch of the third nerve. Attempted adduction movements result in retraction of the globe and narrowing of the lid fissure. The visual handicap is seldom severe. Visual acuity can be normal, and the eye is otherwise normal. Unless the deviation is very large, strabismus surgery is best avoided.

H. Complete Ophthalmoplegia (Sudden): Complete ophthalmoplegia of sudden onset can be due to brain stem vascular disease, Wernicke's encephalopathy, pituitary apoplexy, Miller-Fisher syndrome, myasthenic crisis, bulbar poliomyelitis, diphtheria, botulism, chronic meningitis, and syphilitic or arteriosclerotic basilar aneurysm.

Symptoms & Signs of Extraocular Muscle Palsies

Diplopia occurs when the visual axes are not aligned. This is especially true when the onset of strabismus is after age 6 years (suppression and abnormal retinal correspondence do not develop). Dizziness (dysequilibrium) that disappears with monocular patching is often associated. Head tilt occurs, especially in paresis of the superior oblique muscle, when the patient tilts the head to the opposite side to avoid diplopia by moving the eye out of the field of action of the paralyzed muscle.

Ptosis is caused by weakness or paralysis of the levator muscle. Any extraocular muscle palsy that occurs with minor head trauma (subconcussive injuries) should be investigated for a basal tumor.

SYNDROMES AFFECTING CRANIAL NERVES III, IV, & VI (Fig 15–22)

Peripheral Involvement of Cranial Nerves III, IV, & VI

A. Gradenigo's Syndrome: Gradenigo's syndrome is characterized by pain in the face (from irritation of the trigeminal nerve) and abducens palsy. It is produced by meningeal inflammation at the tip of the petrous bone and occurs most often as a rare complication of otitis media or petrous bone tumors.

B. Orbital Fissure Syndrome: All extraocular peripheral nerves pass through the orbital fissure and can be involved by a traumatic bone fracture in this area or by tumor encroaching on the fissure from the orbital or cranial side.

C. Orbital Apex Syndrome: This is similar to the orbital fissure syndrome with the addition of optic nerve signs and usually greater proptosis. It is caused by an orbital tumor or trauma that damages the optic and extraocular nerves.

Chronic Progressive External Ophthalmoplegia[*]

This rather rare disease involves all 3 extraocular nerves. It is characterized by a slowly progressive inability to move the eyes and often is associated with severe early ptosis and normal pupillary reactions and accommodation. It may begin at any age and progresses over a period of 5–15 years to complete external ophthalmoplegia. This disease is frequently associated with other abnormalities such as pigmentary degeneration of the retina, deafness, cerebellar-vestibular abnormalities, cardiac conduction defects, and peripheral neuropathy. When it includes heart block and retinitis pigmentosa, it is called "ophthalmoplegia plus," or Kearns-Sayre syndrome.

The differential diagnosis includes ophthalmoplegia with motor neuron disease, progressive supranuclear palsy, Möbius's syndrome, spinocerebellar degeneration, Bassen-Kornzweig disease, Refsum's disease, and juvenile sphingolipidosis.

MYASTHENIA GRAVIS

Myasthenia gravis is characterized by abnormal fatigability of striated muscle after repetitive contraction that improves after rest; it often is first manifested by weakness of extraocular muscles. Unilateral fatiguing ptosis is a frequent first sign, with subsequent bilateral involvement of extraocular muscles, so that diplopia is often an early symptom. Unusual ocular presentations include clinical presentations that simulate gaze palsies, internuclear ophthalmoplegias, vertical nystagmus, and progressive external ophthalmoplegia. Generalized weakness of the arms and legs, difficulty in swallowing, weakness of jaw muscles, and difficulty in breathing may follow rapidly in untreated cases. There are no sensory changes.

The disease is not rare, with an incidence of 1:20,000–30,000. It usually affects young adults aged 20–40 years, though it may occur at any age and is often misdiagnosed as hysteria, especially because the weakness can be greater in exciting or embarrassing situations.

The onset may follow an upper respiratory infection, stress, or any injury and has been noted as a transitory condition in newborn infants of myasthenic mothers. The disease has been associated with hyperthyroidism (5%), thyroid abnormalities (15%), autoimmune disease (5%), and diffuse metastatic carcinoma (7%).

The differential diagnosis includes progressive nuclear ophthalmoplegia, brain stem lesions, epidemic encephalitis, bulbar and pseudobulbar palsy, postdiphtheritic paralysis, botulism, multiple sclerosis, and toxic reactions to beta-blockers (eg, propranolol) or penicillamine. Many other drugs may unmask or exacerbate myasthenia gravis. They include lithium, aminoglycoside antibiotics, chloroquine, and phenytoin anticonvulsants.

Substantial neurophysiologic evidence indicates that the orgin of the disease is at the neuromuscular junction, for there is convincing evidence of morphologic changes in the motor end plate on electron microscopy, probably due to antibodies against it and the presynaptic site. A commercial test of anti-acetylcholine receptor antibodies can diagnose the disease.

Most patients merely have thymic hyperplasia, apparent on lateral oblique chest x-rays or CT scan of the mediastinum or noted at surgical removal of the thymus.

Cholinesterase destroys acetylcholine at the myoneural junction, and cholinesterase-inhibiting drugs (neostigmine) markedly improve the condition. The edrophonium chloride (Tensilon) test is used in addition to the neostigmine diagnostic test. Edrophonium, 2 mg (0.2 mL), is given intravenously over 15 seconds. Relief of ptosis constitutes a positive response and confirms the diagnosis of myasthenia gravis. If no response occurs in 30 seconds, an additional 5–7 mg (0.5–0.7 mL) is given. The test is most helpful when marked ptosis is present, but myasthenia can affect any muscle or combination of muscles and significant improvement in function is also helpful. Mildly positive Tensilon tests can occur in neurogenic palsies, however.

Myasthenia gravis is medically treated with pyridostigmine (Mestinon). Topical anticholinesterase drops are not helpful. Ptosis usually responds to treatment, but it is difficult to titrate the cholinesterase inhibitors precisely enough to correct varying weaknesses and strengths in the extraocular muscles. Thymectomy is of benefit for patients with generalized muscle weakness and is done now as soon as the disease becomes generalized.

The course of this chronic disease is not steady, and remissions are frequent, especially if the disease is confined to the extraocular muscles. During a severe exacerbation, the patient may die from paralysis of the muscles of respiration.

The prognosis depends to a great extent upon the patient's response to medication, ability to regulate medication, and thymectomy, which is associated with a 5-year remission rate of 95%. An intelligent

---

[*]External ophthalmoplegia is a general term that denotes inability to move the eyes normally as a result of any nuclear or infranuclear involvement of cranial nerves III, IV, or VI; the pupillary reaction and accommodation are normal.

patient well-instructed about the disease can live a normal life span.

NYSTAGMUS
(Fig 15–31)

Nystagmus is defined as involuntary, rhythmically repeated oscillations of one or both eyes in any or all fields of gaze. The movements are either pendular, with undulating movements of equal speed, amplitude, and duration in each direction; or jerky, with slower movements in one direction (slow component) followed by a rapid return to the original position (fast component).

Nystagmus is classified as grade I, present only with the eyes directed toward the fast component; grade II, present also with the eyes in primary position; or grade III, present even with the eyes directed toward the slow component. The movements may be horizontal, vertical, oblique, rotatory, circular, or a combination of these. The direction may change depending upon the direction of gaze.

The **amplitude** of nystagmus refers to the extent of the movements, and the **rate** refers to the frequency of oscillation. Generally, the faster the rate, the smaller the amplitude and vice versa. Nystagmus is usually conjugate but is occasionally dysconjugate, as in physiologic end-gaze nystagmus, Parinaud's nystagmus, and see-saw nystagmus.

Nystagmus is also occasionally dissociated, as in internuclear ophthalmoplegia, spasmus nutans, see-saw nystagmus, monocular visual loss, acquired pendular nystagmus, and with asymmetric muscle weakness in myasthenia gravis.

Known factors relating to ocular movements, malfunction of which can cause nystagmus, are as follows: The labyrinth exerts influence on eye movements by 2 mechanisms: (1) the otolith apparatus influences torsional eye movements in response to head position, and (2) the semicircular canals influence eye movements in response to acceleration and deceleration. The gaze mechanism influences the supraconnections of extraocular muscle function.

Physiology of Symptoms

Reduced visual acuity is caused by inability to maintain steady fixation. False projection is evident in vestibular nystagmus, where past-pointing is present. Head tilting is usually involuntary, to decrease the nystagmus. The head is turned toward the fast components in jerk nystagmus or set so that the eyes are in a position that minimizes ocular movement in pendular nystagmus. The patient sometimes complains of illusory movement of objects (oscillopsia). This is more apt to be present in nystagmus due to lesions of lower centers, such as the labyrinth, or associated with

the sudden onset of nystagmus in an adult. The apparent movement of the environment occurs during the slow component and causes an extremely distressing vertigo, so that the patient is unable to stand. Head nodding is most apt to accompany congenital nystagmus, spasmus nutans, and miner's nystagmus. Nystagmus is noticeable and cosmetically disturbing except when excursions of the eye are very small.

Classification of Nystagmus
  A. Physiologic nystagmus
    1. End-point nystagmus
    2. Optokinetic nystagmus
    3. Stimulation of semicircular canals
  B. Pathologic nystagmus
    1. Congenital
      a. Poor vision
      b. Congenital
      c. Latent
    2. Spasmus nutans
    3. Downbeat nystagmus
    4. Upbeat nystagmus
    5. Convergence retraction nystagmus
    6. See-saw nystagmus
    7. Horizontal nystagmus
      a. Voluntary
      b. Acquired pendular
      c. Periodic alternating
      d. Gaze-evoked
    8. Vestibular nystagmus

PHYSIOLOGIC NYSTAGMUS

Three types of nystagmus can be elicited in the normal person. Alteration of normal response may be helpful diagnostically.

End-Point (End-Gaze) Nystagmus

Normal individuals have a wide null or quiet zone but can have horizontal nystagmus on end-horizontal gaze (ie, pupillary light reflex just on both corneas); physiologic end-gaze nystagmus disappears as the eyes move a few degrees. It is primarily horizontal but may have a slight torsional component and may be of greater amplitude in the abducting eye.

Optokinetic Nystagmus

This type of nystagmus may be elicited in all normal individuals, most easily by means of a rotating drum with alternating black and white lines; but in fact it may be elicited by any repetitive targets in the visual field, such as telephone poles as seen from the window of a fast-moving car. The slow component follows the object, and the fast component moves rapidly in the opposite direction to fixate on each succeeding object. A unilateral or asymmetric horizontal response usually indicates a parietal lobe tumor. Anterior cerebral (ie, frontal lobe) lesions may inhibit this response only very temporarily when an acute saccadic gaze palsy is present, which suggests the presence of a compensatory mechanism that is much greater than for lesions situated farther posteriorly. Asymmetry of response in the vertical plane suggests a brain stem lesion.

Nystagmus Elicited by Stimulation of Semicircular Canals

Endolymph flow in the semicircular canals inputs into the vestibular nuclei; they then maintain resting vestibular tonus on the oculomotor nuclei via the paramedian pontine reticular formation and the medial longitudinal fasciculus as well as on the cerebellum and cerebral cortex.

A. Bárány Rotating Chair: The horizontal canals are parallel to the floor when the head is tilted 30 degrees forward. Rotation of the subject causes jerk nystagmus in the direction of the turning. The slow component is in the opposite direction—the same as the flow of endolymph in the semicircular canals.

B. Caloric Stimulation: With the subject supine and the head flexed on the chest, cold-water ear irrigation produces nystagmus with the fast component away from the side of irrigation whereas warm water produces nystagmus with the fast component toward the side of irrigation. (Mnemonic device is COWS: cold-opposite, warm-same.) This is named for the obvious or fast phase, but the true component is the slow or vestibular component; the fast or saccadic movement is a corrective movement that occurs in the alert patient with an intact reticular activating system. Hence, a comatose patient with an intact pons will show only the true vestibular component.

PATHOLOGIC NYSTAGMUS

Nystagmus can be thought of as a disorder of the mechanisms that hold the eyes or fixation steady; therefore, the neural systems involved in nystagmus include cerebellovestibular, optokinetic, and pursuit systems. The defective neural system for some nystagmus patterns is delineated.

Congenital Nystagmus

Congenital impairment of vision or visual deprivation due to lesions in any part of the eye or optic nerve can result in pendular nystagmus. Causes include corneal opacity, cataract, albinism, Chédiak-Higashi syndrome, corectopia, achromatopsia, posterior polar chorioretinitis, aniridia, and optic atrophy. It at least in part occurs because of poor fixation.

Pendular nystagmus, which occurs in children with poor vision, has been called "sensory nystagmus"; and jerk nystagmus, which occurs in children with good vision, has been called "motor nystagmus." However, eye movement recordings delineate jerk and pendular wave forms that are irrespective of visual acuity. Jerk nystagmus will be associated with a "foveating or breaking saccade" to achieve good vision;

in pendular nystagmus, the eyes oscillate across the target, but on eye movement recordings a jerk component can be seen.

Congenital nystagmus is present at birth or shortly thereafter. It is usually horizontal and conjugate, but occasionally it can have a vertical vector to the wave form. However, whatever movement is observed on horizontal gaze is mirrored on vertical gaze. Since the lesion is thought to be a defect in horizontal pursuit, horizontal optokinetic nystagmus is absent but vertical optokinetic nystagmus is still present. This latter point differentiates it from poor vision, in which a corresponding absent or deficient optokinetic nystagus is present whether horizontal or vertical repetitive targets are viewed. Most patients with congenital nystagmus have a relatively quiet or "null" zone that can be eccentric to the primary position, and they will adjust a head turn to keep this eccentric position straight ahead. Since this nystagmus is decreased by convergence, many patients will adopt an esotropia, but it is increased by anxiety or increased "effort to see." Mechanical esotropia by prisms or ocular surgery can decrease this "effect to see" and thus improve vision.

Latent Nystagmus

Latent nystagmus is a variant of congenital nystagmus that appears only when one eye is covered, and then both eyes develop nystagmus with the slow phase toward the cover and the fast phase away.

Spasmus Nutans

Spasmus nutans is a bilateral nystagmus in which each eye has a very different amplitude or is dislocated. It is associated with head nodding as a compensatory vestibular mechanism. It is benign, but central nervous system visual disorders must be eliminated. It may appear at about 4 months of age and should resolve by age 3 years or rarely later.

Downbeat Nystagmus

Downbeat nystagmus is associated with cervicomedullary junction abnormalities. It is often evident in the primary position as a slow upward drift with a rapid corrective saccade down. Occasionally it is evident only on oblique gaze down. The mechanism for the eyes "drifting up" may be loss of inhibition on the central vestibular connections to the anterior semicircular canals, a vertical pursuit imbalance, or vestibulocerebellar disease affecting the vertical neural integrators. Disorders known to produce it include not only Arnold-Chiari malformation and basilar invagination but also demyelinating disease, cerebellar atrophy, hydrocephalus, and anticonvulsants.

Upbeat Nystagmus

Upbeat nystagmus occurs in the primary position of gaze and is increased on upgaze or downgaze.

A. Upgaze Nystagmus: Increase of upbeat nystagmus on upgaze is due to disorders of the anterior superior cerebellar vermis. It can also occur in meningitis and secondary to barbiturates, alcohol, and anticonvulsants. It is characterized by a tendency of the eyes to drift down, with corrective saccades upward and increase in amplitude with increasing upward gaze. It may be due to loss of influence of the anterior semicircular canals that mediate upward vestibular tone.

B. Downgaze Nystagmus: On downgaze—rarely seen—a fine upbeat nystagmus has been associated with medullary abnormalities.

Convergence-Retraction Nystagmus

Convergence-retraction nystagmus occurs on attempted upgaze in patients with Parinaud's syndrome from dorsal midbrain lesions. Here the fast phases of the nystagmus are convergent and horizontal. The eyes will not turn upward. They appear to retract during each fast phase of the nystagmus. The nystagmus can best be evoked as the patient watches down-moving stripes on an optokinetic nystagmus tape or drum. Electromyographic studies show co-contraction of extraocular muscles and loss of normal agonist-antagonist reciprocal innervation.

See-Saw Nystagmus

See-saw nystagmus is characterized by rising intorsion of one eye and falling extorsion of the other—then the reverse. Although it is uncommon, it is associated with chiasmatic tumors. The generator of this nystagmus may be the interstitial nucleus of Cajal.

Horizontal Nystagmus

A. Voluntary Nystagmus: Horizontal nystagmus is a high-frequency burst of horizontal oscillations that are saccadic in each direction. This is self-induced by convergence in normals and is an ill-sustained shuddering or shivering movement.

B. Acquired Pendular Nystagmus: This uncommon disorder occurs in multiple sclerosis and other white matter brain stem abnormalities and may be associated with palatal myoclonus. It may be horizontal, vertical, or both. Both vectors—whatever their direction—have the same amplitude. Lesions in the dentato-rubro-olivary connections may be responsible.

C. Periodic Alternating Nystagmus: This is a direction-reversing type of nystagmus in which each direction can take 1–2 minutes before reversing. It occurs in pontomedullary junction abnormalities and has been reported in some cases to be abolished by baclofen.

D. Gaze-Evoked Nystagmus: This type of nystagmus is induced by looking out of the primary position, either horizontally or vertically. Such a movement depends on a neural integrator to correlate pursuit, saccadic, and vestibular input, but if this integrator is defective the eyes cannot be maintained in eccentric gaze out of the primary position and will drift back. Cerebellar diseases, sedatives, and anticonvulsant medications can be associated with gaze-evoked nystagmus and faulty smooth pursuit. Cere-

bellopontine angle neoplasms can produce unilateral gaze paresis with coarse gaze-evoked nystagmus and rapid vestibular nystagmus to the opposite side (due to asymmetric vestibular input).

Vestibular Nystagmus

Vestibular nystagmus is always of the jerk type. The slow component is considered to be a response to impulses originating in the semicircular canals; the fast component is a corrective movement. Vestibular nystagmus is not dependent upon visual stimuli—ie, it is present with the lids closed as well as open and can be elicited in blind individuals also. The vestibular system is inhibited or dampened by visual fixation and can be deconditioned by training, which is why ice skaters stare fixedly after several spinning turns—and another reason why they train. Rotatory movements are especially characteristic of vestibular nystagmus, but horizontal or vertical vestibular nystagmus also occurs.

Physiologic nystagmus elicited by stimulation of the semicircular canals by means of the Bárány chair or caloric stimulation depends upon normal vestibular function.

The following characteristics of vestibular nystagmus demonstrate its origin in labyrinthine and vestibular nerve disease: (1) vertigo, tinnitus, and deafness are apt to be associated; (2) nystagmus is maximal early in the disease and tends to improve or disappear in 2–3 weeks (unless the vestibular nuclei are affected directly, in which case nystagmus may be permanent); and (3) the lesion is always destructive, and its direction (fast component) is away from the side the lesion is on.

Vestibular nystagmus may be due to labyrinthitis, Meniere's disease, trauma (including surgical destruction of one labyrinth); vascular, inflammatory, or neoplastic lesions of the vestibular nerves; lesions of the vestibular nuclei (encephalitis, multiple sclerosis, syringobulbia, poliomyelitis, thrombosis of the posteroinferior cerebellar artery); or cerebellar tumors and abscesses (probably as a result of pressure on the vestibular pathways).

CEREBROVASCULAR DISORDERS OF OPHTHALMOLOGIC IMPORTANCE

Vascular Insufficiency & Occlusion of the Internal Carotid Artery

Amaurosis fugax is fleeting or transient loss of vision, usually associated clinically with carotid occlusive disease, but it can occur with any microembolism or thrombotic disorder, including cardiac valvular disease, impending arterial thrombosis, migraine, hypotension, papilledema, orbital tumors, and hyperviscosity states. In embolization, vision can be lost completely or intermittently, like a curtain rising or falling. In hypotension, the visual field constricts from the periphery to the center.

Perhaps 95% of episodes of amaurosis fugax occur as a result of atherosclerotic lesions of the ipsilateral internal carotid artery. Cerebral and retinal disturbances occur as a result of small emboli breaking loose from the sclerotic plaque and lodging in cerebral or retinal arterioles. (Occlusion of the central retinal artery or a major branch can occur.) These small plaques (Hollenhorst plaques) may be visible with the ophthalmoscope as small glistening yellow spots situated at bifurcations of the retinal arteries. A finding of reduced ophthalmic artery pressure—as determined by ophthalmodynamometry, bruits over the internal carotid artery, and angiography—helps to confirm the diagnosis. Removal of an atherosclerotic plaque by carotid endarterectomy may improve the quality of life for the patient and decrease the likelihood of embolic stroke to the cerebral hemisphere.

Duller white-gray embolic fragments in the retinal blood vessels are the hallmark of calcific emboli from cardiac valvular disease, and gummy white nonreflective plugs neatly filling a blood vessel are platelet-fibrin material that can be from carotid occlusive disease. Most embolic fragments can be seen readily with the ophthalmoscope in the posterior pole, but most will also eventually pass through the retinal microvasculature, and only 10% remain in place. To induce more rapid passage and better visual results, they are treated with a varying combination of aspirin, dipyridamole, CO_2-O_2 mixture, paracentesis and ocular massage, and intravenous acetazolamide. After 24 hours, the clinical picture is usually irreversible, though exceptions to this rule have been reported. Visual acuity better than counting fingers implies a better prognosis with vigorous treatment.

Occlusion of the Middle Cerebral Artery

This disorder may produce severe contralateral hemiplegia, hemianesthesia, and homonymous hemianopia. The lower quadrants of the visual fields (upper radiations) are most apt to be involved. Aphasia may be present if the dominant hemisphere is involved.

Vascular Insufficiency of the Vertebrobasilar Arterial System

Brief episodes of transient bilateral blurring of vision commonly precede a basilar artery stroke. An attack seldom leaves any residual visual impairment, and the episode may be so minimal that the patient or doctor does not heed the warning. The blurring is described as a graying of vision, just as if the house lights were being dimmed at a theater. Episodes seldom last more than 5 minutes—often only a few seconds—and may be associated with other transient symptoms of vertebral-basilar insufficiency. Antiplatelet drugs can decrease the frequency and severity of vertebrobasilar symptoms.

Occlusion of the Basilar Artery

Complete or extensive thrombosis of the basilar artery nearly always causes death. With partial occlusion or basilar "insufficiency" due to arteriosclerosis, a wide variety of brain stem and cerebellar signs may be present. These include nystagmus, supranuclear oculomotor signs, and involvement of cranial nerves III, IV, VI, and VII.

Prolonged anticoagulant therapy has become the accepted treatment of partial basilar artery thrombotic occlusion.

Occlusion of the Posterior Cerebral Artery

Occlusion of the posterior cerebral artery seldom causes death. Occlusion of the cortical branches (most common) causes homonymous hemianopia, usually superior quadrantic. (The artery supplies primarily the visual cortex.) Lesions on the left in right-handed persons can cause aphasia, agraphia, and alexia if they are extensive and include parietal and occipital involvement. Involvement of the occipital lobe and the splenium of the corpus callosum can cause alexia (inability to read) without agraphia (inability to write)—such a patient would not be able to read his own writing. Occlusion of the proximal branches may produce the thalamic syndrome (thalamic pain, hemiparesis, hemianesthesia, choreoathetoid movements) and cerebellar ataxia.

Subdural Hemorrhage

Subdural hemorrhage results from tearing or shearing of the veins bridging the subdural space from the pia mater to the dural sinus. It leads to an encapsulated accumulation of blood in the subdural space, usually over one cerebral hemisphere. It is nearly always caused by trauma to the head. The trauma may be minimal and may precede the onset of neurologic signs by weeks or even months.

In infants, subdural hemorrhage produces progressive enlargement of the head with bulging fontanelles. The diagnosis is established by the finding of bloody spinal fluid on tapping the subdural space and by enlarged head measurements. Ocular signs include strabismus, pupillary changes, papilledema, and retinal hemorrhages.

In adults, the symptoms of chronic subdural hematoma are severe headache, drowsiness, and mental confusion, usually appearing hours to weeks (or even months) after trauma. Symptomatology is similar to that of cerebral tumors. Papilledema is present in 30–50% of cases. Retinal hemorrhages occur in association with papilledema. Ipsilateral dilatation of the pupil is the most common and most serious pupillary sign and is an urgent indication for immediate surgical evacuation of blood. Unequal, miotic, or mydriatic pupils can occur, or there may be no pupillary signs. Other signs, including vestibular nystagmus and cranial nerve palsies, also occur. Many of these signs result from herniation and compression of the brain stem and therefore often appear late with stupor and coma.

Skull films may show a shift of a calcified pineal gland. CT scan or carotid arteriography frequently confirms the diagnosis.

Treatment of acute large subdural hematoma consists of surgical evacuation of the blood; small hematomas may be treated with steroids or simply followed with careful observation. Without treatment, the course of large hematomas is progressively downhill to coma and death. With early and adequate treatment, the prognosis is good.

Subarachnoid Hemorrhage
(Fig 15–32)

Subarachnoid hemorrhage most commonly results from ruptured congenital berry aneurysms of the circle of Willis in the subarachnoid space. It may also result from trauma, birth injuries, intracranial hemorrhage, hemorrhage associated with tumors, arteriovenous malformations, or systemic bleeding disorders.

The most prominent symptom of subarachnoid hemorrhage is sudden, severe headache, usually occipital and often associated with signs of meningeal irritation (eg, stiff neck). Drowsiness, loss of consciousness, coma, and death may occur rapidly once an aneurysm ruptures and produces a subarachnoid hemorrhage. Ocular symptoms are not always present. A posterior communicator-internal carotid aneurysm may produce a third nerve palsy with pupillary involvement by distention of an aneurysmal sac before the aneurysm ruptures and produces a subarachnoid hemorrhage. Oculomotor palsy with associated numbness and pain in the distribution of the ipsilateral trigeminal nerve is pathognomonic of a supraclinoid,

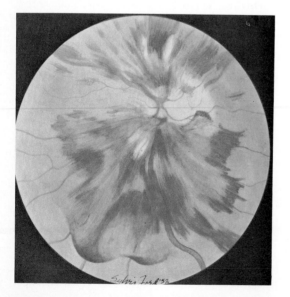

Figure 15–32. Subhyaloid hemorrhage around optic disk associated with subarachnoid hemorrhage. (Drawing.)

internal carotid, or posterior communicating artery aneurysm. Papilledema usually appears late when it does occur and after there has been a subarachnoid hemorrhage. Various types of retinal hemorrhage occur infrequently (preretinal hemorrhages are the most common) and carry a poor prognosis for life when they are both early and extensive, since they reflect rapid severe elevation of increased intracranial pressure. Exophthalmos may occur as a result of extravasation of blood into orbital tissues. Pressure of an aneurysm on the optic nerve may cause blindness in one eye.

Arteriography following injection of radiopaque substances may help to demonstrate and localize the aneurysms. Blood is present in the cerebrospinal fluid.

Ligation of aneurysmal vessels or of parent arterial trunks may be advisable. Supportive treatment, including control of blood pressure, is all that can be done during the acute phase of subarachnoid hemorrhage. Thus, it is important to diagnose the posterior communicator-internal carotid aneurysm when it first produces third nerve palsy with pupillary involvement.

Migraine

Migraine is a common episodic illness of unknown cause and varied symptomatology characterized by severe unilateral headache (which alternates sides), visual disturbances, nausea, and vomiting. The neurologic symptoms that usually precede the headache occur in the vasoconstrictive phase; the headache follows in the vasodilative phase. There is usually a family history of a similar disorder. The disease usually becomes manifest between ages 15 and 30 years. It is more common and more severe in women. Many factors, particularly emotional ones, may predispose or contribute to attacks. Prodromal symptoms are common and include drowsiness, paresthesias, "scintillating" scotomas, blurred vision, and other symptoms. In some patients, homonymous hemianopia can be accurately recorded on the tangent screen during attacks. There are no other objective findings. Visual symptoms usually last only 15–20 minutes.

Ergotamine tartrate, when given early in an attack, is often effective. Once the attack is well under way, treatment is of little value. The headaches last several hours to several days. Bed rest is often helpful though not essential.

PHAKOMATOSES

The phakomatoses (from Gk *phakos* "birthmark" + *-oma* "swelling") are a group of diseases characterized by multiple hamartomas occurring in various organ systems and at variable times.

NEUROFIBROMATOSIS
(Recklinghausen's Disease)

Neurofibromatosis is a generalized hereditary disease characterized by multiple tumors of the skin, central nervous system, peripheral nerves, and nerve sheaths. Other developmental anomalies—particularly of the bones—may be associated. Inheritance is in an autosomal dominant pattern with incomplete penetrance. The incidence is 1:2000 deliveries, and there is no racial predominance. Signs may be present at birth but are activated during pregnancy, puberty, and at menopause. There are 2 clinical manifestations of the disease: central and peripheral. The former is associated with central nervous system tumors and some skin changes; the latter shows mostly skin or other organ tumors.

Clinical Findings

Tumors may occur anywhere in the body, including the eye. Café au lait spots (small pigmented areas of skin) tend to enlarge and darken with age. A few such lesions may occur in 5–10% of the normal population; in neurofibromatosis, however, there are 5 or 6 spots greater than 1.5–2 cm in diameter; they are especially significant if they occur in axillary distribution. Cutaneous neurofibromas occur especially on the trunk and spare the palms and soles.

Tumors of the lids may represent isolated cutaneous neurofibromas and may be associated with glaucoma. Tumors of the optic nerve meninges (meningiomas) and glial cells (astrocytomas) occur also. These can cause papilledema or optic atrophy. There may be iris neurofibromas (like nevi) and enlarged corneal nerves.

Spinal cord neurofibromas occur frequently. The acoustic nerve is the cranial nerve most commonly involved, resulting in the syndrome of the cerebellopontine angle; if bilateral, this syndrome is highly suggestive of neurofibromatosis.

Bone development is affected when the tumor involves periosteum. Pulsating exophthalmos occasionally occurs when an osseous developmental defect of the sphenoid wing of the posterior orbit is present.

Treatment & Prognosis

Orbital or intracranial surgery may be needed to remove tumors for functional or cosmetic reasons.

When lesions are confined to the skin, the prognosis is good. Intracranial and intraspinal lesions are usually multiple and imply a bad prognosis. The disease tends to be fairly stationary, with only slow progression over long periods of time. Neurofibromas of the peripheral nerves also occur and may undergo sarcomatous degeneration.

ANGIOMATOSIS RETINAE CEREBELLI
(Von Hippel-Lindau Disease)

This rare disease occurs most commonly in men in the third decade of life but can appear at any age up to 60 years. Its incidence is 1:10,000, and there is neither gender nor racial predominance. About 25% of patients show autosomal dominant inheritance. The earliest signs are dilatation and tortuosity of the retinal vessels, which later develop into an angiomatous formation with hemorrhages and exudates. A stage of massive exudation, retinal detachment, and secondary glaucoma occurs later and will cause blindness if not treated. The disease is unilateral in 65% of cases. The onset is in the second and third decades, and patients must be followed expectantly with periodic presymptomatic screening because in 25% of cases or less, the retinal angiomatosis is associated with a similar generalized process, most often affecting the cerebellum (hemangioblastoma) and less commonly the pancreas, kidney (renal cell carcinoma), adrenal gland, and other organs. Present evidence suggests that this is all one genetically determined disease showing autosomal dominant inheritance with variable expression.

Treatment & Prognosis

Early treatment of retinal lesions with photocoagulation, diathermy, or cryotherapy—singly or in combination—has been effective in some cases. Cerebral and cerebellar tumors have been removed successfully, but recurrences are not uncommon.

MRI will revolutionize follow-up of these patients, since it can be done without radiation hazard and therefore frequently.

STURGE-WEBER SYNDROME

This uncommon nonfamilial disease with unknown inheritance is recognizable at birth by a characteristic nevus flammeus (port wine stain, or venous angioma) on one side of the face following the distribution of one or more branches of the fifth cranial nerve. There is corresponding angiomatous involvement of the meninges and brain by venous aneurysms on the same side, which cause jacksonian seizures (85%), mental retardation (60%), and cerebral cortical atrophy. Since these cortical lesions calcify, they can be seen on plain skull x-rays after infancy. Unilateral infantile glaucoma on the affected side frequently develops if there is extensive involvement of the conjunctiva with hemangioma of the episclera and anterior chamber anomalies. Lid or conjunctival involvement nearly always implies ultimate intraocular involvement and glaucoma. Forty percent of patients with one port wine stain on the face develop a choroidal hemangioma on the same side. There is at least one cytogenic study reporting trisomy 22.

Treatment & Prognosis

There is no effective treatment for Sturge-Weber syndrome, though the glaucoma can be controlled in rare cases by cyclodiathermy or trabeculectomy with trabeculotomy.

TUBEROUS SCLEROSIS
(Bourneville's Disease)

Tuberous sclerosis is characterized by the triad of adenoma sebaceum, epilepsy, and mental retardation, though about one-third of affected individuals have normal intelligence. Adenoma sebaceum (angiofibromas) occurs in 90% of patients over the age of 4 years, and the number of lesions increases with puberty. These flesh-colored papules are 1–2 mm in diameter and have a butterfly distribution on the nose and alar area and can also occur in the subungual and periungual areas. Ash leaf-shaped, hypopigmented ovals can be present on the skin even of neonates but are best seen under Wood's (ultraviolet) light.

Retinal hamartomas appear as oval or circular white areas in the peripheral fundus and characteristically have a mulberrylike appearance (see Fig 11–23). Histologically, the retinal tumors are composed of hyaline material with areas of calcification and may be degenerated astrocytomas. Renal hamartomas occur in 80% of patients. Subependymal nodules in the periventricular areas of the brain can calcify and appear as candle wax gutterings or drippings on skull x-rays in 25–30% of patients. These nodules can become astrocytomas. Seizures occur in 90% of patients within the first 3 years of life.

The disease is inherited sporadically (80%) or in an autosomal dominant pattern with high penetrance. Vision is generally normal, and progression of the retinal hamartomas is rare. The prognosis for life relates to the degree of central nervous system involvement. In severe cases, death can occur in the second or third decade of life; if there is minimal central nervous system involvement, life expectancy should be normal.

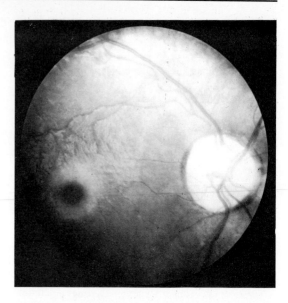

Figure 15–33. Cherry-red spot of Tay-Sachs disease in an 18-month-old child.

Vogt), and adult and GM_1-gangliosidosis (mucolipidosis).

Severe mental and physical deterioration occurs, usually causing death within a few years. The later the onset, the milder the disease. The liver and spleen show increased gangliosides. The striking ocular finding of a cherry-red spot in the macula is seen in congenital and infantile cases (Fig 15–33). Optic atrophy and retinal pigmentary changes are frequently present in the juvenile and adult forms. Extraocular muscle dysfunction is a less frequent finding in all forms.

CEREBROMACULAR DEGENERATION

Genetically determined (autosomal recessive) neuronal lipid storage diseases of the brain may affect the neural elements of the retina as well. The clinical forms are classified mainly according to age at onset. The pathologic changes are present prenatally, with clinical manifestations occurring as a critical level of intraneuronal lipidosis is reached. A definitive diagnosis can be established readily by conjunctival biopsy, rectal biopsy, or appendectomy showing ganglioside accumulation even before clinical signs are present.

Five forms of cerebromacular degeneration (ganglioside lipidosis) are recognized: congenital, infantile (Tay-Sachs), late infantile, juvenile (Spielmeyer-

NIEMANN-PICK DISEASE
(Sphingomyelin-Sterol
Lipidosis)

This entity is quite similar to the ganglioside lipidoses. There is deposition of glycolipid in the ganglion cells of the brain and retina. The spleen, liver, and other reticuloendothelial organs are massively infiltrated with glycolipid. Inheritance is in an autosomal recessive pattern, and 2 clinical forms are recognized. The infantile form is the most common and most severe, with death usually occurring in 2 or 3 years. A cherry-red spot in the macula may be present. The juvenile or adult form is much more benign and usually not associated with ocular findings.

REFERENCES

Anmarkrud N: The value of fluorescein fundus angiography in evaluating optic disc oedema. *Acta Ophthalmol* 1977;**55**:605.

Arnold AC et al: Retinal periphlebitis and retinitis in multiple sclerosis. 1. Pathologic characteristics. *Ophthalmology* 1984;**91**:255.

Asbury AK et al: Oculomotor palsy in diabetes mellitus: A clinicopathological study. *Brain* 1970;**93**:555.

Baker RS, Buncic JR: Sudden visual loss in pseudotumor cerebri due to central retinal artery occlusion. *Arch Neurol* 1984;**41**:1274.

Balkan R, Hoyt CS: Associated neurologic abnormalities in congenital third nerve palsies. *Am J Ophthalmol* 1984; **97**:315.

Baloh RW, Yee RD, Honrubia V: Optokinetic nystagmus and parietal lobe lesions. *Ann Neurol* 1980;**7**:269.

Bever CT Jr et al: Prognosis of ocular myasthenia. *Ann Neurol* 1983;**14**:516.

Boghen DR, Glaser JS: Ischaemic optic neuropathy: The clinical profile and history. *Brain* 1975;**98**:689.

Bogousslavsky J et al: Correlates of brain-stem oculomotor disorders in multiple sclerosis: Magnetic resonance imaging. *Arch Neurol* 1986;**43**:460.

Brown GC, Shields JA: Tumors of the optic nerve head. *Surv Ophthalmol* 1985;**29**:239.

Burde RM et al: Optic neuritis: Etiology? *Surv Ophthalmol* 1980;**24**:307.

Cala LA, Mastaglia FL, Black JL: Computerized tomography of brain and optic nerve in multiple sclerosis: Observations in 100 patients, including serial studies in 16. *J Neurol Sci* 1978;**36**:411.

Caprioli J, Lesser RL: Basal encephalocele and morning glory syndrome. *Br J Ophthalmol* 1983;**67**:349.

Caroll FD: Nutritional amblyopia. *Arch Ophthalmol* 1966;**76**:406.

Caroll WM et al: The incidence and nature of visual pathway involvement in Friedreich's ataxia: A clinical and visual evoked potential study of 22 patients. *Brain* 1980;**103**:413.

Cogan DG: *Neurology of the Ocular Muscles*, 2nd ed. Thomas, 1978.

Cogan DG, Lessell S: Neuro-ophthalmology and medical ophthalmology: A dialogue. (Editorial.) *Arch Ophthalmol* 1976;**94**:393.

Cullen JF, Coleiro JA: Ophthalmic complications of giant cell arteritis. *Surv Ophthalmol* 1976;**20**:247.

Currie J, Lubin JH, Lessell S: Chronic isolated abducens paresis from tumors at the base of the brain. *Arch Neurol* 1983;**40**:226.

Daroff RB, Dell'Osso LF: Periodic alternating nystagmus and the shifting null. *Can J Otolaryngol* 1974;**3**:367.

D'Cruz AA, Ellenberger C: Diagnostic differences in visual field defects. *Neuro-ophthalmology* 1983;**3**:239.

deGroot J, Chusid JG: *Correlative Neuroanatomy*, 20th ed. Appleton & Lange, 1988.

Durelli L et al: High-dose intravenous methylprednisolone in the treatment of multiple sclerosis: Clinical-immunologic correlations. *Neurology* 1986;**36**:238.

Frisén L: Swelling of the optic nerve head: A staging scheme. *J Neurol Neurosurg Psychiatry* 1982;**45**:13.

Gittinger JW et al: Progressive visual loss associated with peculiar disc swelling. *Surv Ophthalmol* 1979;**24**:117.

Glaser JS: *Neuro-ophthalmology*. Harper & Row, 1978.

Green GJ, Lessell S, Loewenstein JI: Ischemic optic neuropathy in chronic papilledema. *Arch Ophthalmol* 1980;**98**:502.

Halliday AM, McDonald WI: Visual evoked potentials. In: *Clinical Neurophysiology*. Stalberg E, Young RR (editors). Butterworths, 1981.

Halmagyi GM et al: Downbeating nystagmus: A review of 62 cases. *Arch Neurol* 1983;**40**:777.

Hardwig P, Robertson DM: Von Hippel-Lindau disease: A familial, often lethal, multisystem phakomatosis. *Ophthalmology* 1984;**91**:263.

Harrington DO: *The Visual Fields: A Textbook and Atlas of Clinical Perimetry*, 5th ed. Mosby, 1981.

Hayreh SS: Anterior ischaemic optic neuropathy. 3. Treatment, prophylaxis, and differential diagnosis. *Br J Ophthalmol* 1974;**58**:981.

Hayreh SS: Optic disc edema in raised intracranial pressure. 5. Pathogenesis. *Arch Ophthalmol* 1977;**95**:1553.

Hoffman HJ: How is pseudotumor cerebri diagnosed? *Arch Neurol* 1986;**43**:167.

Hollenhorst RW: Vascular status of patients who have cholesterol emboli in the retina. *Am J Ophthalmol* 1966;**61**:1159.

Hotchkiss MG et al: Bilateral Duane's retraction syndrome: A clinical-pathologic case report. *Arch Ophthalmol* 1980;**98**:870.

Hoyt WF: Ophthalmoscopy of the retinal nerve fiber layer in neuro-ophthalmologic diagnosis. *Aust J Ophthalmol* 1976;**4**:14.

Huber A: *Eye Signs and Symptoms in Brain Tumors*, 3rd ed. Mosby, 1976.

Johns K et al: Magnetic resonance imaging of the brain in isolated optic neuritis. *Arch Ophthalmol* 1986;**104**:1486.

Johnson KP, Nelson BJ: Multiple sclerosis: Diagnostic usefulness of cerebrospinal fluid. *Ann Neurol* 1977;**2**:425.

Keast-Butler J, Taylor D: Optic neuropathies in children. *Trans Ophthalmol Soc UK* 1980;**100**:111.

Kupersmith MJ et al: Contrast sensitivity loss in multiple sclerosis: Selectivity by eye, orientation, and spatial frequency measured with the evoked potential. *Invest Ophthalmol Vis Sci* 1984;**25**:632.

Leigh RJ, Zee DS: *The Neurology of Eye Movements*. Vol 23 of: *Contemporary Neurology Series*. Davis, 1983.

Leonard TJ, Moseley IF, Sanders, MD: Ophthalmoplegia in carotid cavernous sinus fistula. *Br J Ophthalmol* 1984;**68**:128.

Lessell S: Optic neuropathies. *N Engl J Med* 1978; **299**:533.

Lindenberg R, Walsh FB, Sacks JG: *Neuropathology of Vision: An Atlas*. Lea & Febiger, 1973.

Lowenfeld ID: The Argyll Robertson pupil, 1869–1969: A critical survery of the literature. *Surv Ophthalmol* 1969;**14**:199.

Margalith D, Tze WJ, Jan JE: Congenital optic nerve hypoplasia with hypothalamic-pituitary dysplasia: A review of 16 cases. *Am J Dis Child* 1985;**139**:361.

McDonald WI: The significance of optic neuritis. *Trans Ophthalmol Soc UK* 1983;**103**:230.

Miller NR: Anterior ischemic optic neuropathy: Diagnosis and management. *Bull NY Acad Med* 1980;**56**:643.

Miller NR (editor): *Walsh & Hoyt's Clinical Neuro-ophthalmology*, 4th ed. Vol 1. Williams & Wilkins, 1982.

Minckler DS, Tso MO, Zimmerman LE: A light microscopic, autoradiographic study of axoplasmic transport in the optic nerve head during ocular hypotony, increased intraocular pressure, and papilledema. *Am J Ophthalmol* 1976;**82**:741.

Moseley IF, Sanders DM: *Computerized Tomography in Neuro-ophthalmology.* Saunders, 1982.

Moses RA: *Adler's Physiology of the Eye: Clinical Application,* 7th ed. Mosby, 1980.

Moster ML et al: Isolated sixth-nerve palsies in younger adults. *Arch Ophthalmol* 1984;**102**:1328.

Mumenthaler M: Giant cell arteritis (cranial arteritis, polymyalgia rheumatica). *J Neurol* 1978;**218**:219.

Nadeau SE, Trobe JD: Pupil sparing in oculomotor palsy: A brief review. *Ann Neurol* 1983;**13**:143.

Nikoskelainen E: Later course and prognosis of optic neuritis. *Acta Ophthalmol* 1975;**53**:273.

O'Brien JF: The lysosomal storage diseases. *Mayo Clin Proc* 1982;**57**:192.

Page NG, Sanders MD: Bilateral central scotomata due to intracranial tumour. *Br J Ophthalmol* 1984;**68**:449.

Parkin PJ, Hierons R, McDonald WI: Bilateral optic neuritis: A long-term follow-up. *Brain* 1984;**107**:951.

Paul TO, Hoyt WF: Funduscopic appearance of papilledema with optic tract atrophy. *Arch Ophthalmol* 1976;**94**:467.

Perkin GD, Rose FC: *Optic Neuritis and Its Differential Diagnosis.* Oxford Univ Press, 1979.

Quigley HA, Addicks EM: Quantitative studies of retinal nerve fiber layer defects. *Arch Ophthalmol* 1982;**100**:807.

Richardson JE, Hamilton W: Diabetes insipidus, diabetes mellitus, optic atrophy, and deafness: Three cases of "DIDMOAD" syndrome. *Arch Dis Child* 1978;**52**:796.

Rosenberg RN, Chutorian A: Familial opticoacoustic nerve degeneration and polyneuropathy. *Neurology* 1967;**17**:827.

Rush JA, Younge BR: Paralysis of cranial nerves III, IV, and VI: Cause and prognosis in 1,000 cases. *Arch Ophthalmol* 1981;**99**:76.

Rush JA et al: Optic glioma: Long-term follow-up of 85 histopathologically verified cases. *Ophthalmology* 1982;**89**:1213.

Sanders EA et al: Estimation of visual function after optic neuritis: A comparison of clinical tests. *Br J Ophthalmol* 1986;**70**:918.

Savino PJ et al: Optic tract syndrome: A review of 21 patients. *Arch Ophthalmol* 1978;**96**:656.

Sebag J et al: Optic disc cupping in arteritic anterior ischemic optic neuropathy resembles glaucomatous cupping. *Ophthalmology* 1986;**93**:357.

Smith JL, Hoyt WF, Susac JO: Ocular fundus in acute Leber optic neuropathy. *Arch Ophthalmol* 1973;**90**:349.

Spector RH, Troost BT: The ocular motor system. *Ann Neurol* 1981;**9**:517.

Stanbury JB et al (editors): Disorders of lysosomal enzymes. Pages 751–969 in: *The Metabolic Basis of Inherited Disease,* 5th ed. McGraw-Hill, 1983.

Thompson HS: Pupil in clinical diagnosis (symposium). *Trans Am Acad Ophthalmol Otolaryngol* 1977;**83**:847.

Thompson HS: Pupillary signs in the diagnosis of optic nerve disease. *Trans Ophthalmol Soc UK* 1976;**96**:377.

Thompson HS et al (editors): *Topics in Neuro-ophthalmology.* Williams & Wilkins, 1979.

Toussaint D et al: Clinicopathological study of the visual pathways, eyes, and cerebral hemispheres in 32 cases of disseminated sclerosis. *J Clin Neuro-ophthalmol* 1983;**3**:211.

Trobe JD, Glaser JS, Cassady JC: Optic atrophy: Differential diagnosis by fundus observation alone. *Arch Ophthalmol* 1980;**98**:1040.

Trobe JD, Lorber ML, Schlezinger NS: Isolated homonymous hemianopia: A review of 104 cases. *Arch Ophthalmol* 1973;**89**:377.

Troiano R et al: Effect of high-dose intravenous steroid administration on contrast-enhancing computed tomographic scan lesions in multiple sclerosis. *Ann Neurol* 1984;**15**:257.

Tso MO: Axoplasmic transport in papilledema and glaucoma. *Trans Am Acad Ophthalmol Otolaryngol* 1977;**83**:771.

Wallace DC: A new manifestation of Leber's disease and a new explanation for the agency responsible for its unusual pattern of inheritance. *Brain* 1970;**93**:121.

Wertenbaker C et al: Downbeat nystagmus. *Surv Ophthalmol* 1981;**25**:263.

Williams R, Taylor D: Tuberculous sclerosis. (Review.) *Surv Ophthalmol* 1985;**30**:123.

Womack LW, Liesegang TJ: Complications of herpes zoster ophthalmicus. *Arch Ophthalmol* 1983;**101**:42.

Younge BR, Sutula F: Analysis of trochlear nerve palsies: Diagnosis, etiology, and treatment. *Mayo Clin Proc* 1977;**52**:11.

Zangemeister WH, Mueller-Jensen A: Neuromyelitis optica: Clinical and neurophysiological features. *Neuro-ophthalmology* 1984;**4**:81.

Ocular Disorders Associated With Systemic Diseases

16

Michael D. Sanders, FRCP, FRCS, & Elizabeth M. Graham, MRCP, DO

Examination of the eye provides the ophthalmologist an opportunity to make a unique contribution to the diagnosis of systemic disease. Nowhere else in the body can a microcirculatory system be investigated with such precision, and nowhere else are the results of minute focal lesions so devastating. Most systemic diseases involve the eyes, and therapy demands some knowledge of the vascular, rheologic, and immunologic nature of these diseases.

VASCULAR DISEASE

NORMAL ANATOMY & PHYSIOLOGY

The blood supply to the eye is from the ophthalmic artery, which is the first branch of the internal carotid artery. The first branches of the ophthalmic artery are the central retinal artery and the long posterior ciliary arteries. The retina is therefore perfused by retinal and choroidal vessels that provide contrasting anatomic and physiologic circulations. The retinal arteries correspond to arterioles in the systemic circulation but are thin-walled, with several layers of medial muscle cells. They function as end arteries and feed a capillary bed consisting of small capillaries (7 μm) with tight endothelial junctions. Dependent on this anatomic arrangement is the maintenance of the blood-retina barrier, and this system is autoregulated, since there are no autonomic nerve fibers. Most of the blood within the eye, however, is in the choroidal circulation, which is characterized by a high flow rate, autonomic regulation, and an anatomic arrangement with collateral branching and large capillaries (30 μm), all of which have fenestrations in juxtaposition to Bruch's membrane. Clinical examination of the retinal vessels is facilitated by the use of red-free light, and fluorescein angiography enables us to obtain information about the dynamic and functional aspects of this circulation.

PATHOLOGIC APPEARANCES IN RETINAL VASCULAR DISEASE

Hemorrhages

Retinal hemorrhages result from diapedeses from veins or capillaries, and the morphologic appearances depend upon the size, site, and extent of damage to the vessel (Fig 16–1). Hemorrhages may be caused by any condition that alters the integrity of the endothelial cells. They usually indicate some abnormality of the retinal vascular system, and systemic factors should be considered in relation to (1) vessel wall disease (eg, hypertension, diabetes), (2) blood disorders (eg, leukemia, polycythemia), and (3) reduced perfusion (eg, carotid cavernous fistula, acute blood loss).

A. Preretinal Hemorrhages: These result from damage to the superficial disk or retinal vessels and

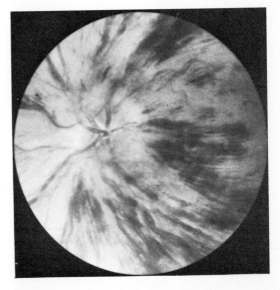

Figure 16–1. Flame-shaped retinal hemorrhages in the nerve fiber layer radiate out from the optic disk. Three days before the photograph was taken, the patient experienced sudden loss of vision, which left him with light perception only.

are usually large, producing a gravity-dependent fluid level.

B. Linear Hemorrhages: These usually small hemorrhages lie in the superficial nerve fiber layers and hence have a characteristic linear appearance, conforming to the alignment of nerve fibers in any particular area of the fundus.

C. Punctate Hemorrhages: Hemorrhages situated deeper in the substance of the retina are punctate and derived from capillaries and smaller venules. The circular appearance is related to the anatomic arrangement of structures in the retina.

D. Subretinal Hemorrhages: These hemorrhages are less common because normally there are no blood vessels between the retina and the choroid. Such hemorrhages are large and red, with a well-defined margin and no fluid level. They are seen in relation to the disk and in any condition where abnormal vessels pass from the choroidal circulation into the retina.

E. Hemorrhages Under the Pigment Epithelium: Hemorrhages situated under the pigment epithelium are usually dark and large, so that they must be differentiated from choroidal melanomas and hemangiomas.

F. White Central Hemorrhages (Roth's Spots): Superficial retinal hemorrhages with pale or white centers are not pathognomonic of any disease process but may arise in a variety of circumstances: (1) retinal infarction (cotton wool spot) with surrounding hemorrhage; (2) retinal hemorrhage in combination with extravasation of white corpuscles (eg, leukemia); and (3) retinal hemorrhage with central resolution.

Neuronal Effects of Focal Retinal Ischemia

The funduscopic appearance of arteriolar occlusion depends on the size of the vessel occluded, the duration of occlusion, and the time course. Occlusion of major arterioles produces a total, hemispheric, or segmental pallid swelling of the retina. Occlusion of a precapillary retinal arteriole produces the pathognomonic appearance of a cotton wool spot (Fig 16–2). This consists of a pale, slightly elevated swelling usually one-fourth to one-half the size of the optic disk. Pathologic examination shows distention of neurons, with cytoid bodies (Fig 16–3); electron microscopy shows the accumulation of axoplasm and organelles. Occlusion of arterioles, whether due to intrinsic vessel wall disease or to intramural factors, may produce these pathognomonic signs.

A. Optic Disk Infarction (Ischemic Optic Neuropathy): Impairment of the blood supply to the optic disk produces sudden visual loss, usually with an altitudinal field defect and pallid swelling of the optic disk. The primary abnormality is complete or partial interruption of the choroidal blood supply to the disk, while the retinal capillaries on the surface of the disk appear dilated. Fluorescein angiography confirms the circulatory alterations (Fig 16–4). Optic disk infarction is often caused by giant cell arteritis in old age and by hypertension and arteriosclerotic disease in middle age.

Investigations should include serum lipids, blood glucose, serologic tests for syphilis, and assessment of blood viscosity by hemoglobin, hematocrit, and fibrinogen determinations. Giant cell arteritis merits measurement of the erythrocyte sedimentation rate and

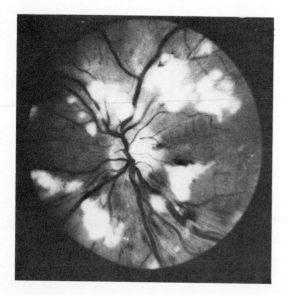
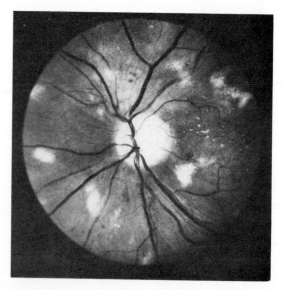

Figure 16–2. Cotton wool spots. **Left:** Numerous cotton wool spots are seen in the posterior pole in a patient with accelerated hypertension. **Right:** One month after hypotensive treatment. Note resolution of the infarcts.

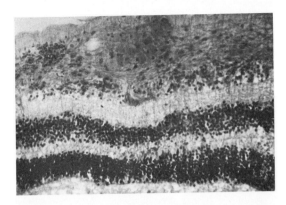

Figure 16–3. Cotton wool spot. Histologic examination shows cytoid bodies and distended neurons in the superficial retinal layers. Deeper retinal layers are normal. (Courtesy of Professor N Ashton.)

temporal artery biopsy on an urgent basis. Corticosteroids are essential in the management of giant cell arteritis, but the results of use of these drugs are equivocal in nonarteritic disorders.

B. Choroidal Infarction: Though the connection has rarely been recognized, certain clinical appearances have been attributed to ciliary vessel occlusion. These include small pale areas in the equatorial region which resolve to leave mottled pigmentary areas (Elschnig's spots) due to necrosis of the pigment epithelium. Larger infarcts may occur, which may be triangular or linear.

C. Retinal Emboli: Transient episodes of monocular visual loss lasting 5–10 minutes are character-

istic of amaurosis fugax. Patients often describe a curtain coming down from above or across their vision, usually with complete return of vision within seconds or minutes. Amaurosis fugax is most commonly due to retinal emboli.

Paresthesias in the contralateral limbs localize the disorder to the carotid artery and suggest involvement of the ophthalmic artery and middle cerebral artery. It is important for the ophthalmologist to auscultate the carotid for a systolic bruit and to search the fundus for emboli. Retinal emboli are of 3 main types:

1. Cholesterol emboli (Hollenhorst plaques)– These usually arise from an atheromatous plaque in the carotid artery and consist of cholesterol and fibrin. They lodge at the bifurcation of retinal arterioles, are refractile, and may appear larger than the vessel that contains them (Fig 16–5).

2. Calcific emboli–Originating from damaged cardiac valves, these emboli lodge within the arteriole, producing complete occlusion and infarction of the distal retina. Calcific emboli are solid and calcified and occur in younger patients with a variety of cardiac lesions.

3. Platelet/fibrin emboli–Most cases of amaurosis fugax are probably due to the transit of platelet aggregates through the retinal and choroidal circulations. The emboli are usually broken up as they traverse the retinal circulation and hence are rarely seen, though occasionally they produce retinal infarction. Arising from abnormalities of the heart or great vessels, they may be reduced by drugs that reduce platelet coagulability (eg, aspirin).

Patients with retinal emboli who are under 40 years of age should undergo cardiac studies (24-hour ECG,

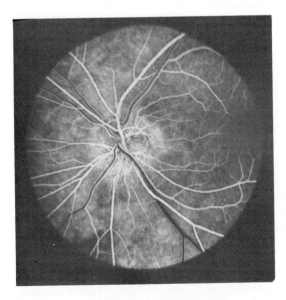

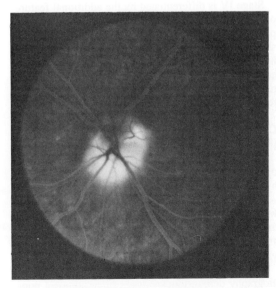

Figure 16–4. Ischemic optic neuropathy. Sudden visual loss in a 48-year-old man produced a complete inferior altitudinal field loss. *Left:* Fluorescein angiography shows impaired filling of the upper part of the disk with dilatation of retinal capillaries at the lower part of the disk. *Right:* Photograph 10 minutes after injection shows leakage of dye mainly at the lower part of the disk.

part of the spectrum of central retinal vein occlusion. Investigations are similar in the 2 conditions, but arterial disease—particularly hypertension—is found more commonly in patients with retinal branch vein occlusion than in those presenting with central retinal vein occlusion.

ATHEROSCLEROSIS & ARTERIOSCLEROSIS

The process of atherosclerosis occurs in larger arteries and is due to fatty infiltration of a patchy nature occurring in the intima and associated with fibrosis. Involvement of smaller vessels (ie, less than 300 μm) by diffuse fibrosis and hyalinization is termed arteriosclerosis. The retinal vessels beyond the disk are less than 30 μm; therefore, involvement of the retinal arterioles should be termed arteriosclerosis, whereas involvement of the central retinal artery is properly termed atherosclerosis.

Atherosclerosis is a progressive change developing in the second decade, with lipid streaks in larger vessels, progressing to a fibrous plaque in the third decade. In the fourth and fifth decades, ulceration, hemorrhages, and thrombosis occur, and the lesion may be calcified. Destruction of the elastic and muscular elements of the media produces ectasia and rupture of the large vessels, though in smaller vessels obstruction is usually seen. The clinical results of atherosclerosis are seen several decades after the onset of the process. Contributing factors to atheroma include hyperlipidemia, hypertension, and obesity.

Arteriosclerosis is characterized by an enhanced light reflex, focal attenuation, and irregularity of caliber. These signs may also be seen in the arterioles of normotensive individuals in middle age. These findings are due to fibrosis and hyalinization as confirmed by fluorescein angiography and histologic examination. In elderly individuals with arteriosclerosis and associated mild hypertension, it is difficult to differentiate the changes of arteriosclerosis from those of hypertension.

Appearance of Retinal Vessels

A normal arteriolar wall is transparent, so that what is actually seen is the column of blood within the vessel. A thin, central light reflection in the center of the blood column appears as a yellow refractile line about one-fifth the width of the column. As the walls of the arterioles become infiltrated with lipids and cholesterol, the vessels become sclerotic. As this process continues, the vessel wall gradually loses its transparency and becomes visible; the blood column appears wider than normal, and the thin light reflex becomes broader. The grayish yellow fat products in the vessel wall blend with the red of the blood column to produce a typical "copper wire" appearance. This indicates moderate arteriosclerosis. As sclerosis proceeds, the blood column-vessel wall light reflection resembles "silver wire," which indicates severe arteriosclerosis; at times, even occlusion of an arteriolar branch may occur.

Red-free light (a white light with a green filter) allows details of hemorrhages, focal irregularity of blood vessels, and nerve fibers to be seen more clearly (Fig 16–8).

HYPERTENSIVE RETINOPATHY

A major contribution to the study of hypertensive retinopathy was made by Wagener and Keith in 1939. They placed patients with hypertensive retinopathy into 4 groups (Figs 16–9 to 16–12). Stages I and II were restricted to arteriolar changes with attenuation and an increased light reflex ("copper" or "silver" wiring). The changes are mild, and subsequent observers have experienced difficulty in differentiating between these 2 groups. More emphasis has been placed on stages III and IV, which include cotton wool spots, hard exudates, hemorrhages, and extensive microvascular changes.

The classification has been of particular value in assessing the prognosis of patients with hypertension. The 5-year survival rate of patients in group I is about 70%; in group IV it is about 1%.

The appearance of the fundus in hypertensive retinopathy is determined by the degree of elevation of the blood pressure and the state of the retinal arterioles. Thus, in young patients with accelerated hypertension, an extensive retinopathy is seen, with hemorrhages, retinal infarcts (cotton wool spots), choroidal infarcts (Elschnig's spots), and occasionally serous detachment of the retina (Fig 16–13). Experimental work on monkeys made hypertensive suggests that ateriolar spasm initially occurs as a response to the high blood pressure and that this is followed by degeneration of the muscle of the blood vessel, with subsequent breakdown of the endothelial cells lining the vessel lumen. Secondary closure of the vessels occurs as a result of infiltration of the wall by plasma and fibrinogen to produce fibrinoid necrosis. The vascular damage is often associated with fibrin degradation products in the plasma, and this may play a part in the vascular changes of accelerated hypertension.

In contrast, elderly patients with arteriosclerotic vessels are unable to respond in this manner, and their vessels are thus protected by the arteriosclerosis. It is for this reason that elderly patients seldom exhibit florid hypertensive retinopathy (Fig 16–14).

Fluorescein angiography has made possible accurate documentation of these microcirculatory changes. In young patients with hypertension, arteriolar attenuation and occlusion are seen, and capillary nonperfusion can be verified in relation to a cotton wool spot, which is surrounded by abnormal dilated capillaries and microaneurysms and demonstrates increased permeability on fluorescein angiography.

Resolution of the cotton wool spots and the arteriolar changes occurs with successful hypotensive

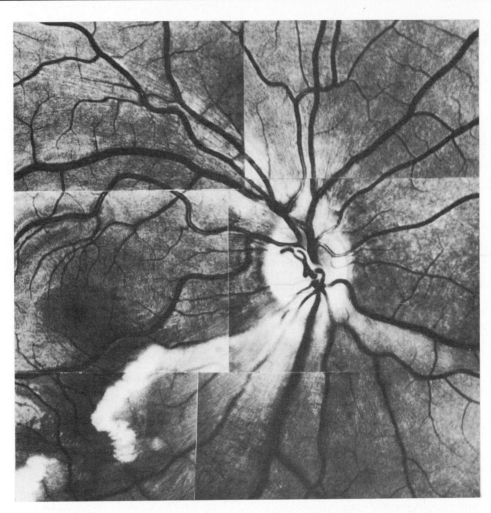

Figure 16–8. Acute retinal infarction. Red-free photograph shows acute arterial occlusion in a congenitally anomalous vessel at the disk. The inferior retina is infarcted, but axoplasm has accumulated beneath the fovea in an irregular pattern owing to preserved neuronal function of the distal ganglion cells.

therapy. In elderly patients, the underlying arteriosclerotic changes are irreversible.

Other Forms of Hypertensive Retinopathy

A severe retinopathy may be seen in advanced renal disease, in patients with pheochromocytoma, and in preeclampsia-eclampsia. All such patients should receive a complete medical workup to establish the nature of the hypertension, including measurement of 24-hour urinary vanillylmandelic acid excretion and occasionally measurement of blood levels of norepinephrine and selective adrenal angiography in cases of suspected pheochromocytoma (Fig 16–15).

CHRONIC OCULAR ISCHEMIA

Reduction in the retinal arteriovenous pressure gradient may produce acute signs of ocular ischemia (see preceding pages) or the less frequently recognized chronic changes.

Carotid Occlusive Disease

Carotid occlusive disease usually presents in middle-aged and elderly patients and is due to involvement of both the carotid artery and its smaller branches. Contributory factors include hypertension, smoking, and hyperlipidemia. In younger patients, rare forms of arteritis may occur (eg, Takayasu's disease).

In anterior segment ischemia, patients develop iritis, intraocular pressure changes, and pupillary abnormalities. In retinal ischemia (see Fig 16–16A), patients show evidence of capillary dilatation and hemorrhages, capillary occlusion, new vessels at the optic disk, and cotton wool patches.

Carotid Cavernous Fistula

Carotid cavernous fistula results from a communication between the carotid artery or its branches and

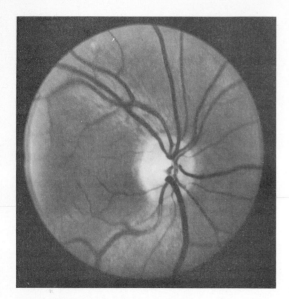

Figure 16–9. Keith-Wagener retinopathy stage I. Minimal vascular changes; a nearly normal fundus.

the cavernous sinus, producing characteristic vascular signs. Direct carotid fistulas are usually acute, florid, and posttraumatic, whereas fistulas from dural vessels are usually chronic, mild, and not associated with trauma. Clinical features include elevated intraocular pressure, dilated conjunctival vessels, dilated retinal vessels with hemorrhages and fluorescein leakage (Fig 16–16B), ophthalmoplegia (usually lateral rectus), and bruit.

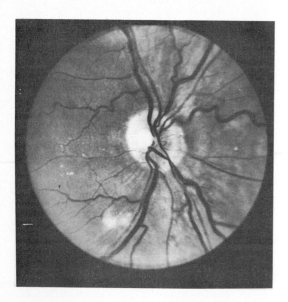

Figure 16–10. Keith-Wagener retinopathy stage II. There is irregularity of caliber of the arterioles and focal attenuation. Signs of retinal vascular disease include hard exudates at the macula, a cotton wool patch below the macula, and grooves in the nerve fiber layer beneath the disk, suggesting previous microinfarcts.

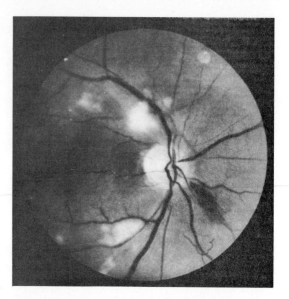

Figure 16–11. Keith-Wagener retinopathy stage III. Marked attenuation of retinal arterioles is apparent, with numerous microinfarcts and a large retinal hemorrhage.

Diagnosis is by angiography but should only be considered at the same time as therapeutic intervention. Closure of the fistula or the feeding vessels by embolization may provide dramatic and permanent recovery.

BENIGN INTRACRANIAL HYPERTENSION

Benign intracranial hypertension is a term used to indicate raised intracranial pressure in the presence of

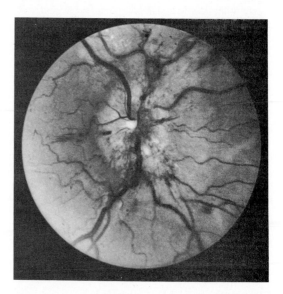

Figure 16–12. Keith-Wagener retinopathy stage IV. This may include the same retinal changes as stage III, but in addition there is disk swelling.

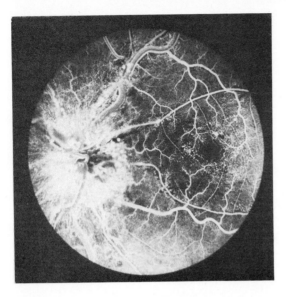

Figure 16–13. Accelerated hypertension. Fluorescein angiogram in a young man showing arteriolar constriction, dilatation of capillaries with microaneurysms, and areas of closure. Marked disk edema is present.

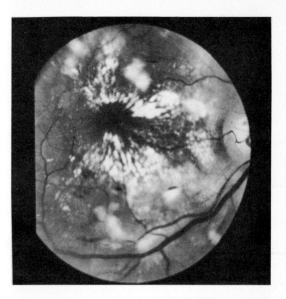

Figure 16–15. Pheochromocytoma. Marked circinate retinopathy with signs of recent retinal infarction and hemorrhages.

normal radiologic studies and normal cerebrospinal fluid. Patients present with headache, tinnitus, and dizziness; obscurations, blurred vision, and diplopia are the ophthalmologic features. Etiologic factors include (1) drug therapy, particularly oral contraceptives, nalidixic acid, tetracyclines, sulfonamides, vitamin A, and prolonged steroid therapy or steroid withdrawal in children; (2) endocrine abnormalities

(thyroid or parathyroid); (3) blood dyscrasia; (4) trauma; and (5) middle ear disease. Frequently, there is no obvious cause; in this (idiopathic) group, the patients are usually young overweight women with irregular menstrual periods. Benign intracranial hypertension is very rare in men, and a thorough search for a precipitating cause is mandatory in these patients.

The cause of the intracranial pressure increase is unknown, although both diminished absorption of cerebrospinal fluid and cerebral edema secondary to abnormality of the cerebral vessels have been suggested.

On examination, visual fields are normal with enlarged blind spots due to gross papilledema. Cerebrospinal fluid pressure is raised and may be as high as 500 mm of water. The aims of treatment are to reduce spinal fluid pressure and prevent permanent visual loss and optic atrophy, which occurs in up to 50% of patients. Treatment includes strict diet, serial lumbar punctures, diuretics (eg, acetazolamide), and occasionally optic nerve sheath decompression or lumboperitoneal shunt procedures.

SUBACUTE INFECTIVE ENDOCARDITIS

Inflammatory changes on the cardiac valves may produce multiple embolization with frequent ocular manifestations. The emboli may arise from vegetations on the cardiac valves and may be composed of platelet and fibrinogen aggregates or calcified endocardial vegetations. Ocular changes therefore are related to transit or obstruction of emboli in the conjunctival, retinal, or choroidal circulatory systems (Fig 16–17). Focal vasculitis due to circulating immune complexes has been demonstrated in the kidney, and similar changes can presumably occur in the eye.

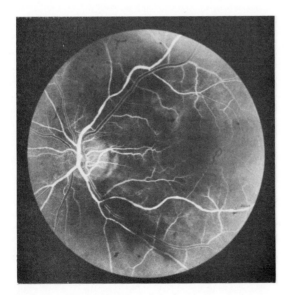

Figure 16–14. Accelerated hypertension. Fluorescein angiogram in an elderly woman showing marked arteriolar constriction and irregularity but few signs of florid retinopathy.

A

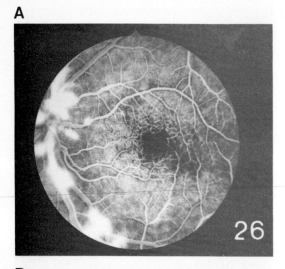

B

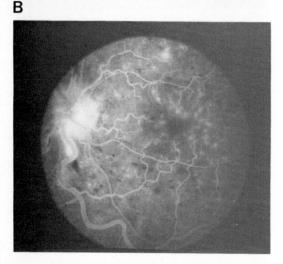

Figure 16–16. ***A:*** Fluorescein angiography of left fundus in a patient with chronic ocular ischemia secondary to Takayasu's disease. Note capillary dilatation, leakage of dye, retinal hemorrhages, cotton-wool spots, and neovascularization of the optic nerve head. ***B:*** Fluorescein angiography, showing leakage at optic disk and macula in a patient with chronic ocular ischemia secondary to dural arteriovenous fistula.

HEMATOLOGIC & LYMPHATIC DISORDERS

PERNICIOUS ANEMIA

Pernicious anemia occurs when lack of intrinsic factor prevents absorption of vitamin B_{12}; the normal intake is 2 μg daily, and normal blood levels are 350 μg/L.

Macrocytic anemia with thrombocytopenia is the classic hematologic abnormality.

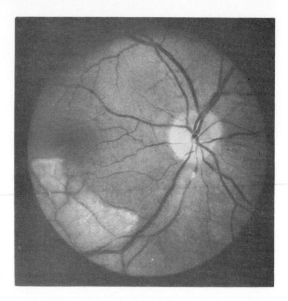

Figure 16–17. Subacute bacterial endocarditis. Calcific embolus impacted in arteriole below the disk, producing a distal area of retinal infarction.

Ocular involvement is rare. Retinal and choroidal hemorrhages can occur as a result of platelet deficiency or if the red blood cell count is less than 2.5 million/μL. The paucity of red cells may produce characteristic pallor of the conjunctiva. Optic neuropathy is present in 5% of cases. Ophthalmoplegia occurs rarely.

Treatment is by intramuscular injection of hydroxocobalamin (vitamin B_{12}), 1000 μg weekly for 2 months and monthly thereafter for life.

ACUTE MASSIVE HEMORRHAGE

Complete and sudden permanent blindness occurs rarely following acute massive hemorrhage, most commonly if bleeding is from the gastrointestinal tract or uterus. Such loss of vision is usually due to ischemic optic neuropathy (infarction of the disk). Though common prior to the use of blood transfusion, this type of blindness is rarely seen today.

DISSEMINATED INTRAVASCULAR COAGULATION

Disseminated intravascular coagulation, an acquired coagulation disorder, is characterized by clotting in small blood vessels throughout the body, particularly the renal cortex, heart, and brain. Occlusion of the choroidal vessels occurs, producing hemorrhage, thinning of the pigment epithelium, and serous retinal detachments. The inner retina and its blood supply may be affected in neonates but not in adults.

LEUKEMIA

The ocular changes of leukemia occur primarily in those structures with a good blood supply, including the retina, the choroid, and the optic disk (Fig 16–18). Changes are most common in the acute leukemias, where hemorrhages are seen in the nerve fiber and preretinal layers. Visual loss may occur when the hemorrhage occurs at the macula, and some hemorrhages may have white centers. If the white blood cell count is excessively elevated, retinal evidence of hyperviscosity syndrome (see below) may occur, with dilatation of the retinal arteries and veins, microaneurysms, and deep punctate hemorrhages.

Infiltration by leukemic cells may also occur in the retina, producing irregular pale areas, or in the choroid, causing pigmentary mottling. Infiltration at the optic disk is characteristic of acute lymphoblastic leukemia of infancy, in which blindness usually results.

HYPERVISCOSITY SYNDROMES

Increased viscosity results in a reduced flow of blood through the eye. This produces a characteristic appearance in the fundus of dilatation of the arteries and veins, which appear darker than normal, and retinal hemorrhages, microaneurysms, and areas of capillary closure (Fig 16–19). The main factors that contribute to blood viscosity are the red blood cells and plasma constituents, notably fibrinogen and the immunoglobulins. Polycythemia (high red cell count), either primary or secondary, may produce a hyperviscosity syndrome; the other main causes are macroglobulinemia (high IgM concentration) and multiple myeloma. Reduction of the abnormalities producing hyperviscosity can reverse the retinal changes.

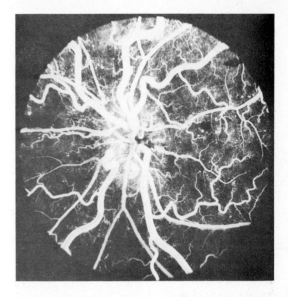

Figure 16–19. Hyperviscosity syndrome. Dilated arteries and veins, with hemorrhages and microaneurysms in a patient with hyperviscosity due to elevated IgM levels.

SICKLE CELL DISEASE

Sickle cell hemoglobinopathies are heritable disorders in which the normal adult hemoglobin is replaced by sickle hemoglobin in the red cell. This causes "sickle-shaped" deformity of the red cell on deoxygenation. Various types of sickling are described: sickle cell anemia (SS), sickle cell hemoglobin C (SC), and sickle cell thalassemia.

Ocular abnormalities include conjunctival changes, with "comma-shaped capillaries," and retinal

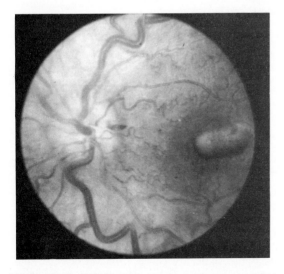
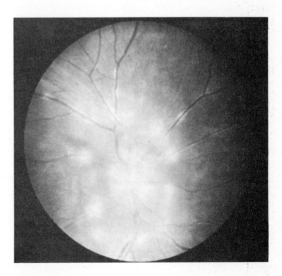

Figure 16–18. *Left:* Retinal changes in chronic myeloid leukemia, where dilated veins and hemorrhages may be seen. *Right:* In acute lymphoblastic leukemia, infiltration of the disk may be seen.

changes, including arterial occlusions, neovascular patterns (sea fan), and extensive capillary closure (Fig 16–20). Vitreous hemorrhage may result from bleeding arising from neovascular membranes, and choroidal occlusive phenomena have also been reported.

MALIGNANT LYMPHOMA

Lymphocytes are now divided into T and B subsets. Lymphomas of T cell origin (eg, Hodgkin's disease) do not usually involve the eye or orbit. B cell lymphomas may be undifferentiated, histiocytic, mixed, or malignant. They characteristically affect the eye and orbit and may be associated with systemic involvement. Orbital involvement may be seen in the conjunctiva, the lacrimal gland, or within the muscle cone. Orbital lymphoma represents a common cause of proptosis in the elderly. Rarely, malignant lymphoma may present as posterior uveitis of the eye, progressing to multiple cerebral lymphomas. Diagnosis may be difficult to make, even with the use of vitreous biopsy, vitrectomy, and sophisticated monoclonal antibody diagnostic techniques.

NEOPLASTIC DISEASE
(Fig 16–21)

Increasing age is associated with an increasing incidence of malignant disease. Thus, the ophthalmologist encounters these diseases more frequently in elderly people and must be familiar with the broad spectrum of their manifestations.

Neoplastic disease may involve the eye and optic pathways by direct spread or by metastatic effects.

The effect of the metastases depends upon the size and site of the metastasis and the site of the primary lesion. The most frequent primary tumor metastasizing to the eye is carcinoma of the breast in women and bronchial carcinoma in men, followed by neoplasms of the genitourinary and intestinal tracts and, less frequently, tumors of the kidney, thyroid, and prostate and malignant melanoma.

Metastatic Effects
A. Conjunctiva: Direct spread may occur from an iris or ciliary body melanoma. Subconjunctival hemorrhage occurs with bleeding disorders secondary to neoplasia (eg, liver failure, disseminated intravascular coagulation).

B. Sclera: Metastatic deposits are rare. Jaundice indicates biliary obstruction (eg, due to carcinoma of the head of the pancreas).

C. Iris, Ciliary Body, and Choroid: Melanoma deposits are common in all of these structures, and metastases from primary breast tumors are often seen in the choroid. These are often multiple, bilateral, and asymptomatic unless situated near the macula. Choroidal metastases probably represent the commonest choroidal neoplasm.

Uveitis sometimes occurs secondary to these metastases.

D. Vitreous: Neoplastic disease associated with immunologic disturbance (eg, reticulum cell sarcoma, carcinoma, lymphoma) may present initially as posterior uveitis.

Vitreous hemorrhage may occur directly from choroidal or retinal neoplasm or secondary to retinal neovascularization.

Amyloidosis, which may follow slow-growing tumors, produces strands in the vitreous.

E. Retina: Retinal detachment is a complication of choroidal metastases. Retinal vascular occlusion occurs secondary to hematologic abnormalities resulting from distant carcinomas (eg, pancreas, renal cell carcinoma); more rarely, photoreceptor degeneration may occur.

F. Orbit: Direct invasion from lacrimal adenocarcinoma or from carcinoma of the paranasal sinuses and nasopharynx will produce proptosis and painful ophthalmoplegia (known as the orbital apex syndrome due to involvement at the orbital fissure of cranial nerves II, III, IV, and VI). Compression of the optic nerve may produce central scotomas with disk edema or optic atrophy.

G. Extraocular Muscles: Orbital apex syndrome is discussed above. Discrete metastases of the extraocular muscles are rare. Meningeal carcinomatosis may produce nuclear palsies of the extraocular muscles or sixth nerve palsy secondary to raised intracranial pressure.

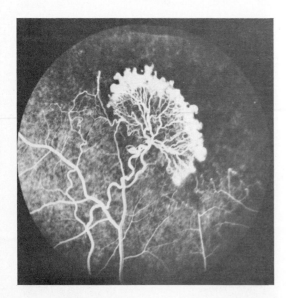

Figure 16–20. Sickle cell disease. Fluorescein angiogram of equatorial "sea fan," with extensive capillary closure peripheral to the fan.

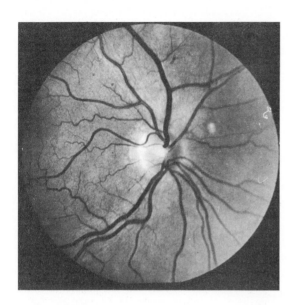

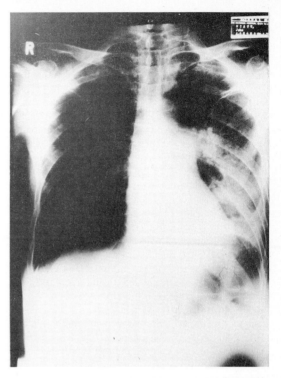

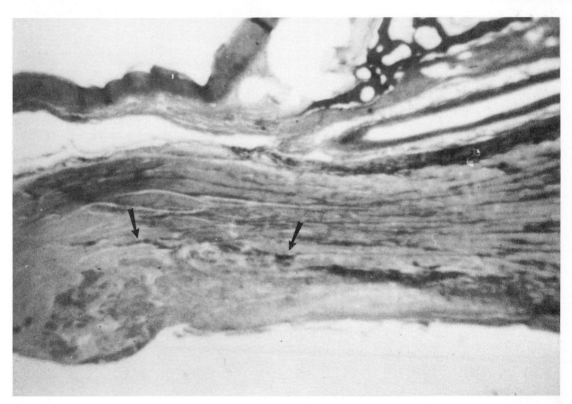

Figure 16–21. Neoplastic disease. ***Top left:*** Normal fundus of a patient with rapid visual loss in his only eye. ***Top right:*** Chest x-ray showed left lower lobe consolidation and a hilar mass. ***Bottom:*** Carcinoma of the bronchus was confirmed at autopsy, and metastasis was found in the optic nerve in the region of the canal (arrows).

H. Optic Nerve: Direct infiltration or compression of the optic nerve sheath from metastases or meningiomas results in progressive visual loss and optic atrophy. A carcinomatous optic neuropathy is reported in association with meningeal carcinomatosis when the visual loss is thought to have a vascular cause.

I. Optic Chiasm: Metastatic deposits characteristically present in patients with diabetes insipidus, because the highly vascular posterior pituitary is more susceptible to hematogenous spread of tumor cells. These patients therefore present with bitemporal field defects in addition to polyuria and polydipsia. Symptoms of dysfunction of the anterior pituitary or suprasellar extension to the chiasm may occur later.

J. Optic Tract, Optic Radiation, and Optic Cortex: Neoplasms in this area produce characteristic hemianopic field defects (see Chapter 14). These are associated with different symptoms (eg, temporal lobe epilepsy) according to the site of the neoplasm.

Nonmetastatic Effects

Uveitis occurs in patients with immunologic disturbances.

The myasthenic (Eaton-Lambert) syndrome occurs in patients with bronchial carcinoma and is characterized by fatigable weakness of skeletal muscles and, very rarely, ptosis and ophthalmoplegia. The electromyographic findings are diagnostic: The action potential of the motor unit is reduced in the resting muscle after a single maximal stimulus but increases after 4 seconds of tetanic stimulation.

Cerebellar degeneration occurs most commonly in women with ovarian carcinoma. The characteristic features include ataxia, dysarthria, and nystagmus.

METABOLIC DISORDERS

DIABETES MELLITUS

Diabetes mellitus is a complex metabolic disorder that also involves the small blood vessels, often causing widespread damage to many body tissues, including the eyes.

The ocular complications of diabetes are dependent not only upon impaired carbohydrate metabolism but also upon as yet undefined complexes of factors, and these may occur before the characteristic findings of glycosuria, hyperglycemia, polyuria, and polydipsia become manifest. The ocular complications occur approximately 20 years after onset despite apparently adequate diabetic control. Improved treatment measures (eg, improved insulins, antibiotics) that have lengthened the life span of diabetics have actually resulted in a marked increase in incidence of retinopathy and other ocular complications. Diabetes has be-

come the most common cause of blindness in younger people throughout the world. The visual outlook for adult (maturity onset) diabetics is considerably better than for juvenile diabetics.

The possibility of diabetes should be considered in all patients with unexplained retinopathy, cataract, extraocular muscle palsy, optic neuropathy, or sudden changes in refractive error. Absence of glycosuria or a normal fasting blood glucose level does not exclude a diagnosis of diabetes. Postprandial blood glucose determinations and glucose tolerance tests may be required. Rarely, the diabetic ocular change may become evident before there is demonstrable evidence of impaired glucose tolerance.

Retinopathy
(Figs 16–22 to 16–25)

Diabetic retinopathy is a common cause of blindness and now accounts for almost one-fourth of blind registrations in the western world.

Metabolic and hematologic factors are important in the development of diabetic retinopathy. Atheroma may be associated, and higher triglyceride and insulin levels are found in diabetics with atherosclerosis. Contributory rheologic factors include elevated blood viscosity and abnormal leukocyte and platelet function. The glycosylated hemoglobin HbA_{1c} increases the affinity of the blood for oxygen and is increased in diabetics to 12% from the normal level of 3.6% of total hemoglobin. The level of HbA_{1c} can be correlated with blood lipid concentrations and provides a measure of the efficacy of treatment.

HLA typing may be important in detecting diabetics who are vulnerable to severe diabetic retinopathy: (1) Increased incidence of HLA-A1 and HLA-B8 occurs in juvenile diabetes with microangiopathy; (2) HLA-B8, when occurring alone, is associated with severe diabetic retinopathy.

The presence and degree of retinopathy seem to be more closely related to the duration of the disease than to its severity. Control plays only a minor role (if any) in the onset, once the process is well under way.

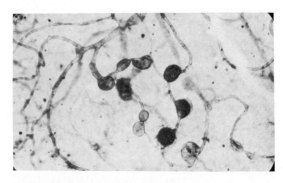

Figure 16–22. Diabetic retinopathy stage I. Trypsin-digested whole mount showing microaneurysms of the retinal capillaries.

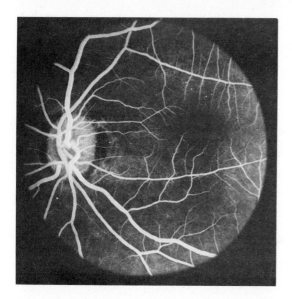

Figure 16–23. Diabetic retinopathy. Fluorescein angiogram shows earliest stage with microaneurysm in the macular region.

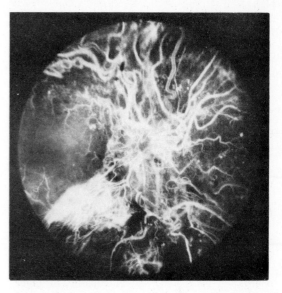

Figure 16–25. Proliferative diabetic retinopathy. Fluorescein angiogram shows extensive growth of vessels into the vitreous with marked fluorescein leakage.

The juvenile diabetic develops a severe form of retinopathy within 20 years in 60–75% of cases, even if under good control. The retinopathy often begins in stage IV and progresses to stage V. In older diabetic patients, retinopathy usually begins in stage I and seldom progresses beyond stage III. Macular degeneration may reduce the central visual acuity markedly in the later stages.

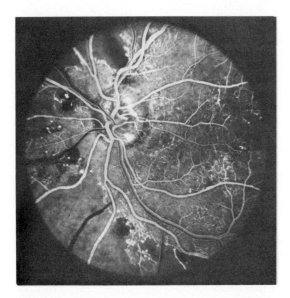

Figure 16–24. Diabetic retinopathy. Fluorescein angiogram shows florid retinopathy of diabetes with extensive areas of capillary closure, dilated capillaries with microaneurysms, and early new vessel formation at the optic disk.

The details of characteristics and treatment of diabetic retinopathy are presented in Chapter 14.

Lens Changes

A. True Diabetic Cataract (Rare): Bilateral cataracts occasionally occur with a rapid onset in severe juvenile diabetes. The lens may become completely opaque in several weeks. The process starts as snow-white areas in the cortex—posterior subcapsular and some anterior subcapsular opacities that progressively involve more and more cortex—which finally become confluent to make the entire lens opaque.

B. Senile Cataract in the Diabetic (Common): Typical senile nuclear sclerosis, posterior subcapsular changes, and cortical opacities occur earlier and more frequently in diabetics.

C. Sudden Changes in the Refraction of the Lens: Especially when diabetes is not well controlled, changes in blood glucose levels cause changes in sugar alcohols of the lens that in turn cause changes in refractive power by as much as 3 or 4 diopters. This results in blurred vision. Such changes do not occur when the disease is well controlled.

Iris Changes

Glycogen infiltration of the pigment epithelium and sphincter and dilator muscles of the iris may cause diminished pupillary responses. The reflexes may also be altered by the autonomic neuropathy of diabetes.

Rubeosis iridis is common in severe juvenile diabetes. Numerous small intertwining blood vessels develop on the anterior surface of the iris. Spontaneous hyphema may occur. The formation of peripheral anterior synechiae is aided by the vascularization of anterior chamber structures, eventually blocking aqueous outflow sufficiently to cause secondary glaucoma.

Extraocular Muscle Palsy
(Fig 16–26)

This common occurrence in diabetes is manifested by a sudden onset of diplopia caused by paresis of an extraocular muscle. This may be the presenting sign and is due to infarction of the nerve. When the third nerve is involved, pain may be a prominent symptom. Differentiation from a posterior communicating aneurysm is important; in diabetic third nerve palsy, the pupil is usually spared. Recovery of ocular motor function usually occurs within a year and frequently within 6–8 weeks. The fourth and sixth nerves may be similarly involved.

Optic Neuropathy

Visual loss is usually due to infarction of the optic disk or nerve. A characteristic telangiectatic pattern is visible at the optic disk in some younger diabetics with sudden visual loss. There is also a form of optic neuropathy that is associated with diabetes insipidus, diabetes mellitus, and deafness.

GOUT

Inflammatory changes in the eye, as in the joints, are due to the deposition of monosodium urate. This usually occurs in the conjunctiva and episclera, presenting as an acute and uncomfortable red eye. Less frequently, the sclera may be involved, and this can be associated with anterior uveitis, which is responsive to topical corticosteroid and cycloplegic therapy.

ENDOCRINE DISEASES

Disturbances of the endocrine glands have a number of important ocular manifestations. By far the most important of these are due to disturbances of the thyroid gland, although parathyroid and pituitary abnormalities also produce significant ocular changes.

THYROID GLAND DISORDERS

1. GRAVES' DISEASE

The general term Graves' disease has been used to describe patients with hyperthyroidism due to an autoimmune process. Patients with the eye signs of Graves' disease but without clinical evidence of hyperthyroidism are referred to as having ophthalmic Graves' disease. Apart from signs of hyperthyroidism, patients may have pretibial myxedema and clubbing of the fingers, and when these signs occur in com-

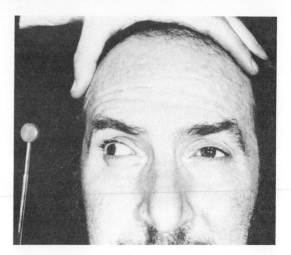

Figure 16–26. Pupil-sparing third nerve palsy in diabetes mellitus. Sudden painful ophthalmoplegia, left ptosis, failure of adduction, and normal pupillary responses.

bination with the ocular signs, the condition is termed thyroid acropachy.

Sophisticated diagnostic tests provide accurate diagnosis of thyroid disease (Table 16–2). These include the ability to recognize T_3 toxicosis and the ability to assess the hypothalamopituitary axis with the use of the TRH test.

Table 16–2. Thyroid function tests.

	Hyper-thyroid	Hypo-thyroid	Comments
Plasma T_4	+	−	
T_3 resin uptake	−	+	Thyopac technique. Other tests may vary.
Free thyroxine index	+	−	
Plasma TSH levels	−	+	In pituitary hypothyroidism, TSH is reduced.
Response to TRH	Absent	Exaggerated	Absent in pituitary hypothyroidism.
Autoantibodies	May be present	May be present (Hashimoto's)	

T_3 assay: A patient who is clinically hyperthyroid but with normal plasma T_4 may have T_3 thyrotoxicosis and raised plasma T_3 levels; the TRH test will show a hypothyroid response.

Clinical Findings

Patients may present with nonspecific complaints such as dryness of the eyes, discomfort, or prominence of the eyes. The American Thyroid Association has graded the ocular signs in order of increasing severity from 0 (no signs or symptoms) to 6 (sight loss due to optic nerve involvement). Class 3 involvement is proptosis greater than 22 mm.

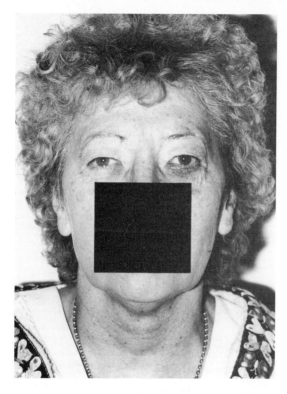
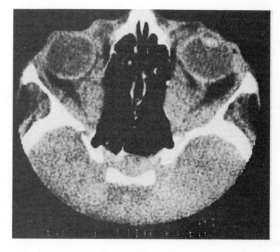

Figure 16–27. Thyroid ophthalmopathy. *Left:* Proptosis, visual loss, and ophthalmoplegia occurred in this elderly woman with a history of thyroid disease. *Right:* CT scans showed gross thickening of the ocular muscles, particularly in relation to the orbital apex. The increased intraorbital pressure is producing convexity of the medial orbital wall.

Class	Signs
0	No signs or symptoms
1	Only signs, which include upper lid retraction, with or without lid lag, or proptosis to 22 mm. No symptoms.
2	Soft tissue involvement
3	Proptosis > 22 mm
4	Extraocular muscle involvement
5	Corneal involvement
6	Sight loss due to optic nerve involvement

Lid retraction may be unilateral or bilateral and may be accompanied by impaired elevation of the eyes. Lid retraction appears to be pathognomonic of thyroid disease, particularly when associated with exophthalmos. The pathogenesis of lid retraction is not completely understood. Some features suggest overactivity of the sympathetic system, particularly the reversal of the retraction following administration of guanethidine eye drops. However, the absence of any pupillary dilatation has led to alternative explanations, and spasm of the striated levator palpebrae superioris muscle has been suggested.

A. Exophthalmos: (Fig 16–27.) The degree of exophthalmos may be extremely variable. Measurements using the Hertel or Krahn exophthalmometer range from minimal (20 mm) to excessive (28 mm or more). The condition is usually asymmetric and may be unilateral, and it is important clinically to assess the resistance to manual retropulsion of the globe. The increase in orbital contents that produces the exophthalmos is largely due to an increase in the bulk of the ocular muscles. Visualization of the ocular muscles is now possible with the advent of the CT scan (Fig 16–27), which can differentiate exophthalmos from an intraconal orbital tumor. In some cases, thickening of the ocular muscles may be restricted to certain muscles only (eg, medial or inferior rectus muscles).

B. Ophthalmoplegia: This is seen more commonly in ophthalmic Graves' disease, which usually affects older people and may be grossly asymmetric. Limitation of elevation is the most frequent finding, and this is mainly due to adhesions between the inferior rectus and inferior oblique muscles. Confirmation may be gained by measuring the intraocular pressure on elevation, when a substantial increase in the intraocular pressure suggests tethering. Often there is mild limitation of ocular movements in all positions of gaze. Patients complain of diplopia, which may be relieved by corticosteroid treatment, may spontaneously return to normal, or, if it remains static for 6–12 months, can frequently be relieved by surgical correction of one or more extraocular muscles.

C. Retinal and Optic Nerve Changes: Compression of the globe by the orbital contents may produce elevation of the intraocular pressure and retinal or choroidal striae. The optic disk may become swollen and progress to visual loss from optic atrophy. Optic neuropathy associated with Graves' disease occasionally occurs as a result of compression and ischemia of the optic nerve as it traverses the tense orbit.

D. Corneal Changes: In some patients, a superior limbic keratoconjunctivitis may be seen, though this is not specific for thyroid disease. In severe exophthalmos, corneal exposure and ulceration may occur.

Pathogenesis of the Ocular Signs

The main feature is gross distention of the ocular muscles due to the deposition of mucopolysaccharides. The mucopolysaccharides are strongly hygroscopic, which accounts for the increased water content of the orbits. There is an increase in the orbital connective tissue, with numerous fibroblasts, and the tissues are infiltrated by lymphocytes and plasma cells.

The pathogenesis of Graves' disease remains unknown, though an immunologic disorder involving both cellular and humoral elements has been implicated. Long-acting thyroid stimulator (LATS) is unlikely to be of significance in humans, because it is not always found in patients with ocular signs. There has, however, been good correlation between hyperthyroidism and human-specific thyroid stimulator, previously known as LATS protector, although this correlation is not seen in patients with Graves' disease. Thyroid autoantibodies against thyroglobulin and the microsome fraction of thyroid cells are frequently found in Hashimoto's disease and less often in Graves' disease. There are now thought to be 2 pathogenetic components to Graves' disease: (1) immune complexes of thyroglobulin-antithyroglobulin bind to extraocular muscles and produce a myositis; and (2) exophthalmos-producing substance acts with ophthalmic immunoglobulins to displace thyroid-stimulating hormones from the retro-orbital membranes, which results in the increase of retro-orbital fat.

Cellular immunity is also abnormal in Graves' disease. Lymphocytes from patients show increased migration inhibition. The total T lymphocyte count in peripheral blood may be abnormal, and there may be differences in the subpopulations of T cells. Patients with reduced T lymphocyte counts respond well to treatment with corticosteroids, but those with increased counts failed to improve with steroids. The finding of thyroid autoantibodies in a number of patients adds further credence to the immunologic theory of pathogenesis of this disorder.

Treatment

A. Medical Treatment: Medical treatment includes adequate control of the hyperthyroidism as a primary measure. However, thyroid ophthalmopathy may occur in the euthyroid or hypothyroid states. Severe cases with visual loss, disk edema, or corneal ulceration merit urgent medical treatment with corticosteroids in high doses (eg, prednisolone, 100 mg);

low doses are ineffective. Plasmapheresis is occasionally used with good results in the treatment of refractory cases of malignant exophthalmos, but full immunosuppression must follow plasmapheresis to prevent rebound increase of immunoglobulins and recurrence of disease. Immunosuppressive agents (eg, azathioprine) may play a supportive role and allow a lower maintenance dose of corticosteroids. In most cases, medical treatment produces adequate control, and surgical decompression is now performed less frequently. Guanethidine (Ismelin) eye drops, 10%, may produce temporary resolution of the lid retraction, which may be useful for cosmetic reasons.

B. Surgical Treatment: The lid retraction may be cosmetically improved by section of Müller's muscle (Henderson's operation) or by a lateral tarsorrhaphy. The latter may also provide some protection for the cornea. Decompression of the orbit may be performed from an intracranial approach (Krönlein's operation) with removal of the superior and lateral walls of the orbit. Currently in favor is antral decompression, in which the inferior and medial walls of the orbit are removed. Finally, if troublesome diplopia persists, ocular muscle surgery is often effective.

2. HYPOTHYROIDISM (Myxedema)

Significant ocular signs are not common in myxedema. Edema of the lids and periorbital tissue is commonly encountered. Thin superficial corneal opacities and small, flaky, white opacities in the lens cortex, neither of which seriously interferes with vision, may be present. Optic neuritis, with eventual optic atrophy and serious visual disability, occurs very rarely.

PARATHYROID GLAND DISORDERS

1. HYPOPARATHYROIDISM

Occasionally at thyroidectomy, the parathyroid glands are removed inadvertently, causing hypoparathyroidism. Spontaneous cases, although rare, should be suspected in young patients with cataracts. The blood calcium decreases, and serum phosphates are increased. Tetany may ensue and can be severe enough to cause generalized convulsions. The ocular manifestations consist of blepharospasm and twitching eyelids. Small, discrete, punctate opacities of the lens cortex develop that may eventually require lens extraction. Treatment with calcium salts, calciferol, and dihydrotachysterol usually prevents further development of lens opacities, but any that have occurred prior to treatment remain.

2. HYPERPARATHYROIDISM

In hyperparathyroidism, deposition of calcium may rarely occur in soft tissue. "Metastatic" calcification of the cornea and conjunctiva may be an early sign of the hypercalcemia encountered in this disorder.

VITAMINS & EYE DISEASE

Vitamins are organic complexes that are essential for normal growth and maintenance of life. Vitamins A, D, and K are fat-soluble; vitamins B and E are water-soluble. Abnormal intake may produce systemic effects and ocular manifestations.

VITAMIN A

Vitamin A (retinol) is found in fish oil and liver, and its precursor (carotene) is found in plants, vegetables, and cream. The normal daily requirement is 5000–7000 IU, and the normal blood level is 50–70 IU/L.

1. VITAMIN A DEFICIENCY

Symptoms and signs of vitamin A deficiency do not occur until the blood level drops below 50 IU/L. Vitamin A is essential for the maintenance of epithelium throughout the body, and deficiency produces changes in (1) the corneal and conjunctival epithelia **(xerophthalmia)** (Fig 16–28) and (2) retinal function **(night blindness).** Deficiency is due to dietary factors in underdeveloped countries (eg, seasonal, pregnancy) and more commonly to malabsorption in developed countries (eg, blind loop syndrome, massive gut resection).

Pathology

The conjunctival and corneal epithelia become dry and thickened; under the microscope, keratinized epithelium has replaced the normal columnar epithelium.

In the cornea, there is degeneration of Bowman's membrane and infiltration of the stroma with inflammatory cells and fluid. Yellow spots form in the cornea, and progression may result in hypopyon or perforation.

Clinical Findings

The damaged epithelium may produce dry, irritable eyes and blurred or distorted vision in severe cases. On examination, there are white foamy areas in the conjunctival tissue exposed by the palpebral apertures called Bitot's spots (Fig 16–29).

Xerosis of the corneal epithelium occurs in 2 stages: **prexerosis,** a loss of luster and reduction in corneal sensitivity; and **true xerosis,** an extension of conjunctival xerosis onto the cornea. Microscopic study of the scrapings from Bitot's spots shows large, keratinized epithelial cells with pale, indistinct cytoplasm and fragmented nuclei. The normal columnar conjunctival epithelium is keratinized and squamous. Xerosis bacilli (nonpathogenic diphtheroids originally thought to be the cause of xerosis) are numerous.

In severe cases, perforation of the cornea and subsequent loss of the eye can occur. Bilateral corneal scarring is common.

Night blindness is an early symptom and rarely severe. The fundi are normal, showing no pigmentary change, although yellow spots are occasionally seen in the retinal periphery.

The mechanism of any relationship between vitamin A deficiency and retinitis pigmentosa is not known.

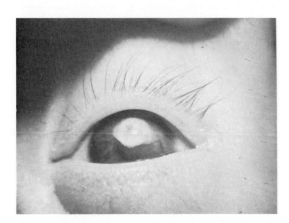

Figure 16–28. Keratomalacia. Case of xerophthalmia in a 5-month-old child.

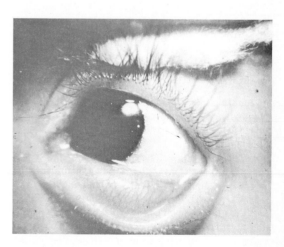

Figure 16–29. Xerophthalmia. Bitot's spot is seen as a foamy, white, wedge-shaped area with the base at the limbus.

Treatment

Both night blindness and xerophthalmia can be cured with adequate doses of vitamin A (eg, 20,000 IU/d). Recently, topical application of retinoic acid has been beneficial.

2. HYPERVITAMINOSIS A

Vitamin A intoxication has produced benign intracranial hypertension. These patients present with bilateral papilledema that may resolve months after ceasing ingestion.

VITAMIN B

The vitamin B complex is subdivided into 8 groups, but only vitamin B_1 and vitamin B_2 will be discussed here. Pernicious anemia (vitamin B_{12} deficiency) is discussed on p 288.

Vitamin B₁ Deficiency

Vitamin B_1 (thiamine) is found in animal and vegetable matter. The normal daily requirement is 1 mg, and the normal plasma levels are 21 μg/L.

Deficiency produces **beriberi,** characterized by high-output cardiac failure resulting in pleural and peritoneal effusions; in addition, peripheral neuritis is seen.

Seventy percent of patients have ocular abnormalities. Epithelial changes in the conjunctiva and cornea produce dry eyes and blurred vision. Visual loss with centrocecal scotomas may also be due to optic atrophy, and ocular motor palsies may be seen.

Treatment is by correction of dietary deficiency with liver, whole wheat bread, cereals, eggs, and yeast, or with parenteral injection of thiamine, 50 mg, or parenteral multivitamin preparation. **Wernicke's syndrome** of ophthalmoplegia, ptosis, and nystagmus is usually due to thiamine deficiency associated with alcoholism, although it can occur in other malnutrition states.

Vitamin B₂ Deficiency

Vitamin B_2 (nicotinic acid and riboflavin) is found in animals and vegetables, particularly liver, yeast, and wheat germ. The minimal daily requirement is 12–15 mg.

Nicotinic acid deficiency (pellagra) is quite common in alcoholics and is characterized by dermatitis, diarrhea, and dementia. Ocular involvement is rare, and optic neuritis or retinitis may develop.

Riboflavin deficiency has been said to cause a number of ocular changes. Rosacea keratitis, vascularization of the limbal cornea, seborrheic blepharitis, and secondary conjunctivitis have all been attributed to riboflavin deficiency, but these conditions seldom respond to riboflavin therapy. Optic atrophy is at times caused by ariboflavinosis. Definite riboflavin-deficient conditions respond well to dried (brewer's) yeast, 25–30 g 3 times daily.

VITAMIN C

Vitamin C (ascorbic acid) is found in fresh citrus fruits and green vegetables. The daily requirement is 50–100 mg, and the normal plasma level is 6.32 mg/L.

In vitamin C deficiency (scurvy), hemorrhages may develop in a variety of sites, eg, skin, mucous membranes, body cavities, the orbits, and subperiosteally in the joints. Hemorrhages may also occur into the lids, subconjunctival space, anterior chamber, vitreous cavity, and retina.

Treatment of vitamin C deficiency is with proper diet, particularly adequate amounts of citrus juice. Supplements of ascorbic acid, 200–300 mg/d orally, or sodium ascorbate injection, 0.5–1 g intravenously or intramuscularly daily in divided doses, will help correct vitamin C deficiency rapidly.

VITAMIN D

Vitamin D Deficiency

Children with rickets may develop zonular cataracts due to hypocalcemia.

Hypervitaminosis D

Calcium deposites in the cornea (forming band keratopathy) and in the conjunctiva are the most common ocular changes. Strabismus, epicanthal folds, osteosclerosis of orbital bones, nystagmus, papilledema, sluggish pupillary reaction, iritis, and cataract are less common ocular findings. The incidence of these changes has declined substantially since the content of vitamin D in milk and other foodstuffs has been subject to government regulation.

GRANULOMATOUS DISEASES

Many of the so-called granulomatous infectious diseases, including tuberculosis, sarcoidosis, brucellosis, leprosy, and toxoplasmosis, undergo a chronic course with frequent exacerbations and remissions. The eye is often involved, particularly by anterior uveitis. The following paragraphs deal with other ocular complications of these systemic diseases.

TUBERCULOSIS

Ocular tuberculosis results from endogenous spread from systemic foci. The incidence of eye involvement is less than 1% in known cases of pulmonary tuberculosis.

Tuberculosis of the Uveal Tract

A. Iritis (Anterior Uveitis): Many cases of granulomatous uveitis are said to be tuberculous, although very few cases have been established. At times only the anterior segment of the eye is involved. A few patients develop cells in the vitreous cavity with the picture of central retinal vein thrombosis. This may be associated with a high platelet count and may represent a hypersensitivity "erythema nodosum" reaction in the retina. Local treatment of iritis with mydriatics and corticosteroids is indicated. Systemic tuberculosis therapy is useful in the treatment of established cases of tuberculous uveitis.

B. Miliary Tuberculosis: In this usually fatal form of tuberculosis, many small discrete yellowish nodules are visible ophthalmoscopically in the posterior pole of the eye.

C. Solitary Tubercles: These occur as gray isolated masses about the size of the optic disk in the posterior fundus and usually cause minimal functional disturbance. The tubercles may be the first sign of an impending generalized uveitis. Solitary tubercles are occasionally seen in the iris or ciliary body.

Occasionally, orbital periostitis has occurred because of a tubercle.

SARCOIDOSIS
(Fig 16–30)

Sarcoidosis is a multisystem disease, with pulmonary, ocular, cutaneous, and reticuloendothelial system manifestations. The pulmonary changes include hilar lymphadenopathy, although pulmonary fibrosis may occur in the later stages. Erythema nodosum is seen in some cases, and sarcoid infiltration of the skin also occurs. Hepatosplenomegaly and lymphadenopathy are important signs of generalized systemic involvement.

Clinical Findings

Enlargement of the parotid glands occurs and, when associated with uveitis, is called **Heerfordt's syndrome.** Enlargement of lacrimal and salivary glands (**Mikulicz's syndrome**) also occurs.

A granulomatous uveitis with large mutton fat keratic precipitates and posterior synechiae is the commonest ocular manifestation. Sarcoid nodules may also be seen in the conjunctiva. Recent reports have suggested that granulomatous involvement of the retina, choroid, and optic disk may be seen more frequently than heretofore recognized. There are also reports that vitreous inflammation and involvement of the pars plana may be due to sarcoidosis. Neurologic sarcoidosis may produce visual loss from optic nerve involvement, and ocular motor and other cranial nerve palsies may be seen.

Pathogenesis & Diagnosis

The immunologic basis of sarcoidosis is not fully understood, but there is a depression of cell-mediated immunity and hyperactivity of humoral immunity. Lymphopenia is common, and the distribution of T lymphocytes is abnormal. The T cell count in peripheral blood is reduced, although there is some evidence that it is raised in other organs (eg, lungs). There is no correlation between immunologic abnormalities and clinical status. The diagnosis depends on clinical suspicion and confirmation by biopsy. Tissue

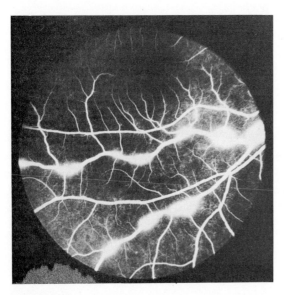
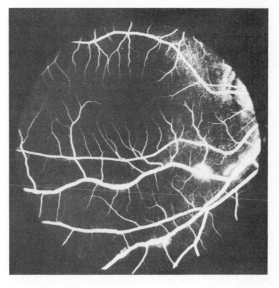

Figure 16–30. Sarcoidosis. Focal periphlebitis is a feature of ocular sarcoid and responds dramatically to corticosteroids. *Left:* Before treatment. *Right:* After treatment.

that has been biopsied includes the conjunctiva, liver, and scalene lymph node. Transbronchial biopsy is a useful technique that confirms the diagnosis in 85% of cases. If biopsy confirmation is not available, the Kveim test should be performed. This test consists of the intradermal injection of sarcoid material and then, after a period of 6 weeks, biopsy of the area, which, if positive, shows a granulomatous reaction with giant cells. Unfortunately, this test is less specific than transbronchial biopsy and is positive in only 20% of patients presenting with uveitis who later develop sarcoidosis. The Mantoux test should also be performed, though it is usually negative. Serum angiotensin-converting enzyme is produced by epithelioid cells, and raised levels may be found in sarcoidosis. This is an excellent test for assessing disease activity but not for diagnosis. Angiotensin-converting enzyme levels may also be high in tuberculosis, leprosy, primary biliary cirrhosis, experimental allergic alveolitis, and Hodgkin's disease.

Gallium scan is a helpful diagnostic test in sarcoidosis. Radioactive gallium is absorbed by activated macrophages and may localize in inflammatory foci, eg, lacrimal and salivary glands. Increased uptake in the lacrimal gland may also occur in Sjögren's syndrome, leukemia, and lymphoma.

Treatment

The uveitis is controlled by corticosteroids and mydriatics applied topically. The development of new vessels in the retina may require photocoagulation. The systemic disease is controlled by the administration of oral corticosteroids.

EALES'S DISEASE

This disease was originally reported to occur in young men in a poor general state of health who experienced recurrent vitreous hemorrhages from areas of retinal neovascularization. However, such symptoms are also known to occur in tuberculosis, sarcoidosis, systemic lupus erythematosus, sickle cell disease, and diabetes. Extensive investigations are therefore indicated to exclude these conditions in patients with consistent clinical features. If test results are negative, Eales's disease is then appropriate as a diagnosis arrived at by exclusion. Photocoagulation of the new vessels can reduce the chance of further vitreous hemorrhage.

LEPROSY
(Hansen's Disease)

Leprosy is a chronic granulomatous disorder caused by *Mycobacterium leprae,* an acid-fast bacillus. It is estimated that 12–15 million people in the world have leprosy and that of this number, 20–50% (2.4 to 6 or 7 million) have ocular involvement. In tropical countries, the infection is endemic.

Three major types of leprosy are recognized: lepromatous, tuberculoid, and dimorphous. The type any given patient will develop depends upon the individual's immunity to the organism and the number of invading organisms. Thus, a person with minimal or no cell-mediated immunity and in whom the organisms are numerous (multibacillary) develops lepromatous leprosy, whereas a person with strong resistance and few organisms (paucibacillary) develops tuberculoid leprosy. The eye may be affected in any type of leprosy, but ocular involvement is more common in the lepromatous type. Ocular lesions are due to direct invasion by *M leprae* of the ocular tissues or of the nerves supplying the eye and adnexa. Since the organism appears to grow better at lower temperatures, infection is more apt to involve the anterior segment of the eye than the posterior segment.

Clinical Findings

The early clinical signs of ocular leprosy are lagophthalmos, loss of the lateral portions of the eyebrows and eyelashes (madarosis), conjunctival hyperemia, and superficial keratitis (Fig 16–31), with interstitial keratitis—beginning typically in the superior temporal quadrant of the cornea—often supervening.

Scarring of the cornea from interstitial or exposure keratitis (or both) causes blurred vision and often blindness. Granulomatous iritis with lepromas (iris pearls) is common, and a low-grade iritis associated with iris atrophy and a pinpoint pupil may also occur. Hypertrophy of the eyebrows with deformities of the lids and trichiasis are late changes, and exposure keratitis, typically in the inferior and central cornea, can result from facial nerve palsy and absence of corneal sensation.

Ocular leprosy can be diagnosed on the basis of characteristic signs combined with a characteristic skin biopsy.

Treatment

The best drugs for treating leprosy are the sulfones, which are bacteriostatic, and clofazimine and rifampin, which are bactericidal. In multibacillary infec-

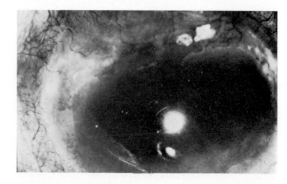

Figure 16–31. Leprosy keratitis, left eye. (Courtesy of W Richards.)

tions, it is now recommended that the 2 types of drugs be used together. Since the host may harbor the organisms for years, long-term therapy is necessary. Drug reactions such as erythema nodosum leprosum may require corticosteroids or clofazimine for adequate control. Granulomatous iritis may be benefited by topical atropine and corticosteroids; low-grade iritis with iris atrophy is benefited by topical phenylephrine and epinephrine.

SYPHILIS

Congenital Syphilis

Manifestations of syphilis acquired in utero or at birth include mental deficiency, saddle nose, rhinitis, Hutchinson's teeth, alopecia, exanthemas, deafness, and bone lesions. The most common eye lesion is interstitial keratitis (see p 121). Chorioretinitis unassociated with interstitial keratitis occurs fairly often. There are many small yellow dots and pigment clumps in the peripheral fundus, giving the typical "salt and pepper" appearance. In other cases, the chorioretinitis occurs as larger isolated patches or may have the appearance of retinitis pigmentosa. Syphilitic conjunctivitis or dacryoadenitis is rare.

Congenital syphilis is treated with large doses of penicillin.

Acquired Syphilis

Ocular chancre (primary lesion) occurs rarely on the lid margins and follows the same course as a genital chancre.

Iritis and iridocyclitis occur in the secondary stage of syphilis along with the rash in about 5% of cases. The iritis is acute, with fibrous exudates in the anterior chamber.

Other less common ocular manifestations of acquired syphilis are interstitial keratitis and chorioretinitis, which occur much less frequently in acquired than in congenital syphilis; chorioretinitis usually is widespread and often involves the disk, producing posterior uveitis (Fig 16–32).

Most cases of syphilis can now be diagnosed by the Venereal Disease Research Laboratory (VDRL) or *Treponema pallidum* hemagglutination (TPHA) tests. Further tests include the *T pallidum* immobilization (TPI) test and the fluorescent treponemal antibody (FTA-ABS) test. The latter test can indicate whether a recent infection has occurred. The increasing incidence of syphilis requires the use of these tests in all patients with unexplained uveitis, vitritis, retinal vasculitis, ischemic optic neuropathy, or ocular motor nerve palsies. Treatment consists of systemic penicillin in very high dosage, with systemic corticosteroids.

Neuro-ophthalmologic Considerations

Neurosyphilis may be asymptomatic or may present as meningovascular syphilis, tabes dorsalis, or general paralysis of the insane. **Meningovascular**

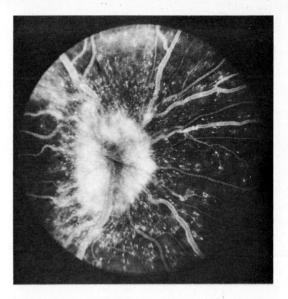

Figure 16–32. Secondary syphilis. Bilateral visual loss occurred in a 24-year-old man. Late fluorescein photographs showed disk leakage with dilatation and leakage of peripapillary capillaries.

syphilis particularly involves the base of the brain and may produce cerebrovascular accidents (midbrain or pontine syndromes) or cranial nerve palsies. **Tabes dorsalis** occurs 20–30 years after the initial infection and typically is associated with lightning pains, ataxia, absent deep tendon reflexes, and loss of posterior columnar function. In 90% of cases, there are Argyll Robertson pupils, bilaterally small pupils that fail to constrict to light but constrict normally to accommodation. Optic atrophy is seen in 20% of cases. **General paralysis of the insane** is now an uncommon manifestation and represents progressive loss of cortical function due to chronic meningoencephalitis. Cranial nerve palsies, Argyll Robertson pupils, and optic atrophy are rare features.

When serologic tests and examination of cerebrospinal fluid suggest active treponemal infection, a 21-day course of penicillin should be given.

BRUCELLOSIS

During the chronic stage of this disease, ocular involvement by the endogenous route is fairly common. Iritis is the most frequent ocular complication. The uveitis is not always granulomatous; if nongranulomatous, the inflammation tends to subside in a short time. Less common complications include choroiditis, generalized uveitis, and nummular keratitis, which has the same clinical appearance as epidemic keratoconjunctivitis. These lesions usually heal well but occasionally ulcerate, and they can develop into chronic keratitis with periodic exacerbations and remissions.

Other ocular complications of brucellosis, including

scleritis, are rarely seen. Cases of ocular brucellosis may respond to tetracycline and streptomycin, although the organism develops resistance easily. The iritis is treated locally by mydriatics. Corticosteroids are sometimes of value locally but are contraindicated systemically.

TOXOPLASMOSIS

This disease is of great ocular importance. The organism is a protozoal parasite that infects a great number of animals and birds and has worldwide distribution. Although there have not been a great many proved human cases, toxoplasmosis is probably the most common cause of posterior chorioretinitis.

Congenital Toxoplasmosis (Fig 16–33)

Infection occurs in utero, and one-third of infants born to mothers who acquired toxoplasmosis during pregnancy—particularly during the third trimester—will be affected.

The disease is recognized after birth by the typical posterior polar chorioretinitis, which is usually seen in the inactive stage. A number of cases also show cerebral or cerebellar calcification by x-ray, although only a minority show signs of central nervous system disease such as convulsions, mental deficiency, hemiplegia, or paraplegia. The congenital form is nearly always arrested by the time it can be diagnosed.

Congenital toxoplasmosis is perhaps the most common cause of posterior uveitis. A focal choroiditis is seen, usually in the posterior pole, and an active lesion is often related to an old healed lesion. Episodes of posterior uveitis and chorioretinitis usually represent a reactivation of a congenital infection. Rarely, panuveitis may occur, or papillitis progressing to optic atrophy. Isolated anterior uveitis does not occur. Pe-

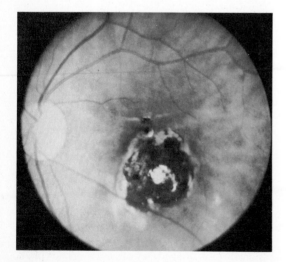

Figure 16–33. Healed toxoplasmic chorioretinitis. Note scaring in left macular area.

ripheral vision is preserved, but because the macula is involved in at least 50% of cases, central vision is reduced.

Treatment with systemic corticosteroids reduces inflammation but does not prevent scar formation. Subconjunctival or retrobulbar injection of corticosteroids is contraindicated, because it may cause severe exacerbation of disease. Clindamycin may be considered in acute cases, although pseudomembranous colitis is an infrequent complication of this treatment.

Acquired Toxoplasmosis

Acquired toxoplasmosis affects young adults and is characterized by general malaise, lymphadenopathy, sore throat, and hepatosplenomegaly similar to that seen in infectious mononucleosis. Toxoplasmic retinochoroiditis may rarely follow acquired systemic toxoplasmosis.

VIRAL DISEASES

HERPES SIMPLEX

The most common manifestation of herpes simplex is fever blisters on the lips. The most common and serious eye lesion is herpes simplex (dendritic) keratitis (see p 121). Vesicular skin lesions can also appear on the skin of the lids and the lid margins. Herpes simplex may cause iridocyclitis and may rarely cause severe encephalitis. (Corticosteroids should not be employed in early stages.)

There are 2 morphologic strains of the virus: type 1 and type 2. Ocular infections are usually produced by type 1, whereas genital infections are caused by type 2.

Retinitis due to herpes simplex virus type 1 occurs in adults suffering from herpes encephalitis or in immunosuppressed patients. Severe occlusive retinal vasculitis develops, followed by retinal necrosis and detachment. Type 1 antigens have been found in all layers of the retina, pigment epithelium, and choroid. Intravenous acyclovir prevents spread of the disease, and prophylactic retinal buckling may be useful.

Herpes simplex virus type 1, varicella-zoster virus, and cytomegalovirus have all been implicated in **acute retinal necrosis syndrome,** which produces a similar clinical picture but affects healthy young individuals.

HERPES ZOSTER (See Chapter 15.)

POLIOMYELITIS

Bulbar poliomyelitis severe enough to cause lesions of the third, fourth, or sixth cranial nerve is usually fatal. Any type of internal or external ophthalmoplegia may result in survivors. Supranuclear abnormalities ("gaze" palsies, paralysis of convergence or divergence) are rare residual defects. Optic neuritis is rarely present. Treatment is purely symptomatic, although occasionally a residual extraocular muscle imbalance can be greatly improved by strabismus surgery.

GERMAN MEASLES
(Rubella)

Maternal rubella during the first trimester of pregnancy causes congenital anomalies, including serious heart disease, genitourinary disorders, and many serious ocular diseases, in about 10% of infants. The most common eye complication is cataract, which is bilateral in 75% of cases. The embryonal and fetal nuclei of the lens are usually opaque, and visual acuity is often below 20/200. Other congenital ocular anomalies are frequently associated with the cataracts, eg, uveal colobomas, searching nystagmus, microphthalmos, strabismus, retinopathy, and infantile glaucoma. Congenital cataract, especially if bilateral, may require surgical removal, but the prognosis is always guarded, since other ocular anomalies are often present that may not be recognized until the cataract is removed. Many physicians have felt that therapeutic abortion is advisable if rubella occurs during the first trimester of pregnancy, since the rate of serious congenital anomalies is so high.

Cataract surgery should be delayed until at least age 2, since the live virus is present in ocular tissues for many months after birth. The results of early surgery are unsatisfactory in a very high percentage of cases.

HEPATITIS B

The hepatitis B virus is transmitted primarily via blood transfusion or improperly sterilized syringes, needles, or scalpels. Infections produce a mild acute hepatitis; uveitis with disk edema is a rare complication. The virus has been implicated in the pathogenesis of glomerulonephritis and polyarteritis nodosa via immune complex formation, but there is no evidence for a similar association with idiopathic inflammatory eye disease.

MEASLES
(Rubeola)

Acute conjunctivitis is common early in the course of measles. Koplik's spots can occur on the conjunctiva. There may also be an associated epithelial keratitis.

Interest has recently been shown in the slow virus of measles, which produces an encephalitis (**subacute sclerosing panencephalitis**). Ocular signs include disk edema and macular changes due to neuroretinal involvement. The prognosis is extremely poor.

The treatment of the eye complications of measles is symptomatic unless there is secondary infection, in which case local antibiotic ointment is used.

MUMPS

The most common ocular complication of mumps is dacryoadenitis. A diffuse keratitis with corneal edema resembling the disciform keratitis of herpes simplex occurs rarely. It usually clears completely within 2–3 weeks. Other less common eye complications of mumps include episcleritis, iridocyclitis, choroiditis, and optic neuritis, all of which tend to heal with little or no residual damage. Mumps encephalitis can cause a wide variety of neuro-ophthalmologic abnormalities that may be permanent, including internal and external ophthalmoplegia, pupillary abnormalities, and gaze palsies. Convalescent serum and gamma globulin may help to modify the disease; otherwise, treatment is symptomatic.

CHICKENPOX
(Varicella)

Swollen lids, conjunctivitis, vesicular conjunctival lesions, and (rarely) optic neuritis may occur as part of the clinical picture of chickenpox.

INFECTIOUS MONONUCLEOSIS

Although this fairly common disease is often looked upon as benign and self-limited, there is increasing evidence that significant complications are not rare. The disease process can affect the eye directly, causing nongranulomatous uveitis, scleritis, conjunctivitis, retinitis, or papillitis. Complete recovery is usual, but residual visual loss can result. The central nervous system may also be involved, causing infranuclear muscle palsies, nystagmus, and pupillary abnormalities. No specific therapy is available, although gamma globulin has been used with questionable benefit.

CYTOMEGALIC INCLUSION
DISEASE

Infection with cytomegalovirus, a member of the herpesvirus group, may range from a subclinical infection to classic manifestations of cytomegalic inclusion disease. The virus most frequently affects newborn infants and compromised hosts, and the disease can be acquired or congenital. The clinical findings in the newborn infant may include prematurity, hepatosplenomegaly, jaundice, and microcephaly. The ocular findings include focal necrotizing retinitis and choroiditis with perivascular infiltrates and retinal hemorrhages. Other reported ocular findings include microphthalmia, cataract, optic atrophy, and optic disk malformation.

Histopathologic examination of the retinal and choroidal lesion shows large inclusion-bearing cells characteristic of cytomegalovirus infections. There is disruption of the normal architecture of the retina and choroid, with evidence of necrosis and mononuclear and perivascular infiltration. Calcifications in the retina may be observed.

Laboratory studies include isolation of the virus from a fresh urine specimen, from a throat swab, or from a liver biopsy. Serologic tests, complement-fixing antibodies, and indirect FA tests may become positive. The evaluation of cord serum IgM and IgA in newborn infants is helpful as a nonspecific aid in the diagnosis of congenital cytomegalic inclusion disease.

The differential diagnosis in the congenital disease should include toxoplasmosis, rubella, herpesvirus hominis or herpes simplex infection, and syphilis.

Ganciclovir is the drug of choice for cytomegalic inclusion retinitis. It halts the progression of the disease without eradicating the virus. (See section on Acquired Immune Deficiency Syndrome, below.)

FUNGAL DISEASE

CANDIDIASIS

The introduction of modern surgical and immunosuppressive methods of treatment to clinical medicine has resulted in a marked increase in the number of people with compromised immune systems and, therefore, an increase in the susceptibility of these patients to a large number of opportunistic pathogens that were previously considered saprophytes. *Candida albicans* is one of the most important opportunistic fungi.

Many factors are responsible for this apparent emergence of *Candida* as an important opportunistic organism. These factors include the increasing long-term use of corticosteroids and cytotoxic agents, widespread use of antibiotics, abdominal surgery, prolonged use of indwelling intravenous catheters and hyperalimentation, widespread abuse of intravenous narcotic drugs, infusion of glucose solutions, diabetes, debilitating diseases, malnutrition, and malignant diseases.

The ocular involvement accompanies systemic *Candida* infection and candidemia in approximately two-thirds of cases. The initial *Candida* lesion is a focal necrotizing granulomatous retinitis with or without choroiditis, characterized by fluffy white exudative lesions associated with cells in the vitreous overlying the lesion. Such lesions may spread to in-

volve the optic nerve and other ocular structures. Endophthalmitis, panophthalmitis, Roth's spots, papillitis, and exudative retinal detachment may occur. Spread into the vitreous cavity may result in the formation of a vitreous abscess. Anterior uveitis occurs with cells and flare in the anterior chamber, and a hypopyon may form.

Treatment consists of vitrectomy and systemic administration of amphotericin B, flucytosine, and ketoconazole.

ACQUIRED IMMUNODEFICIENCY SYNDROME (AIDS)

Acquired immune deficiency syndrome is now known to be caused by a retrovirus called human immunodeficiency virus (HIV). The virus infects mature T helper cells, leading to immunosuppression, the severity of which depends on the balance between the rates of destruction and replacement of T cells. The persistent immunodeficiency leads to opportunistic infections. The virus has been recovered from various body fluids, including blood, semen, saliva, tears, and cerebrospinal fluid. It has also been isolated from brain tissue, suggesting potential neurotropism. The viral envelope undergoes continuous structural change, so that antibodies are rendered ineffective and the development of a vaccine is extremely difficult. The virus responsible for virtually all cases of infection in the Western World is HIV-1, but at least one similar virus (HIV-2) has now been identified in western Africa. HIV-2 also causes illness, but its pathogenicity may be less. These 2 viruses have similar core proteins but different envelope proteins, and so antibody tests for HIV-1 may not necessarily identify infections with HIV-2.

The virus is thought to have originated in the green monkey, native to central Africa, and then to have traversed the species barrier. The virus has spread from Africa to many other parts of the world, including Haiti and the USA. So far, 73% of adult cases have occurred in homosexual or bisexual men, 17% in intravenous drug abusers, 3% in recipients of blood or blood product transfusions (1% of these were patients with hemophilia or other blood coagulation disorders), and 1% in persons who have had heterosexual contact with an AIDS carrier or patient. Seventy-one percent of pediatric cases have occurred congenitally in children whose parents had AIDS or were at increased risk for AIDS.

Transmission & Prevention of AIDS

Transmission of the AIDS virus (HIV) is primarily by exchange of bodily fluids during sexual contact or through the use of contaminated needles by intravenous drug abuse. Transmission may also occur when contaminated blood products are transfused. The virus is not transmitted by casual contact, but because it is found in tears, conjunctival cells, and blood, health workers must take reasonable precautions when handling infectious waste or in contact with body fluids.

The virus can be inactivated readily in vitro by common disinfectants, including isopropanol, ethanol, glutaraldehyde, and sodium hypochlorite, or by heat inactivation at 60 °C for brief periods. The Centers for Disease Control has published specific guidelines for preventing transmission of the virus in tears. Gloves should be worn when exposure is anticipated, and any skin exposure must be followed by hand washing with soap and water. Tonometer heads should be disinfected for 5–10 minutes and then rinsed thoroughly and dried.

Routine screening for the detection of antibodies against HIV by ELISA is now available. This is a specific and sensitive test that is used to screen all blood donors. The test can also be performed on blood taken from cadavers and thus provides valuable screening for corneal donors. However, screening cannot always exclude infected donors, since antibodies may not develop for several weeks after infection.

Clinical Findings

The spectrum of clinical disease is wide, presumably due to the degree of immunologic damage and the frequency and nature of opportunistic infections. Typically, an acute flulike illness occurs a few weeks after infection, followed months later by weight loss, fever, diarrhea, lymphadenopathy, and encephalopathy. In Third World countries, patients often develop tuberculosis, malaria, or bacterial pneumonia. Ocular involvement occurs in 50–70% of cases. The commonest findings are retinal microvasculopathy with cotton-wool spots and hemorrhages and conjunctival vasculopathy characterized by comma vessels, sludging of the blood, and linear hemorrhages (Fig 16–34). The cause of these findings is unknown, but they are sometimes associated with increased plasma viscosity and may represent immune complex deposition.

The hallmark of the acquired immune deficiency syndrome is the high incidence of infections, which are frequently multiple, opportunistic, and severe. The eye is involved in 30% of cases, and both the anterior segment and the retina may be affected. Viral opportunistic infections of the retina are most common, particularly cytomegalovirus retinitis. This typically presents as a hemorrhagic necrotic retinopathy spreading from vascular arcades and associated with arteriolar occlusions. The vitreous is quiet; retinal detachment may occur. Diagnosis is usually based on circumstantial evidence of positive antibody titers in blood, urine, or cerebrospinal fluid. Ocular fluids and retinal specimens are rarely examined. The treatment of choice is ganciclovir, a virostatic drug that stops progression of disease but does not eradicate the virus from the eye. Maintenance therapy is thus required, which brings the attendant problems of long-term intravenous therapy; neutropenia is the most important side effect.

Herpes simplex retinitis begins in the peripheral retina, advances to involve the entire fundus, and is associated with arteriolar occlusion. The retinitis almost always occurs concurrently with herpes simplex encephalitis, and this serves to distinguish herpes simplex from cytomegalovirus retinitis, which is rarely complicated by encephalitis. Treatment is with acyclovir, but maintenance therapy is again required.

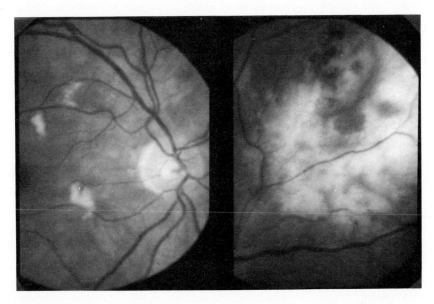

Figure 16–34. Retinal changes in AIDS. Multiple cotton wool spots **(left)** and retinal necrosis with hemorrhage **(right)** due to opportunistic infection. (Courtesy of R Marsh.)

Toxoplasma chorioretinitis is usually bilateral, acquired (congenital infections are rarely reactivated in AIDS), and associated with substantial vitreous reaction; candidal endophthalmitis is rarely seen except in drug addicts. More unusual organisms that occasionally produce retinitis include *Cryptococcus*, herpes zoster, *Mycobacterium avium-intracellulare*, *Haemophilus influenzae*, and *Sporothrix schenkii*.

Herpes zoster ophthalmicus is a common presenting feature of HIV infection and may be very severe, with anterior segment necrosis and ophthalmoplegia. Herpes simplex, molluscum contagiosum, and Kaposi's sarcoma frequently affect the eyelids and surrounding tissues.

Neuro-ophthalmologic problems are divided into those related directly to HIV infection of the brain, such as optic neuropathy and intranuclear ophthalmoplegia, and those caused by cerebral abscesses or encephalitis.

Zidovudine (AZT) is the drug of choice for retrovirus infection and is used in the majority of HIV-infected patients. It may eventually modify the need for prophylaxis or maintenance treatment of opportunistic infections.

MULTISYSTEM AUTOIMMUNE DISEASES

This ill-defined group of diseases is characterized by widespread inflammatory damage of connective tissue with deposition of fibrinoid tissue in the ground substance. There is evidence that an autoantibody reaction against normal tissue antigens produces tissue damage. Ocular involvement is frequent in most collagen diseases.

SYSTEMIC LUPUS ERYTHEMATOSUS

Discoid lupus erythematosus is localized to the skin region on either side of the nose, conforming to the characteristic "butterfly" distribution. There are no generalized features.

Systemic or disseminated lupus erythematosus is a multisystem disease including "butterfly skin lesions," pericarditis, Raynaud's phenomenon, renal involvement, arthritis, anemia, and central nervous system signs. Almost any ocular structure can be involved, but scleritis, conjunctivitis, and keratoconjunctivitis sicca (in 25% of cases) are predominant. Uveitis rarely occurs, and retinal involvement produces signs of arteriolar occlusion, probably a manifestation of arteritis. The fundus picture may be complicated by a hypertensive retinopathy, which in severe cases can cause capillary occlusion or even proliferative retinopathy.

Pathogenesis & Diagnosis

The disease is an immunologic disorder marked by the presence of circulating immune complexes. Diagnostic tests include anti-DNA antibodies and mitochondrial type V antibodies. Active disease is associated with raised circulating immune complexes and reduced fractions of complement.

Vascular occlusion in systemic lupus erythematosus may be associated with anticardiolipin antibodies.

Treatment

Systemic steroids and sometimes immunosuppressives may be very effective therapeutically.

DERMATOMYOSITIS

This rare disease occurs frequently in children. Characteristically there is a degenerative subacute inflammation of the muscles, sometimes including the extraocular muscles. The lids are commonly a part of the generalized dermal involvement and may show marked swelling and erythema. Retinopathy—consisting of multiple white, irregular opacities appearing much like cotton wool patches—as well as flame-shaped hemorrhages may occur. High doses of systemic corticosteroids will frequently effect a remission that continues even after cessation of therapy. The ultimate prognosis is poor, however.

SCLERODERMA

This rare chronic disease is characterized by widespread alterations in the collagenous tissues of the mucosa, bones, muscles, skin, and internal organs. Men and women between 15 and 45 years of age are affected. The skin in local areas becomes tense and "leathery," and the process may spread to involve large areas of the limbs, rendering them virtually immobile. The skin of the eyelids is often involved. Iritis and cataract occur less frequently. Retinopathy similar to lupus erythematosus and dermatomyositis may be present. Systemic corticosteroid treatment has improved the prognosis substantially, and retinopathy usually improves or disappears.

POLYARTERITIS NODOSA

This collagen disease affects the medium-sized arteries, most commonly in men. There is intense inflammation of all the muscle layers of the arteries, with fibrinoid necrosis. The main clinical features are fever of unknown origin, weight loss, nephritis, hypertension, acute abdominal symptoms, pulmonary signs, peripheral neuropathy, and muscle pain with wasting. Cardiac involvement is common, although death is usually caused by renal dysfunction.

Ocular changes are seen in 20% of cases and consist of episcleritis and scleritis. When the limbal vessels

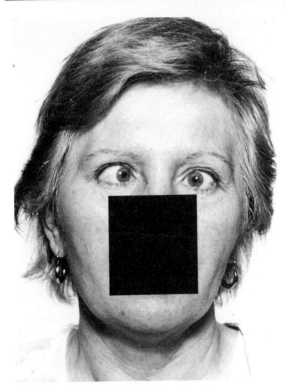

Figure 16–35. Polyarteritis nodosa. Bilateral sixth nerve palsies.

are involved, guttering of the peripheral cornea may occur. The commonest ocular signs are seen in the retinal circulation, where cotton wool spots and hemorrhages reflect retinal arteritis. The central artery may be involved, and if the disk vessels are affected, disk edema results. Ophthalmoplegia may result from arteritis of the vasa nervorum (Fig 16–35). Systemic corticosteroids are of some value, but the long-term prognosis is uniformly bad.

WEGENER'S GRANULOMATOSIS

This granulomatous process shares certain clinical features with polyarteritis nodosa. The 3 diagnostic criteria are (1) necrotizing granulomatous lesions of the respiratory tract, (2) generalized necrotizing arteritis, and (3) renal involvement with necrotizing glomerulitis.

There is a spectrum of disease ranging from classic Wegener's granulomatosis, with the 3 features described above, to a more benign form, termed necrotizing sarcoidal granulomatosis.

Ocular complications occur in 50% of cases, and proptosis owing to orbital granulomatous involvement occurs with associated ocular muscle or optic nerve involvement (Fig 16–36). If the vasculitis affects the eye, conjunctivitis, episcleritis, scleritis, uveitis, and

retinal vasculitis may occur. Nasolacrimal duct obstruction is a rare complication.

It has been suggested that there is a partial cell-mediated immunodeficiency, and therapy with combined corticosteroids and immunosuppressives (particularly cyclophosphamide) often produces a satisfactory response.

RHEUMATOID ARTHRITIS

Rheumatoid arthritis is a disease of middle and old age and is 3 times more common in women than in men. Uveitis is a rare complication, but scleritis and episcleritis are comparatively common. The scleritis may herald exacerbation of the systemic disease, tends to occur with widespread vasculitis, and may lead to scleromalacia perforans.

Corticosteroid drops are helpful in episcleritis or anterior uveitis, but systemic treatment (corticosteroids plus indomethacin or phenylbutazone) is necessary for scleritis. Operative procedures (subconjunctival injection, scleral biopsy) on the sclera are contraindicated, since risks are involved. Keratoconjunctivitis sicca is present in 15% of cases.

JUVENILE RHEUMATOID ARTHRITIS (Still's Disease)

Ocular complications occur 3 times more frequently in girls, and particularly when few joints are affected, of which the knee is the most common. The systemic disease appears to be disproportionately mild in chil-

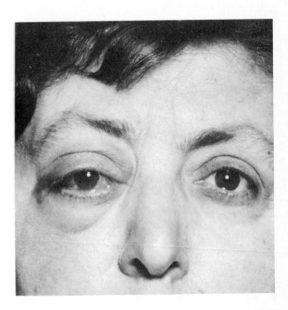

Figure 16–36. Classic Wegener's granulomatosis with proptosis, ptosis, and ophthalmoplegia. The condition has remained static for 10 years with use of corticosteroids and cyclophosphamide.

dren with severe visual loss, and diagnosis and treatment may therefore be delayed. Ocular involvement may occur before joint involvement. A chronic insidious uveitis with a high incidence of anterior segment complication develops (eg, posterior synechiae, cataract, secondary glaucoma, band-shaped keratopathy). Antinuclear antibodies are positive in 88% of patients with juvenile rheumatoid arthritis who develop uveitis, whereas they are positive in only 30% of the group as a whole.

SJÖGREN'S SYNDROME

Sjögren's syndrome is a systemic disorder with diverse features. The disease is characterized by the clinical triad of keratoconjunctivitis sicca (see p 00), xerostomia or dryness of the mouth, and a connective tissue disease, usually rheumatoid arthritis. It is more common in females. The onset of ocular symptoms occurs most frequently during the fourth, fifth, and sixth decades. Lymphoid proliferation is a prominent feature of Sjögren's syndrome and may involve the kidneys, the lungs, or the liver, causing renal tubular acidosis, pulmonary fibrosis, or liver cirrhosis. Lymphoreticular malignant disease such as reticulum cell sarcoma may complicate the benign course of Sjögren's syndrome many years after the onset.

The histopathologic changes of the lacrimal glands consist of lymphocytic infiltration and occasional plasma cells leading to atrophy and destruction of the glandular structures. These changes are part of the generalized polyglandular affection in Sjögren's syndrome, resulting in dryness of the eyes, mouth, skin, and mucous membranes.

Because of the relative inaccessibility of the lacrimal gland, the labial salivary gland biopsy serves as an important diagnostic procedure in patients with suspected Sjögren's syndrome.

The tear lysozyme level is absent or reduced in over 90% of patients.

Tubuloreticular viruslike structures resembling the unenveloped nucleocapsids of paramyxovirus have been observed in the renal biopsy and in the capillary endothelial cells and infiltrating lymphocytes of the labial salivary glands in patients with Sjögren's syndrome. Although the pathogenesis is not yet clear, there is increasing evidence that immunologic and viral factors interact in a susceptible host to account for the disease process.

ANKYLOSING SPONDYLITIS

Ankylosing spondylitis is a disease occurring mainly in men 16–40 years of age. There is almost always uveitis occurring at some stage in the disease, which is intermittent, exudative, and may be accompanied by scleritis. There is a strong association with HLA-B27. There is an antigenic cross-reactivity between HLA-B27 and *Klebsiella pneumoniae,* and ac-

tive uveitis in ankylosing spondylitis patients is associated with the presence of this organism in the feces.

REITER'S DISEASE

The diagnosis of Reiter's disease is based on a triad of signs that includes urethritis, conjunctivitis, and arthritis. Scleritis, keratitis, and uveitis may also be seen in addition to conjunctivitis. The disease has a high correlation with HLA-B27 antigen.

BEHÇET'S DISEASE

Behçet's disease consists of the clinical triad of relapsing iritis and aphthous and genital ulceration (Fig 16–37). Ocular signs occur in 75% of cases; the uveitis is severe, occasionally associated with hypopyon. Posterior uveitis is common, and retinal periphlebitis and papillitis may occur. Treatment is difficult, and the prognosis is poor. Systemic corticosteroids and azathioprine or chlorambucil constitute the most satisfactory regimen, but cyclosporine may also be beneficial.

Exacerbation of the disease coincides with a raised erythrocyte sedimentation rate, raised IgG (with fall in IgA in the acute phase and a later rise of IgA in the convalescent phase), and raised C9 levels with C-reactive protein. Fibrinolytic studies may also be abnormal, particularly in patients developing major vein thrombosis and retinal vein thrombosis.

UVEITIS WITH INFLAMMATORY BOWEL DISEASE

Scleral, episcleral, and uveal tract involvement may be seen in both ulcerative colitis and Crohn's disease. Conversely, bowel symptoms may be seen in patients with ankylosing spondylitis.

HUMAN LEUKOCYTE ANTIGENS

Histocompatibility antigens are unique markers on the surfaces of all nucleated cells. The human leukocyte A system is the major group of such antigens.

The genes responsible for the formation of these antigens are found in 5 adjacent loci on each of the pair of chromosome 6. Therefore, each cell in a heterozygous individual can contain up to 10 different antigens.

The 5 loci are named A, B, C, D, and DR. Humoral antibodies that can be detected by serologic methods are bound to antigens at loci A, B, and C. Cross-reactivity occurs when an antiserum to one particular antigen reacts weakly with another antiserum. This may account for some of the associations of specific disorders with different HLA antigens. The antigen

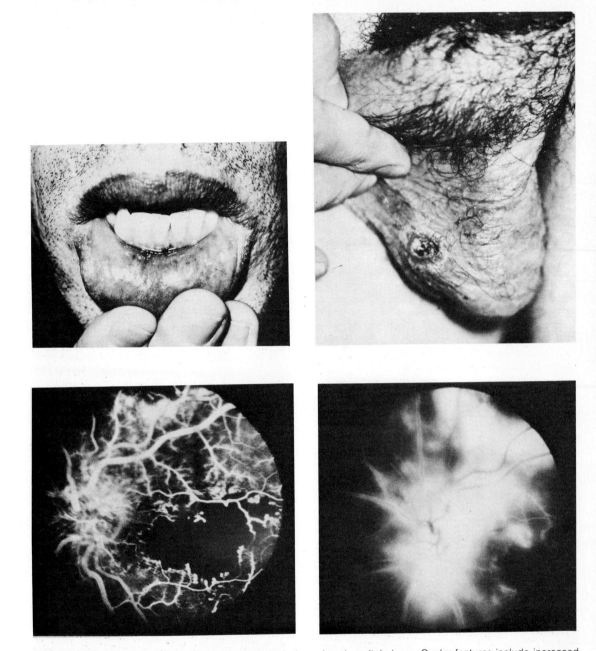

Figure 16–37. Behçet's disease. Clinical features include oral and genital ulcers. Ocular features include increased capillary permeability and areas of retinal ischemia and infiltration. Marked leakage of capillaries is seen in the late stages of fluorescein angiography *(bottom right)*.

controlled by locus D can be detected by mixed lymphocyte culture when donor lymphocytes are incubated with lymphocytes of the proposed recipient and blastic transformation and division occur.

Some groups of HLA appear to be inherited together, eg, HLA-A8, HLA-B1, and HLA-Dw3, and are called haplotypes. This occurs because the different antigens are close together on a gene and therefore inherited "en bloc." This phenomenon is called linkage disequilibrium, because there is a reduction in the normal genetic transfer that occurs during meiosis.

The association between different HLA haplotypes (ie, different HLA groups inherited together) and specific diseases is well known. Ninety percent of people with ankylosing spondylitis have HLA-B27. A person with HLA-B27 is 100 times more likely to develop ankylosing spondylitis than a person without this haplotype. However, only 5% of people who do possess HLA-B27 actually develop ankylosing spondylitis.

Table 16–3. Association of HLA types with systemic diseases.

Behçet's disease	HLA-B5
Juvenile diabetic retinopathy	HLA-B8 (without A1)
Myasthenia gravis	HLA-DR3
	HLA-B8
Thyrotoxicosis	HLA-Dw3
	HLA-B8
Multiple sclerosis	HLA-DR3
	HLA-Dw2
Ankylosing spondylitis	HLA-B27
Reiter's disease	HLA-B27
Acute anterior uveitis	HLA-B27
Rheumatoid arthritis	HLA-DR4
	HLA-Dw4

Other associations are listed in Table 16–3.

The HLA-D-related (HLA-DR) locus is the most important in immunologically mediated conditions; it codes for class II cell surface antigens that are expressed on a restricted population of cells, including macrophages, activated T cells, B cells, and vascular endothelial cells and thymocytes.

The serum level of other immunoregulatory proteins is also genetically determined and may indicate disease susceptibility (eg, α_1-antitrypsin levels are increased in patients with retinal vasculitis).

HERITABLE CONNECTIVE TISSUE DISEASES

MARFAN'S SYNDROME
(Arachnodactyly)
(Fig 16–38)

The most striking feature of this rare syndrome is increased length of the long bones, particularly of the fingers and toes. Other characteristics include scanty subcutaneous fat, relaxed ligaments, and, less commonly, other associated developmental anomalies, including congenital heart disease and deformities of the spine and joints. Ocular complications are often seen—in particular, dislocation of the lenses, usually superiorly and nasally. Less common ocular anomalies include severe refractive errors, megalocornea, cataract, uveal colobomas, and secondary glaucoma. There is a high infant mortality rate. Removal of a dislocated lens may be necessary. The disease is genetically determined, nearly always as an autosomal dominant, often with incomplete expression, so that mild, incomplete forms of the syndrome are seen. Several reports have correlated cytogenetic changes with Marfan's syndrome.

MARCHESANI'S SYNDROME

This is a rare hereditary disorder characterized by multiple skeletal and ocular abnormalities, which it transmitted as an autosomal recessive trait. Patients are short and stocky, with well-developed muscles. The hands and feet are characteristically spade-shaped; in childhood, x-rays show delayed carpal and tarsal ossification. Ocular complications include spherophakia and ectopia lentis, which give rise to lenticular myopia, iridodonesis, and glaucoma. The prognosis for vision is usually poor because the glaucoma resists all forms of treatment.

OSTEOGENESIS IMPERFECTA
(Brittle Bones & Blue Scleras)

This rare autosomal dominant syndrome is characterized by multiple fractures, blue scleras, and, less commonly, deafness. The disease is usually manifest soon after birth. The long bones are very fragile, fracturing easily and often healing with fibrous bony union. The bones become more fragile with age. The very thin sclera allows the blue color imparted by the underlying uveal tract to show through. There is often no visual functional impairment. Occasionally, abnormalities such as keratoconous, megalocornea, and corneal or lenticular opacities are also present that do interfere with visual function.

Ophthalmologic treatment is seldom necessary.

HEREDITARY METABOLIC DISORDERS

MUCOPOLYSACCHARIDOSES

Mucopolysaccharides are long glycoside polymers consisting of a chain of 100 sugar residues attached to a protein core. The polymers are either dermatan or heparan sulfate, and in the mucopolysaccharidoses there is defective breakdown of those polymers due to enzyme deficiency, resulting in the deposition of mucopolysaccharide in the tissues and an elevated urinary excretion.

There are 6 clearly defined disorders of mucopolysaccharide metabolism (I–VI) that all used to be grouped together and called **gargoylism.**

Corneal clouding occurs in **Hurler's syndrome** (type I) (Fig 16–39), **Scheie's syndrome** (type I), **Morquio's disease** (type IV), and **Maroteaux-Lamy syndrome** (type V A + B) and noticeably not in **Hunter's syndrome** (type I), the only X-linked inherited variety; the others are all autosomal recessive. Other ocular features are megalocornea, buphthalmos, pigmentary retinopathy, and optic atrophy.

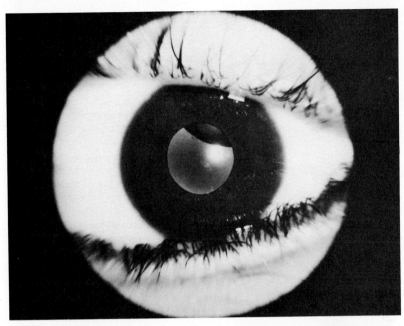

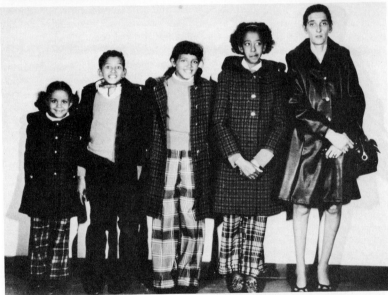

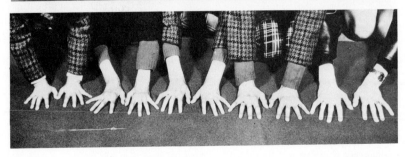

Figure 16–38. Marfan's syndrome. Familial expression of arachnodactyly and upward dislocation of the lens.

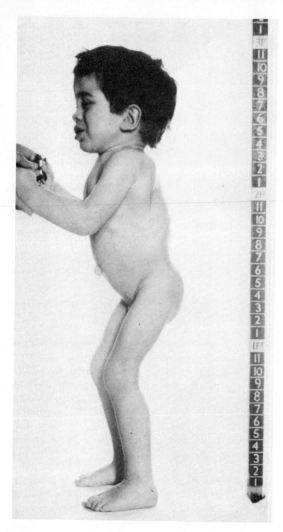

Figure 16–39. Clinical features of Hurler's syndrome include gargoylism, gibbus, and umbilical hernia.

HEPATOLENTICULAR DEGENERATION (Wilson's Disease)

This rare autosomal recessive disease of young adults, characterized by abnormal copper metabolism, causes changes in the basal nuclei, cirrhosis of the liver, and a pathognomonic corneal pigmentation called the Kayser-Fleischer ring. The ring appears as a green or brown band peripherally and deep in the stroma near Descemet's membrane and may only be visible with a slit lamp. The disease is progressive and often results in death by age 40.

Treatment with penicillamine has resulted in sustained clinical improvement in some cases.

CYSTINOSIS

This rare autosomal recessive derangement of amino acid metabolism causes widespread deposition of cystine crystals throughout the body. Dwarfism, nephropathy, and death in childhood from renal failure are the rule. Cystine crystals can be readily seen in the conjunctiva and cornea, where fine particles are seen predominantly in the outer third of the corneal stroma.

There is no treatment.

ALBINISM

Generalized albinism is a disease affecting the metabolism of melanin and is inherited as an autosomal recessive trait. The skin and hair are white, and there is a generalized lack of pigment throughout the body that is apparent from birth. The eyebrows and lashes are white. The irides appear reddish, and the pupil appears red. The fundus is red, with a prominent choroidal vessel pattern, since the pigment epithelium of the retina is deficient. Photophobia is prominent. The macula is often poorly developed, greatly impairing visual function, and this often causes an associated searching nystagmus that reduces visual acuity to about 20/200.

HOMOCYSTINURIA

Homocystinuria is a rare autosomal recessive disorder of amino acid metabolism characterized clinically by mental retardation, downward dislocation of the lenses of the eyes, and genu valgum. The plasma homocystine and methionine levels are elevated. Patients with homocystinuria have deficiency of cystathionine synthesase. Urinary excretion of homocystine is increased, and the nitroprusside test of the urine is positive. Thrombosis of medium-sized arteries is common, often resulting in early death from cerebrovascular, coronary, or renal vascular occlusions. These are relatively common during general anesthesia and are due to excess platelet aggregation. Dietary therapy is possible with either a high-pyridoxine diet or a low-methionine diet with added cystine, or a combination of these two.

GALACTOSEMIA

Galactosemia is a rare autosomal recessive disorder of carbohydrate metabolism that becomes clinically manifest soon after birth by feeding problems, vomiting, diarrhea, abdominal distention, hepatomegaly, jaundice, ascites, cataracts, mental retardation, and elevated blood and urine galactose levels. Dietary exclusion of milk and all foods containing galactose and lactose for the first 3 years of life will prevent the clinical manifestations and will result in improvement of existing abnormalities. Even the cataract changes, which are characterized by vacuoles of the cortex, are reversible in the early stage.

Identification of the carrier state is possible by finding a 50% reduction of galactose-6-phosphatase.

MISCELLANEOUS SYSTEMIC DISEASES WITH OCULAR MANIFESTATIONS

VOGT-KOYANAGI-HARADA SYNDROME (Fig 16–40)

Bilateral uveitis associated with alopecia, poliosis, vitiligo, and hearing defects, usually in young adults, has been termed Vogt-Koyanagi disease. When the choroiditis is more exudative, serous retinal detachment occurs, and the complex is known as Harada's syndrome. There is a tendency toward recovery of visual function, but this is not always complete. Corticosteroids have a favorable effect upon the disease. Local corticosteroids and mydriatics are indicated.

ERYTHEMA MULTIFORME (Stevens-Johnson Syndrome)

Erythema multiforme is a serious mucocutaneous disease that occurs as a hypersensitivity reaction to drugs or food. Children are most susceptible. The manifestations consist of generalized maculopapular rash, severe stomatitis, and purulent conjunctivitis, sometimes leading to symblepharon and occlusion of the lacrimal gland ducts **(dry eye syndrome).** In severe cases, corneal ulcers, perforations, panophthalmitis can destroy all visual function. Systemic corticosteroid treatment often favorably influences the course of the disease and usually preserves useful visual function. Secondary infection with *Staphylococcus aureus* is common and must be vigorously treated by local antibiotics instilled into the conjunctival sac. Frequently there is marked reduction of tear formation that can be helped by instillation of artificial tears.

GIANT CELL ARTERITIS (Including Temporal or Cranial Arteritis)

This is a disease of elderly patients (over age 60). Medium-sized arteries are involved, particularly the intima of the vessels. Branches of the external carotid system are frequently involved, though pathologic studies have shown more diffuse arterial involvement. Polymyalgia rheumatica may precede or accompany the disease. Patients feel ill and have excruciating pain over the temporal or occipital arteries. Visual loss due to an ischemic optic neuropathy is frequent, and a few cases have a central retinal artery occlusion. Visual loss may also be due to cortical blindness. Other central nervous system signs include cranial nerve palsies and signs referable to brain stem lesions. The diagnosis is confirmed by a high erythrocyte sedimentation rate (ESR) and a positive temporal artery biopsy. In

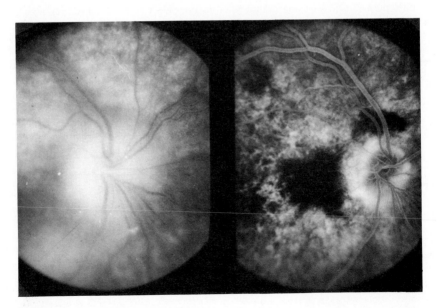

Figure 16–40. Vogt-Koyanagi-Harada syndrome. Acute pigment epithelial disease with disk swelling and cells in the vitreous *(left).* Three months later, disk swelling has subsided and pigment epithelial damage is seen *(right).*

early stages of the disease, the ESR may be normal, but usually it is 80–100 mm in the first hour. It is important to make the diagnosis early, because immediate systemic corticosteroids produce dramatic improvement. The disease activity is monitored by the erythrocyte sedimentation rate and the clinical state. The corticosteroid dose may have to be maintained for several years and should be kept below 5 mg prednisolone daily if possible, since with higher doses the survival rate is markedly reduced.

IDIOPATHIC ARTERITIS OF TAKAYASU (Pulseless Disease)

This disease, found most frequently in young women and occasionally in children, is a polyarteritis of unknown cause with increased predilection for the aorta and its branches. Manifestations may include evidence of cerebrovascular insufficiency, syncope, absence of pulsations in the upper extremities, and ophthalmologic changes compatible with chronic hypoxia of the ocular structures. Ophthalmodynamometry may be of value by demonstrating decreased carotid blood flow on one or both sides. The disease is sometimes associated with rheumatoid arthritis, which supports the idea that it is a collagen disease.

Thromboendarterectomy, prosthetic graft, and systemic corticosteroid therapy have been reported to be successful.

LAURENCE-MOON-BIEDL SYNDROME

Obesity, mental deficiency, polydactyly, hypogonadism, and retinitis pigmentosa form the complete syndrome. The retinal changes are not always typical of retinitis pigmentosa and may be present soon after birth or develop during adolescence. This rare syndrome is genetically determined and follows an autosomal recessive pattern with a high rate of consanguinity. The heterozygous state may be identified by mild incomplete evidences of the disease. It is interesting that a single abnormal gene can account for such a multiplicity of clinical findings.

ROSACEA (Acne Rosacea)

This disease of unknown cause is primarily dermatologic, beginning as a hyperemia of the face associated with acneiform lesions and eventually causing hypertrophy of tissues (such as rhinophyma). Chronic blepharitis due to staphylococcal infection or seborrhea is often present. Rosacea keratitis develops in about 5% of cases. Episcleritis, scleritis, and nongranulomatous iridocyclitis are rare ocular complications.

Topical corticosteroids help in controlling keratitis or iridocyclitis, but there is no specific therapy.

LOWE'S SYNDROME

This rare syndrome consists of cerebral defects, mental retardation, and ocular anomalies associated with dwarfism due to renal dysfunction (a congenital defect of reabsorption in the renal tubules, causing aminoaciduria). The eye findings include congenital cataract, infantile glaucoma, and nystagmus. All cases reported to date have occurred in males, suggesting X-linked inheritance. Early mortality rates are high.

LYME DISEASE

Lyme disease is a vector-mediated multisystem illness caused by the spirochete *Borrelia burgdorferi*. The usual vectors are small ixodid ticks that have a complex 3-host life cycle involving multiple mammalian and avian species.

The disease has 3 major stages. Initially, in the area of the tick bite, there develops the characteristic skin lesion of erythema chronicum migrans, often accompanied by regional lymphadenopathy, malaise, fever, headache, myalgia, and arthralgia. Several weeks to months later there is a period of neurologic and cardiac abnormalities. After a few more weeks or even years, rheumatologic abnormalities develop—initially, migratory musculoskeletal discomfort, but later a frank arthritis that may recur over several years.

Conjunctivitis is a frequent finding in the first stage. Cranial nerve palsies—particularly of the seventh but also of the third, fourth, or sixth cranial nerves—often occur in the neurologic phase. Other ophthalmologic abnormalities that have been reported include uveitis, ischemic optic neuropathy, optic disk edema, bilateral keratitis, and choroiditis with exudative retinal detachments.

Laboratory diagnosis is by demonstration of specific IgM and IgG antibodies in serum or cerebrospinal fluid. The spirochetes may also be isolated from these sources.

Tetracycline and penicillin are effective both in curing the initial infection and preventing late complications.

IMMUNOSUPPRESSIVE AGENTS USED IN EYE DISEASE

Immunosuppressive agents are used to suppress inflammatory reactions within the eye, particularly those affecting the uveal tract but also the sclera, retina, and optic nerve. Frequently, the cause of inflammation is not known, and, hence, the use of these drugs is empirical. All patients must have a full medical examination before treatment is started. Special consideration must be given to patients with infections and blood diseases, and regular blood counts must be performed during the course of treatment.

Corticosteroids (eg, prednisolone) are the mainstay of immunosuppressive treatment in ophthalmology. High doses (eg, 60 mg of prednisolone daily) may be required to control inflammation, and there is a high incidence of side effects. Weight gain, acne, and hirsutism are common; peptic ulceration, myopathy, osteoporosis, and avascular necrosis are less frequently encountered. Alternate-day regimens produce fewer side effects in some patients. Azathioprine may be added as a corticosteroid-sparing drug. Ideally, the patient should be given only 40 mg/d for 3 consecutive months, and the dosage should then be reduced to 10 mg/d. The total course should not last for more than 3 years. Intravenous methylprednisolone (1 g/d given over 3 hours in dextrose saline for 3 days) is an effective method of controlling exacerbations in patients already taking high doses of corticosteroids.

Cyclosporine is an immunosuppressive agent isolated from the fermentation products of a fungus that was recovered from Norwegian soil. It has an effective immunomodulating action and causes suppression of T helper cells. It is a useful alternative drug for refractory sight-threatening noninfectious inflammatory eye disease in patients who have not responded to corticosteroids or in whom the optimal therapeutic dose of corticosteroids is associated with intolerable side effects. The recommended oral daily dose is 5 mg/kg. The most important side effect is renal toxicity, but liver toxicity may also occur. Close surveillance and monitoring of kidney and liver functions are mandatory on every patient receiving cyclosporine therapy. The drug should not be given to hypertensive patients. Reduction of the daily dose may be associated with troublesome rebound of the ocular inflammation.

Fortunately, cytotoxic agents are rarely indicated in the mangement of inflammatory eye disease, except in severe cases of Behçet's syndrome and Wegener's granulomatosis. These drugs and their important side effects are listed in Table 16–4. Cytotoxic agents are sometimes used in the treatment of myasthenia gravis (see Fig 16–41 and Chapter 15).

OCULAR COMPLICATIONS OF CERTAIN SYSTEMICALLY ADMINISTERED DRUGS (See also Chapter 26.)

AMIODARONE

Amiodarone is a benzofuran derivative used to treat cardiac dysrhythmias, particularly Wolff-Parkinson-White syndrome, and angina pectoris. Most patients develop small punctate deposits in the basal cell layer of the corneal epithelium. The severity of keratopathy is related to the total daily dose and is mild at a dose of less than 200 mg daily. The deposits rarely interfere with vision, and although they progress with continued treatment, even in low dosage, they always resolve completely when treatment is stopped (Fig 16–42).

Table 16–4. Cytotoxic agents used in the management of inflammatory eye disease.

Drug	Daily Dose (mg/kg)	Maximum Length of Treatment	Specific Indications	Side Effects
Azathioprine	2.5–3	18 months	Corticosteroid-sparing	Bone marrow depression (usually leukopenia, but may be anemia, thrombocytopenia, and bleeding) (irreversible in elderly patients). Skin rashes, drug fever, nausea and vomiting, sometimes diarrhea. Hepatic dysfunction (raised liver enzymes, mild jaundice). Lymphoma.
Chlorambucil	0.05–0.2	2½ years (4 g)	Behçet's disease	Moderate depression of peripheral blood count. Excessive doses produce severe bone marrow depression with leukopenia, thrombocytopenia, and bleeding. Lymphoma. Prevent cystitis with adequate hydration. Chlorambucil: Leukemia may occur. Large doses near puberty may cause infertility. Cyclophosphamide: Nausea and vomiting acutely. Alopecia and hemorrhagic cystitis occasionally. Infertility may occur.
Cyclophosphamide	1.25–2.5	3 years	Wegener's granulomatosis	
Colchicine	0.01–0.03	5 years	Behçet's disease	Occasionally nausea, vomiting, abdominal pain, diarrhea. Rarely, hair loss, bone marrow depression, peripheral neuritis, myopathy.

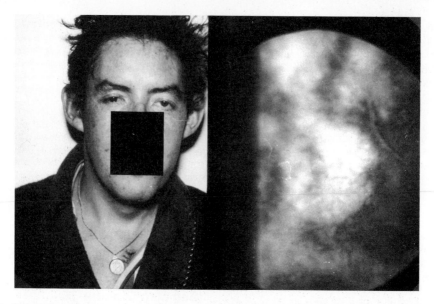

Figure 16–41. Retinitis in an immunosuppressed patient. **Left:** This patient with myasthenia gravis underwent thymectomy and received long-term immunosuppression with cytotoxic agents. **Right:** He developed retinal necrosis and Ramsay Hunt syndrome following infection with herpes zoster.

ANTICHOLINERGICS
(Atropine & Related Synthetic Drugs)

All of these drugs, when given preoperatively or for gastrointestinal disorders, may cause blurred vision in presbyopic patients because of a direct action on accommodation. They also tend to dilate the pupils, so that in patients with narrow anterior chamber angles there is the added threat of angle-closure glaucoma. This is the cause of angle-closure glaucoma (frequently attributed to ''nervousness'') occasionally seen in patients hospitalized for general surgery.

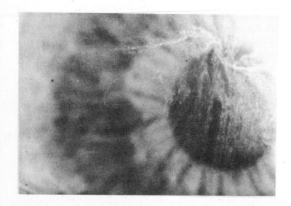

Figure 16–42. Amiodarone keratopathy. (Courtesy of DJ Spalton.)

ANTIDEPRESSANTS

Tricyclic antidepressants and monoamine oxidase inhibitors have an anticholinergic effect and theoretically may exacerbate open-angle glaucoma or provoke an attack of angle-closure glaucoma. However, this is rare in clinical practice, and if a patient is already receiving treatment for open-angle glaucoma, the medication will overcome any effect of the antidepressants.

CHLORAMPHENICOL

Chloramphenicol, in addition to the possibility of causing severe blood dyscrasias, hepatic and renal disease, and gastrointestinal disturbances, can sometimes cause optic neuritis. This is especially true in children. Bilateral blurred vision with central scotomas occurs. Stopping the drug does not always restore vision.

Despite the possibility of toxic optic neuropathy, choroamphenicol may still be required for the treatment of bacterial endophthalmitis. The drug is generally not administered for more than 1 week.

CHLOROQUINE

Originally employed as an antimalarial drug, chloroquine has also been widely used in the treatment of many collagen diseases, especially systemic lupus erythematosus and rheumatoid arthritis, and skin diseases, including discoid lupus erythematosus and sarcoidosis. With high dosage—often 250–750 mg daily administered for months or years—serious ocular toxicity has occurred. Corneal changes were described first and consisted of diffuse haziness of the epithelium and subepithelial area, occasionally sufficient to simulate an epithelial dystrophy. These changes cause only mild blurring of vision and are reversible upon drug withdrawal. Similar changes have been described in patients receiving quinacrine. Minimal corneal involvement is not necessarily an indication for discontinuance of chloroquine therapy. Corneal changes have been reported in about 30% of patients on long-term chloroquine treatment.

A less common but more serious ocular complication of long-term chloroquine therapy is retinal damage, causing loss of central vision as well as constriction of peripheral visual fields. Pigmentary changes and edema of the macula, marked alteration of the retinal vessels, and in some cases peripheral pigmentary changes can be seen ophthalmoscopically. Fluorescein fundus photography aids greatly in establishing early diagnosis or evaluating the extent of macular involvement. Visual field examination reveals central scotomas and peripheral field constriction. There are also changes in the electroretinogram, dark adaptation, and color vision. The damage is always bilateral and is usually equal in both eyes. The visual loss is irreversible and may even progress after cessation of therapy. No treatment is of any value.

Long-term chloroquine therapy must be undertaken only upon urgent indications. These patients should be examined by an ophthalmologist every 3–4 months. Between examinations, patients should make a rough test of visual acuity once weekly.

CHLOROTHIAZIDE

Xanthopsia (yellow vision) has been reported in patients taking this oral diuretic.

CONTRACEPTIVES, ORAL

Although numerous reports suggest that in predisposed individuals oral contraceptives can provoke or precipitate ophthalmic vascular occlusive disease or optic nerve damage, it is difficult to establish a definite cause and effect relationship. Optic neuritis, retinal arterial or venous thrombosis, and pseudotumor cerebri have been described in patients taking oral contraceptives. Since there is some uncertainty regarding the possibility of such ocular complications, oral contraceptives should be used only by healthy women with no history of vascular, neurologic, or ocular disease.

CORTICOSTEROIDS

It has been clearly demonstrated that long-term systemic corticosteroid therapy can cause chronic open-angle glaucoma and cataracts and can provoke and worsen attacks of herpes simplex keratitis. Locally administered corticosteroids are much more potent in this respect and have the added disadvantage of causing fungal overgrowth if the corneal epithelium is not intact. Steroid-induced subcapsular lens opacities cause some impairment of visual function but usually do not progress to advanced cataract. Cessation of therapy will arrest progression of the lenticular opacities, but the changes are irreversible.

Systemic corticosteroids may also cause papilledema associated with pseudotumor cerebri, both during administration and shortly after withdrawal.

DIGITALIS

Blurred vision and disturbed color vision are said to be the most common ocular complications of digitalis toxicity, although the actual incidence of such symptoms in patients receiving digitalis is extremely low. The purified glycosides of digitalis probably produce fewer of the toxic ocular symptoms than the whole leaf.

Visual acuity may be decreased. Objects may appear yellow (xanthopsia) or, less commonly, green, brown, red, "snowy," or white. The patient may complain of photophobia and flashes of light. Scotomas and, very rarely, transient and permanent amblyopia have been described. The toxic effects of digitalis may be due to direct effects on the retinal reception cells or retrobulbar neuritis, or they may be of central origin.

ETHAMBUTOL

Ocular complications are rare unless the daily dose is greater than 25 mg/kg, but they do occur because the drug is often used in resistant cases of tuberculosis. Optic neuropathy affecting the papillomacular bundle produces centrocecal scotoma and reduced color vision. A chiasmal pattern of involvement may also be seen. Visual loss is dose-dependent and may improve over 6 months after cessation of the drug.

OXYGEN

Premature infants who are given any concentration of oxygen in excess of that in the air may develop retinopathy of prematurity (retrolental fibroplasia). These infants should receive only the amount of oxygen necessary for survival. The incidence of the condition was considerably reduced in the 1960s with rigid restriction of oxygen, but despite continued restriction, the incidence has recently risen again. This may be due to prematurity itself (with advanced medical techniques, smaller infants are surviving); the condition is found in 40–77% of infants weighing less than 1 kg. The clinical features are described in Chapter 11. Vitamin E given daily reduces the severity but not the incidence of retinopathy of prematurity.

In adults, administration of hyperbaric oxygen (3 atmospheres) can cause constriction of the retinal arterioles. In one reported case, a patient with an old inactive retrobulbar neuritis exposed to 100% oxygen at 2 atmospheres of pressure developed almost complete loss of visual field in 2 hours.

PHENOBARBITAL & PHYENYTOIN

Ocular complications relate to oculomotor involvement, producing nystagmus and weakness of convergence and accomodation. The nystagmus may persist for many months after cessation of the drug, and the degree of oculomotor abnormality is related to drug dosage. Early abnormalities include disturbance of smooth pursuit.

PHENOTHIAZINES

The phenothiazines usually exert an atropinelike effect on the eye so that the pupils may be dilated, especially with large doses. Of greater clinical significance, however, are the pigmentary ocular changes, which include pigmentary retinopathy and pigment deposits on the corneal endothelium and anterior lens capsule. The corneal and lens pigmentation may cause blurring of vision, but the pigment deposits usually disappear several months after the drug is discontinued. In pigmentary retinopathy, there is a diminution of central vision, night blindness, diffuse narrowing of the retinal arteries, and occasionally severe blindness.

The piperidine group (eg, thioridazine) has a higher risk of causing pigmentary retinopathy, and the maximum daily dose should not exceed 600 mg. The retinal changes are partly reversible under normal circumstances, but in some patients more severe irreversible changes occur at the "safe" dosage level.

The dimethylamine group (eg, chlorpromazine) rarely produces retinal pigmentary changes.

The piperazine group (eg, trifluoperazine) does not produce these retinal complications.

All of these drugs can produce an extrapyramidal syndrome that may involve eye movements. Large doses can provoke profound hypotension, which may produce ischemic optic neuropathy.

Patients receiving large dosages or prolonged treatment with phenothiazines should be questioned regarding visual disturbances and should have periodic ophthalmoscopic examinations.

QUININE & QUINACRINE

Quinine and quinacrine, when used in the treatment of malaria, may cause bilateral blurred vision, sometimes following a single dose. There is constriction of the visual field and, rarely, total blindness. The tendency is toward partial recovery, although usually there are permanent peripheral field defects. The ganglion cells of the retina are affected first, presumably as a result of vasoconstriction of the retinal arterioles. Varying degrees of retinal edema occur early. Optic atrophy is a late finding.

SALICYLATES

Hypersensitivity reactions are common with aspirin taken at therapeutic dosage levels, producing angioneurotic edema and conjunctivitis. Withdrawal of the drug usually results in improved visual function, but complete recovery is rare.

SEDATIVE TRANQUILIZERS

When taken regularly, the so-called minor tranquilizers can decrease tear production by the lacrimal gland, thus resulting in ocular irritation because of dry eyes. Tear production returns to normal when the tranquilizers are discontinued.

The principal drugs in this group are meprobamate, chlordiazepoxide, and diazepam.

FETAL EFFECTS OF DRUGS

The visual pathways of the fetus are occasionally affected by drugs taken by the mother during pregnancy.

Phenytoin may cause optic nerve hypoplasia.

Pigmentary retinopathy has been reported in a child of a mother taking **busulfan** for acute myeloid leukemia.

Warfarin is teratogenic and may produce a hypoplastic nose, stippled epiphyses, and skeletal abnormalities. Affected children may present with recurrent sticky eyes from obstruction of the nasolacrimal duct secondary to malformation of the nose. Other ocular abnormalities include optic atrophy, microphthalmia, and lens opacities. (**Heparin** does not produce these abnormalities, since it is a large molecule that does not cross the placenta.)

REFERENCES

Arruga J, Sanders MD: Ophthalmologic findings in 70 patients with evidence of retinal embolism. *Ophthalmology* 1982;**89:**1336.

Baum J et al: Bilateral keratitis as a manifestation of Lyme disease. *Am J Ophthalmol* 1988;**105:**75.

Bergsma D, Bron AJ, Cotlier E (editors): *The Eye and Inborn Errors of Metabolism.* AR Liss, 1976.

Bialasiewicz AA et al: Bilateral diffuse choriditis and exudative retinal detachments with evidence of Lyme disease. *Am J Ophthalmol* 1988;**105:**419.

Brewerton DA: The histocompatibility antigen (HLA 27) and acute anterior uveitis. *Trans Ophthalmol Soc UK* 1974;**94**:735.

Centers for Disease Control: Recommendations for preventing possible transmission of human T-lymphotropic virus type III/lymphadenopathy-associated virus from tears. *MMWR* 1985;**34**:533.

Cogan DG: *Ophthalmic Manifestations of Systemic Vascular Disease.* Saunders, 1974.

Diabetic Retinopathy Study Group: Preliminary report on effects of photocoagulation therapy. *Am J Ophthalmol* 1976;**81**:383.

Edwards JE Jr et al: Ocular manifestations of *Candida* septicemia: Review of seventy-six cases of hematogenous *Candida* endophthalmitis. *Medicine* 1974;**53**:47.

Eva PR, Pascoe PT, Vaughan DG: Refractive change in hyperglycaemia: Hyperopia, not myopia. *Br J Ophthalmol* 1982;**66**:500.

Fay MT et al: Atypical retinitis in patients with the acquired immunodeficiency syndrome. *Am J Ophthalmol* 1988;**105**:483.

Ferry AP, Font RL: Carcinoma metastatic to the eye and orbit. *Arch Ophthalmol* 1975;**93**:472.

Finkel MF: Lyme disease and its neurologic complications. *Arch Neurol* 1988;**45**:99.

Fraunfelder FT: *Drug-Induced Ocular Side-Effects and Drug Interactions.* Lea & Febiger, 1976.

Fujikawa LS et al: Isolation of human T-cell leukemia/lymphotropic virus type III (HTLV-III) from the tears of a patient with acquired immunodeficiency syndrome (AIDS). *Lancet.* [In press.]

Gass JDM, Olson CL: Sarcoidosis with optic nerve and retinal involvement. *Arch Ophthalmol* 1976;**94**:945.

Holland GN et al: Ocular toxoplasmosis in patients with the acquired immunodeficiency syndrome. *Am J Ophthalmol* 1988;**106**:653.

James DG, Spiteri MA: Behçet's disease. *Ophthalmology* 1982;**89**:1279.

Kaplan HJ, Waldrep JC: Immunologic insights into uveitis and retinitis: The immunoregulatory circuit. *Ophthalmology* 1984;**91**:655.

Keltner JL: Giant-cell arteritis: Signs and symptoms. *Ophthalmology* 1982;**89**:1101.

Keltner JL et al: Dural and carotid cavernous sinus fistulas: Diagnosis, management, and complications. *Ophthalmology* 1987;**94**:1585.

Leonard TJ, Moseley IF, Sanders MD: Ophthalmoplegia in carotid cavernous sinus fistula. *Br J Ophthalmol* 1984;**68**:128.

Martin LS, McDougal JS, Loskoski SL: Disinfection and inactivation of the human T lymphotropic virus type III/lymphadenopathy-associated virus. *J Infect Dis* 1985;**152**:400.

O'Connor GR: Factors related to the initiation and recurrence of uveitis. *Am J Ophthalmol* 1983;**96**:577.

Orcutt JC, Page NGR, Sanders MD: Factors affecting visual loss in benign intracranial hypertension. *Ophthalmology* 1984;**92**:1303.

Passo MS, Rosenbaum JT: Ocular syphilis in patients with human immunodeficiency virus infection. *Am J Ophthalmol* 1988;**106**:1.

Rahi AHS, Barner A: *Immunopathology of the Eye.* Blackwell, 1976.

Rose FC (editor): *The Eye in General Medicine.* Chapman & Hall, 1983.

Sadun AA et al: Assessment of visual impairment in patients with Alzheimer's disease. *Am J Ophthalmol* 1987;**104**:113.

Sanders MD, Hoyt WF: Hypoxic ocular sequelae of carotid-cavernous fistulae. *Br J Ophthalmol* 1969;**53**:82.

Schuman JS et al: Acquired immunodeficiency syndrome (AIDS). *Surv Ophthalmol* 1987;**31**:384.

Spire B et al: Inactivation of lymphadenopathy associated virus by chemical disinfectants. *Lancet* 1984;**2**:899.

Sturrock GD, Mueller HR: Chronic ocular ischaemia. *Br J Ophthalmol* 1984;**68**:716.

Walsh JB: Hypertensive retinopathy: Description, classification, and prognosis. *Ophthalmology* 1982;**89**:1127.

Watson PG, Hazleman BL (editors): *The Sclera and Systemic Disorders.* Saunders, 1976.

17 Immunologic Diseases of the Eye

G. Richard O'Connor, MD & Khalid F. Tabbara, MD

The eye is frequently considered to be a special target of immunologic disease processes, but proof of the causative role of these processes is lacking in all but a few disorders. In this sense, the immunopathology of the eye is much less clearly delineated than that of the kidney, the testis, or the thyroid gland. Because the eye is a highly vascularized organ and because the rather labile vessels of the conjunctiva are embedded in a nearly transparent medium, inflammatory eye disorders are more obvious (and often more painful) than those of other organs such as the thyroid or the kidney. The iris, ciliary body, and choroid are the most highly vascularized tissues of the eye. The similarity of the vascular supply of the uvea to that of the kidney and the choroid plexus of the brain has given rise to justified speculation concerning the selection of these 3 tissues, among others, as targets of immune complex diseases (eg, serum sickness).

Immunologic diseases of the eye can be grossly divided into 2 major categories: antibody-mediated and cell-mediated diseases. As is the case in other organs, there is ample opportunity for the interaction of these 2 systems in the eye.

ANTIBODY-DEPENDENT & ANTIBODY-MEDIATED DISEASES

Before it can be concluded that a disease of the eye is antibody-dependent, the following criteria must be satisfied: (1) There must be evidence of specific antibody in the patient's serum or plasma cells. (2) The antigen must be identified and, if feasible, characterized. (3) The same antigen must be shown to produce an immunologic response in the eye of an experimental animal, and the pathologic changes produced in the experimental animal must be similar to those observed in the human disease. (4) It must be possible to produce similar lesions in animals passively sensitized with serum from an affected animal upon challenge with the specific antigen.

Unless all of the above criteria are satisfied, the disease may be thought of as *possibly* antibody-

dependent. In such circumstances, the disease can be regarded as antibody-mediated if only one of the following criteria is met: (1) if antibody to an antigen is present in higher quantities in the ocular fluids than in the serum (after adjustments have been made for the total amounts of immunoglobulins in each fluid); (2) if abnormal accumulations of plasma cells are present in the ocular lesion; (3) if abnormal accumulations of immunoglobins are present at the site of the disease; (4) if complement is fixed by immunoglobulins at the site of the disease; (5) if an accumulation of eosinophils is present at the site of the disease; or (6) if the ocular disease is associated with an inflammatory disease elsewhere in the body for which antibody dependency has been proved or strongly suggested.

HAY FEVER CONJUNCTIVITIS

This disease is characterized by edema and hyperemia of the conjunctiva and lids (Fig 17–1) and by itching and watering of the eyes. There is often an associated itching sensation in the nose as well as rhinorrhea. The conjunctiva appears pale and boggy because of the intense edema, which is often rapid in onset. There is a distinct seasonal incidence, some

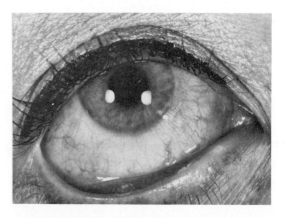

Figure 17–1. Hay fever conjunctivitis. Note edema and hyperemia of the conjunctiva. (Courtesy of M Allansmith and B McClellan.)

patients being able to establish the onset of their symptoms at precisely the same time each year. These times usually correspond to the release of pollens by specific grasses, trees, or weeds.

Immunologic Pathogenesis

Hay fever conjunctivitis is one of the few inflammatory eye disorders for which antibody dependence has been definitely established. It is recognized as a form of atopic disease with an implied hereditary susceptibility. IgE (reaginic antibody) is believed to be attached to mast cells lying beneath the conjunctival epithelium. Contact of the offending antigen with IgE triggers the release of vasoactive substances, principally leukotrienes and histamine, in this area, and this in turn results in vasodilatation and chemosis.

The role of circulating antibody to ragweed pollen in the pathogenesis of hay fever conjunctivitis has been demonstrated by passively transferring serum from a hyersensitive person to a nonsensitive one. When exposed to the offending pollen, the previously nonsensitive individual reacted with the typical signs of hay fever conjunctivitis.

Immunologic Diagnosis

Victims of hay fever conjunctivitis show many eosinophils in Giemsa-stained scrapings of conjunctival epithelium. They show the **immediate** type of response, with wheal and flare, when tested by scratch tests of the skin with extracts of pollen or other offending antigens. Biopsies of the skin test sites have occasionally shown the full-blown picture of an **Arthus reaction,** with deposition of immune complexes in the walls of the dermal vessels. Passive cutaneous anaphylaxis can also be used to demonstrate the presence of circulating antibody.

Treatment

Systemically administered antihistaminics such as diphenhydramine or tripelennamine are effective, particularly when given prophylactically during the season of greatest exposure. Sustained-release capsules of antihistaminics such as Ornade (chlorpheniramine maleate) are preferred by some. Locally applied antihistaminics such as Prefrin-A drops contain both an antihistaminic agent (pyrilamine) and a vasoconstrictor (phenylephrine). Where conjunctival edema is severe and of sudden onset, epinephrine drops (1:100,000) instilled into the conjunctival sac may help to reduce the edema quickly. Corticosteroids applied locally offer some relief. Topical use of cromolyn (disodium cromoglycate; Opticrom), a stabilizer of the mast cell, appears to be effective in the treatment of certain types of immediate hypersensitivity reactions.

Immunotherapy with gradually increasing doses of subcutaneously injected pollen extracts or other suspected allergens appears to reduce the severity of the disease in some individuals if started well in advance of the season. The mechanism is presumed to be production of blocking antibodies in response to the injection of small, graded doses of the antigen. This procedure cannot be recommended routinely, however, in view of the generally good results and relatively few complications of antihistamine therapy. Acute anaphylactoid reactions have occasionally resulted from overzealous immunotherapy.

VERNAL CONJUNCTIVITIS & ATOPIC KERATOCONJUNCTIVITIS

These 2 diseases also belong to the group of atopic disorders. Both are characterized by itching and lacrimation of the eyes but are more chronic than hay fever conjunctivitis. Furthermore, both ultimately result in structural modifications of the lids and conjunctiva.

Vernal conjunctivitis characteristically affects children and adolescents; the incidence decreases sharply after the second decade of life. Like hay fever conjunctivitis, vernal conjunctivitis occurs only in the warm months of the year. Most of its victims live in hot, dry climates. The disease characteristically produces giant ("cobblestone") papillae of the tarsal conjunctiva (Fig 17–2). The keratinized epithelium from these papillae may abrade the underlying cornea, giving rise to complaints of foreign body sensation.

Atopic keratoconjunctivitis affects individuals of all ages and has no specific seasonal incidence. The skin of the lids has a characteristic dry, scaly appearance. The conjunctiva is pale and boggy. Both the conjunctiva and the cornea may develop scarring in the later stages of the disease. Atopic cataract has also been described. Staphylococcal blepharitis, manifested by scales and crusts on the lids, commonly complicates this disease.

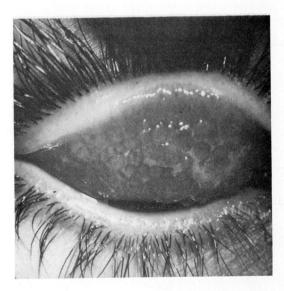

Figure 17–2. Giant papillae ("cobblestones") in the tarsal conjunctiva of a patient with vernal conjunctivitis.

Immunologic Pathogenesis

Reaginic antibody (IgE) is fixed to subepithelial mast cells in both of these conditions. Contact between the offending antigen and IgE is thought to trigger degranulation of the mast cell, which in turn allows for the release of vasoactive amines in the tissues. It is unlikely, however, that antibody action alone is responsible, since—at least in the case of papillae of vernal conjunctivitis—there is heavy papillary infiltration by mononuclear cells. Hay fever and asthma occur much more frequently in patients with vernal conjunctivitis and atopic keratoconjunctivitis than in the general population. Of the criteria outlined above (see p 320) for demonstration of *possibly* antibody-dependent diseases, (2), (5), and (6) have been met by atopic keratoconjunctivitis.

Immunologic Diagnosis

As in hay fever conjunctivitis, patients with atopic keratoconjunctivitis and vernal conjunctivitis generally show large numbers of eosinophils in conjunctival scrapings. Skin testing with food extracts, pollens, and various other antigens reveals a wheal-and-flare type of reaction within 1 hour of testing, but the significance of these reactions is not established.

Treatment

Local instillations of corticosteroid drops or ointment relieve the symptoms. However, caution must be observed in the long-term use of these agents because of the possibility of steroid-induced glaucoma and cataract. Corticosteroids produce less dramatic relief in vernal conjunctivitis than in atopic keratoconjunctivitis, and the same can be said of the antihistamines. Cromolyn seems to be useful in treating both atopic and vernal conjunctivitis. It may also allow dosages of corticosteroids to be reduced. Recently, topical administration of 1% cyclosporine eye drops has been found to be effective in the treatment of severe vernal keratoconjunctivitis. Plasmapheresis has relieved the symptoms of patients with atopic keratoconjunctivitis. This therapeutic modality, however, is still investigational.

Avoidance of known allergans is helpful; such objects as duck feathers, animal danders, and certain food proteins (egg albumin and others) are common offenders. Specific allergens have been much more difficult to demonstrate in the case of vernal disease, although some workers feel that such substances as rye grass pollens may play a causative role. Installation of air conditioning in the home or relocation to a cool, moist climate is useful in vernal conjunctivitis if economically feasible.

RHEUMATOID DISEASES AFFECTING THE EYE

The diseases in this category vary greatly in their clinical manifestations depending upon the specific disease entity and the age of the patient. Uveitis and scleritis are the principal ocular manifestations of the rheumatoid diseases. **Juvenile rheumatoid arthritis** affects females more frequently than males and is commonly accompanied by iridocyclitis of one or both eyes. The onset is often insidious, the patient having few or no complaints and the eye remaining white. Extensive synechia formation, cataract, and secondary glaucoma may be far-advanced before the parents notice that anything is wrong. The arthritis generally affects only one joint (eg, a knee) in cases with ocular involvement.

Ankylosing spondylitis affects males more frequently than females, and the onset is in the second to sixth decades. It may be accompanied by iridocyclitis of acute onset, often with fibrin in the anterior chamber (Fig 17–3). Pain, redness, and photophobia are the initial complaints, and synechia formation is common.

Rheumatoid arthritis of adult onset may be accompanied by acute scleritis or episcleritis (Fig 17–4). The ciliary body and choroid, lying adjacent to the sclera, are often involved secondarily with the inflammation. Rarely, serous detachment of the retina results. The onset is usually in the third to fifth decade, and women are affected more frequently than men.

Reiter's disease affects men more frequently than women. The first attack of ocular inflammation usually consists of a self-limited papillary conjunctivitis. It follows, at a highly variable interval, the onset of nonspecific urethritis and the appearance of inflammation in one or more of the weight-bearing joints. Subsequent attacks of ocular inflammation may consist of acute iridocyclitis of one or both eyes, occasionally with hypopyon (Fig 17–5).

Immunologic Pathogenesis

Rheumatoid factor, an IgM autoantibody directed against the patient's own IgG, may play a major role in the pathogenesis of rheumatoid arthritis. The union of IgM antibody with IgG is followed by fixation of

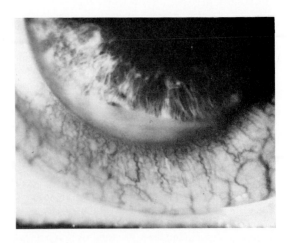

Figure 17–3. Acute iridocyclitis in a patient with ankylosing spondylitis. Note fibrin clot in anterior chamber.

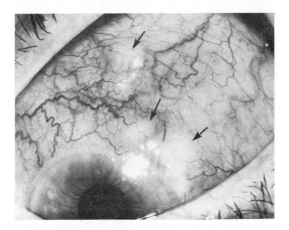

Figure 17–4. Scleral nodules in a patient with rheumatoid arthritis. (Courtesy of S Kimura.)

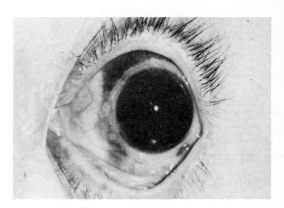

Figure 17–6. Scleral thinning in a patient with rheumatoid arthritis. Note dark color of the underlying uvea.

complement at the tissue site and the attraction of leukocytes and platelets to this area. An occlusive vasculitis, resulting from this chain of events, is thought to be the cause of rheumatoid nodule formation in the sclera as well as elsewhere in the body. The occlusion of vessels supplying nutriments to the sclera is thought to be responsible for the "melting away" of the scleral collagen that is so characteristic of rheumatoid arthritis (Fig 17–6).

While this explanation may suffice for rheumatoid arthritis, patients with the ocular complications of juvenile rheumatoid arthritis, ankylosing spondylitis, and Reiter's syndrome usually have negative tests for rheumatoid factor, so other explanations must be sought.

Outside the eyeball itself, the lacrimal gland has been shown to be under attack by circulating antibodies. Destruction of acinar cells within the gland and invasion of the lacrimal gland (as well as the

salivary glands) by mononuclear cells result in decreased tear secretion. The combination of dry eyes (keratoconjunctivitis sicca), dry mouth (xerostomia), and rheumatoid arthritis is known as Sjögren's syndrome (see Chapter 16).

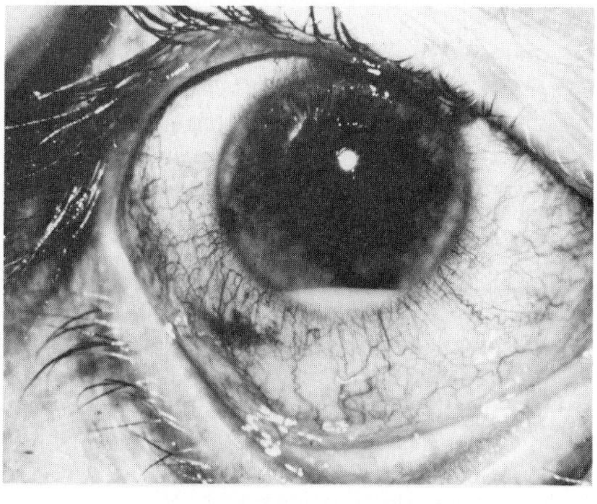

A growing body of evidence indicates that the immunogenetic background of certain patients accounts for the expression of their ocular inflammatory disease in specific ways. Analysis of the HLA antigen system shows that the incidence of HLA-B27 is significantly greater in patients with ankylosing spondylitis and Reiter's syndrome than could be expected by chance alone. It is not known how this antigen controls specific inflammatory responses.

Immunologic Diagnosis

Rheumatoid factor can be detected in the serum by a number of standard tests involving the agglutination of IgG-coated erythrocytes or latex particles. Unfortunately, the test for rheumatoid factor is not positive in the majority of isolated rheumatoid afflictions of the eye.

The HLA types of individuals suspected of having ankylosing spondylitis and related diseases can be determined. HLA-B27 is associated with ankylosing spondylitis and Reiter's syndrome. X-ray of the sacroiliac area is a valuable screening procedure that may show evidence of spondylitis prior to the onset of low back pain in patients with the characteristic form of iridocyclitis.

Treatment

Patients with uveitis associated with rheumatoid disease respond well to local instillations of corticosteroid drops (eg, dexamethasone 0.1%) or ointments. Orally administered corticosteroids must occasionally be resorted to for brief periods. Salicylates given orally in divided doses with meals are thought to reduce the frequency and blunt the severity of recurrent attacks. Atropine drops (1%) are useful for the relief of pho-

Figure 17–5. Acute iridocyclitis with hypopyon in a patient with Reiter's disease.

tophobia during the acute attacks. Shorter-acting mydriatics such as phenylephrine 10% should be used in the subacute stages to prevent synechia formation. Corticosteroid-resistant cases, especially those causing progressive erosion of the sclera, have been treated successfully with immunosuppressive agents such as chlorambucil. Nonsteroidal anti-inflammatory agents such as piroxicam (Feldene) are useful in the symptomatic treatment of scleritis.

OTHER ANTIBODY-MEDIATED EYE DISEASES

The following antibody-mediated diseases are infrequently encountered by the practicing ophthalmologist.

Systemic lupus erythematosus, associated with the presence of circulating antibodies to DNA, produces an occlusive vasculitis of the nerve fiber layer of the retina. Such infarcts result in cytoid bodies or "cotton wool" spots in the retina (Fig 17–7).

Pemphigus vulgaris produces painful intraepithelial bullae of the conjunctiva. It is associated with the presence of circulating antibodies to an intercellular antigen located between the deeper cells of the conjunctival epithelium.

Cicatricial pemphigoid is characterized by subepithelial bullae of the conjunctiva. In the chronic stages of this disease, cicatricial contraction of the conjunctiva may result in severe scarring of the cornea, dryness of the eyes, and ultimate blindness. Pemphigoid is associated with local deposits of tissue antibodies directed against one or more antigens located in the basement membrane of the epithelium.

Lens-induced uveitis is a rare condition that may be associated with circulating antibodies to lens proteins. It is seen in individuals whose lens capsules have become permeable to these proteins as a result of trauma or other disease. Interest in this field dates back to Uhlenhuth (1903), who first demonstrated the organ-specific nature of antibodies to the lens. Witmer showed in 1962 that antibody to lens tissue may be produced by lymphoid cells of the ciliary body.

CELL-MEDIATED DISEASES

This group of diseases appears to be associated with cell-mediated immunity or delayed hypersensitivity. Various structures of the eye are invaded by mononuclear cells, principally lymphocytes and macrophages, in response to one or more chronic antigenic stimuli. In the case of chronic infections such as tuberculosis, leprosy, toxoplasmosis, and herpes simplex, the antigenic stimulus has clearly been identified as an infectious agent in the ocular tissue. Such infections are often associated with delayed skin test reactivity following the intradermal injection of an extract of the organism.

More intriguing but less well understood are the granulomatous diseases of the eye for which no infectious cause has been found. Such diseases are thought to represent cell-mediated, possibly autoimmune processes, but their origin remains obscure.

OCULAR SARCOIDOSIS

Ocular sarcoidosis is characterized by a panuveitis with occasional inflammatory involvement of the optic nerve and retinal blood vessels. It often presents as iridocyclitis of insidious onset. Less frequently, it occurs as acute iridocyclitis, with pain, photophobia, and redness of the eye. Large precipitates resembling drops of solidified "mutton fat" are seen on the corneal endothelium. The anterior chamber contains a good deal of protein and numerous cells, mostly lymphocytes. Nodules are often seen on the iris, both at the pupillary margin and in the substance of the iris stroma. The latter are often vascularized. Synechiae are commonly encountered, particularly in patients with dark skin. Severe cases ultimately involve the posterior segment of the eye. Coarse clumps of cells ("snowballs") are seen in the vitreous, and exudates resembling candle drippings may be seen along the course of retinal vessels. Patchy infiltrations of the choroid or optic nerve may also be seen.

Infiltrations of the lacrimal gland and of the conjunctiva have been noted on occasion. When the latter are present, the diagnosis can easily be confirmed by biopsy of the small opaque nodules.

Immunologic Pathogenesis

Although many infectious or allergic causes of sarcoidosis have been suggested, none has been con-

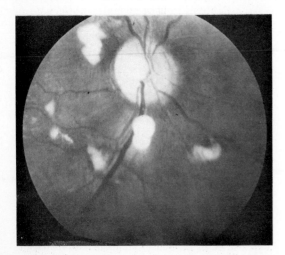

Figure 17–7. "Cotton wool" spots in the retina of a patient with lupus erythematosus.

firmed. Noncaseating granulomas are seen in the uvea, optic nerve, and adnexal structures of the eye as well as elsewhere in the body. The presence of macrophages and giant cells suggests that particulate matter is being phagocytosed, but this material has not been identified.

Patients with sarcoidosis are usually anergic to extracts of the common microbial antigens such as those of mumps, *Trichophyton, Candida,* and *Mycobacterium tuberculosis.* As in other lymphoproliferative disorders such as Hodgkin's disease and chronic lymphocytic leukemia, this may represent suppression of T cell activity such that the normal delayed hypersensitivity responses to common antigens cannot take place. Meanwhile, circulating immunoglobins are usually detectable in the serum at higher than normal levels.

Immunologic Diagnosis

The diagnosis is largely inferential. Negative skin tests to a battery of antigens to which the patient is known to have been exposed are highly suggestive, and the same is true of the elevation of serum immunoglobulins. Biopsy of a conjunctival nodule or scalene lymph node may provide positive histologic evidence of the disease. X-rays of the chest reveal hilar adenopathy in many cases. Elevated levels of serum lysozyme or serum angiotensin converting enzyme may be detected.

Treatment

Sarcoid lesions of the eye respond well to corticosteroid therapy. Frequent instillations of dexamethasone 0.1% eye drops generally bring the anterior uveitis under control. Atropine drops should be prescribed in the acute phase of the disease for the relief of pain and photophobia; short-acting pupillary dilators such as phenylephrine should be given later to prevent synechia formation. Systemic corticosteroids are sometimes necessary to control severe attacks of anterior uveitis and are always necessary for the control of retinal vasculitis and optic neuritis. The latter condition often accompanies cerebral involvement and carries a grave prognosis.

SYMPATHETIC OPHTHALMIA & VOGT-KOYANAGI-HARADA SYNDROME

These 2 disorders are discussed together because they have certain common clinical features. Both are thought to represent autoimmune phenomena affecting pigmented structures of the eye and skin, and both may give rise to meningeal symptoms.

Clinical Features

Sympathetic ophthalmia is an inflammation in the second eye after the other has been damaged by penetrating injury. In most cases, some portion of the uvea of the injured eye has been exposed to the at-mosphere for at least 1 hour. The uninjured or "sympathizing" eye develops minor signs of anterior uveitis after a period ranging from 2 weeks to several years. Floating spots and loss of the power of accommodation are among the earliest symptoms. The disease may progress to severe iridocyclitis with pain and photophobia. Usually, however, the eye remains relatively quiet and painless while the inflammatory disease spreads around the entire uvea. Despite the presence of panuveitis, the retina usually remains uninvolved except for perivascular cuffing of the retinal vessels with inflammatory cells. Papilledema and secondary glaucoma may occur. The disease may be accompanied by vitiligo (patchy depigmentation of the skin) and poliosis (whitening) of the eyelashes.

Vogt-Koyanagi-Harada syndrome consists of inflammation of the uvea of one or both eyes characterized by acute iridocyclitis, patchy choroiditis, and serous detachment of the retina. It usually begins with an acute febrile episode with headache, dysacusis, and occasionally vertigo. Patchy loss or whitening of the scalp hair is described in the first few months of the disease. Vitiligo and poliosis are commonly present but are not essential for the diagnosis. Although the initial iridocyclitis may subside quickly, the course of the posterior disease is often indolent, with long-standing serous detachment of the retina and significant visual impairment.

Immunologic Pathogenesis

In both sympathetic ophthalmia and Vogt-Koyanagi-Harada syndrome, delayed hypersensitivity to melanin-containing structures is thought to occur. Although a viral cause has been suggested for both of these disorders, there is no convincing evidence of an infectious origin. It is postulated that some insult, infectious or otherwise, alters the pigmented structures of the eye, skin, and hair in such a way as to provoke delayed hypersensitivity responses to them. Soluble materials from the outer segments of the photoreceptor layer of the retina have recently been incriminated as possible autoantigens. Patients with Vogt-Koyanagi-Harada syndrome are usually Orientals, which suggests an immunogenetic predisposition to the disease.

Histologic sections of the traumatized eye from a patient with sympathetic ophthalmia may show uniform infiltration of most of the uvea by lymphocytes, epithelioid cells, and giant cells. The overlying retina is characteristically intact, but nests of epithelioid cells may protrude through the pigment epithelium of the retina, giving rise to **Dalen-Fuchs nodules.** The inflammation may destroy the architecture of the entire uvea, leaving an atrophic, shrunken globe.

Immunologic Diagnosis

Skin tests with soluble extracts of human or bovine uveal tissue are said to elicit delayed hypersensitivity responses in these patients. Several investigators have recently shown that cultured lymphocytes from patients with these 2 diseases undergo transformation to lymphoblasts in vitro when extracts of uvea or rod outer segments are added to the culture medium. Circulating antibodies to uveal antigens have been found in patients with these diseases, but such antibodies are to be found in any patient with long-standing uveitis, including those suffering from several infectious entities. The spinal fluid of patients with Vogt-Koyanagi-Harada syndrome may show increased numbers of mononuclear cells and elevated protein in the early stages.

Treatment

Mild cases of sympathetic ophthalmia may be treated satisfactorily with locally applied corticosteroid drops and pupillary dilators. The more severe or progressive cases require systemic corticosteroids, often in high doses, for months or years. An alternate-day regimen of oral corticosteroids is recommended for such patients in order to avoid adrenal suppression. The same applies to the treatment of patients with Vogt-Koyanagi-Harada disease. Occasionally, patients with long-standing progressive disease become resistant to corticosteroids or cannot take additional corticosteroid medication because of pathologic fractures, mental changes, or other reasons. Such patients may become candidates for immunosuppressive therapy. Oral cyclosporine has been used successfully for both conditions. More recently, cyclosporine has shown promise in the treatment of steroid-resistant uveitis.

OTHER DISEASES OF CELL-MEDIATED IMMUNITY

Giant cell arteritis (temporal arteritis) (see Chapter 16) may have disastrous effects on the eye, particularly in elderly individuals. The condition is manifested by pain in the temples and orbit, blurred vision, and scotomas. Examination of the fundus may reveal extensive occlusive retinal vasculitis and choroidal infarcts. Atrophy of the optic nerve head is a frequent complication. Such patients have an elevated sedimentation rate. Biopsy of the temporal artery reveals extensive infiltration of the vessel wall with giant cells and mononuclear cells.

Polyarteritis nodosa (see Chapter 16) can affect both the anterior and posterior segments of the eye. The corneas of such patients may show peripheral thinning and cellular infiltration. The retinal vessels reveal extensive necrotizing inflammation characterized by eosinophil, plasma cell, and lymphocyte infiltration.

Behçet's disease (see Chapter 16) has an uncertain place in the classification of immunologic disorders. It is characterized by recurrent iridocyclitis with hypopyon and occlusive vasculitis of the retinal vessels. Although it has many of the features of a delayed hypersensitivity disease, dramatic alterations of serum complement levels at the very beginning of an attack suggest an immune complex disorder. Furthermore, high levels of circulating immune complexes have

recently been detected in patients with this disease. Most patients with eye symptoms are positive for HLA-B51, a subtype of HLA-B5.

Contact dermatitis of the eyelids represents a significant though minor disease caused by delayed hypersensitivity. Atropine, perfumed cosmetics, materials contained in plastic spectacle frames, and other locally applied agents may act as the sensitizing hapten. The lower lid is more extensively involved than the upper lid when the sensitizing agent is applied in drop form. Periorbital involvement with erythematous, vesicular, pruritic lesions of the skin is characteristic.

Phlyctenular keratoconjunctivitis (Fig 17–8) represents a delayed hypersensitivity response to certain microbial antigens, principally those of *M tuberculosis*. It is characterized by acute pain and photophobia in the affected eye, and perforation of the peripheral cornea has been known to result from it. The disease responds rapidly to locally applied corticosteroids. Since the advent of chemotherapy for pulmonary tuberculosis, phlyctenulosis is much less of a problem than it was 30 years ago. It is still encountered occasionally, however, particularly among American Indians and Alaskan Eskimos. Other pathogens such as *Staphylococcus aureus* and *Coccidioides immitis* have also been implicated in phlyctenular disease.

CORNEAL GRAFT REACTIONS (Fig 17–9)

Blindness due to opacity or distortion of the central portion of the cornea is a remediable disease. If all other structures of the eye are intact, a patient whose

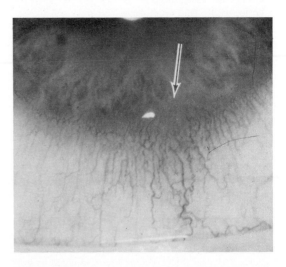

Figure 17–8. Phlyctenule (arrow) at the margin of the cornea. (Courtesy of P Thygeson.)

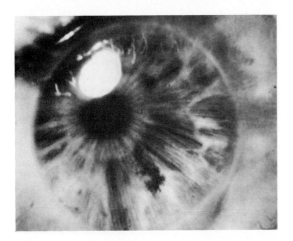

Figure 17–9. A cornea severely scarred by chronic atopic keratoconjunctivitis into which a central graft of clear cornea has been placed. Note how distinctly the iris landmarks are seen through the transparent graft. (Reproduced, with permission, from Stites DP et al [editors]: *Basic & Clinical immunology*, 5th ed. Lange, 1984.)

vision is impaired solely by corneal opacity can expect great improvement from a graft of clear cornea into the diseased area. Trauma, including chemical burns, is one of the most common causes of central corneal opacity. Others include scars from herpetic keratitis, endothelial cell dysfunction with chronic corneal edema (including pseudophakic bullous keratopathy and Fuchs' dystrophy), keratoconus, and opacities from previous graft failures. All of these conditions represent indications for penetrating corneal grafts, provided the patient's eye is no longer inflamed and the opacity has been allowed maximal time to undergo spontaneous resolution (usually 6–12 months). It is estimated that approximately 10,000 corneal grafts are performed in the USA annually. Of these, about 90% can be expected to produce a beneficial result.

The cornea was one of the first human tissues to be successfully grafted. The fact that recipients of corneal grafts generally tolerate them well can be attributed to (1) the absence of blood vessels or lymphatics in the normal cornea and (2) the lack of presensitization to tissue-specific antigens in most recipients. Reactions to corneal grafts do occur, however, particularly in individuals whose own corneas have been damaged by previous inflammatory disease. Such corneas may have developed both lymphatics and blood vessels, providing afferent and efferent channels for immunologic reactions in the engrafted cornea.

Although attempts have been made to transplant corneas from other species into human eyes (xenografts), particularly in countries where human material is not available for religious reasons, most corneal grafts have been taken from human eyes (allografts). Except in the case of identical twins, such grafts always represent the implantation of foreign tissue into a donor site; thus, the chance for a graft rejection due to an immune response to foreign antigens is virtually always present.

The cornea is a 3-layered structure composed of a surface epithelium, an oligocellular collagenous stroma, and a single-layered endothelium. Although the surface epithelium may be sloughed and later replaced by the recipient's epithelium, certain elements of the stroma and all of the donor's endothelium remain in place for the rest of the patient's life. This has been firmly established by sex chromosome markers in corneal cells when donor and recipient were of opposite sexes. The endothelium must remain healthy in order for the cornea to remain transparent, and an energy-dependent pump mechanism is required to keep the cornea from swelling with water. Since the recipient's endothelium is in most cases diseased, the central corneal endothelium must be replaced by healthy donor tissue.

A number of foreign elements exist in corneal grafts that might stimulate the immune system of the host to reject this tissue. In addition to those mentioned above, the corneal stroma is regularly perfused with IgG and serum albumin from the donor, although none—or only small amounts—of the other blood proteins are present. While these serum proteins of donor origin rapidly diffuse into the recipient stroma, these substances are theoretically immunogenic.

Although the ABO blood antigens have been shown to have no relationship to corneal graft rejection, the HLA antigen system probably plays a significant role in graft reactions. HLA incompatibility between donor and recipient has been shown by several authors to be significant in determining graft survival, particularly when the corneal bed is vascularized. It is known that most cells of the body possess these HLA antigens, including the endothelial cells of the corneal graft as well as certain stromal cells (keratocytes). The epithelium has been shown by Hall and others to possess a non-HLA antigen that diffuses into the anterior third of the stroma. Thus, while much foreign antigen may be eliminated by purposeful removal of the epithelium at the time of grafting, that amount of antigen which has already diffused into the stroma is automatically carried over into the recipient. Such antigens may be leached out by soaking the donor cornea in tissue culture for several weeks prior to engraftment.

Both humoral and cellular mechanisms have been implicated in corneal graft reactions. It is likely that early graft rejections (within 2 weeks) are cell-mediated reactions. Cytotoxic lymphocytes have been found in the limbal area and stroma of affected individuals, and phase microscopy in vivo has revealed an actual attack on the grafted endothelial cells by these lymphocytes. Such lymphocytes generally move inward from the periphery of the cornea, making what is known as a "rejection line" as they move centrally. The donor cornea becomes edematous as the endothelium becomes compromised by an accumulation of lymphoid cells.

Late rejection of a corneal graft may occur several weeks to many months after implantation of donor tissue into the recipient eye. Such reactions may be antibody-mediated, since cytotoxic antibodies have been isolated from the serum of patients with a history of multiple graft reactions in vascularized corneal beds. These antibody reactions are complement-dependent and attract polymorphonuclear leukocytes, which may form dense rings in the cornea at the sites of maximum deposition of immune complexes. In experimental animals, similar reactions have been produced by corneal xenografts, but the intensity of the reaction can be markedly reduced either by decomplementing the animal or by reducing its leukocyte population through mechlorethamine therapy.

Treatment

The mainstay of the treatment of corneal graft reactions is corticosteroid therapy. This medication is generally given in the form of frequently applied eye drops (eg, prednisolone acetate, 1%, hourly) until the clinical signs abate. These clinical signs consist of conjunctival hyperemia in the perilimbal region, a cloudy cornea, cells and protein in the anterior chamber, and keratic precipitates on the corneal endothelium. The earlier treatment is applied, the more effective it is likely to be. Neglected cases may require systemic or periocular corticosteroids in addition to local eye drop therapy. Occasionally, vascularization and opacification of the cornea occur so rapidly as to make corticosteroid therapy useless, but even the most hopeless-appearing graft reactions have occasionally been reversed by corticosteroid therapy. Oral cyclosporine has been used successfully in the treatment of corneal graft rejection.

Patients known to have rejected many previous corneal grafts are managed somewhat differently, particularly if disease affects their only remaining eye. An attempt is made to find a close HLA match between donor and recipient. Pretreatment of the recipient with immunosuppressive agents such as azathioprine has also been resorted to in some cases. Although HLA testing of the recipient and the potential donor is indicated in cases of repeated corneal graft failure or in cases of severe corneal vascularization, such testing is not necessary or practicable in most cases requiring keratoplasty.

REFERENCES

Braude LS, Chandler JW: Corneal allograft rejection: The role of the major histocompatibility complex. *Surv Ophthalmol* 1983;**27**:290.

Chandler JW, Gillette TE: Immunologic defense mechanisms of the ocular surface. *Ophthalmology* 1983;**90**:585.

Foulks GN et al: Histocompatibility testing for keratoplasty in high-risk patients. *Ophthalmology* 1983;**90**:239.

Friedlaender MH: *Allergy and Immunology of the Eye.* Harper & Row, 1979.

Friedlaender MH, O'Connor GR: Eye diseases. Chap 33, pp 610–618, in: *Basic & Clinical Immunology,* 6th ed. Stites DP, Stobo JD, Wells JV (editors). Appleton & Lange, 1987.

Freidlaender MH, Okumoto M, Kelley J: Diagnosis of allergic conjunctivitis. *Arch Ophthalmol* 1984;**102**:1198.

Gillette TE, Chandler JW, Greiner JV: Langerhans cells of the ocular surface. *Ophthalmology* 1982;**89**:700.

Jakobiec FA, Lefkowitch J, Knowles DM II: B- and T-lymphocytes in ocular disease. *Ophthalmology* 1984;**91**:635.

Kaplan HJ, Waldrep JC: Immunologic insights into uveitis and retinitis: The immunoregulatory circuit. *Ophthalmology* 1984;**91**:655.

Mehra RM et al: Chlorambucil in the treatment of iridocyclitis in juvenile rheumatoid arthritis. *J Rheumatol* 1981;**8**:141.

Mondino BJ, Brown SI: Immunosuppressive therapy in ocular cicatricial pemphigoid. *Am J Ophthalmol* 1983;**96**:453.

Nichols CW et al: Conjunctival biopsy as an aid in evaluation of the patient with suspected sarcoidosis. *Ophthalmology* 1980;**87**:287.

Nussenblatt RB: HLA and ocular disease. Proceedings of the Immunology of the Eye Workshop 1. Steinberg GM, Gery I, Nussenblatt RB (editors). *Immunology Abstracts* 1980;**Spr Suppl**:25.

O'Connor GR (editor): *Immunologic Diseases of the Mucous Membranes: Pathology, Diagnosis, and Treatment.* Masson, 1980.

O'Connor GR, Chandler JW (editors): *Advances in Immunology and Immunopathology of the Eye.* Masson, 1985.

Potts AM: The relation of immunology to the study of eye disease. Pages 335–338 in: *Year Book of Ophthalmology 1978.* Hughes WF (editor). Year Book, 1978.

Rahi AHS, Garner A: *Immunopathology of the Eye.* Blackwell, 1976.

Rao NA et al: The role of the penetrating wound in the development of sympathetic ophthalmia: Experimental observations. *Arch Ophthalmol* 1983;**101**:102.

Reed CE, Friedlaender MH: Immunologic aspects of diseases of the eye. *JAMA* 1982;**258**:2692. [Special issue.]

Rocklin RE et al: Generation of antigen-specific suppressor cells during allergy desensitization. *N Engl J Med* 1980;**302**:1213.

Sacks EH et al: Lymphocytic subpopulations in the normal human conjunctiva: A monoclonal antibody study. *Ophthalmology* 1986;**93**:1276.

Salisbury JD, Gebhardt BM: Suppression of corneal allograft rejection by cyclosporin A. *Arch Ophthalmol* 1981;**99**:1640.

Silverstein AM, O'Connor GR (editors): *Immunology and Immunopathology of the Eye.* Masson, 1979.

Smolin G, O'Connor GR: *Ocular Immunology,* 2nd ed. Lea & Febiger, 1986.

Theodore FH, Bloomfield SE, Mondino BJ: *Clinical Allergy and Immunology of the Eye.* Williams & Wilkins, 1983.

Wong VG, Anderson RR, McMaster PRB: Endogenous immune uveitis: The role of serum sickness. *Arch Ophthalmol* 1971;**85**:93.

Special Subjects of Pediatric Interest   18

Paul Riordan-Eva, FRCS, MA, MB, BChir

The immediate examination of the newborn infant consists of a brief observation of color, responses, extremities, and digits, and a quick inspection of body surfaces. The more complete examination is done in the nursery.

Because the development of the eye often reflects organ and tissue development of the body as a whole, many congenital somatic defects are mirrored in the eye. A careful eye examination soon after birth may suggest the need for further investigative procedures. Subjective response is limited to the following response to a moving light. The instruments required for the ocular examination of the newborn are a good hand light, an ophthalmoscope, a loupe for magnification, and a portable slit lamp if required.

External Inspection

The eyelids are inspected for growths, deformities, lid notches, and symmetric movement with opening and closing of the eyes. The absolute and relative size of the eyeballs is noted, as well as position and alignment. Spontaneous and elicited conjugate eye movements may also be examined. The size and luster of the corneas are noted, and the anterior chambers are examined for clarity and iris configuration. The size, position, and light reaction of the pupils are also noted.

Ophthalmoscopic Examination

With undilated pupils, some information can be obtained by use of the ophthalmoscope in a dimly lighted room. Ideally, however, all newborns should be examined with an ophthalmoscope through dilated pupils. Ophthalmoscopic examination will demonstrate any corneal, lens, or vitreous opacities as well as abnormalities in the fundus. Preretinal hemorrhages have been reported in 30–45% of newborns, usually clearing completely within a few weeks and leaving no permanent visual dysfunction.

THE NORMAL EYE IN INFANTS & CHILDREN

Tests for Visual Acuity

In the early years, visual acuity should be appraised as part of each general "well child" examination. It is best not to wait until the child is old enough to respond to visual charts, since these may not furnish accurate information until school age. Estimations of vision should be made in the first few days by as-

---

> **PEDIATRIC EYE EXAMINATION SCHEDULE**
>
> **Hospital Nursery**
> External eye examination and ophthalmoscopic examination through dilated pupils as outlined in the text. Two drops of sterile 5% homatropine and 2.5% phenylephrine in each eye are instilled 1 hour prior to examination. Special emphasis should be placed on the optic disks and maculas; detailed examination of the peripheral retinas is not necessary.
>
> **Age 6 Months**
> Test ocular fixation and ocular movement.
>
> **Age 4**
> Visual acuity test with illiterate "E" chart and stereopsis by the random dot "E" test to rule out amblyopia. Visual acuity should be normal 20/20–20/30.
>
> **Age 5–16**
> Test visual acuity at age 5. If normal, test visual acuity with the Snellen chart every 2 years until age 16. Color vision should be tested at age 8–12. No other routine eye examination (eg, ophthalmoscopy) is necessary if visual acuity is normal and the eyes appear normal upon inspection.

---

certaining the pupillary responses to light, which rules out complete dysfunction of the eyes. In later weeks, light fixation reflexes can be elicited—single and bilateral reflexes first, and then binocular following and converging reflexes. A good response consists of prompt fixation and following reflexes, equal in each eye, with the light reflex centered in the pupil when the source is near the examiner's eye.

These indirect inferences about the status of the developing sensory systems can now be augmented by the quantitative techniques of optokinetic nystagmus, forced-choice preferential looking methods, and visually evoked potentials (see Chapter 2). These tests have demonstrated that normal adult visual acuity is attained by about 2 years of age (Table 18–1).

During the growing years, the parents' observations of the child's clumsiness, awareness of surroundings, and apparent sharpness of vision are valuable aids. From about age 4 on, it becomes possible to elicit subjective responses by use of the illiterate "E" chart. Usually, at the first or second grade level, the regular Snellen chart may be employed.

Table 18–1. Development of visual acuity (approximate).

Age	Visual Acuity
2 months	20/400
6 months	20/100
1 year	20/50
2 years	20/20

Eyeball

In the newborn, the eye is relatively larger in comparison with body size than in later life. However, the anteroposterior diameter, which determines the focusing of the eye, is relatively short (averaging about 17.3 mm). This would produce a marked hyperopia if it were not for the greater curvature of the lens at this time.

Cornea

The cornea of the newborn is also relatively large and reaches adult size by about 2 years of age. It is flatter than the adult cornea, however, and the curvature is greater at the periphery than in the center, whereas the opposite is true in the adult.

Lens

At birth the lens is more globular than in adulthood, and its greater refractive power compensates for the shortness of the eye. The lens grows throughout life as new fibers are added to the periphery, and this causes it to flatten. The consistency of the lens material changes throughout life from a soft plasticlike material to the glassy consistency seen in old age. This accounts for the gradual loss in power of accommodation with advancing age.

Refractive State

About 80% of children between the ages of 2 and 6 years are hyperopic, 5% myopic, and 15% emmetropic. About 10% have refractive errors that require correction before age 7 or 8. Hyperopia remains relatively static or gradually diminishes until 19 or 20 years of age. Myopia often develops between age 6–9 and increases throughout adolescence, with the greatest change at the time of puberty. Astigmatism is congenital and remains relatively constant throughout life. Transient refractive changes are well documented in the neonatal period.

Iris

At birth there is little or no pigment on the anterior surface of the iris. The posterior pigment layer shows through the translucent tissue, usually giving the effect of a bluish or slate-gray color. As the pigment begins to appear on the anterior surface, the iris assumes its definitive color. If considerable pigment is deposited, the eyes become brown. Less pigmentation results in blue, gray, hazel, or green eyes. It may take 1–2 years for the pigmentary deposits to occur; in the meantime it is impossible to ascertain the ultimate color of the eyes.

Pupil

In the newborn, the pupil is situated slightly to the nasal side of and below the center of the cornea. Because of the refractive power of the cornea in the neonatal period, the pupil appears larger than it actually is. The apparent diameter varies between 2.5 and 5.5 mm and averages about 4 mm. In infancy, the pupil is smaller than at birth. Congenital underdevelopment of the dilator muscle is common in children with congenital cataracts. The pupillary reflexes appear at about the fifth fetal month and are active by the sixth month. At about age 1 the pupil begins to widen, and it reaches its greatest diameter during adolescence. It again becomes smaller with advancing age. Myopes have larger pupils than hyperopes.

Normal pupils are round and regular and constantly move in response to changes in lighting and upon focusing. Anisocoria, a difference in the size of the 2 pupils, is often a normal finding; in the absence of neurologic abnormalities, it requires no further special diagnostic consideration.

Position

During the first month of life, eye movements may be poorly coordinated and there may be some doubt about the straightness of the eyes. By 3 months of age, however, the binocular reflexes are well developed; any deviation noted after that time should be investigated. Stereoacuity can be shown to develop in most infants beginning at 3 months of age. If strabismus is suspected after age 3 months, referral to an ophthalmologist is indicated.

Nasolacrimal System

The fetal development of the nasolacrimal passages begins as cords of cells that usually hollow out about the time of birth. Because there may normally be a few weeks' delay in duct formation, failure of tear production in the first few weeks does not necessarily indicate any difficulty; failure of the ducts to function by 6 months of age, however, needs attention.

Optic Nerve

By term, some fibers in the optic nerve near the globe begin to become myelinated, but the amount of myelin surrounding individual nerves increases dramatically during the ensuing months and may continue to increase up to the age of 2 years.

The Normal Ocular Fundus of Infants & Children

The ophthalmoscopic appearance of the normal fundus in an infant differs greatly from that of an adult. Most of the differences are due to the distribution of pigments.

In premature infants, remnants of the tunica vasculosa lentis are frequently visible with the ophthalmoscope, either in front of the lens, behind the lens, or in both positions. The remnants are usually absorbed by the time the infant has reached term, but rarely they remain permanently and appear as a complete or partial "cobweb" in the pupil. At other times remnants of the primitive hyaloid system fail to absorb completely, leaving a cone on the optic disk that projects into the vitreous and is called Bergmeister's papilla.

Physiologic cupping of the disk is usually not seen in premature infants and is rarely seen at term; if seen then, it is usually very slight. In such cases the optic disk will appear gray, resembling optic nerve atrophy. This relative pallor, however, gradually changes to the normal adult pink color at about 2 years of age.

The foveal light reflection is absent in infants. Instead, the macula has a bright "mother-of-pearl" appearance with a suggestion of elevation. This is more pronounced in black infants. At 3–4 months of age, the macula becomes slightly concave and the foveal light reflection appears.

The peripheral fundus in the infant is gray, in contrast to the orange-red fundus of the adult. In white infants the pigmentation is more pronounced near the posterior pole and gradually fades to almost white at the periphery. In black infants there is more pigment in the fundus and a gray-blue sheen is seen throughout the periphery. In white infants a white periphery is normal and should not be confused with retinoblastoma. During the next several months, pigment continues to be deposited in the retina, and usually at about 2 years of age the adult color is evident.

CONGENITAL EYE DEFECTS

Most congenital ocular defects are genetically determined. Examples include congenital ptosis, refractive errors, aniridia, strabismus, retinitis pigmentosa, and arachnodactyly (Marfan's syndrome). Absence of a positive family history is no proof that the defect is not in the germ plasm (see Chapter 19).

Other congenital defects may be caused by interference with the development of the embryo, such as the multiple defects associated with rubella infection of the mother during the first 3 months of pregnancy. In this instance the infant may suffer from any or all of the following: cataracts, heart disease, deafness, microcephaly, microphthalmos, and mental deficiency. Eye defects are common in cerebral palsy.

Anophthalmos

This is a rare condition in which one or both eyeballs are absent or rudimentary. There may be either a congenital absence of any ocular structure or an arrest of development to the point where only histologic evidence is present. The eyelids are usually present. They are often adherent at the margins but can be separated. Anophthalmos may be associated with a chromosomal variation and there may be associated intracranial anomalies.

Congenital Cystic Eye

This is a developmental abnormality resulting from complete or partial failure of invagination of the primary optic vesicle. The eye is variable in size and is usually associated with some degree of neuroglial proliferation. The malformation occurs at about the fourth week of embryonic life.

Cyclopia

Cyclopia, which is a rare midline fusion of developing eye structures together with generalized anterior brain and skull defects, is usually not compatible with life since it is transmitted by a recessive lethal gene.

Palpebral Colobomas

A unilateral cleft of one upper lid is the most common type of palpebral coloboma. Bilateral clefts or fissures can occur in lower as well as upper lids and may be associated with other malformations of the face or globe. No specific embryonic maldevelopment has been established as being causative. Large defects require early repair to avoid corneal ulceration due to exposure.

Microphthalmos

In microphthalmos, one or both eyes are markedly smaller than normal. Many other ocular abnormalities may be present also, eg, cataract, glaucoma, aniridia, and coloboma. Somatic abnormalities are also often present, eg, polydactyly, syndactyly, clubfoot, polycystic kidneys, cystic liver, cleft palate, and meningoencephalocele. Microphthalmos is nearly always genetically determined—most frequently as a recessive but occasionally as a dominant trait.

Corneal Defects

There may be partial or complete opacity of the corneas such as is found in congenital glaucoma, faulty development of the cornea with persistent corneal-lens attachments, birth injuries, intrauterine inflammation, interstitial keratitis, and mucopolysaccharide depositions of the cornea as in Hurler's syndrome. The most frequent cause of opaque corneas in infants and young children is congenital glaucoma. In most instances, the eye is larger than normal (macrophthalmos, hydrophthalmos, buphthalmos). Birth injuries may cause extensive corneal opacities with edema as a result of rupture of Descemet's membrane. These usually clear spontaneously.

Megalocornea is an enlarged cornea with normal function usually transmitted as an X-linked recessive trait. It must be differentiated from infantile glaucoma. There are usually no associated defects.

Iris & Pupillary Defects

Misplaced or ectopic pupils are frequently observed. The usual displacement is upward and laterally (temporally) from the center of the cornea. Such displacement is occasionally associated with ectopic lens, congenital glaucoma, or microcornea. Multiple pupils are known as **polycoria.** A true pupil must constrict on exposure to light, indicating a sphincter muscle. Congenital miosis is due to a poorly developed dilator muscle. Little change in pupillary size is noted after instillation of a mydriatic. Congenital mydriasis is characterized by large and inactive pupils and underdeveloped sphincter muscles and must be differentiated from mydriasis due to juvenile paresis and pineal tumor. **Coloboma of the iris** indicates incomplete closure of the fetal ocular cleft and usually occurs below and nasally. It may be associated with coloboma of the lens, choroid, and optic nerve. **Aniridia** (absence of the iris) is a rare abnormality, frequently associated with secondary glaucoma (see p 200) and due to an autosomal dominant hereditary pattern. Various abnormalities in the shape of the pupils have been described but are not necessarily significant. Persistent mesodermal remnants usually appear as threadlike bands running across the central pupillary space and attached to the lesser circle of the iris. They rarely have clinical significance or interfere with visual acuity.

The color of the iris is determined largely by heredity. Abnormalities in color include **albinism** (see p 312), due to the absence of normal pigmentation of the ocular structures and frequently associated with poor visual acuity and nystagmus; and **heterochromia,** which is a difference in color in the 2 eyes that may be a primary developmental defect with no functional loss or may be secondary to an inflammatory process.

Lens Abnormalities

The lens abnormalities most frequently noted are cataracts, although there may be faulty development, forming colobomas, or subluxation, as seen in Marfan's syndrome.

Any lens opacity that is present at birth is a congenital cataract, regardless of whether or not it interferes with visual acuity. Congenital cataracts are often associated with other conditions. Maternal rubella during the first trimester of pregnancy is a common cause of congenital cataract. Other congenital cataracts have a hereditary background.

If the opacity is small enough so that it does not occlude the pupil, adequate visual acuity is attained by focusing around the opacity. If the pupillary opening is entirely occluded, however, normal sight does not develop, and the poor fixation may lead to nystagmus and amblyopia. Good visual results have been reported with both monocular and binocular cataracts receiving early surgery and aphakic correction. Thus, early referral to an ophthalmologist is indicated.

Choroid & Retina

Gross defects of the choroid and retina are visible with the ophthalmoscope. The choroidal structures may show congenital colobomas, usually in the lower nasal region, which may also include the iris and all or part of the optic nerve. Posterior polar chorioretinal scarring is a pigmentary disturbance often caused by intrauterine toxoplasmosis. Other congenital lesions of the choroid and retina include drusen, aneurysms, optic nerve malformations, medullated nerve fibers, hereditary macular degeneration, and those associated with intrauterine infections.

DEVELOPMENTAL BODY DEFECTS ASSOCIATED WITH OCULAR DEFECTS

Albinism

Congenital deficiency of pigment may involve the entire body (complete albinism) or a part of the body (incomplete albinism). When incomplete albinism involves only the eye, function may be normal or impaired. In complete ocular albinism, there is usually an abnormal development of the macula, a significant refractive error, nystagmus, and severe photophobia. The eyebrows and eyelashes are white, the conjunctiva is hyperemic, the irides are gray or red, and the pupil appears red. Treatment consists of relieving photophobia with tinted glasses or opaque contact lenses with a clear central area 2–3 mm in diameter.

Marfan's Syndrome

A congenital disorder of mesodermal origin that is nearly always transmitted as an autosomal dominant trait; the major features are (1) long, thin fingers and toes (arachnodactyly), (2) generalized relaxation of ligaments, (3) generalized muscular underdevelopment, (4) bilateral dislocation of the lenses (ectopia lentis), (5) abnormalities of the heart and, occasionally, aortic aneurysm, (6) high-arched palate, and (7) other deformities of the sternum, thorax, and joints.

The lenses are usually dislocated and visual acuity suffers because the patient is not seeing through the lens centers. Cataracts frequently develop in the subluxated lenses. Cataract surgery may become necessary but has a less favorable prognosis than routine cataract surgery.

Osteogenesis Imperfecta

This rare affliction is characterized by increased fragility of the bones and laxity of the ligaments, with frequent fractures and dislocations, dental defects, deafness, and blue scleras. The blue color is darker in the anterior parts of the scleras over the ciliary bodies. It is thought to be due to abnormal thinness of the sclera and remains unchanged throughout life. Cataracts, megalocornea, and keratoconus may also be present. It nearly always occurs as an autosomal dominant trait.

Hurler's Syndrome

This is a rare condition due to autosomal recessive inheritance in which there is infiltration of mucopolysaccharides into the tissues, especially the liver, spleen, lymph nodes, pituitary gland, and corneas. Other ocular signs include slight ptosis, larger thickened eyelids, and strabismus (esotropia). The corneas show a diffuse haziness, which progresses to a milk-white opacity. Glaucoma may eventually develop. There is no satisfactory treatment.

Oxycephaly
(Acrocephaly, Tower Skull, Steeple Head)

This deformity is evident at birth but is often attributed to normal distortion during delivery and is seldom diagnosed at the time of delivery. It is characterized by a high, dome-shaped or pointed skull, high forehead, bulging temporal fossae, flattened cheekbones, shallow orbits, a high, narrow palatal arch, and synostosis of the cranial suture. Syndactyly may also be present. The ocular signs include exophthalmos (due to flatness of the orbits), wide separation of the eyes, and exotropia. Closure of the eyelids may be difficult or impossible. Loss of vision may follow increased intracranial pressure. Nystagmus is common. Various operative procedures have been devised for the relief of intracranial pressure. If vision is to be preserved, surgery must be performed before optic atrophy has progressed. The syndrome is due to an autosomal dominant gene of weak penetrance.

Acrobrachycephaly

In this abnormality the head is wide, whereas in oxycephaly it is narrow. Acrobrachycephaly is caused by premature closure of the coronal sutures. Growth occurs only laterally and vertically, and the anteroposterior diameter is short. The ocular signs are similar to those of oxycephaly.

Other abnormalities involving the development of the skull are scaphocephaly (increased anteroposterior diameter due to premature closure of the sagittal suture) and plagiocephaly (asymmetric flattening, usually due to premature closure of a single coronal suture).

Craniofacial Dysostosis
(Crouzon's Disease)

This rare hereditary deformity, due to an autosomal dominant gene, is characterized by exophthalmos, atrophy of the maxilla, enlargement of the nasal bones, abnormal increase in the space between the eyes (ocular hypertelorism), optic atrophy, and bony abnormalities of the region of the perilongitudinal sinus. The palpebral fissures slant downward (in contrast to the upward slant of Down's syndrome). Strabismus and nystagmus are also present. The strabismus is secondary to both structural anomalies of the muscles and orbital angle anomalies.

Laurence-Moon-Biedl Syndrome

This syndrome includes retinitis pigmentosa, polydactyly, obesity, hypogenitalism, and mental retardation. It is inherited as an autosomal recessive.

POSTNATAL PROBLEMS

The most common ocular disorders of children are external infections of the conjunctiva and eyelids (bacterial conjunctivitis, sties, blepharitis), strabismus, ocular foreign bodies, allergic reactions of the conjunctiva and eyelids, refractive errors (particularly myopia), and congenital defects. Since it is more difficult to elicit an accurate history of causative factors and subjective complaints in children, it is not uncommon to overlook significant ocular disorders (espeically in very young children). Aside from the altered frequency of occurrence of the types of ocular disorders, the causes, manifestations, and treatment of eye disorders are about the same for children as for adults. Certain special problems encountered more frequently in infants and children are discussed below.

Ophthalmia Neonatorum
(Conjunctivitis of the Newborn)

Conjunctivitis in the newborn may be of chemical, bacterial, chlamydial, or viral origin. *Chlamydia* is now the commonest identifiable infectious cause of neonatal conjunctivitis in the USA. Differentiation is sometimes possible according to the timing of presentation, but appropriate smears and cultures are essential. Chemical conjunctivitis caused by the silver nitrate drops instilled into the conjunctival sac at birth is most apparent during the first or second day of life. Inclusion blennorrhea due to chlamydial infection has its onset between the fifth and 14th days; the presence of typical inclusion bodies in the epithelial cells of a conjunctival smear confirms this diagnosis. Bacterial conjunctivitis, usually due to *Staphylococcus aureus*, *Haemophilus* species, pneumococcus, enterococcus, *Neisseria gonorrhoeae*, or *Pseudomonas* species (the last 2 being the most serious because of potential corneal damage), presents between the second and fifth days after birth. Provisional identification of the causative organism may be made from conjunctival smears. Herpes simplex virus produces characteristic giant cells and viral inclusions on cytologic examination.

Silver nitrate conjunctivitis is usually self-limited. In inclusion blennorrhea, systemic therapy with erythromycin is more effective than topical therapy and aids in the eradication of concurrent nasopharyngeal carriage, which may predispose to the development of pneumonitis. Gonococcal conjunctivitis necessitates parenteral therapy with aqueous crystalline benzylpenicillin given intravenously for penicillin-sensitive strains, and cefotaxime given intravenously with topical erythromycin for penicillinase-producing strains. In all cases due to *Chlamydia* or gonococci, both parents should also be given systemic treatment. Other types of bacterial conjunctivitis require topical instillation of antibacterial agents, such as sodium sulfacetamide, bacitracin, or tetracycline, as soon as results of smears are known. Herpetic keratoconjunctivitis usually resolves spontaneously but may require antiviral therapy, particularly when associated with disseminated infection.

Silver nitrate solution (1%) should be contained in sealed single-use disposable containers. Because of the possibility of chemical conjunctivitis and the lack of effectiveness of silver nitrate against *Chlamydia*, some authorities advocate use of topical erythromycin or tetracycline instead for prophylaxis. Instillation of silver nitrate or an antibiotic is still required in most states in the USA.

Antenatal diagnosis and treatment of maternal genital infections should prevent many cases of neonatal conjunctivitis. The presence of active maternal genital herpes at the time of delivery is an indication for elective cesarean section.

Retinopathy of Prematurity (Retrolental Fibroplasia)

In the early stages of retinopathy of prematurity, demarcated areas of avascularity develop in the peripheral retina. These are followed by extraretinal fibrovascular proliferation and retinal detachment. Supplemental oxygen therapy in neonatal intensive care units was strongly implicated as a causative factor in the original epidemic of 1943–1953. There was a marked reduction in the incidence of disease once oxygen therapy was more carefully controlled. A recent resurgence has been noted by many ophthalmologists, particularly in premature infants of very low birth weight (< 1000 g). The causative factors in these cases are as yet unclear. (See also Chapter 11 and discussion of oxygen in Chapter 16).

Congenital Glaucoma

Congenital glaucoma (see Chapter 12) may occur alone or in association with many other congenital lesions. Early recognition is essential to prevent permanent blindness. Involvement is often bilateral. The most striking symptom is extreme photophobia. Early signs are corneal haze or opacity, increased corneal diameter, and increased intraocular pressure. Since the outer coats of the eyeball are not as rigid in the child, the increased intraocular pressure expands the corneal and scleral tissues. Useful vision may be preserved by early diagnosis and medical and surgical treatment by an ophthalmologist.

Leukocoria (White Pupil)

Parents will occasionally see a white spot through the infant's pupil (leukocoria). Although retinoblastoma must be ruled out, the opacity is more often due to cataract, retrolental fibroplasia, persistence of the tunica vasculosa lentis, or corneal scarring.

Retinoblastoma

This rare malignant tumor of childhood is fatal if untreated. Two-thirds of cases occur before the end of the third year; rarely, cases have been reported in later childhood, adolescence, and even (very rarely) in adults. In about 30% of cases, retinoblastoma is bilateral. Development of the tumor is thought to occur because of the loss, from both members of the chromosome pair, of the normally protective dominant allele at a single locus within chromosomal band 13q14. This is caused by mutations, either in the somatic retinal cells alone (nonheritable retinoblastoma) or in the germ line cells as well (heritable ret-

inoblastoma). In heritable retinoblastoma, children of survivors have a nearly 50% chance of having the disease, and it is more apt to be bilateral in succeeding generations. Parents who have produced one child with retinoblastoma run a 4–7% risk of producing the disease in each subsequently born child. Retinoblastoma is usually not discovered until it has advanced far enough to produce an opaque pupil. Infants and children with presenting symptoms of strabismus should be examined carefully to rule out retinoblastoma, since a deviating eye may be the first sign of the tumor.

Enucleation is the treatment of choice in nearly all unilateral cases of retinoblastoma. Additional discussion, including other possible methods for treatment, is presented on p 392.

Strabismus

Strabismus is present in about 2% of children. Its early recognition is often the responsibility of the pediatrician or the family physician. Occasionally, childhood strabismus has neurologic significance. Treatment of strabismus is best started at the age of 6 months to ensure development of the best possible visual acuity and a good cosmetic and functional result (binocular vision). The idea that a child may outgrow crossed eyes should be discouraged. Neglect in the treatment of strabismus may lead to undesirable cosmetic effects, psychic trauma, and amblyopia (see below) in the deviating eye. Strabismus is covered in depth in Chapter 13.

Amblyopia

Amblyopia is decreased visual acuity of one eye (uncorrectable with lenses) in the absence of organic eye disease.

Normal development of the physiologic mechanisms of the retina and visual cortex is determined by postnatal visual experience. Monocular deprivation due to any cause, congenital or acquired, during a critical period of development (probably lasting up to age 10 in humans) prevents the establishment of normal vision in the involved eye. Reversal of this effect is possible only within a much more limited time period, which decreases with increasing age from a few months to only a few weeks. Early suspicion and prompt referral for treatment of the underlying condition are important in preventing amblyopia.

The most common causes of amblyopia are strabismus, in which the image from the deviated eye is suppressed to prevent diplopia, and anisometropia, in which an inability to focus the eyes simultaneously causes suppression of the image of one eye. Both of these conditions are treatable. (See Chapter 13.)

Since poor visual function in a young child may go unnoticed, routine testing of visual acuity at age 4 is essential in reducing the number of cases of amblyopia.

REFERENCES

Atkinson J et al: Screening for refractive errors in 6–9 month old infants by photorefraction. *Br J Ophthalmol* 1984;**68**:105.

Balkan R, Hoyt CS: Associated neurologic abnormalities in congenital third nerve palsies. *Am J Ophthalmol* 1984;**97**:315.

Banks MS: Infant refraction and accommodation. *Int Ophthalmol Clin* 1980;**20**:205.

Beller R et al: Good visual function after neonatal surgery for congenital monocular cataracts. *Am J Ophthalmol* 1981;**91**:559.

Cameron JH, Cameron M: Visual screening of pre-school children. *Br Med J* 1978;**2**:1693.

Campbell PB et al: Incidence of retinopathy of prematurity in a tertiary newborn intensive care unit. *Arch Ophthalmol* 1983;**101**:1686.

Farrell SA et al: Prenatal diagnosis of retinal detachment in a Walker-Warburg syndrome. *Am J Med Genet* 1987;**28**:619.

Fulton, AB, Hansen RM, Manning KA: Measuring visual acuity in infants. *Surv Ophthalmol* 1981;**25**:325.

Gallie BL, Phillips RA: Retinoblastoma: A model of oncogenesis. *Ophthalmology* 1984;**91**:667.

Garner A: An international classification of retinopathy of prematurity. *Br J Ophthalmol* 1984;**68**:690.

Hall SM, Pugh AG, Hall DMB: Vision screening in the under-5s. *Br Med J* 1982;**285**:1096.

Halloran SL et al: Accuracy of detection of the retinoblastoma gene by esterase D linkage. *Arch Ophthalmol* 1985;**103**:1329.

Hammerschlag MR et al: Erythromycin ointment for ocular prophylaxis of neonatal chlamydial infection. *JAMA* 1980;**244**:2291.

Harley RD (editor): *Pediatric Ophthalmology*, 2nd ed. Saunders, 1983.

Hoskins HD, Shaffer RN, Hetherington J: Anatomical classification of the developmental glaucomas. *Arch Ophthalmol* 1984;**102**:1331.

Hoyt CS, Nickel BL, Billson FA: Ophthalmological examination of the infant. *Surv Ophthalmol* 1982;**26**:177.

Kalina RE: Examination of the premature infant. *Ophthalmology* 1979;**86**:1690.

Mayer DL, Fulton AB, Rodier D; Grating and recognition acuities of pediatric patients. *Ophthalmology* 1984;**91**:947.

Michalski A, Leonard JV, Taylor DS: The eye and inherited metabolic disease: A review. *J R Soc Med* 1988;**81**:286.

Mukai S et al: Linkage of genes for human esterase D and hereditary retinoblastoma. *Am J Ophthalmol* 1984;**97**:681.

Nelson LB: *Pediatric Ophthalmology: Major Problems in Clinical Pediatrics.* Vol 25. Saunders, 1984.

Nelson LB (editor): *Symposium on Pediatric Ophthalmology: The Pediatric Clinics of North America.* Vol 30. Saunders, 1983.

Ophthalmia neonatorum today. (Editorial.) *Lancet* 1984;**2**:1375.

Pierce JM, Ward ME, Seal DV: Ophthalmia neonatorum in the 1980s: Incidence, aetiology and treatment. *Br J Ophthalmol* 1982;**66**:728.

Repka MX, Miller NR: Optic atrophy in children. *Am J Ophthalmol* 1988;**106**:191.

Rice NSC, Taylor D: Congenital cataract: A cause of preventable blindness in children. (Editorial.) *Br Med J* 1982;**285**:581.

Skarf B, Hoyt CS: Optic nerve hypoplasia in children: Association with anomalies of the endocrine and CNS. *Arch Ophthalmol* 1984;**102**:62.

Wybar K, Taylor D (editors): *Paediatric Ophthalmology: Current Aspects.* Marcel Dekker, 1983.

Genetic Aspects

Taylor Asbury, MD, & Paul Riordan-Eva, FRCS, MA, MB, BChir

Genetic influences are being described in an increasing number of diseases, and a primary causative role for genetic defects is being more clearly defined in many instances. Thus, it becomes increasingly important to understand the principles of genetic transmission. Much of the background work in clinical genetics has been done in ophthalmology. The eye seems to be unusually prone to genetically determined disease, and an accurate diagnosis of ocular disease can usually be arrived at on the basis of careful clinical examination.

Clinicians can estimate the risk of occurrence of many genetically determined diseases (usually the rare but severe ones), but the familial incidence of many other diseases also known to be genetically determined still cannot be accurately predicted.

Mechanisms of Inheritance

An individual's genetic identity (**genotype**) is carried by **chromosomes,** which are composed of DNA. There are 23 pairs of chromosomes in the nucleus of the normal human somatic cell. Twenty-two of these pairs are somewhat similar (homologous) and are therefore termed **autosomal.** The 23rd pair is composed of the **sex chromosomes** (X and Y). In the female this pair is homologous (XX), whereas in the male it is heterologous (XY). A number of agents (quinacrine mustard, trypsin, Giemsa's stain) produce morphologic banding of human chromosomes that permits their identification and classification into a number of groups.

Each chromosome is composed of many small functional units termed **genes,** which are situated at specific sites (**loci**) along the length of the chromosome. Genes are thus also arranged in pairs. The alternate forms of a gene at a locus controlling a particular characteristic are known as **alleles.** There are commonly 2 alternate forms, but there may be more. When the alleles at a particular locus are the same, the individual is said to be homozygous, and when they are different, heterozygous.

Genes exert their effects by controlling the production of proteins within the cell cytoplasm. Complementary copies of the DNA constituting specific genes are formed with RNA, and these are used to direct protein synthesis. The mechanisms regulating gene expression are complex.

DNA recombinant technology using isolated human DNA fragments inserted into bacterial cells has led to the identification of the DNA sequences and protein products of specific genes. Linkage studies and DNA probes have identified the position of specific gene loci and carriers for certain mutant genes.

The **gametes** (spermatozoon and ovum) are produced by a special type of cell division called **reduction-division meiosis,** in which the 23 pairs of chromosomes dissociate, each daughter cell receiving one chromosome of each pair. One of each pair passes into each daughter cell as a random occurrence. Exchange of chromosomal material (**translocation**) between the members of each pair also occurs. At fertilization, each chromosome of the spermatozoon joins its corresponding chromosome of the ovum to produce a cell with 46 chromosomes of unique genetic consitution. All cell divisions after fertilization (**mitosis**) involve duplication and separation of all the chromosomes to produce cells with the constant number of 46 chromosomes and identical genetic constitution.

The expression of the genotype in physical characteristics is known as the **phenotype.** The inheritance of certain characteristics of the human phenotype, such as eye color, can be explained on the basis of interaction between the 2 alleles at a single chromosomal locus. Each allele determines the development of one form of the particular characteristic. In the homozygous individual, this form is correspondingly expressed. In the heterozygous individual, one allele is said to be **dominant** because it determines the phenotype, while the other is **recessive** (not expressed). This is the basis of **mendelian inheritance,** from which are derived many of the terms used to describe patterns of inheritance. The inheritance of many phenotypic characteristics, however, cannot easily be classified in this way. This has led to modifications of the original mendelian concepts, including variable expression and variable penetration of genes. Recent improvements in the understanding of gene regulation and expression, as well as recognition of the role of environmental factors, have demonstrated why this model breaks down. Nevertheless, the framework of mendelian inheritance is still of immense value in clinical genetics as a means of describing modes of inheritance and estimating the risk of transmission of certain genetically determined abnormalities. The major alternative patterns of inheritance are those due to chromosomal abnormalities and those described as multifactorial, involving multiple genes or major environmental influences.

MENDELIAN INHERITANCE

Mendelian inheritance can be divided into 3 main groups: autosomal dominant, autosomal recessive, and X-linked recessive.

Autosomal Dominant Inheritance

An abnormal dominant gene produces its specific abnormality even though its paired gene (allele) is normal. Males and females are affected alike and, being heterozygous, have a theoretical 50% chance of passing along the affected gene (and therefore the abnormality) to each of their offspring, even when mated to genotypically normal individuals (Fig 19–1).

Given a particular group of pedigrees, autosomal dominant inheritance is established if the following conditions are met: (1) Males and females are equally affected. (2) Direct transmission has occurred over 2 or more generations. (3) About 50% of individuals in the pedigrees are affected.

Quite a large number of uncommon but serious diseases with ocular manifestations are transmitted in this way: forms of juvenile glaucoma, Marfan's syndrome, congenital stationary night blindness (Fig 19–2), osteogenesis imperfecta, neurofibromatosis, Lindau-Von Hippel disease, and tuberous sclerosis. The process of natural selection tends to keep most of these serious diseases at a low incidence in the general population, since many of these people are unable to produce children even if they do manage to live to the age of reproduction.

Dominant disease may be more or less severe from generation to generation depending upon its **expression;** a disease with "variable expression" is one that can occur in a mild or severe form. An example is neurofibromatosis, in which genotypically affected individuals may have merely café au lait spots or may have many serious manifestations. One cannot predict if or when the disease will be more serious (with central nervous system tumors or optic nerve gliomas) in a succeeding generation. If the genetic pattern is present but there is no evidence of the disease, one says that its **penetrance** is reduced. It may be quite difficult to differentiate dominant inheritance with reduced penetrance from recessive inheritance (see below). Those pedigrees which demonstrate neither a definite autosomal dominant nor a definite recessive pattern are properly classified as irregular dominants (dominant inheritance with variable expression) or incomplete recessives (carrier state identifiable clinically).

In certain diseases such as hemoglobin S disease, there is a clearly defined intermediate phenotype that corresponds to the heterozygous individual. This is known as **codominant inheritance.**

Autosomal Recessive Inheritance

Abnormal recessive genes must lie in pairs (duplex state) to produce manifest abnormality. Thus, each parent must contribute one recessive abnormal gene. Each parent is clinically unaffected (genotypically affected but phenotypically normal), since a normal dominant gene makes the abnormal gene recessive (Fig 19–3).

It is difficult to establish that a given disease results from autosomal recessive inheritance. Some of the criteria used to establish recessive inheritance are the following:

(1) Occurrence of the same disease in collateral branches of the family.

(2) History of consanguinity. The higher the rate of consanguinity in the pedigrees of a given disease, the more likely the disease is to be recessive and the rarer the occurrence of the disease in the general population. Consanguinity creates greater opportunities for the genes to lie in the duplex state, inasmuch as an individual with 2 related parents can receive the same affected gene from each, a common ancestor having originally passed on the affected gene.

(3) The occurrence of the disease in about 25% of siblings. This only holds for groups of pedigrees. There is a 25% chance that the 2 abnormal genes will be passed on to one individual. There is a 50% chance that a normal gene will modify the affected gene. In this case, the individual is a carrier of the disease (just like the parents) but is not affected with the disease (ie, genotypically affected but phenotypically normal). In the remaining 25% of siblings, 2 normal genes lie together and the abnormal gene is completely lost (ie, the individual is genotypically normal). Although a number of pedigrees are required to definitely establish recessive inheritance, even a single pedigree is suggestive if more than one sibling is similarly affected without antecedent history.

Many disease processes have been definitely established as resulting from autosomal recessive inheritance, and many others are suspected of having

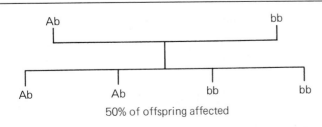

A = Abnormal dominant gene
b = Normal gene lying at same position in the paired chromosome cells

50% of offspring affected

Figure 19–1. Autosomal dominant inheritance.

Note: Individuals assumed to have genotypically-ly normal mates are not shown in the diagram.

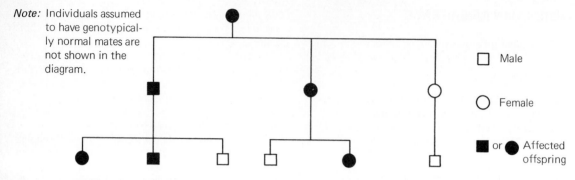

Male

Female

or ● Affected offspring

Figure 19–2. Pedigree of congenital stationary night blindness (abnormal dominant gene).

such a genetic background. Included among the definite cases are Laurence-Moon-Biedl syndrome and inborn errors of metabolism such as oculocutaneous albinism (Fig 19–4), galactokinase deficiency, and Tay-Sachs disease.

X-Linked (Sex-Linked) Recessive Inheritance

The sex chromosomes are one of the 23 pairs of human chromosomes. Identical chromosomes appear in females; these have been labeled designate X chromosomes. One such chromosome appears with a dissimilar mate in the male; this smaller chromosome has been labeled the Y chromosome. Therefore, XX is female and XY is male.

The criteria for X-linked inheritance are (1) that only males are affected, (2) that the disease is transmitted through carrier females to half of the sons, and (3) that there is no father-to-son transmission.

Many of the genes of the X chromosome are unopposed by a gene of the Y chromosome. Abnormalities of these genes cause disease in the male, whereas in the female an abnormal recessive gene of the sex chromosome is masked by its normal allele. Therefore, nearly all of the X-linked diseases are manifested in males, whereas the disease is passed through the female. A male and his maternal grandfather are affected, and the intervening female is the carrier.

Among the important eye diseases with an X-linked genetic pattern are color blindness (Fig 19–5), ocular albinism, and one type of retinitis pigmentosa.

Females have a mosaic of somatic cells consisting of cell groups with one X chromosome functioning and cell groups with the other X chromosome functioning (Lyon hypothesis). When the female is a carrier of an X-linked disease, this mosaicism is occasionally detectable. Such is the case in female carriers of ocular albinism, in whom groups of pigmented and albino retinal pigment epithelial cells are visible ophthalmoscopically.

CHROMOSOMAL ABNORMALITIES

When mitosis is interrupted in metaphase, the chromosomes can be spread on a slide, counted, and photographed. These cytogenetic studies have made possible the classification of chromosomes into 7 groups based upon characteristics such as size and the position of the centromere. The groups contain as few as 2 or as many as 7 chromosomes, with the chromosomes of any group being indistinguishable from each other. The study of cytogenetics has also established that some clinical states can be correlated with an abnormal number of chromosomes, most frequently one more (trisomy) or occasionally one less (monosomy) than the normal number of 46. A few of the more common syndromes are summarized briefly below. Since the addition or subtraction of an entire gene is obviously a major genetic abnormality, these syndromes are characterized by many and extensive deformities. Many such abnormal fertilizations result in early abortions and stillbirths.

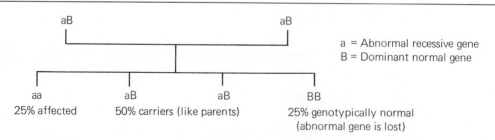

a = Abnormal recessive gene
B = Dominant normal gene

Figure 19–3. Mating of 2 carriers.

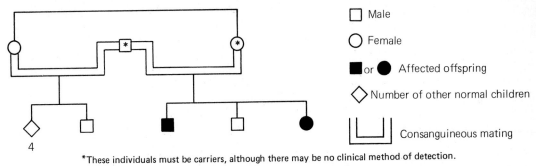

	Male
	Female
or ●	Affected offspring
◇	Number of other normal children
⊔	Consanguineous mating

*These individuals must be carriers, although there may be no clinical method of detection.

Figure 19–4. Pedigree of oculocutaneous albinism. In this case a man married successively 2 sisters, his first cousins.

1. SYNDROMES ASSOCIATED WITH AN ABNORMAL NUMBER OF CHROMOSOMES

Trisomy 13 (Patau's Syndrome)

Anophthalmos, microphthalmos, retinal dysplasia, optic atrophy, coloboma of the uvea, and cataracts are the major eye anomalies; cerebral defects, cleft palate, heart lesions, polydactyly, and hemangiomas are the more severe nonophthalmic changes. Cytogenetically, there is an extra chromosome indistinguishable from group 13–15. Death by age 6 months is the rule.

Trisomy 18 (Edward's Syndrome)

The main features of this rare syndrome are mental and physical retardation, congenital heart defects, and renal abnormalities. Corneal and lenticular opacities, unilateral ptosis, and optic atrophy have been described.

Trisomy 21 (Down's Syndrome)

Although Down's syndrome is a fairly common and well-known entity, the hereditary pattern was long ill-defined. Waardenburg originally suggested that Down's syndrome was a chromosomal problem in 1932. Cytogenetic studies in 1958 revealed an extra chromosome indistinguishable from chromosome 21. The principal manifestations are small stature, a flattened, round, mongoloid facies, saddle nose, thick lower lip, large tongue, soft, seborrheic skin, smooth hair, obesity, small genitalia, short fingers, a simian fold, congenital heart anomalies, mental retardation, and frequent psychic disturbances. The ocular signs include hyperplasia of the iris, narrow palpebral fissures with Oriental slant, frequent strabismus, epicanthus, frequent cataract, high myopia (33%), and Brushfield (silver-gray) spots on the iris.

The incidence of Down's syndrome is significantly increased in children born to older women, particularly those past age 35.

2. ABNORMALITIES INVOLVING SEX CHROMOSOMES

Turner's syndrome is a monosomy (45 chromosomes). For some reason, the affected female receives only one X chromosome. Clinically, growth retardation, rudimentary ovaries and female genitalia, amenorrhea, pterygium colli, epicanthus, cubitus valgus, and ptosis occur. Of particular ophthalmic in-

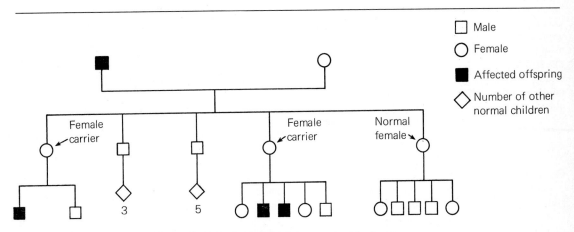

	Male
	Female
■	Affected offspring
◇	Number of other normal children

Figure 19–5. Pedigree of red-green color blindness.

terest is the high incidence of color blindness (8%). This is the same frequency as for males (female incidence, 0.4%) and is readily explained by the fact that the normally recessive gene is unopposed and is expressed just as in the male.

Klinefelter's syndrome is a trisomy involving the X chromosomes. These phenotypical males have 47 chromosomes: the normal 44 autosomes and 3 sex chromosomes, XXY. These individuals are sterile, with small testes, have a eunuchoid physique, and frequently gynecomastia. The ocular finding of interest is the very rare occurrence of color blindness, since the recessive X chromosome is masked by a normal dominant (as in the normal female).

OTHER GENETIC CONSIDERATIONS

Genetic Counseling

Valuable advice can often be given to families concerned with the possibilities of transmitting serious disease to future generations. This entails a working knowledge of basic genetic principles and sensitive counseling skills. A careful history of the pedigree in question is very important, as a single disease may have more than one mode of transmission (eg, retinitis pigmentosa has 3 or more basic patterns). On the other hand, careful inquiries about maternal health during pregnancy may suggest that the anomaly—eg, congenital cataracts—is developmental and therefore unrelated to the genes.

Consanguineous mating increases the prevalence of autosomal recessive traits, and the most likely explanation for 2 individuals' having the same recessive gene is the fact that they are related.

Prenatal Diagnosis

In some cases it is possible to offer families at risk for a specific hereditary disease the option of prenatal diagnosis. This may involve searching for chromosomal abnormalities or specific structural protein defects such as enzyme deficiencies. Currently, techniques are being devised to identify abnormalities at the gene level using DNA linkage studies (eg, in X-linked retinitis pigmentosa) or DNA probes. Prenatal diagnosis by testing amniotic fluid cells obtained by amniocentesis at 14–16 gestational weeks has become a safe and practical procedure. The list of hereditary diseases that can be diagnosed with this method is rapidly increasing. There is, however, a 3-week delay before results of cytogenetic analysis become available. Chorionic villus sampling has certain advantages: It can be undertaken at 8–12 gestational weeks, and results are known within 24 hours. Its overall safety is still being determined.

Genetic Carrier State

Recognition of the genetic carrier state makes possible more accurate prediction of possible disease transmission and helps to establish the genetic nature of a disease by providing an occasion for examination of relatives of affected individuals. Detection is possible in many diseases. There are 3 types:

(1) Autosomal dominant diseases in which the disease appears in a mild or subclinical form (low expression). Because the offspring of such individuals still have the theoretical 50% chance of passing on the disease process, the recognition of this carrier state is important in genetic counseling.

(2) Autosomal recessive diseases with heterozygous manifestations. Affected genes that are normally balanced by a normal allele may cause minor subclinical abnormalities which disclose the presence of the abnormal gene. One can predict the 25% possibility of occurrence of some autosomal recessive diseases if the carrier state can be recognized in both potential mates.

(3) Female carrier in X-linked recessive disease. Subclinical evidence of the disease in daughters of affected fathers differentiates carriers from noncarriers in a number of X-linked recessive diseases (often quite obvious in tapetoretinal degenerative conditions).

Mutation

Mutation occurs when a gene undergoes alteration in the germ cell as a result of spontaneous chemical change within the gene and the change is manifested by a new characteristic. The causes of the change are not well understood, but such extrinsic environmental factors as heat, x-rays, and exposure to radioactive materials may induce it. Most often the new characteristic is unfavorable (ie, disease-producing), but some mutations are favorable and account for the evolution of species (Darwin).

Certain mutations occur repeatedly in specific genes and cause specific disease. Hemophilia, which follows an X-linked pattern, and retinoblastoma, in which a single locus on chromosome 13 q is involved, are examples of disease occurring as a result of mutation. Very few individuals with severe abnormalities reproduce, so that the incidence of such diseases is dependent almost entirely upon mutation. Mutations causing less severe diseases are inherited as dominant, recessive, or X-linked traits depending upon the type of mutated gene.

Retinoblastoma

Recent advances in our understanding of the genetic basis of retinoblastoma illustrate many of the points discussed above. Retinoblastoma is a malignant tumor of retinal photoreceptors (see p 331) seen in childhood. Most cases are sporadic, without transmission to subsequent generations, but a significant proportion are familial. The "two-hit" hypothesis of oncogenesis for this and other hereditary cancers proposes that tumor development is a recessive trait at the cellular level and that 2 separate mutations are necessary to produce the required homozygous state. In retinoblastoma, the relevant mutation is deletion at the chromosomal locus 13q14. In sporadic cases, both mutations occur in the somatic cells of the retina, and for that reason the disease is not genetically transmissible. In familial cases, the first mutation is present in the germ cells, and the second develops in retinal cells.

Predisposition for tumor development is inherited as an autosomal dominant trait, being present in 50% of children of retinoblastoma patients. Nine out of 10 individuals who inherit the germ cell mutation develop the tumor. Familial cases tend to be bilateral and multifocal and to have onset at an early age, whereas sporadic cases are unilateral, unifocal, and appear later. Individuals who inherit the germ cell mutation are also known to have a greatly increased risk for development of independent second primary tumors—particularly osteosarcoma—in later life.

Present practice consists of regular screening of all siblings and children of retinoblastoma patients for the development of retinoblastoma. This necessitates frequent general anesthesia for ophthalmoscopy. It would be advantageous to be able to restrict the screening procedure to individuals truly at risk, ie, those who have inherited the germ cell mutation.

All bilateral cases and those with a family history can be assumed to be familial; unilateral cases may be familial or sporadic. Cases without a family history may be sporadic or may be the first of a series of familial cases following de novo mutation in the germ line. However, these features are not sufficient to reliably identify only those with the germ line mutation.

Fortunately, the necessary process of gene tracking is now becoming possible both by gene linkage studies, using the esterase-D protein, which has a gene locus close to that of the retinoblastoma gene; and by DNA probes for the esterase-D and retinoblastoma genes. These techniques are also applicable to prenatal diagnosis, using chorionic villus sampling. Consequently, it is theoretically possible to identify exactly which retinoblastoma cases are familial and to determine even before birth which siblings or children also possess the germ cell mutation, thus allowing termination of the pregnancy or a much more specific childhood screening program.

GLOSSARY OF GENETIC TERMS*

Abiotrophic disease: Genetically determined disease which is not evident at birth but which becomes manifest later in life.

Acquired: Not hereditary; contracted after birth or in utero.

Alleles: Paired genes or partner genes; genes occupying the same locus on homologous (paired) chromosomes and which, therefore, normally segregate

from each other during the reduction-division of mitosis.

Autosomes: The chromosomes (22 pairs of autosomes in humans) other than the sex chromosomes.

Chromosome: A small threadlike or rodlike structure into which the nuclear chromatin separates during mitosis. The number of chromosomes is constant for any given species (23 pairs in humans: 22 pairs of autosomes and one pair of sex chromosomes).

Congenital: Existing at or before birth; not necessarily hereditary.

Dominant: Designating a gene whose phenotypic effect largely or entirely obscures that of its allele.

Familial: Pertaining to traits, either hereditary or acquired, which tend to occur in families.

Gamete (germ cell): A cell that is capable of uniting with another cell in sexual reproduction (ie, the ovum and spermatozoon).

Gene: A unit of heredity which occupies a specific locus in the chromosome which, either alone or in combination, produces a single characteristic. It is usually a single unit that is capable of self-duplication or mutation.

Genetic carrier state: A condition wherein a given hereditary characteristic is not manifest in one individual but may be genetically transmitted to the offspring of that individual.

Genotype: The hereditary constitution, or combination of genes, that characterizes a given individual or a group of genetically identical organisms.

Germ cell: See Gamete, above.

Hereditary: Transmitted from ancestor to offspring through the germ plasm.

Heterozygous: Having 2 members of a given hereditary factor pair that are dissimilar, ie, the 2 genes of an allelic pair are not the same.

Homozygous: Having 2 members of a given hereditary factor pair that are similar, ie, the 2 genes of an allelic pair are identical.

Meiosis: A special type of cell division occurring during the maturation of sex cells, by which the normal diploid set of chromosomes is reduced to a single (haploid) set, 2 successive nuclear divisions occurring, while the chromosomes divide only once.

Mitosis: Cell division in which daughter nuclei receive identical components of the number of chromosomes characteristic of the species.

Mutation: A transformation of a gene, often sudden and dramatic, with or without known cause, into a different gene occupying the same locus as the original gene on a particular chromosome; the new gene is allelic to the normal gene from which it has arisen.

Penetrance: The likelihood or probability that a gene will become morphologically (phenotypically) expressed. The degree of penetrance may depend upon acquired as well as genetic factors.

Phenotype: The visible characteristics of an individual or those which are common to a group of apparently identical individuals.

Recessive: Designating a gene whose phenotypic effect is largely or entirely obscured by the effect of its allele.

Sex chromosome: The chromosome or pair of chromosomes that determines the sex of the individual. (In the human female, the sex chromosome pair is homologous, XX; in the male, heterologous, XY.)

*Modified from Krupp MA et al: *Physician's Handbook*, 21st ed. Lange, 1985.

Sex linkage: See X linkage, below.
Somatic cells: Cells incapable of reproducing the organism.
Trisomy: The existence of 3 chromosomes of one variety, rather than the normal pair of chromosomes.

X linkage: The pattern of inheritance of genes located on the X chromosome.
Zygote: The cell formed by the union of 2 gametes in sexual reproduction.

REFERENCES

Albert DM, Dryja TP: Recent studies of the retinoblastoma gene. (Editorial.) *Arch Ophthalmol* 1988; **106:**181.

Bergsma D (editor): *Birth Defects Compendium,* 2nd ed. AR Liss, 1979.

Cavenee WK et al: Prediction of familial predisposition to retinoblastoma. *N Engl J Med* 1986;**314:**1201.

Cowell JK et al: Retinoblastoma: Clinical and genetic aspects: A review. *J R Soc Med* 1988;**81:**220.

Duke-Elder S: *System of Ophthalmology.* Vol 7. Mosby, 1962.

Edlin G: *Genetic Principles: Human and Social Consequences.* Jones & Bartlett, 1984.

François J: "Counseling" in ophthalmology. *Ann Ophthalmol* 1976;**8:**265.

François J: *Heredity in Ophthalmology.* Mosby, 1961.

Gilbert F: Retinoblastoma and cancer genetics. (Editorial.) *N Engl J Med* 1986;**314:**1248.

Green JS, Johnson GL: Hereditary diseases as causes of blindness in Newfoundland: Preliminary report. *Can J Ophthalmol* 1983;**18:**281.

Hu DN: Prevalence and mode of inheritance of major genetic eye diseases in China. *J Med Genet* 1987; **24:**584.

Keith CG: *Genetics and Ophthalmology.* Churchill Livingstone, 1978.

Kinnear PE, Jay B, Witkop CJ Jr: Albinism. *Surv Ophthalmol* 1985;**30:**75.

McKusick VA: *Mendelian Inheritance in Man,* 6th ed. Johns Hopkins Univ Press, 1983.

Mets MB, Maumenee IH: The eye and the chromosome. *Surv Ophthalmol* 1983;**28:**20.

Mukai S et al: Linkage between the X-linked retinitis pigmentosa locus and the L1.28 locus. *Am J Ophthalmol* 1985;**100:**225.

Rennie WA (editor): *Goldberg's Genetic and Metabolic Eye Diseases,* 2nd ed. Little, Brown, 1986.

Stanbury JB et al: *The Metabolic Basis of Inherited Disease,* 5th ed. McGraw-Hill, 1983.

Tabbara KF, Badr IA: Changing pattern of childhood blindness in Saudi Arabia. *Br J Ophthalmol* 1985;**69:**312.

Ullman S, Nelson LB, Jackson LG: Prenatal diagnostic techniques: Chorionic villus sampling. *Surv Ophthalmol* 1985;**30:**33.

Waardenburg PJ, Franceschetti A, Klein D: *Genetics and Ophthalmology.* 2 vols. Thomas, 1961, 1963.

Wiggs J et al: Prediction of the risk of hereditary retinoblastoma using DNA polymorphisms within the retinoblastoma gene. *N Engl J Med* 1988;**318:**151.

Trauma

20

Taylor Asbury, MD, & Khalid F. Tabbara, MD

Ocular trauma is a common cause of unilateral blindness in children and young adults; persons in these age groups sustain the majority of severe ocular injuries. Young adults—especially men—are the most likely victims of penetrating ocular injuries. Domestic accidents, batteries, and motor vehicle accidents are the most common circumstances in which ocular injury occurs.

Eye injuries incurred during athletic activity are becoming more common with the increasing popularity of indoor court games. A recent survey found racquetball to exceed other sports in generating ocular injuries, followed by tennis, baseball, basketball, and soccer. Hyphemas and corneal abrasions were the most common injuries sustained, and over 14% of patients had permanent partial or total visual loss.

Initial Examination of Ocular Trauma

Examination begins with the history, which should include an estimate of visual acuity prior to and immediately following the injury. It should be noted whether any visual loss was progressive or sudden. An intraocular foreign body must be suspected if the patient was hammering metal on metal. Injuries in a child that are said to have occurred late at night or several days earlier or a history that is not appropriate for the injury sustained may indicate child abuse. In all cases of ocular trauma, the ''uninjured'' eye should also be carefully examined.

Visual acuity must be measured and recorded before the injured eye is examined. (The eye should be tested again upon recovery from injury and a refraction performed if vision is below normal. This record may have legal significance.) If visual loss is severe, check for light projection, 2-point discrimination, and the presence of an afferent pupillary defect. Test ocular motility and periorbital skin sensation, and palpate for defects in the bony orbital rim. At the bedside, the presence of enophthalmos can be determined by viewing the profiles of the corneas from over the brow. If a slit lamp is not available in the emergency room, a penlight, loupe, or direct ophthalmoscope set on + 10 (black numbers) can be used to examine the inner surfaces of the lids and the anterior segment.

The anterior surface of the cornea is examined for foreign materials or wounds, regularity, and luster. The bulbar conjunctiva is inspected for hemorrhage, foreign material, or tears. The depth and clarity of the anterior chamber are noted. The size, shape, and light reaction of the pupil should be compared with the other eye. If the eyeball is undamaged, the lids, palpebral conjuctiva, and fornices are carefully inspected, including inspection after eversion of the upper lid. A moist cotton-tipped applicator is used to sweep away foreign material from the conjunctival fornices. The direct and indirect ophthalmoscopes are used to view the lens, vitreous, optic disk, and posterior retina. Photographic documentation may be appropriate with external trauma.

Immediate Management of Ocular Trauma

If there is obvious rupture of the globe, avoid further manipulation until the patient has been given general anesthesia. No cycloplegic agents or topical antibiotics should be applied prior to surgery. A Fox shield (or the bottom third of a paper cup) is taped over the eye, and parenteral broad-spectrum antibiotics are started. Analgesics, antiemetics, and tetanus antitoxin are given as needed, with restriction of food and fluids. Induction of general anesthesia should not include the use of depolarizing neuromuscular blocking agents, because these transiently increase pressure on the globe, thus increasing any tendency to extrusion of intraocular contents. Small children may also be better examined with the aid of a short-acting general anesthetic.

In severe injuries it is important for the nonspecialist to bear in mind the possibility of causing further damage by unnecessary manipulation.

Caution: Topical anesthetics, dyes, and other medications placed in an injured eye *must be sterile*. Both tetracaine and fluorescein can be autoclaved repeatedly without impairment of their pharmacologic properties. Individually packaged sterile fluorescein strips are preferred. Most ophthalmic solutions are now available in individual disposable sterile units, which significantly reduces the risk of infection.

ABRASIONS & LACERATIONS OF THE LIDS

Particulate matter should be removed from abrasions of the lids to reduce skin tattooing. The wound is then irrigated with saline and covered with an antibiotic ointment and sterile dressing. Avulsed tissue is cleaned and reattached. Because of the excellent vascularity of the lids, there is a good chance that such tissues will heal without requiring later plastic surgery.

Many lacerations of the lid do not involve the margins and may be sutured in the same way as other lacerations of the skin. If the margin of the lid is involved, however, precautions must be taken to prevent marginal notching. The most effective technique is to freshen the lacerated edges by vertical incisions perpendicular to the lid margins through the full height of the tarsus. These vertical incisions should not be parallel but should be slightly inclined so as to converge at the margin. This results in a slight elevation at the lid edge, which on healing flattens and avoids a notch. The incisions are then joined by a "V," thus forming a pentagonal wedge. The conjunctiva and tarsus are closed by interrupted gut sutures, anatomically reapproximating the layers, with conjunctiva and tarsus posteriorly and skin and orbicularis muscle anteriorly. Several partial-thickness sutures are passed through the exposed tarsal edges. The sutures should not be exposed on the conjunctival side. The edges of the skin are closed with interrupted 6–0 silk or monofilament suture. The lid margin is carefully aligned with two 7–0 silk sutures: one in the posterior margin through the orifices of the meibomian glands and the other in the anterior lid margin through the lash line. The sutures are tied and allowed to remain about 5 mm long. They are placed under the skin closure sutures to prevent their abrading the cornea. Skin grafting can be delayed 1–2 days by keeping exposed tissues moist and covered with antibiotics and a sterile dressing.

If primary repair is not effected within 24 hours, edema may necessitate delayed closure. The wound should be cleansed well and antibiotics administered. After swelling has subsided, repair may be performed. Debridement should be minimized, especially if the skin is not lax.

Lacerations near the inner canthus frequently involve the canaliculi. Early repair is desirable, since the tissue becomes more difficult to identify with swelling. The upper canaliculus is rarely essential to

lacrimal drainage but can often serve as the sole excretory path when the lower one has been destroyed. It is always preferable to repair lacerations of the canaliculi to prevent stricture.

Sharp lacerations through the distal canaliculus can be repaired with a Veirs rod stent or other modifications. Avulsions or proximal canalicular lacerations require silicone nasocanalicular intubation with Quickert probes (Fig 20–1). Various methods of intubating a single canaliculus have been recently described that serve to avoid the risky and traumatic use of pigtail probes. Note that crepitus indicates a sinus fracture, usually ethmoidal, and swelling can signal orbital or preseptal cellulitis.

FOREIGN BODIES ON THE SURFACE OF THE EYE & CORNEAL ABRASIONS

Foreign bodies on the surface of the eye may give a foreign body sensation that can be felt during eye and lid movement, and corneal epithelial defects may cause a similar sensation. Fluorescein will stain the exposed basement membrane of an epithelial defect and can highlight aqueous leakage from penetrating wounds (Seidel's test). A pattern of vertical scratch marks on the cornea indicates particles embedded on the conjunctival surface of the upper lid. Contact lens overwear produces edema of the central cornea epithelium and frequently stippling of the epithelium.

Simple corneal epithelial defects are treated with antibiotics, a cycloplegic agent of intermediate duration (scopolamine, 0.25%), and a pressure patch to immobilize the lids. For removal of foreign matter, a topical anesthetic can be given and a spud or fine-gauge needle used to remove the material during slit lamp exmaination. A cotton-tipped applicator should not be used because it rubs off a large area of epithelium, often without removing the foreign body. Metallic rings surrounding copper or iron fragments (Fig 20–2) can be removed with a battery-operated drill with a burr tip. Deeply embedded inert materials (eg, glass, carbon) may be allowed to remain in the cornea. If removal of deeply embedded fragments is necessary or if there is an aqueous leak requiring sutures or cyanoacrylate glue, the procedure should be undertaken in an operating room, where the anterior chamber can be re-formed (if necessary) under sterile conditions and the surgery performed under the microscope.

Following removal of a foreign body, an antibiotic ointment such as polymyxin B-bacitracin or gentamicin should be instilled 3 times a day into the conjunctival sac to prevent infection. If the wound is extensive, an eye bandage can be used to minimize movement of the lid over the injured area. The wound should be inspected daily for evidence of infection until it is completely healed.

Never give a topical anesthetic solution to the patient for repeated use after a corneal injury, as this

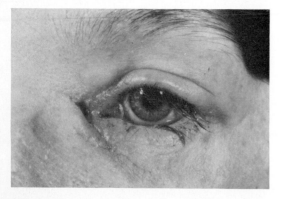

Figure 20–1. Laceration of upper and lower canaliculi and medial canthal region. Silicone tube encircling puncta. (Courtesy of J Sullivan.)

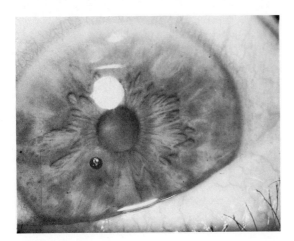

Figure 20–2. Metallic corneal foreign body. (Courtesy of A Rosenberg.)

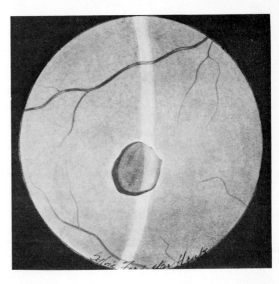

Figure 20–3. Hole in retina, macular area, posttraumatic.

delays healing and masks further damage and can lead to permanent corneal scarring. Steroids should be avoided while an epithelial defect exists. Because corneal abrasions are a frequent complication of general anesthesia, care should be taken to avoid this injury during induction and throughout the procedure by taping the lids closed. Recurrent epithelial erosions sometimes follow corneal injuries and are treated with patching or a bandage contact lens.

PENETRATING INJURIES & CONTUSIONS OF THE EYEBALL

Rupture of the eyeball can occur with sharp penetrating injuries or a blunt contusive force. A blunt object produces a rise in orbital and intraocular pressure, with deformation of the globe. Decompression occurs when the eye wall ruptures or the orbital contents herniate into adjacent sinuses (blowout fracture). The superonasal limbus is the most common site of rupture (contrecoup effect—the lower temporal quadrant being most exposed to trauma).

While most penetrating injuries cause a marked loss of vision, injuries due to small high-velocity particles generated by grinding or hammering might present with only mild pain and blurring. Other signs include hemorrhagic chemosis, conjunctival laceration, a shallow anterior chamber with an eccentrically placed pupil, hyphema, and vitreous hemorrhage. The intraocular pressure can be low, normal, or, rarely, slightly elevated.

In addition to rupture of the wall, contusive forces to the eyeball can result in motility disorders, subconjunctival hemorrhage, corneal edema, aqueous cell and flare, hyphema and angle-recession glaucoma, traumatic mydriasis, rupture of the iris sphincter, iridodialysis, paralysis of accommodation, lens dislocation, and cataract. Injuries sustained by posterior structures include vitreal and retinal hemorrhages, ret-

inal edema (commotio retinae, or Berlin's edema), retinal holes, vitreous base avulsions, retinal detachment, choroidal rupture, and optic nerve contusion (Figs 20–3 and 20–4).

Many of these injuries cannot be seen on external observation. Some, such as cataract, may not develop for many days or weeks following the injury.

Treatment

Except for injuries involving rupture of the eyeball itself, most of the effects of contusion of the eye do not require immediate definitive treatment. However, any injury severe enough to cause intraocular hemorrhage involves the danger of delayed secondary

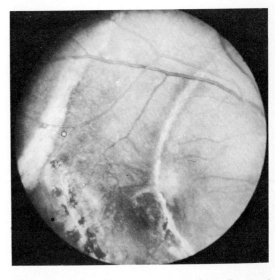

Figure 20–4. Choroidal tears. (Photo by Diane Beeston.)

hemorrhage from a damaged uveal vessel, which may cause intractable glaucoma and permanent damage to the eyeball. The further management of these cases is described in the section below on hyphema.

In the closure of anterior segment wounds, microsurgical techniques should be used. Corneal tissue is accurately realigned with 10–0 nylon sutures to form a watertight closure. To minimize astigmatism, centrally placed corneal sutures should be of short length and more closely spaced than those positioned near the limbus. An incarcerated iris or ciliary body exposed for less than 24 hours can be reposited in the globe by introducing a cyclodialysis spatula through a limbal stab incision and sweeping the tissue into position. If this cannot be achieved or if the tissue has been exposed for more than 24 hours, then the prolapsing tissue should be excised at the level of the wound lip. Any excised tissue should be sent for pathologic examination. Cultures are taken for investigation of possible bacterial infection. Lens remnants and blood are removed by anterior vitrectomy. Viscoelastic materials (sodium hyaluronate), air, or saline injected into the anterior chamber will help realign the edges and prevent uveal incarceration by providing support during wound closure.

Scleral wounds are closed with an interrupted 7–0 or 8–0 nonabsorbable suture. The rectus muscles may be temporarily disinserted to provide better exposure. Posterior scleral exit wounds in a double penetrating injury are self-sealing, and generally no attempt is made at closure.

The prognosis for traumatic retinal detachments is poor because of the macular injury, giant retinal tears, and formation of intravitreal fibrocellular membranes that occur with penetrating injury. Such intravitreal membranes generate sufficient contractile force to detach the retina. Vitrectomy is effective in their treatment, but the timing of this procedure remains controversial. Early vitrectomy is indicated for endophthalmitis. In noninfected cases, delaying surgery for 10–14 days may decrease the risk of intraoperative hemorrhage and permit a posterior vitreous detachment to develop, making surgery technically easier.

Vitreoretinal surgery in the presence of large corneal wounds can be done through a temporary Landers-Foulks keratoprosthesis, to avoid damaging a corneal graft. Primary enucleation or evisceration should only be considered when the globe is completely disorganized. The remaining eye is susceptible to sympathetic ophthalmia whenever penetrating ocular trauma occurs, particularly if there has been damage to the uveal tissues; fortunately, this complication occurs very rarely.

In a prospective study to determine the prognosis of penetrating ocular trauma, it was found that penetrating injuries caused by sharp objects resulted in a better visual outcome than those caused by blunt objects. Visual outcome was better for lacerations less than 10 mm long and in patients with initial visual acuity greater than 20/200. Injuries limited to the anterior segment had a better prognosis than those involving the posterior segment.

INTRAOCULAR FOREIGN BODIES (Fig 20–5)

Foreign bodies that have become lodged within the eye should be identified and localized as soon as possible. Particles of iron or copper must be removed to prevent later disorganization of ocular tissues by degenerative changes (siderosis from iron and chalcosis from copper). Some of the newer alloys are more inert and may be tolerated. Other kinds of particles, such as glass or porcelain, may be tolerated indefinitely and are usually better left alone.

A complaint of discomfort in the eye with blurred vision and a history of striking steel upon steel should arouse a strong suspicion of an intraocular foreign body. The anterior portion of the eye, including the cornea, iris, lens, and sclera, should be inspected with a loupe or slit lamp in an attempt to localize the wound of entry. Direct ophthalmoscopic visualization of an intraocular foreign body may be possible. An orbital soft tissue x-ray must be taken to verify the presence of a radiopaque foreign body as well as for medicolegal reasons.

Various radiologic methods have been used to localize intraocular foreign bodies, including the geometric method of Sweet or the Comberg contact lens (containing a post and ring). Ultrasonography and coronal CT scan of the orbits are the best available methods for precisely locating fragments relative to orbital structures. The Berman metal locator, an electronic instrument, is useful in pinpointing an intraocular foreign body located near one of the accessible areas of the eyeball. The wand of the instrument can be sterilized and passed posteriorly over the exposed field at surgery. The instrument has been particularly useful in locating nonmagnetic foreign bodies.

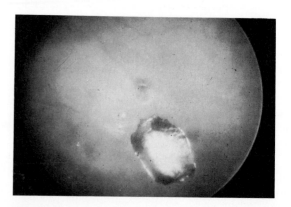

Figure 20–5. Ophthalmoscopic view of intraocular metallic (iron) foreign body in vitreous.

Treatment

If the foreign body is anterior to the lens zonules, it should be removed through an incision into the anterior chamber at the limbus. If it is located behind the lens and anterior to the equator, it should be removed through the area of the pars plana that is nearest to the foreign body because less retinal damage is caused in that manner. If the foreign body is posterior to the equator, it is best removed via the pars plana by vitrectomy and intraocular forceps, thus avoiding major choroidal hemorrhages from incisions of the wall of the eyeball posteriorly. This method is used for both magnetic and nonmagnetic foreign bodies. Special forceps are available for grasping spherical pellets.

Any damaged area of the retina must be treated with diathermy, photocoagulation, or endolaser coagulation to prevent retinal detachment.

HYPHEMA

Contusive forces will frequently tear the iris vessels and damage the anterior chamber angle. Blood in the aqueous may settle out in a visible layer. Acute glaucoma occurs when the filtration meshwork is blocked by fibrin and cells or when clot formation produces pupillary block.

Treatment

Patients with visible hyphemas filling more than 5% of the anterior chamber should be hospitalized for 5 days of bed rest, and patching of the affected eye. If signs of iritis develop, cycloplegic drops are added. The eye is examined daily for secondary bleeding, glaucoma, or corneal blood staining from iron pigment. Glaucoma management includes the use of ocular timolol 0.25% or 0.5% applied twice a day; acetazolamide, 250 mg orally 4 times a day, and hyperosmotic agents (mannitol, glycerol, or sorbitol).

Rebleeding occurs in 16–20% of cases within 2–3 days. This complication carries a high risk of glaucoma and corneal staining. The use of oral aminocaproic acid to stabilize clot formation may reduce the risk of rebleeding. A dose of 100 mg/kg every 4 hours up to a maximum of 30 g/d for 5 days is a good regimen.

The hyphema must be surgically evacuated if the intraocular pressure remains elevated (> 35 mm Hg for 7 days or 50 mm Hg for 5 days) to avoid optic nerve damage or if corneal staining occurs. If the patient has hemoglobinopathy, optic atrophy is likely to develop much more readily and operation should be considered much earlier. Vitrectomy instruments are used to excise the central clot and lavage the anterior chamber. The mechanized probe and irrigation port are introduced anterior to the limbus through clear cornea, to avoid damage to the iris and lens. No attempt is made to extract the clot from the anterior chamber angle or from iris tissue. A peripheral iridectomy is then performed. Another means of clearing

the anterior chamber is by viscoelastic evacuation. A small limbal incision is made to inject the sodium hyaluronate (Amvisc, Healon), and a larger incision 180 degrees away allows the hyphema to be pushed out.

Late-onset glaucoma may follow months to years later as a result of trabecular meshwork damage (angle recession). With rare exceptions, corneal blood staining clears slowly over a period of up to 1 year.

BURNS OF THE EYE

Chemical Burns

All chemical burns must be treated as ophthalmic emergencies. If possible, a tap-water lavage should be started at the site of injury before the patient is transported. In the emergency room, obtain a brief history and perform a brief examination; then begin copious irrigation of the ocular surfaces, including the conjunctival fornices. Sterile isotonic saline (several liters per injured eye) can be conveniently instilled with standard intravenous tubing. A lid speculum and even local anesthetic infiltration of the lids may be necessary to overcome blepharospasm. Give analgesics and topical anesthetic and cycloplegic agents. Use a moist cotton-tipped applicator to remove particulate matter from the fornices. Sometimes a jeweler's forceps is useful for this step. Watch for respiratory distress due to soft tissue swelling of the upper airways. The pH can be checked by placing a strip of indicator paper in the fornix; resume irrigation if it is not between 7.3 and 7.7. After lavage, apply an antibiotic ointment and a pressure dressing.

Alkali rapidly penetrates into deep tissues and will continue to cause damage long after the injury is sustained; therefore, prolonged lavage and repeated pH checks are needed. Acids form a barrier of precipitated tissue that tends to limit further damage. Alkali burns cause an immediate rise in the intraocular pressure owing to contraction of the sclera. A secondary rise occurs 2–4 hours later owing to release of prostaglandin; this increases blood flow to the iris, ciliary processes, and choroid. An intense uvetis develops, which is difficult to monitor through the opaque cornea. Treatment is with topical steroids, antiglaucoma agents, and pupillary dilation during the first 2 weeks. Beyond 2 weeks, steriods are used with caution because they can increase loss of corneal tissue (melting) by the collagenases present in the inflammatory response. A trial with collagenase inhibitors (acetylcysteine) may prove beneficial.

Corneal exposure and persistent epithelial defects are treated with artificial lubricants, tarsorrhaphy, and a bandage contact lens. Long-term complications include angle-closure glaucoma, corneal scarring, symblepharon, entropion, and keratitis sicca. Competency of the conjunctival and scleral vasculature has been shown to be of prognostic value. A greater loss of perilimbal epithelium and increased scleral blanching correspond to a poorer prognosis.

Thermal Burns

Thermal burns of the lids are treated with topical antibiotics and sterile dressings. If corneal damage is sustained, the extensive lid swelling initially makes pressure patching unnecessary. At 2–3 days, ectropion and lid retraction begin. Tarsorrhaphies and moisture chambers fashioned from plastic wrap then protect the cornea. Full-thickness skin grafts are delayed until skin contraction is no longer progressing.

Ultraviolet irradiation, even in moderate doses, often produces a superficial keratitis that is quite painful, although recovery occurs within 12–36 hours without complications. Pain often comes on 6–12 hours after exposure. This type of injury occurs following exposure to an electric welding arc without the protection of a filter. Many "flash burns" are caused by careless exposure in the mistaken belief that the eyes can be burned in this way only when looking directly at the arc. A short circuit in a high-voltage line may cause the same type of injury, as well as exposure to the reflections from snow without protective sunglasses (snow blindness).

In severe cases of "flash burn," instillation of a sterile topical anesthetic may be necessary for examination. A mydriatic (eg, homatropine hydrobromide, 2–5%) should be used. Systemic sedation or narcotics are preferable to topical anesthetics, which interfere with corneal healing. Patching and cold compresses are indicated to relieve discomfort.

Infrared exposure rarely produces an ocular reaction. ("Glassblower's cataract" is rare today but once was common among workers who were required to watch the color changes in molten glass in furnaces without proper filters.) Radiant energy from viewing the sun or an eclipse of the sun without an adequate filter, however, may produce a serious burn of the macula, resulting in permanent impairment of vision. Persons using hallucinogenic drugs such as LSD have been particularly prone to solar macular burns.

Excessive exposure to radiation (x-ray) produces cataractous changes that may not appear for many months after the exposure. The same risk if inherent in exposure to nuclear radiation.

INJURIES INVOLVING THE ORBIT & ITS CONTENTS

Orbital Fractures

Orbital fractures can have concurrent facial trauma, and the appropriate consulting services should be notified. Fractures of the maxilla are classified by the Le Fort system: type I is below the orbital floor; type II passes through the nasal and lacrimal bones in addition to the maxilla forming the medial orbital floor; and type III involves the medial and lateral walls and the orbital floor in the presence of separation of the facial skeleton from the cranium. Orbital roof fractures are rare and are generally caused by penetrating injuries. If visual loss is progressing in the presence of

an optic canal fracture, steroids and surgical decompression may be necessary. When visual loss is sudden and complete, however, recovery is less likely. Carotid-cavernous sinus fistulas are associated with orbital apex fractures, and the orbit should therefore be auscultated for bruits.

Tripod fractures of the zygoma involve the orbital floor but in the absence of dislocation may not need surgical repair. Zygomatic arch fractures do not involve the orbit. Telescoping fractures of the frontal process of the maxilla and the lacrimal and ethmoid bones produce a saddle-nose deformity with telecanthus and lacrimal system obstruction.

When the orbital entrance receives a blow, the compressive forces can fracture the thin medial and inferior walls, with prolapse and entrapment of soft tissues. This force may be transmitted by the soft tissues or directly through the bone without producing an orbital rim fracture. If the blowout is large, enophthalmos of the globe may develop immediately. Alternatively, this may occur at a later time, when the swelling subsides and atrophy or scarring of the soft tissues develops.

Diplopia can be caused by direct neuromuscular damage or swelling of orbital contents. It must be differentiated from entrapment within the fracture of the inferior oblique and rectus muscles or adjacent tissues. This is done by testing forced ductions and noting the presence of pain on attempted upgaze or downgaze. When entrapment is present, passive movement of the eye with forceps is restricted. Sufficient time should pass to allow for spontaneous improvement in eye movements with the resolution of swelling. Sensation is tested in the distribution of the infraorbital nerve. A series of plain x-ray films of the bony orbit should include a Waters view x-ray to show the maxillary sinus (antral) roof. These x-rays may reveal bony defects, an air-fluid level in the sinus, or herniated soft tissues. Only when interpretation of these films is equivocal should CT scan be performed.

The indications for surgical repair of the blowout fracture are (1) persistent diplopia within 30 degrees of the primary position of gaze in the presence of entrapment; (2) enophthalmos of 2 mm or more; or (3) a large fracture (half the orbital floor), which is likely to develop late enophthalmos. Delaying surgery for 1–2 weeks helps the surgeon to assess whether the diplopia will resolve without intervention. Longer delays decrease the likelihood of successful repair of enophthalmos and strabismus.

Surgical repair is usually accomplished via an infraciliary or transconjunctival route, although transantral and infraorbital approaches are also done. The periorbita is incised and elevated to expose the fracture site in the floor and medial walls. Herniated tissue is pulled back into the orbit, and the defect is covered by an alloplastic implant, with care being taken not to damage the infraorbital neurovascular bundle. Complications include blindness, diplopia, extrusion of the implant, or displacement of the implant to press against the lacrimal sac, causing obstruction and dacryocystitis. Other complications include hemorrhage, infection, lower eyelid retraction, and infraorbital anesthesia. Subsequent procedures for strabismus and ptosis may be needed.

Penetrating Injury of the Orbit

Penetrating injuries of the orbital tissue may be produced by flying missiles or sharp instruments. Radiopaque foreign bodies can be localized by x-ray methods similar to those used in locating foreign bodies within the eye. Most orbital foreign bodies are best left alone.

Contusions of the Orbit

Contusion injuries to the orbital contents may result in hemorrhage or subsequent atrophy of the tissue, with enophthalmos. Traumatic paresis of the extraocular muscles occasionally occurs in this way but is usually transient.

Pulsating Exophthalmos Following Orbital Injury

Pulsating exophthalmos occasionally follows a penetrating or contusion injury to the orbital contents that has caused a shunt between the arterial and venous channels, so that the pulse is transmitted into the orbital tissues. (This condition may develop spontaneously but is more frequently traumatic in origin.) A common site of involvement is a fracture through the cavernous sinus.

Pulsating exophthalmos occasionally requires ligation of the carotid artery on the side of the fistula.

PREVENTION OF INJURIES TO THE EYE DURING ATHLETIC ACTIVITY

Persons who engage in athletic activities while wearing prescription lenses made of glass or plastic are at increased risk from shattered lens fragments. The eyewear most effective in preventing injuries consists of polycarbonate lenses in polyamide frames with a posterior retention rim. Solid wraparound frames should be used (rather than hinged frames) because they better withstand lateral blows. Eye guards without lenses do not always prevent a ball from compressing itself between the upper and lower rims and striking the eye. Protection is particularly indicated for those playing racquetball, handball, and squash.

REFERENCES

Bartholomew RS: Viscoelastic evacuation of traumatic hyphaema. *Br J Ophthalmol* 1987;**71**:27.

Batra YK, Bali IM: Corneal abrasions during general anesthesia. *Anesth Analg* 1977;**56**:363.

Bhimani S et al: Computed tomography in penetrating injury to the eye. Am J Ophthalmol 1984;**97**:583.

Bloom SM, Gittinger JW Jr, Kazarian EL: Management of corneal contact thermal burns. *Am J Ophthalmol* 1986; **102**:536.

Bolling JP, Wesley RE: Conservative treatment of orbital roof blow-in fracture. *Ann Ophthalmol* 1987;**19**:75.

Braverman DE, Brown RE Jr; Externalized silicone tube in single canalicular intubation. *Am J Ophthalmol* 1987; **103**:335.

de Juan E Jr et al: Evaluation of vitrectomy in penetrating ocular trauma: A case-control study. *Arch Ophthalmol* 1984;**102**:1160.

Deutsch TS, Feller DB: *Paton and Goldberg's Management of Ocular Injuries,* 2nd ed. Saunders, 1985.

Glynn RJ, Seddon JM, Berlin BM: The incidence of eye injuries in New England adults. *Arch Ophthalmol* 1988;**106**:785.

Goldfarb MS, Hoffman DS, Rosenberg S: Orbital cellulitis and orbital fractures. *Ann Ophthalmol* 1987; **19**:97.·

Green K, Paterson CA, Siddiqui A: Ocular blood flow after experimental alkali burns and prostaglandin administration. *Arch Ophthalmol* 1985;**103**:569.

Grove AS Jr: Computed tomography in the management of orbital trauma. *Ophthalmology* 1982;**89**:433.

Harris GJ, Fuerste FH: Lacrimal intubation in the primary repair of midfacial fractures. *Ophthalmology* 1987;**94**:242.

Hawes MJ, Dortzbach RK: Surgery on orbital floor fractures: Influence of time of repair and fracture size. *Ophthalmology* 1983;**90**:1066.

Kennedy RH, Brubaker RF: Traumatic hyphema in a defined population. *Am J Ophthalmol* 1988;**106**:123.

Koval R et al: The Israeli ocular injuries study: A nationwide collaborative study. *Arch Ophthalmol* 1988;**106**:776.

Kutner B et al: Aminocaproic acid reduces the risk of secondary hemorrhage in patients with traumatic hyphema. *Arch Ophthalmol* 1987;**105**:206.

Mauriello JA Jr, Fiore PM, Kotch M: Dacryocystitis: Late complication of orbital floor fracture repair with implant. *Ophthalmology* 1987;**94**:248.

Mitchell GC et al: A two-year prospective study of penetrating ocular trauma at the Wilmer Ophthalmological Institute. *Ann Ophthalmol* 1987;**19**:104.

Moreira CA Jr, Debert-Ribeiro M, Belfort R Jr: Epidemiological study of eye injuries in Brazilian children. *Arch Ophthalmol* 1988;**106**:781.

Morgan SJ; Chemical burns of the eye: Causes and management. *Br J Ophthalmol* 1987;**71**:854.

Shock JP, Adams D: Long-term visual acuity results after penetrating and perforating ocular injuries. *Am J Ophthalmol* 1985;**100**:714.

Sternberg P Jr et al: Ocular BB injuries. *Ophthalmology* 1984;**91**:1269.

Uusitalo RJ, Ranta-Kemppainen L, Tarkkanen A: Management of traumatic hyphema in children: An analysis of 340 cases. *Arch Ophthalmol* 1988;**106**:1207.

Williams DF et al: Results and prognostic factors in penetrating ocular injuries with retained intraocular foreign bodies. *Ophthalmology* 1988;**95**:911.

21

Optics & Refraction

David L. Guyton, MD

Measurement and correction of refractive errors are essential features of the functional examination of the eye, conferring the benefits of clear optical imagery as well as a measure of best-corrected visual acuity.

A knowledge of basic geometric optics is necessary for understanding refractive errors and their correction. Simplified approximation techniques—such as the use of thin lens optics and the concept of vergence—make ophthalmic optics relatively easy. Trigonometric ray tracing techniques are required for precise optical analysis.

A summary of relevant geometric optics will be followed here by definitions of various types of refractive error and by some discussion of methods for their measurement and correction.

GEOMETRIC OPTICS

Light & Refraction

Light rays appear to bend—or be refracted—when they cross optical interfaces at other than perpendicular incidence. Consideration of the speed of light and its wave properties helps to understand this phenomenon.

A. Speed of Light and Refractive Index: The speed of light in a vacuum is a fundamental constant of nature: approximately 3×10^8 m/s. Light slows down, however, when entering transparent media. The speed of light in a vacuum divided by the speed of light in the medium is called the refractive index (n) of the medium. The refractive index of any medium is always greater than 1, being essentially 1.00 for air; 1.33 for water, aqueous, and vitreous; 1.37 for the cornea; 1.49 for polymethylmethacrylate; and 1.52 for spectacle crown glass.

B. Refraction Illustrated With Wave Fronts: Although for simplification light is thought of as traveling in the form of rays, it actually travels as an electromagnetic wave, with the frequency of vibration determining the color of the light. The frequency of vibration remains constant when light enters a transparent medium, but the speed decreases. Therefore, each wave

front tends to catch up with the one that preceded it, shortening the wavelength of the light inside the medium. When wave fronts of light strike the transparent medium at an angle (Fig 21–1), the wavelength not only decreases but the wave fronts actually change their direction—the phenomenon of refraction.

C. The Laws of Refraction: The first law of refraction states that the incident ray, the refracted ray, and the normal to the surface all lie in the same plane. The second law of refraction (Snell's law) gives mathematical expression to the actual amount of bending that occurs, involving the sines of the angles of incidence and refraction as measured from the normal to the surface. Note in Fig 21–2 that the light ray is bent toward the normal when traveling from a lower to a higher refractive index and away from the normal when traveling from a higher to a lower refractive index.

D. Critical Angle and Total Internal Reflection: A ray of light in air approaching a water or glass surface at *any* angle of incidence will always be partially captured by the surface (a portion is reflected),

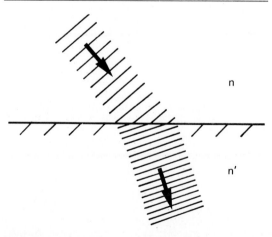

Figure 21–1. Refraction of light as it enters a transparent medium of higher refractive index m'.

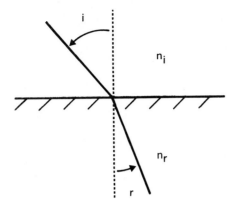

Figure 21–2. Snell's law ($n_i \sin i = n_r \sin r$) describes the exact amount of refraction that occurs.

with the captured (refracted) portion diving into the water or glass in conformity with Snell's law. A ray of light already in the water or glass, on the other hand, can escape from the surface only if its angle of incidence is less than the so-called **critical angle** for the interface (Fig 21–3). As the critical angle is approached, the angle of refraction approaches 90 degrees, with the escaping light ray just grazing across the surface of the water or glass. If the critical angle is exceeded, total internal reflection occurs, with the angle of reflection equaling the angle of incidence.

In the eye, total internal reflection occurring at the tear-air interface prevents a direct view of the angle of the anterior chamber. To allow rays of light from the anterior chamber angle to escape from the eye, the critical angle for the tear-air interface must be increased by applying a plastic or glass goniolens to the tear surface. A second example of total internal reflection in ophthalmology is transmission of light along a fiberoptic tubule, where the angle of incidence is so great that light is multiply reflected along the tubule with very little light loss.

Prisms

A prism exists whenever a transparent piece of material has nonparallel flat surfaces. A prism in cross-section has an apex and a base (Fig 21–4).

A. Net Angle of Deviation: Refraction of light generally occurs at both surfaces of prisms—unless of course the light is perpendicular to one of the surfaces. The deviations occurring at the 2 surfaces may be different—may in fact be in opposite directions—but the net deviation is always toward the base of the prism. The amount of net deviation is not constant but rather is dependent on the angle of incidence of the light (ie, upon the tilt of the prism with respect to the light). The minimum angle of deviation occurs when the light is bent equally at the 2 surfaces. This is the **position of minimum deviation** for the prism. Prisms are calibrated according to defined angles of incidence (Fig 21–4).

B. Prism Diopter (Unit of Prism Power): The power of prisms, in prism diopters ($^\Delta$), is defined as the deviation of a light ray in centimeters, measured 100 cm from the prism (Fig 21–5). Angles can also be measured in prism diopters. Each degree is approximately equal to 2^Δ, but the strict relationship is a trigonometric one, and the approximation only holds for angles less than 45 degrees, or 100^Δ.

C. Displacement of Images by Prisms: As shown in Fig 21–6, if a prism is introduced into the path of light rays converging to form an image, both the light rays and the image are displaced toward the base of the prism (upper diagram). Real images, like real light rays, are displaced toward the bases of prisms. On the other hand, if we look through a prism at an object, the image we see is a virtual image (lower diagram), located by drawing imaginary extensions of the rays of light backward, and this virtual image appears to be displaced toward the apex of the prism. A virtual image formed by a prism, therefore, is displaced toward its apex. Note that the light rays follow exactly the same paths in both cases but travel in opposite directions.

D. Prismatic Effect of Lenses: A lens has no prismatic power at its optical center. Prismatic power is encountered, however, as one moves away from

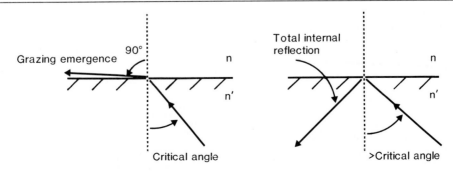

Figure 21–3. The critical angle and total internal reflection.

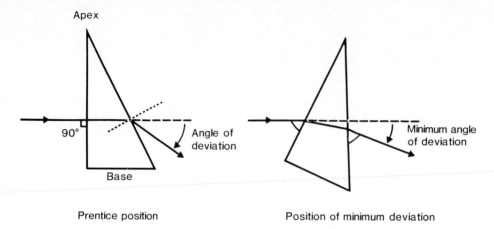

Figure 21–4. Calibration of prisms. Glass prisms and spectacle prisms are calibrated according to the Prentice position, whereas plastic prisms are calibrated according to the position of minimum deviation.

the optical center. According to Prentice's rule, the amount of prism power—in prism diopters—is equal to the number of centimeters of displacement from the center multiplied by the dioptric power of the lens. For example, 1 cm below the optical center of a +3.00 D lens, the prismatic power is equal to 3^Δ base-up. For a −3.00 D lens, the prismatic power at this location would be 3^Δ base-down.

E. Induced Prism in Anisometropia: Different refractive errors in the 2 eyes may be corrected by spectacle lenses, but this requires lenses of different powers. With the eyes looking straight ahead through the optical centers, there is no net prism effect, but in downgaze in the reading position a net vertical prismatic deviation is experienced. The net amount of induced prism can be calculated from Prentice's rule. The patient may be unable to compensate for more than 2^Δ or 3^Δ of net vertical prism and may need to drop the chin for reading, use contact lenses, or have glasses prescribed with a **slab-off prism** to compensate for this problem. (A lens ground with a slab-off prism has prism power only in the reading segment.) If anisometropia develops slowly, however, most patients' oculomotor systems adapt automatically to the induced prism in downgaze, and no optical compensation is required.

F. Fresnel Prisms: Conventional prisms used in spectacle lenses can be bulky, heavy, and cosmetically disfiguring. Light-weight plastic Fresnel prisms are available as Press-On prisms. They consist of side-by-side narrow strips of prisms (Fig 21–7) and are preferable to conventional prisms at least for temporary use. Press-On prisms are available in powers from 0.5^Δ to 30^Δ and are fixed to the back of a spectacle lens by pressing them against the lens under water. Dirt collects in the grooves between the strips of prisms, however, and light scattered from the grooves and from the dirt can decrease visual acuity. For this reason, Fresnel prisms are generally used only for temporary purposes.

G. Chromatic Effect of Prisms: Because the refractive index of transparent materials is slightly different for different wavelengths of light, white light is dispersed into its component colors by prisms. The refractive index for blue light is higher than that for red light, and blue rays are therefore bent more strongly than red rays (Fig 21–8). For a given material, the amount the refractive index varies with wavelength is called the **dispersion** of the material.

H. Chromatic Aberration of Lenses: Lenses also refract blue rays more strongly than red rays, resulting in chromatic aberration (Fig 21–9). The human eye has between 1.5 and 3.0 D of chromatic aberration, depending upon which portion of the visible light spectrum is used for measurement. The eye sees best in yellow light. Side-by-side red and green filters are sometimes used as the red-green (or "duochrome") test to determine the final sphere in clinical

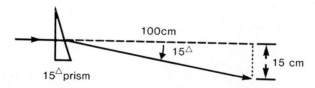

Figure 21–5. Power of a prism in prism diopters.

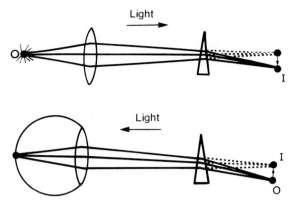

Light →

Light ←

Figure 21–6. Displacement of images by prisms.

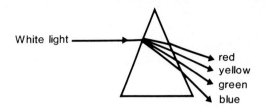

Figure 21–8. Chromatic effect of prisms.

refraction. When the focus of black letters is balanced between the red and green halves of the chart (a chromatic difference of about 0.50 D), yellow light will fall exactly on the retina.

Vergence & Lenses

In secondary school and college physics, lenses were described as having focal lengths and powers, and the lens formula was derived as a function of focal length:

$$1/p + 1/f = 1/q$$

where p was the object distance, f the focal length, and q the image distance. In ophthalmic optics, we gain a better intuitive understanding of the effect of lenses on light by treating the subject in reverse, using the concept of vergence.

A. Vergence: Vergence is a measure of the amount of spreading apart (or coming together) of a bundle of light rays coming from (or heading toward) a *single point*. The direction in which light is traveling must be specified so it will be known whether a bundle

of rays is converging or diverging (Fig 21–10). In ophthalmic optics, we usually speak of light as traveling from left to right, but the direction must in every case be specified and never assumed. Rays of light coming together in the direction of light travel are said to have convergence, or positive vergence, and rays of light spreading apart in the direction of light travel are said to have divergence, or negative vergence. If the rays in a bundle of light are all parallel with each other, the light has zero vergence. If light from every point of a finite-sized object (such as the sun) has zero vergence, the light from the object as a whole is said to be collimated.

B. The Diopter as Unit of Vergence: The vergence of a bundle of light rays is measured in diopters, having the dimensions of reciprocal meters. Vergence in diopters is equal to the reciprocal of the distance in meters to the point where the bundle of light rays would intersect if extended in either direction. Instead of adopting a sign convention according to the direction in which distances are measured, it is easier to assign a plus sign (+) to light that is converging and a minus sign (−) to light that is diverging (Fig 21–11). As the point of crossing is approached, the vergence of the light rays approaches infinity; and infinitely far from the point of crossing, with the light rays appearing parallel, the vergence approaches zero. Note that vergence always changes along the direction of light travel, except that the zero vergence of parallel rays remains constant. Fig 21–12 shows biconvex and biconcave lenses introduced into bundles of light having zero vergence. Both lenses change the vergence of the light, the biconvex lens adding plus vergence and the biconcave lens adding minus vergence. Each lens adds a particular amount of vergence to light no

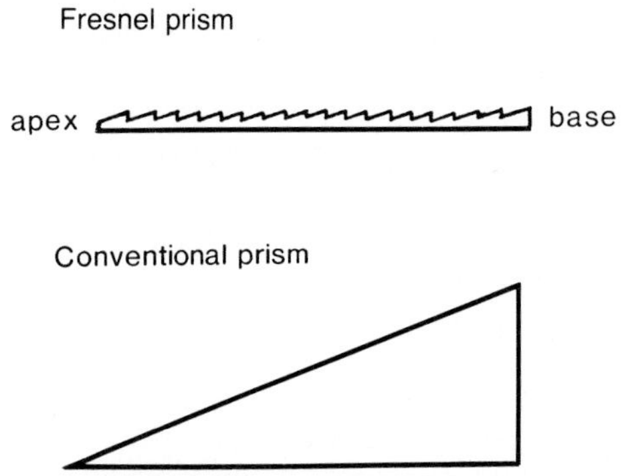

Fresnel prism

apex ⟨⟨⟨⟨⟨⟨⟨⟨⟨⟨⟨ base

Conventional prism

Figure 21–7. The Fresnel prism.

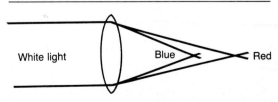

Figure 21–9. Chromatic aberration of lenses. Achromatic lenses may be made by cementing together plus and minus lenses of different refractive index.

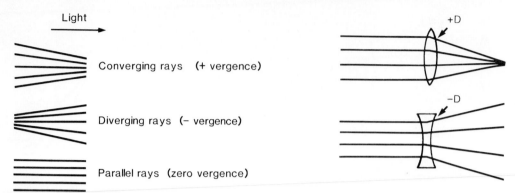

Figure 21–10. Vergence of light.

Figure 21–12. Lens power (D) is equal, in diopters, to the amount of vergence added to the light by the lens.

matter what the vergence to begin with. We therefore can define the **power** of the lens in terms of the amount of vergence it adds to light. Let us express (all in diopters), the vergence of the light entering the lens by U, the power of the lens by D, and the vergence of the light leaving the lens by V. From the definition of the power of the lens, therefore, we have the basic **vergence formula:**

U	+	D	=	V
Vergence of light entering the lens		Amount of vergence added to the light by the lens (power of the lens)		Vergence of light leaving the lens

C. Vergence Calculations: The location of images along the optical axis can easily be found by applying the vergence formula (Fig 21–13). These calculations are always performed in meters, though in ophthalmic optics distances are often specified in centimeters.

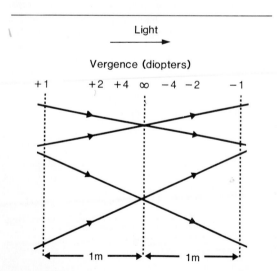

Figure 21–11. Vergence of light as measured in diopters, the reciprocal of the distance in meters to the point of crossing.

D. Multiple Lens Systems: The location of the final image formed by a multiple lens system is determined by calculating the location of the image formed by the first lens; this image becomes the object for the second lens—and so on, for each lens in the system. For this calculation to be correct, the lenses must be taken in order.

E. Real Versus Virtual Objects and Images: A virtual image is sometimes defined as one that cannot be formed on a screen. This definition is inadequate, and a more general definition—one that covers both objects and images—is needed. As illustrated in Fig 21–14, rays incoming to an optical system are designated as object rays. After the optical system has acted upon the incoming light, the outgoing rays are designated as the image rays. The object rays exist only on the incoming side of the optical system, and the image rays exist only on the outgoing side of the system.

The image rays may be converging, parallel, or diverging. If they are converging, they come to a focus on the outgoing side of the optical system and form a **real image.** If they are parallel, they form an image at infinity, defined as neither real nor virtual. If they are diverging, they do not form an image at all but seem to come from a **virtual image** located on the incoming side of the optical system. An image formed on the same side of the optical system as the image rays, therefore, is called a **real image,** whereas an image located by imaginary extensions of the image rays backward to the incoming side of the system is called a **virtual image.**

A similar analysis holds for real and virtual objects. An object on the same side as the object rays is a real object, and diverging rays from the object strike the optical system. If the object rays are converging, however—as often happens within multiple lens systems—the object is virtual and is located by imaginary extensions of the object rays to the outgoing side of the system.

Fig 21–13 provides examples of both real and virtual objects and images. In the upper illustration, both object and image are real. In the lower illustration, both object and image are virtual.

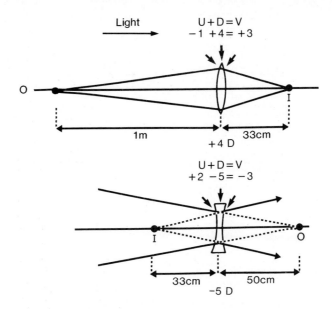

Figure 21–13. Vergence calculations.

F. Conjugate Planes: When an optical system forms an image of an object, the plane of the image is said to be **conjugate** to the plane of the object. If the object is then placed in the image plane and the light is turned around, an image of the object will be formed in the original object plane (Fig 21–15). For any given optical system, there are an infinite number of pairs of conjugate planes.

Direct ophthalmoscopy provides an example of conjugate planes. The patient's retina is conjugate to the examiner's retina. If the direction of light were reversed, the patient would see a clear image of the examiner's retina. The concept of conjugate planes will be particularly important in understanding the optical correction of refractive errors.

G. Object-Image Movement: If an object is moved along the axis of an optical system, the image or images formed of that object always move in the same direction relative to the light path. Alternatively, lenses may be added to move images. Introducing a

plus lens into an optical system causes all images formed downstream from the lens to be pulled **against the light;** and introducing a **minus** lens causes all downstream images to move **in the direction of the light.** For example, a plus lens added to an eye will pull images on the retina into the vitreous (against the light), and a minus lens added to the eye will cause retinal images to move "behind" the retina, in the direction of light travel.

Graphic Analysis of Lens Effects

Exact analysis of the optical effects of lenses requires trigonometric ray tracing techniques. An introduction to such techniques may be found in the chapter on optics and refraction in the eleventh edition of this text, written by Dr Orson White. To simplify our understanding of ophthalmic optics, however, we will

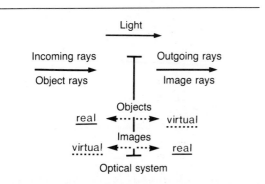

Figure 21–14. Real and virtual objects and images.

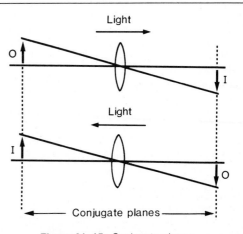

Figure 21–15. Conjugate planes.

Light →

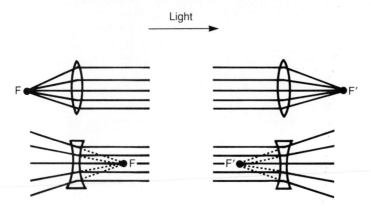

Figure 21–16. The primary and secondary focal points of plus and minus ideal thin lenses.

use algebraic approximations devised by Karl Friedrich Gauss in the early 1800s.

Gaussian optics starts with 2 assumptions: (1) infinitely thin lenses described by their optical centers and 2 focal points, and (2) paraxial light rays (those near the optical axis) forming such small angles with each other and with the optical axis that the sines and tangents of the angles are equal to the angles themselves expressed in radians. Thick lenses, in Gaussian optics, may be approximated by mathematical thin lens equivalents. The vergence formula $U + D = V$ is one of the approximations of Gaussian optics.

A. Focal Points and Focal Lengths: Each ideal thin lens in Gaussian optics has 2 focal points equidistant—if the lens is in air—from the optical center (Fig 21–16). The **primary focal point** is that point along the optical axis where an object must be placed to form an image at infinity. The **secondary focal point** is that point along the optical axis where parallel incident rays are brought to focus. Note that when one is burning leaves with a magnifying glass, the sun's rays are brought to focus—by definition—at the secondary focal point of the lens.

The focal length of the ideal thin lens is the distance from the optical center of the lens to each of the focal points. As can be seen from examination of Figs 25–12 and 25–16 and from the vergence formula, the focal length of a lens in meters is equal to the reciprocal of its power in diopters. For example, a $+5.00$ D lens has a focal length of $\frac{1}{5}$ m, or 20 cm.

B. Ray Tracing: Any number of rays may be traced through an optical system, connecting known pairs of conjugate points, in order to locate images (Fig 21–17). Graphic ray tracing can be an entertaining exercise, but for practical purposes only one ray—the central ray–needs to be drawn. This is because the axial location of the image can first be found with the vergence formula, and the size and orientation of the image can then be determined simply by tracing the central ray.

C. The Central Ray: The central ray passes undeviated from the tip of the object through the center of the lens, extending to infinity in both directions

(Fig 21–18). Because the central ray is one of the light rays from the tip of the object, the tip of the image *must* be on the central ray as well. Therefore, the tip of the image is located precisely by the intersection of the central ray with the image plane as located by the vergence formula.

Note in Fig 21–18 that if the image is on the side of the lens opposite to the object, it must be inverted; and if it is on the same side, it must be erect with respect to the object. Note further that the central ray forms similar triangles extending from the lens to the object and to the image. It is easily seen that the transverse magnification produced—ie, the image height divided by the object height (I/O)—is equal to the image distance divided by the object distance (v/u).

To trace images through multiple lens systems, the vergence formula is applied to each lens in succession—along with the central ray for each lens in succession—until the final image is located and its size and orientation are determined.

D. Thick Lenses: A thick lens may be treated in Gaussian optics as if the optical center had been split into 2 **nodal points** (n and n') (Fig 21–19). The thick

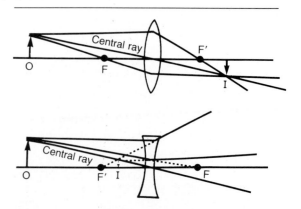

Figure 21–17. Ray tracing through plus and minus lenses.

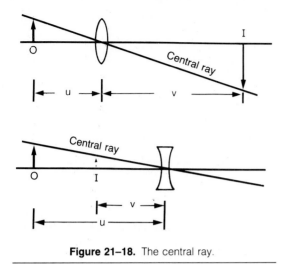

Figure 21–18. The central ray.

lens is further described by 2 **principal planes** (H and H'), which pass through the nodal points if the refractive media on both sides of the lens are the same. Light rays incident on the first principal plane are treated as if they jump over to the second principal plane where all of the refraction occurs (Fig 21–19). The central ray for the thick lens passes from the tip of the object to the first nodal point, then emerges from the second nodal point parallel to the original direction. The true focal lengths are measured from the principal planes to the focal points (F and F'), but the front and back focal lengths are measured from the front and back surfaces of the lens to the appropriate focal points. The back vertex power as measured with a lensmeter corresponds to the reciprocal of the back focal length. In ophthalmic optics, this theory of thick lenses is used to understand the optics of the human eye.

Magnification

Various types of magnification are used in ophthalmic optics, the most common being transverse (the same as linear or lateral) and angular.

A. Transverse (Linear, Lateral) Magnifica-

tion: Transverse magnification—the height of the image divided by the height of the object (I/O)— is easily determined using similar triangles formed by the central ray, as in Fig 21–18. Transverse magnification is thus equal to image distance divided by object distance (v/u).

B. Angular Magnification: Objects or images at infinity must be either infinitely small or infinitely large. Transverse magnification is meaningless in both cases. An infinitely large image or object can have a finite angular size, however, so angular magnification can be used whenever an image or object is at infinity. Angular magnification is equal to the angle subtended by the image divided by the angle subtended by the object.

When only the image *or* the object is at infinity, a fixed reference point must be chosen for determination of angular magnification. For example, when a single plus lens is used as a simple magnifier, the object is placed in the focal plane of the lens, and the image viewed through the lens is seen at infinity. The reference distance for viewing the object without the lens was chosen long ago, arbitrarily, as 25 cm, so that the angular magnification of a simple magnifier is defined as the angle subtended by the image at infinity divided by the angle subtended by the object when held 25 cm from the eye. Mathematically, it turns out that this defined magnification of the simple magnifier is equal to the dioptric power of the plus lens divided by 4.

Direct ophthalmoscopy may be thought of as use of the optical system of the patient's eye as a simple magnifier to view the patient's retina. With the average power of a patient's emmetropic eye being + 60 diopters, the defined angular magnification of direct ophthalmoscopy is therefore 60/4, or 15X.

The magnification of telescopes, which are customarily used to view objects at infinity, is specified in terms of angular magnification. Telescopes are important in ophthalmic optics because the ordinary spectacle lens, in combination with the error lens of the eye, forms either a Galilean telescope or a reverse Galilean telescope. Because the magnification of telescopes is approximately equal to the power of the

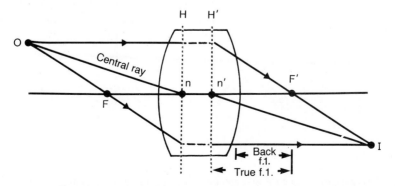

Figure 21–19. Description of a thick lens in Gaussian optics.

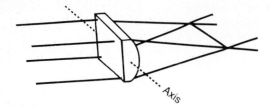

Figure 21–20. A planocylindric lens with axis in the horizontal meridian.

eyepiece divided by the power of the objective, it can be determined that the magnifying power of a spectacle lens, in combination with the error lens of the eye, is approximately 2% magnification per diopter of spectacle lens power. Plus spectacle lenses form ordinary Galilean telescopes and provide magnification, while minus spectacle lenses form reverse Galilean telescopes and cause minification.

Astigmatic Lenses

Lenses with spherical surfaces form point images. Astigmatic lenses, whose surfaces are curved differently in different meridians, do not form point images. Astigmatism is common in the human eye.

A. Cylindric Lenses: The simplest form of astigmatic lens is a planocylinder (Fig 21–20). This lens has one flat surface and one cylindric surface, as if cut from the side of a cylinder of glass. The **axis** of the planocylindric lens is parallel to the axis of the hypothetical cylinder of glass from which the lens was cut. There is no optical power acting in the meridian of the axis (the horizontal meridian in Fig 21–20). The planocylindric lens has maximum power acting in the meridian 90 degrees away from the axis meridian (the vertical meridian in Fig 21–20).

Every astigmatic lens has 2 principal meridians 90 degrees apart: the meridians of greatest and least refractive power. In the case of a planocylindric lens, the 2 principal meridians are the axis meridian and the meridian 90 degrees away from the axis. Vergence calculations may be performed in each principal meridian for an astigmatic lens. For example, the power acting in the vertical meridian of the planocylindric lens in Fig 21–20 converges the light into a horizontal

focal line. No vergence is added to the light in the horizontal meridian.

Because astigmatic lenses are not radially symmetric about the optical axis, the orientation of the principal meridians of the lens must be specified. The orientation of cylindric lenses is specified by the meridian of the axis according to the diagram in Fig 21–21. By convention, 180 degrees is used for the horizontal meridian.

B. Spherocylindric Lenses: A spherocylindric lens in general is specified by the orientation of the 2 principal meridians (always 90 degrees apart) and the power acting in each. A cross diagram is often used for such specification, as illustrated in Fig 21–22. The arms of the cross diagram are drawn parallel to the principal meridians of the spherocylindric lens. Each principal meridian is labeled with the power acting in that meridian.

The spherocylindric lens is more commonly thought of as the combination of a sphere and a cylinder—either a plus cylinder or a minus cylinder—as illustrated in Fig 21–22. The sum of the powers acting in each principal meridian of the combined lenses must equal the power acting in the respective principal meridian of the original spherocylindric lens. Note that in the longhand notation for the spherocylindric lens, the cylinder is specified by its axis, 90 degrees away from the meridian of maximum power.

The longhand notation is used for writing prescriptions for spherocylindric lenses. Transposition back and forth between the minus cylinder form of the prescription and the plus cylinder form is accomplished by the following 3 steps: (1) The transposed sphere is equal to the algebraic sum of the original sphere and cylinder; (2) the transposed cylinder is the same power as the original cylinder, but with opposite sign; and (3) the transposed axis is changed from the original axis by 90 degrees. This transportation works properly in both directions, as can be confirmed by simple transposition between the 2 longhand notations given in Fig 21–22.

Spherocylindric lenses can be easily combined mathematically if their principal meridians are aligned. If the principal meridians are not aligned, complicated trigonometric formulas are necessary—or the resultant combination can be determined simply by holding the lenses together and reading the value

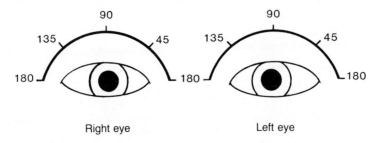

Right eye   Left eye

Figure 21–21. Convention for specifying the orientation of cylinder axes.

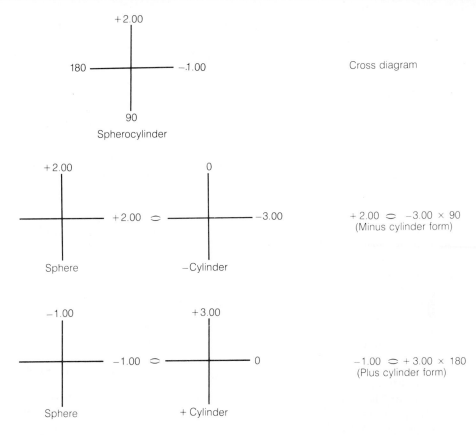

Figure 21–22. Cross diagram and equivalent combinations, including longhand notations, for a spherocylindric lens.

for the combination with a lensmeter. The principal meridians of the combination will always be 90 degrees apart.

C. Conoid of Sturm: The geometric figure formed by the light rays refracted by an astigmatic lens is called the conoid of Sturm, as illustrated in Fig 21–23. In this illustration, the horizontal meridian is the more powerful one, forming the vertical focal line close to the lens; and the vertical meridian is the less powerful one, forming the horizontal focal line farther from the lens. The interval between the 2 focal lines is called the **interval of Sturm.** The 2 focal lines need not be on the same side of the astigmatic lens, since one or both may be virtual focal lines on the incoming side of the lens.

Cross sections of the conoid of Sturm are also shown in Fig 21–23. The cross sections at the focal lines are simply lines, but elsewhere the cross sections are generally ellipses. One of the cross sections between the focal lines is a circle, called the **circle of least confusion.** If the circle of least confusion of an astigmatic eye falls on the retina, images are equally blurred in all directions—hence the term "least confusion." Much of clinical refraction theory is based upon the supposition that best trial-and-error focus with a spherical lens will place the circle of least confusion of the conoid of Sturm on the retina.

Aberrations of Spherical Lenses

Real lenses affect light in a more complicated manner than ideal thin lenses. In addition to chromatic aberration of lenses, which has already been mentioned, there are a number of monochromatic aberrations. For example, spherical lenses refract peripheral rays more strongly than rays near the center (paraxial rays), bringing the peripheral rays to a focus closer to the lens (Fig 21–24). This is called spherical aberration. Spherical aberration produces a characteristic comet-shaped blur called **coma** when the object and image are off the optical axis of the lens system.

Spherical lenses often produce curved images of flat objects. This aberration, called **curvature of field,** is actually helpful in the eye, for the curved image matches fairly closely the curve of the retina.

When a spherical lens is tilted, the lens gains a small astigmatic effect, forming a small conoid of Sturm for each object point. This aberration is called **astigmatism of oblique incidence.** Simply looking in different directions through a spectacle lens yields astigmatism of oblique incidence, but this is minimized by wrapping the lens around the eye in the form of a meniscus lens, with careful selection of the front and back curves by the lens manufacturer. When this

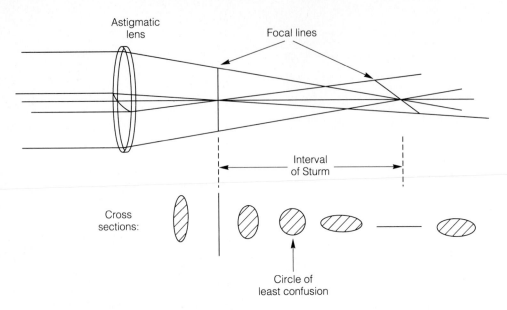

Figure 21–23. The conoid of Sturm, formed by light refracted by an astigmatic lens.

optimization is performed, the lenses are said to have **corrected curves.**

Mirrors

Plane mirrors simply change the direction of light by reflection. Curved mirrors not only change the direction of light but also add vergence in much the same way as lenses. Many of the same optical techniques used with lenses can also be used with mirrors, taking into account the change in the direction of light.

A. Laws of Reflection: There are 2 laws of reflection: The first law states that the incident ray, the normal to the surface, and the reflected ray all lie in the same plane. The second law states that the angle of reflection is equal to the angle of incidence (Fig 21–25).

B. Size of Plane Mirror Required for a Full-Length View: As can be seen in Fig 21–26, one only needs a half-length mirror for a full-length view of oneself, no matter how far the mirror is from the observer. Similarly, holding a plane hand mirror farther from one's face does not increase the amount of face that is seen; the image seen simply becomes smaller, because it moves twice as far away as the mirror.

Light & Vergence Within Refractive Media

The vergence formula, $U + D = V$, is valid only for ideal thin lenses surrounded by air. When the refractive media are *different* on the 2 sides of the lens, the more general lens formula must be applied to each surface separately:

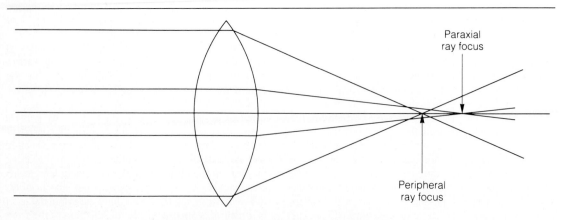

Figure 21–24. Spherical aberration of a biconvex lens.

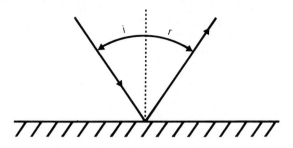

Figure 21–25. Reflection of a light ray.

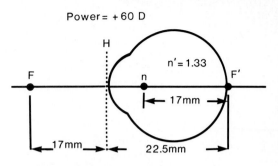

Figure 21–27. The reduced schematic eye.

$$n/u + (n' - n)/r = n'/v$$

where r is the radius of curvature of the surface in meters. Note that when n and n' are equal to 1.00 for air, n/u and n'/v become the U and V of the familiar vergence formula.

THE EYE & ITS OPTICAL CORRECTION

The Optical System of the Eye

The eye's optical system consists of the cornea, the pupil, the crystalline lens, and the fluids surrounding them. For calculation purposes involving images formed on the retina, we often use an approximation for the eye called the **reduced schematic eye.** To further simplify the correction of refractive errors, we speak of the **far point** of the eye rather than having to consider the effect of each of the optical surfaces.

A. Schematic Eye: Gullstrand first determined the average dimensions and optical constants of the human eye. His schematic eye is simplified still further in the reduced schematic eye (Fig 21–27). In the reduced schematic eye, all of the refraction is assumed to occur at the cornea. There is a single principal plane (H) at the cornea and a single nodal point (n) at the center of curvature of the cornea. The eye is filled with fluid of refractive index 1.33, and the nodal point is 17 mm from the retina. The 2 focal lengths (from H to F and from H to F') are different because of the fluid on the posterior side. The equivalent power of the reduced schematic eye is +60 D.

B. Refractive Errors: The refractive state of the eye is often illustrated by parallel rays of light from a point object at infinity coming to focus at or near the retina (Fig 21–28). If this secondary focal point of the eye is on the retina, the eye is said to be **emmetropic;** if it is in front of the retina, the eye is **myopic;** and if the rays of light are intercepted by the retina before coming to focus, the eye is **hyperopic.**

Myopia can occur if the optical system of the eye is too strong (refractive myopia) or if the globe is too long (axial myopia). High myopia is usually of the axial type. Similarly, hyperopia can occur if the refractive power of the eye is too weak (refractive hyperopia, of which aphakia is the extreme example) or if the globe is too short (axial hyperopia, occasionally occurring in congenital disorders of the eye). For axial ametropia, each millimeter of abnormal ocular length causes approximately 3 diopters of refractive error.

In an astigmatic eye, parallel rays of light from infinity come to focus in 2 focal lines rather than in a single focal point. The location of these focal lines with respect to the retina determines the type of astigmatism (Fig 21–29). For example, in simple myopic astigmatism, one focal line is in front of the retina (in the vitreous) and the other is on the retina. Astigmatism is also classified on the basis of orientation of the refractive power (Fig 21–30). An eye that is most powerful in the vertical meridian is said to have **astigmatism with the rule.** It is somewhat more common in young people and is corrected by a plus cylinder with axis within 20 degrees of vertical or a minus

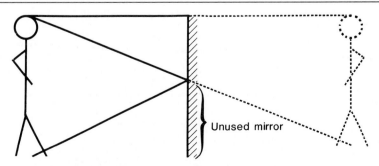

Figure 21–26. The image seen in a plane mirror.

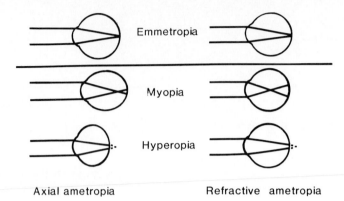

Axial ametropia   Refractive ametropia

Figure 21–28. Spherical refractive errors as determined by the position of the secondary focal point with respect to the retina.

cylinder with axis within 20 degrees of horizontal.

An eye that has its greatest power in the horizontal meridian is said to have **astigmatism against the rule.** This type of astigmatism is more common in older people and is corrected by a plus cylinder with axis within 20 degrees of horizontal or a minus cylinder with axis within 20 degrees of vertical. If the principal meridians of the astigmatism are not within 20 degrees of horizontal and vertical, the astigmatism is termed **oblique.** Oblique astigmatism is further termed **symmetric,** if the correcting cylinder axes are symmetric about the nose, or **asymmetric** if they are not.

In **regular astigmatism,** the power and orientation of the principal meridians are constant across the pupillary aperture. If either the power or the orientation of the principal meridians changes across the pupil, the refraction is irregular—often termed **irregular astigmatism.**

C. Development of Refractive Error: There are both genetic and environmental determinants of refractive error. The relative importance of heredity versus environment is still debated. The average eye is approximately 2 diopters hyperopic at birth by cy-

cloplegic refraction; hyperopia may increase until age 7, but the refractive error then usually begins to change in the direction of myopia. The drift toward myopia is most rapid between ages 7 and 15 but often continues more slowly into the 20s and 30s.

D. Binocular Imbalance (Anisometropia): A difference in refractive errors of the 2 eyes is termed anisometropia. In childhood, differences in spherical refractive error can lead to anisometropic amblyopia, since the 2 eyes always accommodate the same amount, leaving the more hyperopic eye chronically blurred.

Refractive correction of anisometropia often leads to different image sizes on the 2 retinas **(aniseikonia),** with each diopter of spectacle refractive correction changing the image size by approximately 2%. The actual difference between the image sizes in the 2 eyes depends upon whether the refractive error is axial or refractive, however, and the amount of aniseikonia is difficult to determine without special subjective tests. Aniseikonia may be symptomatic simply from the difference in retinal image sizes—or, more commonly, the anisometropic spectacle correction causes

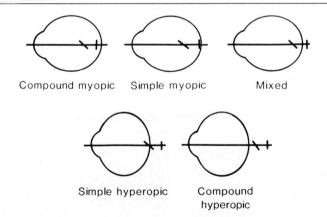

Compound myopic   Simple myopic   Mixed

Simple hyperopic   Compound hyperopic

Figure 21–29. Types of astigmatism, as determined by the positions of the 2 focal lines with respect to the retina.

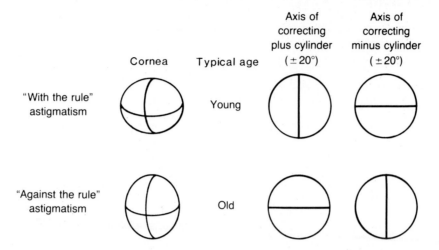

	Cornea	Typical age	Axis of correcting plus cylinder (±20°)	Axis of correcting minus cylinder (±20°)

"With the rule" astigmatism   Young

"Against the rule" astigmatism   Old

Figure 21–30. Types of astigmatism as determined by the orientation of the principal meridians and the orientation of the correcting cylinder axis.

anisophoria or anisotropia in different directions of gaze because of the different prismatic effect induced by the 2 lenses.

Monocular aphakia is an extreme example of anisometropia. Spectacle correction of monocular aphakia produces a difference in image size of approximately 25%. The resulting aniseikonia can be reduced to 6% or 7% if contact lens correction is used instead of spectacle correction, and this lesser amount of image size difference is tolerated by many patients.

E. Far Points and Far Lines: To understand the optical correction of refractive errors, it is helpful to consider the far point of spherical eyes and the far lines of astigmatic eyes. The far point is, by definition, the point on the visual axis of an eye conjugate to the retina when accommodation is completely relaxed. The far point may be located by tracing rays of light out of the eye, beginning from a single point on the retina. The far point of an emmetropic eye is thus at infinity; the far point of a myopic eye is between the eye and infinity; the far point of a hyperopic eye is ''beyond'' infinity, behaving as a virtual far point behind the eye (Fig 21–31). In an astigmatic eye, light

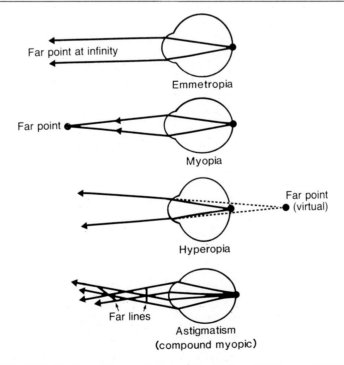

Far point at infinity

Emmetropia

Far point

Myopia

Far point (virtual)

Hyperopia

Far lines

Astigmatism
(compound myopic)

Figure 21–31. Far points and far lines in the various refractive conditions.

from a point on the retina is imaged into a conoid of Sturm, creating 2 far lines instead of a single far point. Each far line is associated with its respective principal meridian, the principal meridian at right angles to the far line.

Because of the principle of conjugacy, a lens that forms an image of infinity at the far point of the patient's eye will provide the exact refractive correction for the eye.

F. Accommodation: Contraction of the ciliary muscle produces increased convexity of the crystalline lens, particularly of the front surface, by mechanisms not completely understood. According to the Helmholtz theory of accommodation, contraction of the ciliary muscle loosens the zonules, and the elasticity of the capsule of the crystalline lens molds the lens into a more spherical shape. Recent investigations, however, suggest that an increase in pressure in the vitreous cavity also plays a role in this molding process.

Traditionally, accommodation has been thought to occur entirely by parasympathetic stimulation of the ciliary muscle, but recent work suggests that the antagonistic role of sympathetic innervation is also important. It has been shown that in the absence of a stimulus for accommodation, the eye does not relax toward the traditional far point but rather relaxes toward a **resting focus** approximately 1 diopter inside the far point (varying with different individuals). From this resting focus position, activation of the sympathetic system drives the eye's point of focus toward the traditional far point, while activation of the parasympathetic system causes increased accommodation. Cycloplegic drugs paralyze the parasympathetic system, allowing the resting sympathetic tone to drive the point of focus to the traditional far point.

The total number of diopters an eye can accommodate, measured from the traditional far point, is called the **amplitude of accommodation,** taking the eye's point of focus from the far point to the near point. The extent of clear vision of an eye, generally stated as being from the far point to the near point (for example, "from 2 m to 50 cm"), is called the **range of accommodation.** The range of accommodation cannot extend beyond infinity, though we often speak of the far point of the hyperope's eye as being "beyond" infinity as a virtual far point behind the eye. The far point, near point, and range of accommodation of hyperopic and myopic eyes are illustrated in Fig 21–32.

Correction of Refractive Errors With Lenses

Refractive errors may be corrected with spectacle lenses, contact lenses, or intraocular lenses. In the measurement of the refractive correction, lenses are often thought of as moving the point of focus inside the eye to the retina. To understand the actual optical correction of the eye, however, it is convenient to use the far point concept.

Because the far point of a myopic or hyperopic eye is conjugate to the retina of that eye, placing an object—or imaging an object—at the far point will cause a clear image of that object to be relayed to the retina. We can thus use a plus or minus lens—as necessary—to form an image of infinity at the far point, correcting the eye for distance. As illustrated in Fig 21–33, the position for the correcting lens is chosen, and the necessary secondary focal length for the lens is then measured by the distance from the position of the lens to the far point of the eye. A minus spectacle lens is thus used for correction of myopia, with its secondary focal point between the correcting lens and infinity; and a plus spectacle lens is used for the correction of hyperopia, with its secondary focal point behind the eye.

For correction of astigmatism, a lens is chosen with principal meridians having the appropriate powers to form an astigmatic image of infinity at the far lines of the astigmatic eye. The secondary focal length of each of the principal meridians is equal to the distance from the astigmatic lens to the respective far line.

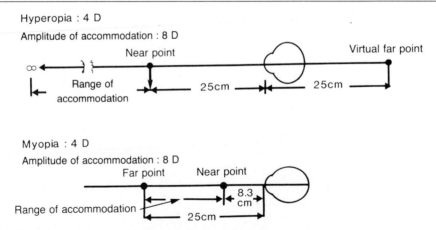

Figure 21–32. Range of accommodation, with far point and near point, in a 4-diopter hyperopic eye **(top)** and a 4-diopter myopic eye **(bottom),** each with an amplitude of accommodation of 8 diopters.

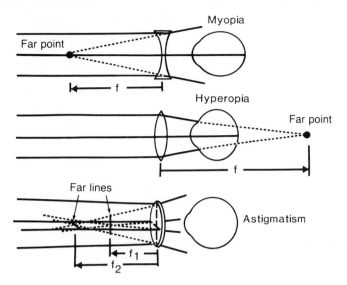

Figure 21–33. The far point concept of refractive correction.

Types of Optical Correction

Spectacle lenses or contact lenses are used to correct most refractive errors except that intraocular lenses have become the favored method to correct aphakia. In addition, various corneal surgical procedures are being developed to permanently change the refractive state of the eye—most of them intended for correction of high refractive errors (see Chapter 6).

A. Spectacle Lenses: Spectacle lenses are manufactured in meniscus form, with the front surface having plus power and the back surface having minus power. The spectacle lens is tilted forward (the **pantoscopic tilt**), as a compromise between distance and near vision, for the purpose of minimizing astigmatism of oblique incidence.

Most bifocal segments are manufactured on the front surface of spectacle lenses, either molded as part of the lens, ground onto the surface, or placed in the form of a fused bifocal segment consisting of a segment of high-index glass embedded in the surface of the spectacle lens. With most bifocal segments manufactured on the front surface, the cylinder, if called for in the prescription, is placed on the back surface (the **minus cylinder form** of spectacle lens). The intermediate reading add in trifocal glasses is customarily half the dioptric power of the full reading add.

Progressive power lenses have progressively increasing plus power incorporated into the lens as the patient looks downward. These lenses have a fairly small zone of clear reading vision, however, with blurred, distorted vision through the right and left lower quadrants of the lens. Progressive power lenses have no image jump and are cosmetically more acceptable than bifocal glasses for some patients.

B. Contact Lenses: The first contact lenses were made of glass, were supported by the sclera, and could be worn for only short periods of time. Lightweight, plastic corneal contact lenses appeared in the late 1940s and rapidly became widely accepted. The original hard contact lenses, made of polymethylmethacrylate, impervious to oxygen and water, are now less commonly dispensed, because gas-permeable rigid contact lenses and soft contact lenses are preferable for the long-term health and stability of the cornea. Gas-permeable rigid contact lenses are made of cellulose acetate butyrate, silicone, or various polymers of silicone with other plastics. They are usually 7.5–9 mm in diameter and move several millimeters with each blink. (This movement is necessary to supply various nutrients in the tears to the corneal epithelium.) Rigid contact lenses, like hard lenses, correct corneal astigmatism by means of the tears, which fill the space between the back surface of the contact lens and the cornea. Rigid lenses and hard contact lenses must be removed during sleep.

Soft contact lenses are made of various hydrogel plastics, contain 40–60% water, and must be kept wet. They are quite pliable, mold themselves to the cornea, and offer little correction for corneal astigmatism unless they are specially designed with toric (astigmatic) surfaces and weighted to keep them from rotating. Soft contact lenses are much larger than hard or rigid lenses, being 13–15 mm in diameter and extending 1 or 2 mm beyond the limbus. Because soft lenses are permeable to water as well as to gases, very little movement of the lenses with blinking is necessary for adequate nourishment of the corneal epithelium. More care is necessary for soft lenses than for hard or rigid lenses, since disinfection after each day's wear requires heat or chemical solutions.

Several types of very thin soft contact lenses are marketed as extended-wear lenses, designed to be worn for a month at a time. Protein deposits develop on these lenses, however, and cleaning sometimes becomes necessary more often than once a month. Disposable contact lenses are now becoming available.

Most contact lenses are fitted for cosmetic purposes, but they are sometimes necessary for athletic activities and for working in steamy or rainy atmospheres. Ophthalmic indications include irregular corneal astigmatism (which can be neutralized by hard or rigid lenses or smoothed out somewhat by soft lenses), bullous keratopathy and recurrent corneal epithelial erosion (soft lenses act as a bandage to minimize or prevent corneal epithelial erosion), and high anisometropic refractive errors such as unilateral aphakia (to equalize retinal image sizes).

Contact lenses are fitted by first measuring the corneal curvature with a keratometer and then choosing the appropriate posterior curve (called the base curve) for the lens. Hard and rigid contact lenses are fitted slightly steeper (more curved) than the corneal principal meridian with the lower keratometer reading. This creates—even with a spherical cornea—a low-power spherical tear lens that prevents the contact lens from riding on and abrading the corneal apex. In addition, with astigmatic corneas, a meniscus tear lens having the shape and power of a minus cylinder fills in the space between the contact lens and the steeper corneal principal meridian, neutralizing the corneal astigmatism.

The desired power of the contact lens is usually determined by refracting over a trial contact lens and adding the overrefraction value to the power of the trial lens. If trial contact lenses are not available, however, the necessary specifications for contact lenses can still be determined—but in this case the powers of the anticipated tear lenses must be taken into account in calculating the final power of contact lens to order.

Soft contact lenses are fitted—according to the manufacturer's charts—by choosing the appropriate base curve for the patient's keratometer readings (''K-readings''). The power of the soft contact lens is generally based upon the spherical equivalent of the patient's refraction. The refraction must of course be calculated for the corneal plane rather than for the spectacle plane, with the difference being significant whenever the refractive correction is greater than 4 or 5 diopters.

Occasionally a hard contact lens placed on an eye with no astigmatism will ''uncover'' astigmatism. This **residual astigmatism** represents lenticular astigmatism that was uncovered when the contact lens neutralized an equal but opposite amount of corneal astigmatism. Such eyes are best corrected with soft contact lenses that will not neutralize the corneal astigmatism significantly.

Several types of bifocal contact lenses are available, the most common type having a central zone for distance vision and a peripheral zone for near vision. When the patient is attending to one distance, rays of light coming through the pupil from the other distance are so far out of focus that they can be ignored—although they do decrease the contrast of the retinal image. Some patients are happy with bifocal contact lenses, but usually only for lower amounts of reading add.

C. Intraocular Lenses: Replacement of the cataractous crystalline lens with an implanted plastic intraocular lens was first performed in 1949. Because its position is close to that of the original crystalline lens, the intraocular lens gives the best available optical correction for aphakia, avoiding the significant magnification and distortion caused by aphakic spectacle lenses. Numerous complications developed from the first intraocular lenses, and it was not until the 1970s that intraocular lens implantation became relatively safe and predictable. Today, well over 90% of cataract extractions are done as a combined procedure with intraocular lens implantation.

Intraocular lenses are made from polymethylmethacrylate, with or without additives that filter out ultraviolet light less than 400 nm in wavelength. The lenses are usually planoconvex, with the convex surface placed anteriorly. Their power is approximately + 60 diopters in air, corresponding to about + 18 to + 20 diopters in aqueous. Today's lenses are supported by plastic loops, or haptics, extending into the angle of the anterior chamber, into the ciliary sulcus behind the iris, or into the capsular bag after extracapsular cataract surgery. Many of the earlier intraocular lenses were supported by the iris, but iris erosion occurred, sometimes with persistent uveitis, and these lenses are now rarely used. If the posterior capsule is at least partially present and the zonules are intact, posterior chamber lenses are generally preferred for implantation today; if not, posterior chamber lenses can be sewn into place or anterior chamber lenses can be implanted. Improper fit of an anterior chamber lens, however, can cause chronic uveitis, glaucoma, and corneal decompensation.

The necessary power for an intraocular lens is calculated using either theoretic or empiric formulas with data supplied by A-scan ultrasonography for the axial length of the eye and by keratometry for the K-readings. The empiric formulas are based on large numbers of results of actual cases and—of the various formulas available—are currently the most widely used. The first empiric formula was the SRK (Sanders-Retzlaff-Kraff) formula:

$$\text{IOL power} = A - 2.5\,L - 0.9\,K$$

where A is a constant peculiar to the particular style and brand of intraocular lens, L is the axial length of the eye in millimeters, and K is the average keratometer reading in diopters.

Special purpose calculators are available to perform these calculations and are often built into A-scan ultrasound equipment. Either an 0.1-mm error in axial length or an 0.25-diopter error in keratometry results in a refraction miscalculation of approximately 0.25 diopter.

METHODS OF CLINICAL REFRACTION

Refractive correction for the eye may be measured by both objective and subjective methods. Although a rough refractive correction for the eye may be determined by the setting on the direct ophthalmoscope necessary to see the retina clearly, the objective method of retinoscopy is far more accurate. Subjective methods of refraction—those requiring the patient's responses to arrive at the final correction—include older techniques using astigmatic dial charts and the cross cylinder testing techniques widely used today.

Retinoscopy

The hand-held streak retinoscope projects a blurred streak of light toward the patient's eye. As the examiner looks through the retinoscope and sweeps the band of light (called the intercept) across the patient's pupil, a red, streak-shaped retinoscopic reflex appears in the pupil (Fig 21–34).

A. Appearance of the Retinoscopic Reflex: The reflex remains parallel to the intercept if the eye has only a spherical error or if the intercept is parallel to one of the principal meridians of the eye's astigmatism. Astigmatism causes misalignment of the reflex with the intercept; and by rotating the intercept from one meridian to the next until the reflex becomes parallel to the intercept, the principal meridians of the astigmatism can be located.

B. Neutralization of Reflex Movement: As the intercept is swept across the patient's pupil, the retinoscopic reflex will move either in the same direction as the intercept (**with movement**), will move in the opposite direction (**against movement**), or will fill the whole pupil and not move at all (**neutralization**). The type of movement depends upon the location of the patient's far point with respect to the retinoscope (Fig 21–35). If the patient's far point is behind the retinoscope, "with" movement is seen, and plus lenses are added before the patient's eye to neutralize the "with" movement. If "against" movement is seen, the far point is between the patient's eye and the retinoscope, and minus lenses are added before the patient's eye. When the far point has been moved to the position of the retinoscope by adding plus or minus lenses, movement of the reflex disappears, with the pupil simply becoming filled with light as the intercept sweeps across it.

C. Compensation for the Working Distance: Once neutralization of the retinoscopic reflex has been achieved, the patient's far point is at the **working distance** of the retinoscopist, usually about $\frac{2}{3}$ m. The spherical correction is then changed approximately 1.50 D in the minus direction to move the patient's far point to the visual acuity chart on the far wall.

D. Automated Retinoscopes: Automated refracting instruments, some of them based on the principle of retinoscopy, have been available since 1974. These instruments use infrared light and determine an objective refraction in a matter of seconds. Alignment of the instrument with the patient's eye is usually critical, however, and young patients accommodate more with the automated instruments than with standard retinoscopy. Although good results can be obtained in normal eyes with automated refractors, these instruments are often unreliable with small pupils, early cataracts, and irregular refractive errors.

Subjective Refraction

Although retinoscopy can often be performed accurately to within 0.50 D, subjective refraction, relying on the patient's responses to different lens choices, is regarded as the standard of accuracy against which other methods must be compared. Reliable responses to subjective techniques can usually be obtained by age 8 providing the patient's ocular media are clear enough—and visual acuity good enough—for the patient to respond to the lens choices.

A. Astigmatic Dials: The first subjective methods for detection and measurement of astigmatism used radiating patterns of black lines on white backgrounds. By adding plus power to fog the patient and then decreasing the plus power slowly until one of the radiating lines came into focus, the principal meridians of the eye's astigmatism could be located. By adding minus cylinder in the appropriate orientation, all the lines could then be made clear, neutralizing the astigmatism. Astigmatic dial methods of refraction

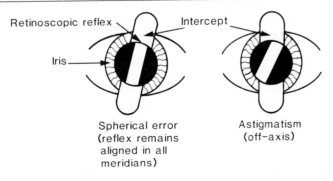

Retinoscopic reflex · Intercept

Iris

Spherical error
(reflex remains
aligned in all
meridians)

Astigmatism
(off-axis)

Figure 21–34. The retinoscopic reflex.

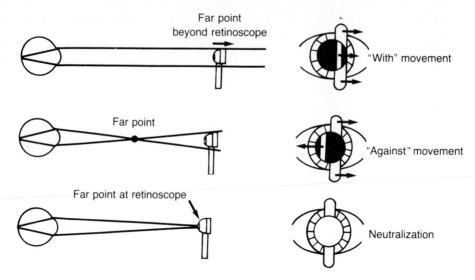

Figure 21–35. Movement of the retinoscopic reflex.

are somewhat cumbersome and can be confusing to some patients; they have generally been superseded by cross cylinder techniques.

B. Cross Cylinder Techniques: The cross cylinder is an astigmatic lens having plus cylinder power in one principal meridian and an equal amount of minus cylinder power in the other. After it is positioned before the eye, the cross cylinder can be abruptly flipped about a meridian 45 degrees away from the principal meridians, thus interchanging the 2 principal meridians. The patient compares visual acuity between the 2 flip choices and responds to the familiar question, "Which is better, 1 or 2?" Although the cross cylinder can be used to detect the presence of astigmatism, it is usually used to refine a previous correction or retinoscopic finding. For example, in Fig 21–36, the cross cylinder is used for the refinement of cylinder power correction. The end point of cross cylinder testing is equal blur with the 2 flip positions, indicating that without the cross cylinder in position the light should be perfectly focused on the retina.

As shown in Fig 21–36, cylinder power is refined with the cross cylinder's principal meridians aligned with the principal meridians of the correcting lens. Cylinder axis, on the other hand, is refined by the same 2-choice procedure, but in this case the principal meridians of the cross cylinder are aligned 45 degrees away from the correcting cylinder axis.

C. Final Refinement of the Sphere: For either the initial adjustment of sphere or the final refinement, the spherical portion of the correction is always changed first in the plus direction. This pulls the image of the visual acuity chart into the vitreous, thus fogging the patient and tending to relax accommodation. Once it is confirmed that the patient's vision blurs with this increased plus sphere, the plus sphere is slowly decreased until best vision is obtained.

D. Reading Adds: With the onset of presbyopia in the mid 40s, plus power must be added to the distance refractive correction to allow comfortable reading vision. The patient's amplitude of accommodation may be measured and analytic methods used to calculate the necessary reading add to leave half the patient's accommodative amplitude in reserve. The usual method for determining reading adds, however, is to estimate the required amount to add from the patient's age and confirm the effect in trial frames.

A reading add of +1.25 D is usually prescribed by age 42–45, progressing to +2.50 D by age 55–60. The reading add can be in the form of a bifocal segment, a progressive power lens, or separate full-frame or half-frame reading glasses. If the patient with bifocal segments is annoyed by blurred imagery at intermediate distances, trifocals can be prescribed, with the intermediate add usually being equal to half the power of the full reading add.

Cycloplegia

The purpose of clinical refraction is to determine the distance refractive correction with the eye's accommodation completely relaxed. The refraction thus determined moves the patient's far point to infinity, allowing complete utilization of the amplitude of accommodation for near vision. Relaxation of accommodation during refraction can usually be achieved in adults simply by the technique of fogging, adding plus power to pull the image of the visual acuity chart into the vitreous. When the patient is fogged, attempts at accommodation simply blur the image more; therefore, the patient's accommodation tends to relax.

Accommodation in children can usually not be fully relaxed by fogging techniques, and pharmacologic paralysis of the ciliary muscle (cycloplegia) is used. A short-acting cycloplegic agent—cyclopentolate

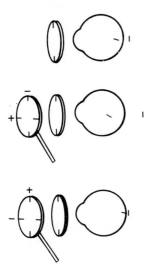

Figure 21–36. Cross cylinder refinement of an astigmatic correction. The residual astigmatism in this eye *(top)* is increased by the first flip position of the cross cylinder *(middle)* and decreased by the second flip position of the cross cylinder *(bottom)*. The second flip position will thus be preferred. Plus cylinder will be added with axis 90, or minus cylinder with axis 180, as called for by the preferred position of the cross cylinder *(bottom),* and the procedure will be repeated, along with repeated refinement of spherical power, until perfect balance between the 2 flip positions of the cross cylinder is achieved.

1%—is commonly used in children, with refraction 30 minutes after administration of the drops. Children with very dark irises, however, may still show accommodation after cyclopentolate, and atropine 0.5% or 1% may be necessary twice a day for 2 or 3 days to achieve full cycloplegia. If atropine toxicity in young children occurs, manifested by fever, flushed face, and rapid pulse, the drops should be discontinued. Sponge baths can be used if necessary to cool the patient, and if toxicity is severe—manifested by delirium—physostigmine can be used to reverse the atropine effect.

Prescribing the Refractive Correction

Much of the art of refraction is in determining the best prescription for the patient based on the old correction, the present refractive findings, and the patient's symptoms and needs.

A. Prescribing for Myopia: Traditionally, the full minus correction has been prescribed for myopia, but the possible implication of prolonged accommodation as a cause of progression of myopia has led some practitioners to undercorrect myopia to the level of 20/25–20/30 binocular visual acuity (about 1.00–1.50 D undercorrected). Atropine and bifocals are sometimes prescribed for patients with rapidly progressing myopia, but the effectiveness of this treatment in slowing or preventing further development of myopia is not universally accepted.

B. Prescribing for Hyperopia: Correction for hyperopia is usually not given unless (1) accommodative esotropia is present that is decreased or eliminated by the hyperopic correction; (2) visual acuity is not developing properly from deficient accommodation in cases of high bilateral hyperopia; or (3) the patient is symptomatic from the sustained accommodation necessary to overcome the hyperopia. For accommodative esotropia or bilateral high hyperopia, full hyperopic correction is usually given, but only partial correction is given in the case of symptoms from accommodative effort, ie, enough correction to relieve symptoms.

C. Prescribing for Astigmatism: Astigmatism in children should usually be corrected if it is more than 1.50 D or if delay of visual acuity development can be demonstrated. If astigmatic correction is given to children, the full cylinder at the correct axis should always be prescribed, since children adapt easily to the optical distortion produced. Adults may not adapt to this distortion, however, and may not tolerate the full astigmatic correction. A walking-around trial with trial frames is helpful in determining whether an adult will tolerate the new prescription long enough to adapt to it. If the patient cannot tolerate the new correction, the cylinder power may have to be arbitrarily reduced or the cylinder axis rotated toward 90 degrees, toward 180 degrees, or toward the previous cylinder axis to lessen the apparent distortion.

REFERENCES

American Academy of Ophthalmology: *Optics, Refraction, and Contact Lenses, 1989.* [Published by the Academy and updated every 3 years.]

Bennett AG, Rabbetts RB: *Clinical Visual Optics.* Butterworths, 1985.

Corboy JM: *The Retinoscopy Book: A Manual for Beginners.* Slack, 1984.

Michaels DD: *Visual Optics and Refraction: A Clinical Approach,* 3rd ed. Mosby, 1985.

Rubin ML: *Optics for Clinicians,* 2nd ed. Triad, 1974.

Southall JPC: *Mirrors, Prisms and Lenses,* 3rd ed. Dover, 1964.

White OW: Optics and refraction. In: *General Ophthalmology,* 11th ed. Vaughan D, Asbury T. Lange, 1986.

Preventive Ophthalmology

Paul Riordan-Eva, FRCS, MA, MB, BChir

The 1980s might be called the decade of preventive medicine. General medicine and all of the specialties have participated in this movement, and ophthalmology has been no exception. Prevention of ocular injuries in industry, in the schools, and in the home has had a long and successful history, but much remains to be done in the fields of infection, genetic disorders, iatrogenic disease, and other special areas.

Much of the responsibility for prevention of nontraumatic ocular disease rests with the pediatrician, the general practitioner, and the internist, but the ophthalmologist has a major role as disseminator of necessary information. Meanwhile, the nonophthalmologist practitioner must be aware of the eye problems that can be treated before visual loss has occurred if detected at an early stage.

Important problems fitting into this category are glaucoma, strabismus, and the complications of such systemic diseases as diabetes, tuberculosis, sarcoidosis, syphilis, and leprosy. It is indeed a tragedy to find hitherto undetected advanced ocular disease in a patient who has been receiving regular medical treatment for another illness. It is hoped that this chapter will give medical students, pediatricians, and general physicians—as well as young ophthalmology residents-in-training—a survey of preventive ophthalmology and that it will alert them to the huge opportunities available to them in sight conservation.

PREVENTION OF THE SEVERE CONSEQUENCES OF UNDIAGNOSED GLAUCOMA

About 1–2% of all people over age 35 have glaucoma. In the USA alone it is estimated that there are at least 300,000 people with undetected glaucoma. About 90% of them have chronic open-angle glaucoma, which does not cause symptoms in the early stages but can ultimately lead to blindness. Patients often do not seek treatment until late in the disease, because there is no pain and the visual acuity (central vision) remains good even when the peripheral fields constrict.

The best way to detect glaucoma is to examine tonometrically all people over 20 every 3 years (or every year if there is a family history of glaucoma). The next most important diagnostic steps are the visual field examination and the ophthalmoscopic examination for pathologic cupping of the optic disk. The visual field examination is normally done on the tangent screen; confrontation field testing in which the examiner's fingers are used as a target will pick up only gross visual field defects.

Tonometry and ophthalmoscopy should be part of every physical examination in the age group over 20. Unfortunately, the overdiagnosis of glaucoma is also a problem. It is also unfortunate that once a patient has been placed on miotics or other antiglaucomatous drugs, it is very difficult to establish the diagnosis of "nondisease."

PREVENTION OF AMBYLOPIA ("Lazy Eye")

Amblyopia can be defined for the purposes of this discussion as diminished visual acuity in one eye in the absence of organic eye disease. Central vision develops from birth to age 6 or 7; if vision has not developed by then, there is little or no chance that it will develop later. In the absence of eye disease, the 2 main abnormalities that will prevent a child from acquiring binocular vision are strabismus and anisometropia.

Strabismus

Esotropia or exotropia in a young child causes double vision. The child quickly learns to suppress the image in the deviating eye and learns to see normally with one eye. Unfortunately, vision does not develop in the unused eye; unless the good eye is patched, sight will never develop in that eye. The child will grow up with one perfectly normal eye that is essentially blind, since it has never developed a functional connection with the visual centers of the brain. This is more likely to occur with esotropia than with exotropia.

Anisometropia

Young children are more concerned with perception of near objects than with those at a distance. If one eye is nearsighted (myopic) and the other farsighted (hyperopic), the child will favor the nearsighted eye. Thus, the farsighted eye will not be used even though it is straight. The result will be the same as in untreated strabismus, ie, monocular blindness due to failure of visual development in an unused eye. The incidence of anisometropia is about 0.75–1%.

Early Diagnosis

The best way to prevent amblyopia is to test the visual acuity of all preschool children. By the time a child reaches school, it is usually too late for occlusion therapy. The parents can perform the test at home with the illiterate "E" chart. This is sometimes known as the "Home Eye Test." Pediatricians and others responsible for the care of small children should test visual acuity no later than age 4.

Photorefraction is said to be useful in screening for anisometropia, ametropia, astigmatism, and strabismus in preschool children. Any child observed to have strabismus after the age of 3 months should be seen by an ophthalmologist.

PREVENTION OF OCULAR INFECTION

In view of its exposure to the environment, the intact eye is remarkably resistant to infection; but once the epithelium of the cornea is breached, microorganisms find susceptible tissues, and even such opportunistic pathogens as *Pseudomonas aeruginosa* may proliferate. Protection of the corneal epithelium thus becomes all-important in the prevention of ocular infection. There are a few bacteria, particularly *Neisseria gonorrhoeae* and *Neisseria meningitidis,* that can proliferate on an intact epithelium, and it is of historical interest that Credé silver nitrate prophylaxis, introduced in 1881, has been responsible for saving thousands of eyes from total visual loss. Even viral infection such as herpes simplex virus infection (a cause of much ocular disability) is in large part dependent on corneal epithelial damage. It is safe to say that the majority of ocular infections, whether bacterial, fungal, chlamydial, or viral in origin, are preventable.

Ophthalmia neonatorum, especially inclusion blennorrhea, is still a problem despite the worldwide use of silver nitrate and other antimicrobial agents at birth. But recent research suggests that the antibiotic erythromycin, instilled in the eye of the newborn, may be effective in controlling not only gonococcal infection but chlamydial infection (inclusion blennorrhea) as well. Systemic erythromycin treatment of pregnant women with cervical chlamydial infections is also effective in reducing the incidence of neonatal chlamydial infections. In view of the high prevalence of gonococcal genital infection in this country and elsewhere, topical prophylaxis cannot be abandoned, but many state laws concerned with it are currently undergoing revision.

Corneal infections in general, particulary hypopyon ulcer, are a major cause of visual loss. It is therefore of first importance to realize that they are in large part preventable. Once the epithelial barrier is breached, the cornea is subject to infection with many pathogens, especially the pneumococcus, and with many opportunistic bacteria and fungi, especially *P aeruginosa, Candida* species, and *Fusarium* species.

The prevention of damage to the corneal epithelium is indisputably the key to the prevention of corneal infection. Fortunately, although direct trauma often occurs, minor abrasions heal so rapidly that infection can only follow a massive inoculation of bacteria or fungi. Such massive inoculations can come from (1) contaminated solutions, (2) dacryocystitis, (3) severe staphylococcal blepharitis, (4) a contaminated contact lens, etc, and all of these can be prevented or treated satisfactorily as called for.

Microbial contamination of contact lenses may occur because of inadequate cleaning and disinfection or contamination of carrying cases. Contact lens solutions—particularly saline made with tablets and other preservative-free solutions—are also commonly contaminated. Contact lenses may cause epithelial damage by abrasion or oxygen deprivation. Extended-wear contact lenses are more commonly associated with corneal infections than daily-wear lenses. All contact lens wearers should be cautioned to report for examination at the first sign of inflammation. Pain, a helpful warning sign, may be absent, since partial corneal anesthesia develops characteristically in contact lens wearers.

Accidental epithelial injury incurred while participating in various sports is also common, and severe epithelial damage may be caused by (1) exposure during coma; (2) ultraviolet light while welding or skiing; or (3) desiccation associated with exophthalmos, facial nerve paralysis, or ectropion of the lower lid, eg, after a severe burn. Many of these damaged eyes have been lost as a result of infection when simple methods of protection have been omitted.

Temporary protection pending definitive therapy can be achieved by patching, tarsorrhaphy, or frequent instillations of ointment or artificial tears; exceptionally, the brief applications of soft contact lenses can be effective.

Intraocular infection is a common sequela to **penetrating injuries** to the eye, particularly those involving a retained foreign body. Prevention of such injuries requires use of protective lenses on a regular basis, not only in industry but also in daily activities. Every individual should be encouraged to have a pair of protective lenses on hand for use around the house to prevent injuries caused by corks from champagne and other bottles, fireworks, power mowers, power drills and other machines, and hazardous chemicals such as those used for opening drains or fertilizing crops (eg, liquids containing ammonia).

Prevention of intraocular infection after **cataract extraction** or other intraocular surgery deserves much attention, since such infections are almost always avoidable. They should in fact never occur in a modern hospital, where committees on infections have the responsibility for preventing them. Fortunately, eye surgery requires such a brief stay in the hospital that colonization of an eye with so-called hospital bacteria is rare indeed.

Most intraocular infections come from (1) contaminated solutions; (2) chronic conjunctival or lid margin infections or chronic dacryocystitis; (3) rarely, aerosols from the noses and throats of surgeons and their assistants; and (4) prolonged surgery. All of these complications can be prevented or minimized. At the time of surgery, the susceptible tissues are exposed for only a short time, and the surgical wound seals rapidly. The eye's local defense mechanisms seem to be able to handle small numbers of microorganisms without difficulty unless compromised by topical corticosteroids or other immunosuppressive drugs.

Since most intraocular surgery is elective, the surgeon has time to assess the patient's immunologic status and to correct any immunodepression due to malnutrition, alcoholism, narcotic addiction, stress, etc. There is also time to make sure that the external eye is not compromised by blepharoconjunctivitis, overt or intermittent dacryocystitis and stenosis, or tear deficiency. Most of these conditions are correctable—or can at least be ameliorated—before surgery.

The bacterial flora of the lids and conjunctiva should be assessed prior to elective intraocular surgery, although not necessarily by means of preoperative cultures. If clinical examination shows normal lid margins and conjunctivas and if there is no history of exudate or gumming of the lids on waking, further examination is unnecessary. But if the external eye is *not* normal, the bacterial flora should be studied for potential pathogens, particularly gram-negative opportunistic pathogens such as *P aeruginosa* and *Proteus* species.

Elimination of such potential pathogens by suitable treatment is mandatory. Antibiotics or antibiotic mixtures used preoperatively cannot be relied upon, and the prolonged use of such agents before surgery tends to inhibit the growth of the normally harmless gram-positive flora. This unfortunately encourages the colonization of both gram-negative bacteria and fungi. There is no substitute for a careful preoperative clinical examination combined with a careful history of previous infection, particularly of intermittent dacryocystitis during the common cold.

If emergency intraocular surgery must be performed in the presence of external eye disease, careful irrigation of the conjunctiva to remove exudate and bacteria-containing mucous threads is indicated. If there is dacryocystitis to deal with, the punct. can be temporarily sealed by cautery.

PREVENTION OF IATROGENIC OCULAR INFECTION

Ophthalmologists have been clearly implicated in the transmission of infectious eye disease. Outbreaks of **epidemic keratoconjunctivitis** have been traced to contamination in the ophthalmologist's office. The adenovirus is transmitted via the ophthalmologist's hands, a tonometer, or solutions contaminated by droppers accidentally rubbed against the infected conjunctiva or lid margin of a patient. Contaminated ophthalmic solutions have also been the source of infection in bacterial corneal ulcers and endophthalmitis following intraocular surgery. *Pseudomonas aeruginosa* used to be a common contaminant of ophthalmic solutions, particularly fluorescein. Instillation of contaminated fluorescein solution to delineate corneal epithelial defects (eg, after removal of a corneal foreign body) may result in severe pseudomonal keratitis and, frequently, loss of the eye.

Other infections can be similarly spread, but their occurrence is not generally recognized. The ophthalmologist should be alert to the possibility that if ophthalmic instruments are improperly sterilized (as by cold sterilization), they may be contaminated with hepatitis B virus. Recent identification of the AIDS virus in tears has suggested a small possibility of transmission by ophthalmologists (see p 62). To date, no such incident has occurred.

Ophthalmologists and their staffs must maintain the highest level of personal hygiene at all times and must use standard sterile technique when appropriate, keeping in mind the possibility of contamination of any solution brought into contact with the eye.

Hands play a major role in the transmission of infection. They should be washed or disinfected (eg, with isopropyl alcohol) before and after the examination of every patient, regardless of whether an ocular infection is thought to be present. Applanation tonometer heads should be wiped clean with a sterile solution after each use and should be thoroughly disinfected at least twice a day and after use on an infected eye. Schiotz tonometers require frequent disinfection because they may harbor organisms within the barrel of the plunger.

Intraocular procedures and injuries to the eye interfere with many of the natural barriers to infection, rendering the eye particularly susceptible. Any surgical ophthalmic procedure or treatment of an injured eye must be performed with strict sterile technique.

Use of contaminated eye solutions should be avoided at all costs. Sterility of solutions is the responsibility of physicians, pharmacists, and pharmaceutical companies, as well as of nurses and even patients.

Single-use disposable vials containing sterile ophthalmic solutions are an absolute requirement in ophthalmic surgery and in treating an injured eye; all operating and emergency rooms should be equipped accordingly. Single-use vials are also the preferred means of administering topical agents to patients in the ophthalmologist's office. The use of multiple-dose containers should be limited to the intact eye. These containers should never be used for other patients after use on an infected eye. The sterility of any ophthalmic solution should be confirmed prior to use. At the time of surgery, the type of solution, its correct formulation, and its sterility should be verified by the surgeon and at least one other person. A useful safeguard is to filter all solutions to be used in intraocular surgery through a membrane (Millipore-type) filter.

PREVENTION OF RADIATION INJURY

Ultraviolet irradiation may cause superficial epithelial keratitis accompanied by pain, redness, and photophobia. The symptoms appear 6–12 hours after exposure to ultraviolet light, eg, while skiing or using an electric welding device. Prevention consists of avoidance of exposure or the wearing of appropriate protective sunglasses or goggles. Chronic exposure to ultraviolet light is suggested but not proved to be a major factor in development of cataract and age-related macular degeneration. The use of ultraviolet filters in spectacle lenses, sunglasses, and intraocular lenses has been advocated for prevention of these disorders.

Solar retinitis (eclipse retinopathy) is a specific type of radiation injury that usually occurs after solar eclipses as a result of direct observation of the sun without an adequate filter. Under normal circumstances, sun-gazing is difficult because of the glare, but cases have been reported in young people who have suffered self-inflicted macular damage by deliberate sun-gazing, perhaps while under the influence of drugs.

The optical system of the eye behaves as a strong magnifying lens, focusing the light onto a small spot on the macula, usually in one eye only, and producing a thermal burn. The resulting edema of the retinal tissue may clear with minimal loss of function, or it may cause significant atrophy of the tissue and produce a defect that is visible ophthalmoscopically as a macular hole. In the latter event, a permanent central scotoma results.

Eclipse retinopathy can easily be prevented by the use of adequate filters when observing eclipses, but the surest way to prevent it is to watch the eclipse on television.

Similar to eclipse retinopathy is the iatrogenic retinal damage that may occur from use of the operating microscope and indirect ophthalmoscope. The risk of damage from the operating microscope can be reduced by the use of filters to block both ultraviolet light and the blue portion of the visible spectrum, light barriers such as an opaque disk placed on the cornea, or air injected into the anterior chamber.

Workers with improperly screened nuclear materials face an increasingly important problem because of the frequent formation of cataracts.

Pterygium is an occupational disease of farmers, sheepherders, and others who live largely outdoors. It is presumably due to exposure (ultraviolet light, desiccation by wind, etc) and can be prevented by wearing protective lenses. This applies also to **basal cell carcinoma** and probably also to **melanoma** of the lids and lid margins. In patients with xeroderma pigmentosum, the eyelids and bulbar conjunctiva frequently develop carcinomas and melanomas, and their development can be minimized, if not prevented entirely, by protective lenses.

PREVENTION OF EXPOSURE KERATITIS

Patients in coma or under prolonged anesthesia who have lid retraction (eg, exophthalmos) or facial nerve paralysis may develop exposure keratitis. This condition can be prevented by patching the eyes, suturing the lids together (tarsorrhaphy), instilling artificial tears, or applying a soft contact lens.

PREVENTION OF XEROPHTHALMIA

Even in the USA, where it should now be all but unknown, occasional cases of xerophthalmia still occur, and in the underdeveloped areas the world over, where nutrition is often poor, it is still common. Vitamin A deficiency disease, in which the eye changes (xerophthalmia and keratomalacia) are the most damaging and often cause blindness (see Chapter 24), is usually the result of a deficient diet associated with poverty. It should be borne in mind, however, that it may also be associated with chronic alcoholism, weight-reducing diets, dietary management of food allergy, or poor absorption from the gastrointestinal tract due to the use of mineral oil or gastrointestinal disease such as chronic diarrhea.

In vitamin A-deficient children, measles may result in severe corneal disease. Because of the eye signs (ie, night blindness, Bitot's spots, or a lackluster corneal epithelium), the ophthalmologist may be the first to recognize vitamin A deficiency. Early recognition and treatment can prevent loss of vision or blindness due to secondary infection and corneal perforation. Treatment of the acute condition may require large intramuscular doses of vitamin A followed by corrective diet and careful analysis of all possible causes.

PREVENTION OF VISUAL LOSS DUE TO DRUGS

All drugs can cause adverse reactions. It is the ophthalmologist's responsibility to prevent visual loss or major ocular disability from drugs used to treat eye diseases.

Ophthalmic drugs should be packaged and labeled so that mistakes are not made by elderly or poorly sighted patients. Atropine and other strong medications may call for color-labeling. On the first visit to a new ophthalmologist, the patient should be asked to bring along any previously prescribed medications in order to avoid duplication and possible overdosage.

Certain ophthalmic drugs have such frequently occurring and damaging side effects that their use requires special monitoring and special warnings to the patient. Atropine and scopolamine, used to dilate the pupil in iridocyclitis, may precipitate acute glaucoma in certain patients with narrow anterior chamber angles. After prolonged use, they can also lead to conjunctivitis and allergic eczema of the eyelids. Many antiglaucoma drugs can produce stenosis of the puncta and shrinkage of the conjunctiva.

Corticosteroids used locally in drop or ointment forms may depress the local defense mechanisms and precipitate corneal ulceration, often fungal. They may also worsen herpetic keratitis and other corneal infections, and on prolonged use may lead to open-angle glaucoma and to posterior polar cataract. Much of the severity of both herpes simplex virus and varicella-zoster virus corneal infections can be blamed on the unwise use of topical corticosteroids. In this situation, short-term improvement has been traded for long-term disaster. Fungal endophthalmitis after cataract surgery is usually the result of the unnecessary use of corticosteroids at the time of the operation and is therefore preventable.

Many drugs used **systematically** have serious ocular side effects, eg, keratopathy, retrobulbar neuritis, retinopathy, and Stevens-Johnson syndrome (erythema multiforme). For this reason, the ophthalmologist must take a careful history of the patient's use of drugs as part of the initial examination. Of special interest are the keratopathy and retinopathy that often follow the use of chloroquine in discoid lupus erythematosus. It is the function of the consulting ophthalmologist to detect any early ocular changes and to inform the dermatologist of them so that he can substitute another medication.

PREVENTION OF GENETIC DISEASES

Until recently, the prevention of genetic disorders received little attention. Now, however, there are genetic counseling centers in many medical centers, and the genetic nature of many disorders that affect the eye is recognized and their transmission better understood than formerly. In conference with internists and pediatricians, it is up to the ophthalmologist to recommend genetic counseling for patients contemplating marriage and children. Patients with histories of childhood diabetes, retinitis pigmentosa, consanguineous mating, retinoblastoma, neurofibromatosis, etc, need genetic counseling to prevent disaster for their offspring.

Some clinical conditions, eg, Down's syndrome (trisomy 21), are associated with an abnormal number of chromosomes or with abnormalities of the sex chromosomes. Prenatal diagnosis can now be made by testing amniotic fluid cells obtained by amniocentesis (a safe and practical procedure), and a positive diagnosis gives the patient the option of abortion.

PREVENTION OF CONGENITAL INFECTIONS

Viral disease of the mother with resultant embryopathy may lead to such ocular anomalies in the offspring as retinopathy, infantile glaucoma, cataract, uveal tract coloboma, etc, and prevention may in some cases be possible. Two viruses, rubella and cytomegalovirus, can be extremely damaging to the infant, and one of them—rubella virus—can be prevented by vaccinations. Once a common childhood disease, rubella led to lifelong immunity, but vaccination is now indicated for susceptible young women approaching childbearing age. Susceptibility can be determined by assessing the antibody content of the young woman's blood. If a mother contracts rubella during early pregnancy, she should be informed of the likelihood of ocular and other abnormalities in her baby, and the arguments for and against abortion should be presented.

Unfortunately, cytomegalovirus (the other virus causing a high incidence of congenital anomalies) continues to be a serious and unsolved threat. No protective vaccine is currently available, though one is currently under study.

Toxoplasmosis is another important cause of congenital infection, leading to (1) chorioretinitis, which may be apparent at birth or may remain subclinical until reactivation occurs later in life; (2) cerebral or cerebellar calcification; (3) hydrocephalus; and occasionally (4) more severe central nervous system abnormalities. Unless the mother is immunocompromised, fetal infection occurs only if she acquires primary infection during pregnancy. This can be prevented by eating only meat that is well cooked, by washing vegetables and fruits, and by wearing gloves when disposing of cat litter or working in the garden so that contact with viable oocysts and tissue cysts is avoided. It has been shown that if acute maternal infection during pregnancy can be identified—such as with the serial serologic tests that are required by law in France and Austria—appropriate antibiotic treatment in those pregnancies allowed to proceed, with adjustments according to whether fetal infection is also present, reduces the incidence of congenital infection and improves the clinical outcome in fetuses that are infected.

PREVENTION OF HERPES SIMPLEX & HERPES ZOSTER

Some progress has been made in the prevention of herpetic disease. The epidemiology of herpes simplex virus type 1 is such that protection of highly susceptible young children (under 5 years of age) from salivary exposure to relatives with labial herpes could conceivably prevent many cases of primary infection, labial or ocular. As for the recurrent disease, many cases can be prevented by modifying the trigger mechanisms—stress, fever, overexposure to sunlight, trauma, etc. Fever, the most frequent trigger, can be reduced by aspirin used at the onset of coryza or other upper respiratory infection, and stress can be minimized by office psychotherapy and, if necessary, by a tranquilizer. The patient with recurrent ocular herpes can be taught to recognize his own trigger mechanisms and to modify them.

The incidence of primary infection of the newborn with herpesvirus type 2 is increasing as genital herpes becomes more common in the United States. A change in the sexual mores of the population would reverse this trend. If maternal herpetic lesions are recognized at the onset of labor, cesarean delivery will prevent exposure of the neonate to the herpesvirus. However, most neonatal infections occur in infants born to mothers with asymptomatic primary or recurrent infections. Identification of such cases would require routine viral cultures in all mothers at the time of delivery—a prohibitively expensive procedure.

Zoster ophthalmicus can be prevented by any means effective in preventing childhood varicella. There is as yet no effective vaccine, but varicella-zoster (VZ) immune globulin is available for immunosuppressed children (eg, with leukemia) who have been exposed to VZ virus. Recurrent infection (zoster) is known to have occurred only in patients immunosuppressed by Hodgkin's disease and other tumors, surgical shock, immunosuppressive drugs (eg, corticosteroids), extreme fatigue, advanced age, etc. Some of these trigger mechanisms, such as stress, may be preventable. Ways of measuring and reducing the immunosuppression of old age—the principal trigger for ophthalmic zoster—are currently under study.

REFERENCES

Baum J, Boruchoff SA: Extended-wear contact lenses and pseudomonal corneal ulcers. (Editorial.) *Am J Ophthalmol* 1986;**101**:372.

Claoué C: Experimental contamination of Minims of fluorescein by *Pseudomonas aeruginosa. Br J Ophthalmol* 1986;**70**:507.

Daffos F et al: Prenatal management of 746 pregnancies at risk for congenital toxoplasmosis. *N Engl J Med* 1988;**318**:271.

Donzis PB et al: Microbial contamination of contact lens care systems. *Am J Ophthalmol* 1987;**104**:325.

Friedlander MH (editor): *Prevention of Eye Disease.* Mary Ann Liebert, Inc., 1988.

Grant WM, Burke JF Jr: Why do some people go blind from glaucoma? *Ophthalmology* 1982;**89**:991.

Hoyt CS: Photorefraction: A technique for preschool visual screening. (Editorial.) *Arch Ophthalmol* 1987;**105**:1497.

Jones DB: Acanthamoeba: The ultimate opportunist? (Editorial.) *Am J Ophthalmol* 1986;**102**:527.

Jordan DR: The potential damaging effects of light on the eye. Part 1. *Canad J Ophthalmol* 1986;**21**:216.

Kaakinen KA, Kaseva HO, Teir HH: Two-flash photorefraction in screening of amblyogenic refractive errors. *Ophthalmology* 1987;**94**:1036.

McCabe R, Remington JS: Toxoplasmosis: The time has come. (Editorial.) *N Engl J Med* 1988;**318**:313.

McDonald HR, Irvine AR: Light-induced maculopathy from the operating microscope in extracapsular cataract extraction and intraocular lens implantation. *Ophthalmology* 1983;**90**:945.

Mondino BJ et al: Corneal ulcers associated with daily-wear and extended-wear contact lenses. *Am J Ophthalmol* 1986;**102**:58.

Morgan KS, Johnson WD: Clinical evaluation of a commercial photorefractor. *Arch Ophthalmol* 1987;**105**:1528.

Prober CG et al: Use of routine viral cultures at delivery to identify neonates exposed to herpes simplex virus. *N Engl J Med* 1988;**318**:887.

Roper-Hall MJ: Prevention of blindness from trauma. *Trans Ophthalmol Soc UK* 1978;**98**:313.

Schachter J et al: Experience with the routine use of erythromycin for chlamydial infections in pregnancy. *N Engl J Med* 1986;**314**:276.

Stenson S: Soft contact lenses are corneal infection. (Editorial.) *Arch Ophthalmol* 1986;**104**:1287.

von Noorden GK: Amblyopia: A multidisciplinary approach. *Invest Ophthalmol Vis Sci* 1985;**26**:1704.

Low Vision

Eleanor E. Faye, MD

In all subspecialties of eye care, patients with irreversible or temporary reduction of vision present a challenge in effective management—not only by medical and surgical treatment but also by helping patients overcome their disabilities.

Patients with impaired visual performance owing to reduced visual acuity uncorrectable by conventional spectacles or contact lenses or to restricted visual field are commonly called **low vision patients.** There may be additional complaints of increased glare sensitivity and abnormalities of color perception, contrast sensitivity, dark adaptation, ocular motility, and fusion.

The many optical and other devices used to improve visual performance in low vision patients are called **low vision aids.** In this chapter, discussion will center on assessment of low vision and provision of low vision aids. Ophthalmologic details about specific entities mentioned will not be discussed.

Since levels of visual performance are most realistically judged according to individual requirements, the term "low vision" may actually denote a wide range of visual impairment from nearly normal to profound loss. In the United States, over 6 million persons are visually impaired but not classified as legally blind.* Over 75% of patients seeking treatment for low vision are age 65 or over. Macular degeneration accounts for about 50% of all cases. Complicated cataract, glaucoma, diabetic retinopathy, optic atrophy, degenerative myopia, and retinitis pigmentosa are other major causes.

Effective low vision management does not place artificial definitions in the way of visual rehabilitation but considers each individual's level of function, visual objectives, and the available low vision aids. Low vision treatment should be started at whatever stage at which a patient experiences difficulty with customary visual tasks. Although progression of impaired vision is the rule, early intervention allows the patient time to adjust to new techniques. An uncertain prognosis is not sufficient reason to delay treatment.

Management of the patient with low vision includes (1) taking a history that incorporates questions about

customary activities; (2) examining the patient for changes in visual acuity, visual field, contrast sensitivity, color perception, and excessive glare; (3) evaluating near vision and reading skills; (4) selection and prescription (or lending) of aids that help achieve visual objectives, with the necessary instruction in their use; and (5) follow-up to ensure adjustment and correct use of the aids or to answer further questions.

HISTORY TAKING

Patients should be asked about the nature of their visual impairment, its duration, and its rapidity of onset. Customary activities that have become tedious or impossible should be specifically discussed. Table 23–1 lists a number of activities that are made difficult or impossible by substandard vision. Individual activities can usually be matched with specific optical and nonoptical aids so that realistic objectives based upon the patient's expectations can be established. Patients should be encouraged to understand the effects of their condition on the visual system. Fears of eventual blindness must be aired and set to rest.

EXAMINATION

Standard refraction may reveal unsuspected refractive errors and is important in prescribing high-add bifocals and in following patients with retinal disease who have intraocular lens implants. Best corrected acuity is measured at 4 m, 2 m, or 1 m with the Lighthouse Ferris-Bailey ETDRS chart, which has lines (each with 5 letters) of 0.1 log unit difference and a convenient Snellen conversion table (Fig 23–1). The 4 m test distance is used for acuity from 4/4 (20/20) to 4/40 (20/200); the 2 m test distance for acuities less than 4/40 (20/200); and the 1 m test distance for acuities less than 2/40 (20/400). Standard Snellen charts may be used at test distances of 3 m (10 ft) or less, but projector charts are not recommended for testing low vision.

One should determine the dominant eye and the preferred eye.

Amsler grids are used to locate central scotomas and to chart their position and density and areas of

---

*Legal blindness—defined as a best corrected visual acuity of 20/200 or less in the better eye or a visual field of 20 degrees or less—affects 1 million individuals in the USA (see Chapter 24).

Table 23–1. Common activities that are adversely affected by visual impairment are listed with suggestions for low vision aids.

Activity	Optical Aids	Nonoptical Aids
Shopping	Hand magnifier	Lighting, color cues
Fixing a snack	Bifocals	Color cues, consistent storage plan
Eating out	Hand magnifier	Flashlight, portable lamp
Identifying money	Bifocal, hand magnifier	Arrange wallet in compartments
Reading print	High power spectacle, bifocal, hand magnifier, stand magnifier, closed circuit television	Lighting, high-contrast print, large print
Writing	Intermediate add hand magnifier, focusable telescope, closed circuit television	Lighting, bold tip pen, black ink
Dialing a telephone	Hand magnifier	Large print dial, hand-printed directory
Crossing streets	Telescope	Cane, ask directions
Finding taxis and bus signs	Telescope	
Reading medication labels	Hand magnifier	Color codes, large print
Reading stove dials	Hand magnifier	Color codes
Thermostat adjustment	Hand magnifier	Enlarged print model
Using a computer	Intermediate add spectacle Telescope	High-contrast color, large print program
Reading signs	Spectacle	Reading slit
Watching sporting event	Telescope	

distortion (Fig 23–2). Note is made of whether the patient sees less distortion monocularly or binocularly to assess any preference for monocular or binocular reading corrections. Central scotomas may also be charted on a tangent screen or Goldmann perimeter. Peripheral fields are best tested on a tangent screen in patients with retinitis pigmentosa and on a Goldmann perimeter in patients with glaucoma and neurologic deficits.

Contrast sensitivity may be assessed both monocularly and binocularly with the Vistech Contrast Sensitivity Vision Test (See Chapter 2). Loss of high-frequency and mid-frequency targets is a predictor of reduced contrast in reading print with low vision optical devices. Superior binocular performance suggests selection of an aid that is used binocularly, eg, base-in prism glasses or binocular reading telescopes. Glare tests are used if lens or corneal opacities complicate other disorders such as glaucoma or macular degeneration to determine whether cataract extraction or keratoplasty might improve acuity. Color identification tests identify difficulty with color cues.

NEAR VISION

Near vision may be evaluated using a combination of single-letter tests and graded text of various sizes. Single letters serve to establish near acuity, graded text to establish reading skills with a selected optical aid. The reciprocal of **distance acuity** may be used to determine the approximate strength of the initial

trial lens for near vision—eg, 20/160 suggests a trial of 8 D of add to read 10-point print.

SELECTION OF AIDS & PATIENT INSTRUCTION

When the dioptric range has been established for the task objectives (the range may be from +3 D to +68 D), the type of low vision device best suited to the individual is selected.

The patient uses various devices under the supervision of a trained instructor until proficiency and efficacy have been established. The mechanics of the aids are reviewed, questions are answered, goals are clarified, and the patient is allowed ample time in a quiet setting to explore the new skills. This may involve one or more sessions and ideally culminates in providing a loaner lens in doubtful cases or prescription of one or more devices. Some patients require home or job trial of an aid before they can be secure. Older patients usually need more adaptation time than younger or congenitally visually impaired persons.

Proper patient instruction is the key to success in management of low vision patients. Prescription of lenses without instruction is successful in only 50% of cases, whereas with instruction the success rate rises to over 90%.

The patient's progress is reviewed after 2 or 3 weeks. Patients are encouraged to call if there are unforeseen problems. Many minor technical difficulties can be solved over the phone.

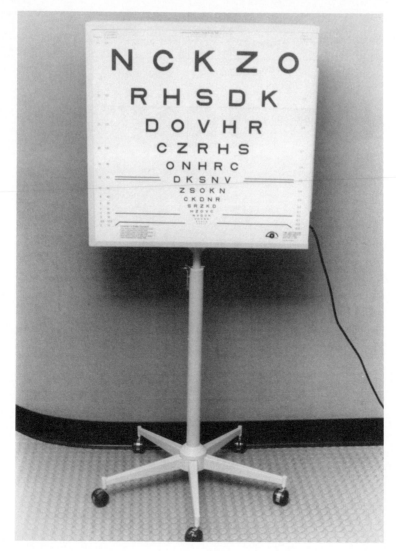

Figure 23–1. Lighthouse modification of the Ferris-Bailey ETDRS chart in a movable light-box.

LOW VISION AIDS

There are 2 basic types of low vision optical aids: (1) convex lens aids such as spectacles, hand magnifiers, and stand magnifiers; and (2) telescopic systems such as spectacle telescopes, clip-on telescopic loupes, and handheld devices. Nonoptical aids include writing aids, large-print publications, improved lighting, yellow filters, and reading stands. Antireflective lenses that absorb specific wavelengths are used to protect eyes from ultraviolet light and glare. Electronic devices include closed-circuit television reading machines and computers.

The practitioner must be familiar with the devices available and the advantages and disadvantages of each in order to provide proper guidance to the instructor and the patient. Prescribing low vision devices requires that both the physician and the instructor also understand how the symptoms of the disorder affect the indications for spectacles, contact lenses, telescopes, intraocular lenses, and low vision magnifying devices.

CONVEX LENS AIDS

Spectacles and hand and stand magnifiers are the mainstays of the low vision practitioner. Various mountings for lenses have inherent advantages and disadvantages. If the patient uses a convex lens in a

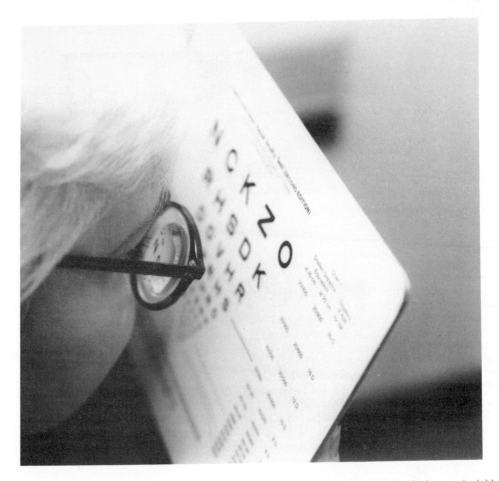

Figure 23–2. Low vision spectacle aid. Patient demonstrates close reading distance (with lenticular spectacle) but with both hands free to hold reading material.

spectacle frame, reading material must be held at the focal distance of the lens, eg, 10 cm for a 10-diopter lens. (Fig 23–2). The closer distances obstruct light, but for a reader the advantage of having both hands free to hold the material outweighs the unfamiliar close reading distance, while lamps can be adjusted to provide sufficient illumination.

Spectacles up to 12 diopters may be used binocularly (with base-in prisms to aid convergence). From 14 to 60 diopters, a monocular aspheric lenticular or doublet lens should be prescribed.

Hand magnifiers are convenient lenses for short-term tasks such as shopping, reading dials and labels, and identifying paper money (Fig 23–3). The advantage of a convex lens held by hand is that a greater working distance is achieved by holding lens and reading material away from the eye. Holding the lens and reading material may be a disadvantage for some patients with neurologic or orthopedic handicaps. Hand magnifiers span a dioptric range of 4–68 diopters. The image from a Rand magnifier is preferably viewed with best corrected distance vision. (Since the image

is coming from infinity, the parallel rays exiting the lens may be viewed without accommodative-effort.)

Stand magnifiers are much like hand magnifiers except that the lens is mounted on a base of predetermined height (Fig 23–4). Because a lens mounting may block light, a lens in an illuminating handle may be the best choice for most patients. Presbyopic patients generally must wear a conventional reading add in conjunction with a fixed-focus stand magnifier.

TELESCOPE SYSTEMS

The telescopic systems generally preferred by patients for distance or intermediate range are hand-held monoculars from $2\times$ to $10\times$ power (Fig 23–5). For patients with complex vocational or hobby require ments, focusable Galilean or Keplerian (internal prism) systems in a spectacle frame are the best choice. The power range for spectacle telescopes is $2\times$ to $8\times$. High powers ($6\times$ to $8\times$) are heavy.

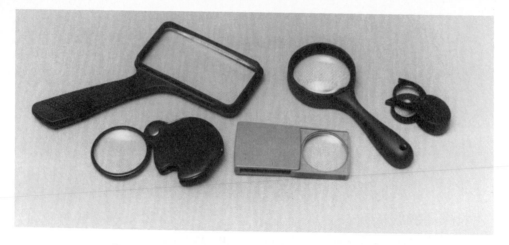

Figure 23-3. Hand magnifiers of various types and strengths.

All optical devices limit the field of vision—spectacles the least and telescopes the most. Therefore, preexisting field limitations of the patient with large central or peripheral scotomas must always be a consideration when prescribing telescopes.

In addition to providing magnifying lenses for reading and telescopes for all ranges of vision from distance to near, the practitioner must consider the importance of symptoms of glare and low contrast for the low vision patient. As a rule, lenses that cut out ultraviolet light below 400 nm, are coated with an antireflective multilayer coating, and are tinted gray to reduce light intensity or amber-yellow to improve contrast are most effective.

Electronic devices, which are more expensive than the average simple reading aid, are worth a trial for persons who have special needs, including needs associated with employment. Viewing written material on a television monitor may facilitate any near task.

MANAGEMENT OF LOW VISION PATIENTS

Treatment plans must take into account the effect of the eye disorder on both visual acuity and visual field. Symptoms of glare, blur, and central or peripheral visual deficits may vary, but they do directly

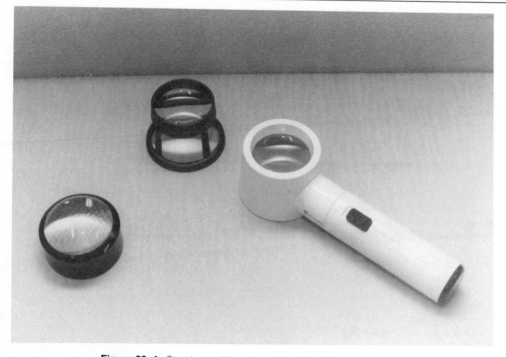

Figure 23-4. Stand magnifiers with and without illumination handle.

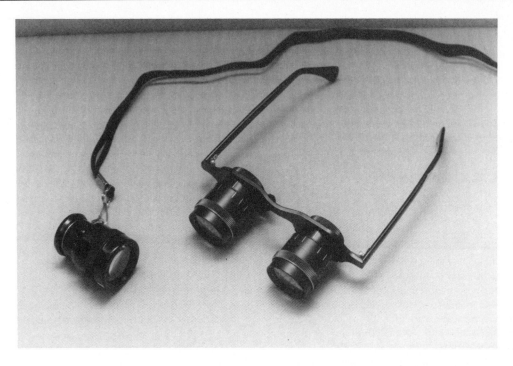

Figure 23–5. Low vision telescopes. **A:** Hand-held monocular telescope. **B:** Spectacle-mounted Galilean focusable telescope.

indicate the strength of the aid required and to some extent the type of aid that can be prescribed as well as the adjustment to the aid.

Low vision problems can be classified in 4 categories: (1) blurred or hazy central and peripheral vision, characteristic of corneal, lens, or vitreous disorders; (2) impaired focal resolution without central scotoma and with normal peripheral acuity, characteristic of macular edema or albinism; (3) central scotomas, characteristic of degenerative or inflammatory macular disorders and optic nerve disease; and (4) peripheral scotomas, characteristic of advanced glaucoma, retinitis pigmentosa, and other peripheral retinal disorders.

1. BLURRED, HAZY VISION

Generalized blurring or haziness of vision may be produced by abnormalities of the ocular media, including a variety of stromal epithelial and corneal endothelial disorders, lens opacities, posterior capsular opacification, vitreous opacities, abnormalities of pupillary size from miosis to aniridia, and retinal edema. Patients also experience glare and dimness of vision with or without photophobia and note reduced contrast perception for stairs, curbs, and objects.

Useful tests of visual function include Snellen visual acuity, glare, and contrast sensitivity tests. A potential acuity meter (PAM) may help differentiate pathologic processes involving the media from those involving the retina.

Treatment

Visual acuity varies markedly with lighting and image contrast. Modification of illumination and attention to details of image enhancement have high priority in treatment. Antireflective lens coatings and neutral gray lenses reduce light intensity, and yellow-amber lenses enhance contrast. Ultraviolet filters should be used, particularly for pseudophakic patients.

Magnification may not be effective, because a magnified image may still be indistinct. Large, bold print may be a better choice—or reading slits of matte plastic or cardboard to reduce glare and outline the text. Contact lenses or keratoplasty for corneal disorders, cataract extraction with or without intraocular lens implantation for lens opacities, and posterior capsulotomy for posterior capsular opacification may also be indicated.

2. IMPAIRED FOCAL RESOLUTION

Macular edema from a variety of disorders and congenital foveal aplasia characteristic of albinism cause impaired focal resolution with normal peripheral acuity. As a rule, visual acuity is in the higher range from 20/50 to 20/200.

Useful tests of visual function include Snellen visual acuity, Amsler grid, and PAM.

Treatment

These patients should have careful refraction for

best possible foveal vision. Characteristically, they respond to reading adds of $+4$ to $+10$ diopters and are proficient readers at the relatively normal reading distances such lenses require. Bifocals should be considered for stable conditions.

Magnifying hand and stand glasses are useful. Amber and antireflective sunglasses improve contrast and reduce glare. Albinos adapt well to hand-held and spectacle-mounted telescopes.

3. CENTRAL SCOTOMAS

The 2 commonest causes of central scotomas are atrophic and exudative (hemorrhagic) age-related macular degeneration, both of which are increasingly common in today's aging society. Other causes are macular holes, myopic macular degeneration, and optic nerve disease.

Patients most often report blurred or distorted central vision (peripheral vision is clear unless cataracts complicate the picture). Difficulty in reading and in discerning facial features are the most common complaints in early stages of macular disease. Dense scotomas are characteristic of the disciform stage of exudative macular disease and optic nerve disease. In the early stages, contrast perception is generally not affected. Travel ability remains relatively normal even in advanced disease.

Useful tests of visual function include Snellen visual acuity, Amsler grid, and contrast sensitivity. Reduced contrast suggests the need for more magnification than predicted from the Snellen visual acuity test.

Treatment

Patients may use eccentric head positions to place images in healthier retinal areas. This technique may be demonstrated to the patient during visual acuity tests or on an Amsler grid.

Magnifying lenses are of benefit. The strength of the prescription is related directly to near visual acuity and contrast as well as to position and density of the scotoma. Patients may use several types of lenses for various tasks, eg, spectacles for reading, and a hand magnifier for shopping. Most patients with macular degeneration learn to use low vision aids successfully, particularly after supportive instruction sessions.

Older patients may require more reinforcement and additional time to adjust. They particularly need reassurance about the remote possibility of blindness.

4. PERIPHERAL SCOTOMA

Peripheral field loss is characteristic of end-stage glaucoma, retinitis pigmentosa, other peripheral retinal diseases, and cerebral vascular disease. While central vision is essential for details, the peripheral field of vision is essential for locating oneself in space, for traveling about safely, and for awareness of potential hazards and objects in the periphery. A person with advanced retinitis pigmentosa may be able to read small print yet need a guide to get around.

Adequate lighting is essential for patients with residual foveal fields. Most patients' photophobia is relieved by amber-orange lenses that block ultraviolet and visible blue light below 527 nm. When contrast perception is reduced by cataract, a combination of contrast sensitivity and glare tests may indicate the best timing for cataract surgery.

When central fields are less than 7 degrees, magnification of an image is not perceived by such a patient as advantageous. Telescopes are therefore not useful, and hand magnifiers and closed-circuit television may be the devices of choice because the amount of magnification can be controlled by the patient. A posterior chamber intraocular lens implant for patients undergoing cataract extraction is essential to maintain normal image size.

TRAINING PROGRAMS

Many practitioners and staff benefit from joint training programs to learn the role of each person in management of low vision patients in a private practice or clinic. Basic setups for a low vision practice are reviewed in a number of publications.

No patient with impaired vision should have to search far and wide for low vision care. Such care should be integrated into every ophthalmologic practice, and practitioners should offer referral to low vision centers for more complex rehabilitation cases.

REFERENCES

Colenbrander A: Dimensions of visual performance. *Trans Am Acad Ophthalmol Otolaryngol* 1977;**83**:332.

Faye EE (editor). *Clinical Low Vision*, 2nd ed. Little, Brown, 1984.

Genensky S et al: Visual environmental adaptation problems of the partially sighted: A final report. Center for the Partially Sighted, Santa Monica Hospital/Medical Center, 1977.

Goodrich GL et al: Training and practice effects in performance with low-vision aids: A preliminary study. *Am J Optom Physiol Opt* 1977;**54**:312.

Jose RT (editor): *Understanding Low Vision*. American Foundation for the Blind, 1983.

Kwitko ML, Weinstock FJ: *Geriatric Ophthalmology*. Grune & Stratton, 1985.

Sekuler R, Kline D, Dismukes K (editors): *Aging and Human Visual Function*. Alan R. Liss, 1982.

ADDITIONAL RESOURCES

Journal of Visual Impairment and Blindness. American Foundation for the Blind. [Monthly periodical.]

National Center for Vision and Aging. The New York Lighthouse. [Information and pamphlets.]

New York Lighthouse: *Catalogue of Low Vision Products*. [Complete stock of low vision aids and products.]

New York Lighthouse Training and Continuing Program for Low Vision Services. The New York Lighthouse. [Professional education programs.]

24

Blindness

Paul Riordan-Eva, FRCS, MA, MB, BChir

In this chapter we shall discuss blindness as a worldwide health problem, with emphasis on avoidable forms of this dread human affliction. The World Health Organization defines visual impairment as shown in Table 24–1. WHO officials encourage investigators and reporting agencies in all countries to report blindness and near blindness according to the categories defined in this table. WHO estimates that there are 28 million blind people in the world today. This figure rises to about 42 million if the criterion is extended to visual acuity of 20/200 or worse.

In the USA, the most widely used definition of partial blindness is that used by the Internal Revenue Service for the purpose of determining who is eligible for tax deductions on that basis: *central visual acuity 20/200 or less in the better eye with best correction, or widest diameter of visual field subtending an angle of no greater than 20 degrees.* An alternative functional definition is *loss of vision sufficient to prevent one from being self-supporting in an occupation, making the individual dependent on other persons, agencies, or devices in order to live.*

"Industrial blindness" is said to be present when a worker can no longer pursue an occupation because of poor vision; "automobile blindness" when vision is so poor that the responsible licensing agency in that state will not issue a driver's license. The term color blindness is a misnomer since this genetically transmitted disorder is not blindness as that term is generally understood and is only a minor handicap to a few people. Loss of vision may affect only the central fields, only the peripheral fields, or only specific portions of the peripheral fields in one or both eyes. Total loss of vision in one eye is said to reduce visual capacity by only 10%, though it makes the other eye infinitely more valuable.

All of the disorders that may cause blindness are discussed more fully in other parts of this book. This chapter is an attempt to summarize some pertinent information about the epidemiology of blindness as a worldwide health problem with emphasis on those categories of blindness that are preventable by the combined efforts of physicians and health agencies.

Measures relevant to rehabilitation of the blind in more developed countries will also be discussed.

Table 24–1. Categories of visual impairment. (Adapted from the International Classfication of Diseases, World Health Organization, 1977.)

Category of Visual Impairment	Visual Acuity (Best Corrected)
Low vision	
1	6/18 3/10 (0.3) 20/70
2	6/60 1/10 (0.1) 20/200
Blindness	
3	3/60 (finger counting at 3m) 1/20 (0.05) 20/400
4	1/60 (finger counting at 1m) 1/50 (0.02) 5/300
5	No light perception

Visual Field

Patients with a visual field radius no greater than 10 degrees but greater than 5 degrees around central fixation should be placed in category 3 and patients with a field no greater than 5 degrees around central fixation in category 4—even if the central acuity is not impaired.

PREVALENCE OF BLINDNESS THROUGHOUT THE WORLD

Table 24–2 lists some countries where fairly reliable data are available about the prevalence of blindness. Even where health statistics are most reliable, the methods of counting the blind are often crude and may be applied according to different criteria in different places and at different times within any extensive geographic area. Furthermore, extrapolations are often made from small sample studies to large populations.

The kind of effort it would take to make a substantial reduction in the prevalence of blindness is almost too vast to contemplate. The same was true years ago when the public health profession set out to eradicate smallpox as one of the scourges of humanity. Smallpox formerly caused much blindness, but it is most unlikely that anyone will ever again be blinded, dis-

Table 24–2. Approximate prevalence of blindness (%). (Estimates based on WHO surveys.)[1]

Chad	3.2–5	Malawi	1
Liberia	3.2	Brazil	0.3
Egypt	2.6	Mexico	0.3
Phillipines	2.1	Australia	0.2
Afghanistan	2	Japan	0.2
Bangladesh	2	USA	0.2
Pakistan	2	UK	0.18
Saudi Arabia	2	Canada	0.15
India	1.5	USSR	0.12
Indonesia	1.3	China	0.1
Chile	1	Germany	0.1

[1] Based on available data, 1969–1980. Some data were only rough estimates when obtained and may have changed markedly since then. In some cases, the survey criteria used did not correspond to WHO definitions. Data taken from Maitchouk IF: Data on blindness: Prevalence and causes throughout the world. In: Lim ASM, Jones BR (editors): World's major blinding conditions. *Vision* 1982;**1**:99. (International Agency for the Prevention of Blindness.)

Table 24–3. Areas of eye afflicted by major blinding diseases.

Anterior segment diseases
Trachoma
Leprosy
Onchocerciasis
Xerophthalmia
Cataract
Herpes simplex keratitis
Posterior segment diseases
Glaucoma
Retinal degeneration
Retinal detachment
Diabetic retinopathy

Note: In general, the anterior segment diseases are more preventable than the posterior segment diseases.

figured, or killed by what was an almost universal public health concern only a few decades ago. Fortunately, it is not necessary in the health professions that success be unqualified and total to earn the label of "success." Eliminating one cause of blindness would be a magnificent victory even if the other causes were unaffected. It is precisely because the numbers are so great that partial success in the effort to treat and prevent blindness must be sought by all available means. WHO estimates that 75% of cases of blindness in developing countries are avoidable.

CAUSES OF BLINDNESS

The leading causes of preventable blindness in the world are trachoma, leprosy, onchocerciasis, and xerophthalmia. Between 6 and 9 million people are blind from trachoma, at least 1 million from leprosy, and 1 million from onchocerciasis. Xerophthalmia is estimated to affect 5 million children each year; 500,000 develop active corneal involvement, and half of these go blind. Although curable, cataract is still responsible for an estimated 17 million cases of blindness worldwide. Glaucoma, retinal detachment, and diabetic retinopathy have not been separately identified in WHO's statistical compilations, but many ophthalmologists believe that each of these disorders would rank ahead of onchocerciasis and xerophthalmia as a cause of blindness. Since some form of treatment is available for all 3 disorders, there is no reason why they should not be included among the avoidable causes of blindness.

Table 24–3 lists areas of the eye afflicted by major blinding diseases.

Trachoma

Trachoma is an infectious disease caused by *Chlamydia trachomatis.* It causes bilateral keratoconjunctivitis that leads to corneal scarring, which, when severe, causes blindness. About 500 million people have trachoma, most of them in Africa, the Middle East, and Asia. It can be prevented by adequate diet, proper sanitary facilities, and education and can be cured by sulfonamides or tetracycline drugs.

Leprosy

Leprosy (Hansen's disease) affects 15–16 million people in the world and has a higher percentage of ocular involvement than any other systemic disease. The type and frequency of ocular involvement differ in different parts of the world, and surveys of leprosy hospitals reveal that 6–90% of patients have ocular involvement. Many investigators feel that all leprosy patients will have ocular manifestations if the disease persists long enough. Reports on the prevalence of blindness among such patients indicate that up to 10% of leprosy patients may be blind from the disease, which means that over 1 million people are blind from leprosy worldwide. Such figures would place leprosy as the second leading cause of blindness resulting from an infectious disease and therefore a greater visual threat than onchocerciasis.

Onchocerciasis

Onchocerciasis (due to *Onchocerca volvulus,* a roundworm) is transmitted by bites of the blackfly *Simulium damnosum* in Africa and other species of *Simulium* in Central and South America. The larvae of the blackfly develop in clear running streams (hence the name river blindness). The adult female harbors the larvae of *O volvulus* and transmits the infection between humans by biting. The parasite larvae develop into mature worms in subcutaneous nodules, and the female produces large numbers of microfilariae, which invade other tissues, including the eye. The major blinding lesion in onchocerchiasis is sclerosing keratitis.

Onchocerciasis is endemic in the greater part of tropical Africa and Central and South America. The most heavily infested zone is the Volta River basin, which extends over parts of Dahomey, Ghama, Ivory Coast, Mali, Niger, Togo, and Upper Volta.

Treatment is discussed in Chapter 8. The best hope for control of the disease is insect eradication and personal protection by screening.

Xerophthalmia

Xerophthalmia is due to hypovitaminosis A. Clinically, there is xerosis of the conjunctiva with characteristic Bitot's spots and softening of the cornea (keratomalacia), which may lead to corneal perforation. Protein malnutrition exacerbates the condition and renders it refractory to treatment. Xerophthalmia is a common cause of blindness in infants, particularly in India, Bangladesh, Indonesia, and the Philippines. Affected infants often do not reach adulthood, dying from malnutrition, pneumonia, or diarrhea.

Xerophthalmia can be prevented by general dietary improvement or vitamin A supplementation. If the problems of distribution and administration were solved, the cost of a quantity of the vitamin sufficient to prevent blindness in 1000 infants would be only about $25.

Cataract

Cataract accounts for 40–80% of cases of blindness in developing countries. As life expectancy increases, there is a continuing rise in the total number of people affected. It is not known why the frequency of cataract in different geographic areas varies so much. Mobile eye camps have aided in management, but there are too few to control the disorder. Many more cataract surgeons are needed in countries such as India and Pakistan.

In most Western countries, the relative prevalence of cataract is low; there is an oversupply of cataract surgeons; and patients at all economic levels have easy access to surgery, which has a 90–95% success rate. Many ophthalmologists, especially in the USA, do not consider cataract to be a cause of blindness in their countries.

Other Causes

Glaucoma, retinal detachment, diabetic retinopathy, and herpes simplex keratitis are discussed in greater detail elsewhere in this text. The incidence of blindness due to glaucoma has decreased in recent years as a result of earlier detection, improved medical and surgical treatment, and a greater awareness and understanding of the disorder by the lay population.

Diabetic retinopathy is an increasingly more common cause of blindness everywhere in the world. Recent advances in surgical treatment (vitrectomy, laser therapy) are of some help, but many patients still suffer from proliferative retinopathy, recurrent vitreous hemorrhages, and eventual bilateral blindness. A vast research effort directed at all aspects of diabetes is in progress, and there is justification for hoping that the next generation of diabetics will benefit greatly from what is being done now.

Hereditary conditions are important causes of blindness but should gradually decrease in incidence in response to the efforts of genetic counselors to increase public awareness of the preventable nature of these disorders.

As is true also in other countries where medical care and social services are widely available, blindness in the USA is to a great extent related to the aging process, and about half of the legally blind people in this country are over age 65. The leading causes of blindness in this age group are degenerative retinal disorders, glaucoma, diabetes, and vascular diseases.

PREVENTION OF BLINDNESS

It should be obvious from the foregoing discussion of the prevalence and causes of blindness that the solution to the problem of blindness lies in prevention rather than treatment. Little has been done where much could be done, particularly in the developing countries, and there, most especially, in children. If a choice must be made, it would be a simple one between (a) spending millions on organ transplant research to keep a few people alive a few years longer and (b) using that money to solve some of the truly desperate problems of the earth's people. In some cases simple remedies are available and are not being used.

Some examples of what can be achieved for modest outlays of scarce funds are as follows:

(1) To cure one person of trachoma in Saudi Arabia: $1.25.

(2) To restore vision to one person in Pakistan blinded by cataracts: $25.

(3) To prevent blindness due to xerophthalmia in one infant in Java: 27 cents.

Recently, on the advice of WHO experts, the World Council for the Welfare of the Blind and several international professional ophthalmic societies and agencies agreed to take the initiative, which led to the establishment in 1974 of the International Agency for Prevention of Blindness (Vision International), with Sir John Wilson, a blind barrister, as president. The aim of this agency is to work with groups formed for the purpose of preventing blindness. Its theme, Foresight Prevents Blindness, was brought into prominent display when WHO celebrated the first World Health Day on April 7, 1976. Its goal was stated as follows: "In every donor country during 1976, every family should be asked—in thanksgiving for sight—to give $10 to save the sight of its fellow countrymen or of the millions in the third world. If we can raise this campaign to that degree of universal appeal, the result could be spectacular."

REHABILITATION OF THE BLIND

Technologic developments in recent years have created new opportunities for richer and more productive lives for blind people. In assessing these advances it is necessary to be aware of the blind population one is dealing with. Different categories of the blind have different needs, and some blind people simply cannot benefit from some of the more glamorous technical achievements. It has been said that over half of the blind people in the USA are over age 65. The elderly widowed housewife may need or want no more than mobility training in home care and a steady supply of Talking Books. A young person facing blindness in later life due to retinitis pigmentosa requires the full range of social services, including educational assessment, job rehabilitation, and psychologic counseling. The physician's role is to know what referral sources are available and how to use them skillfully. This means personally investigating the quality of services offered. Medical social workers, public health nurses, and counseling services and agencies serving the blind and visually handicapped are common sources of reliable information.

Braille

This remarkably effective system of reading for the blind was introduced in 1825. The braille characters consist of raised dots arranged in 2 columns of three. The system is so simple that a blind child can quickly learn to read braille, and proficient readers can learn to read braille as fast as they can talk. The system has been adapted to musical notation and technical and scientific uses also. An international braille code was introduced in 1951.

Braille is used less commonly now than formerly, since many blind people prefer auditory aids both for informational and recreational purposes. Braille continues to be essential on tags attached to items in common personal use even for people who do not wish to use it for reading.

All paper money in the Netherlands and Switzerland is braille-printed to show the denomination.

Mobility Training

Many state commissions for the blind offer a wide variety of mobility training courses, either directly or in cooperation with private agencies. The courses are offered on an outpatient and residential basis and have varied objectives according to the special needs of the people who apply for help. The curriculum commonly includes self-care, home functions, and mobility within the community.

Guide Dogs

The popular concept of the guide dog is somewhat unrealistic and no doubt colored by the natural affection most people have for these handsome animals. The guide dog is not trained to think and thus help its master function better in a strange and hostile world; its major function is to obey commands, and its usefulness is therefore directly related to the competence of its master. It may be said that a cane is not much of a companion, but neither does it have to be fed or housed or taken to the veterinarian when it gets sick. Older patients have trouble with the dogs because considerable physical strength is required to hold them in check. Guide dogs are most useful for students and professional men and women in good health who lead fairly well organized lives. At this time less than 2% of blind people in the USA use guide dogs. Sonar sensor canes may ultimately be a better answer to the mobility problem even for those who are now using a dog successfully.

Electronic Devices

Optacon is an electronic device that converts visual images of letters into tactile forms. It is easily portable and can be used with almost any kind of reading matter. Auditory aids are becoming increasingly important (eg, talking calculators, clocks, paper money identifiers).

FINANCIAL ASSISTANCE PROGRAMS

It is unfortunate that over half of the blind people in the USA are essentially dependent upon Social Security and whatever local supplemental aid may be available to them. For the younger blind population, rehabilitation programs are commonly administered at the state level by a division of the department of education specifically set up to serve blind people in the state. Some of these programs are better than others, and all physicians should support efforts to increase the effectiveness of such programs in their geographic area of influence. The programs are of wide scope and offer preliminary counseling followed by academic or vocational training as the circumstances warrant. Once a realistic vocational objective has been established, full financial support is commonly available. This single resource is probably the most crucial referral available to the ophthalmologist, particularly in the case of young patients. Counseling services are available as early as the junior high school years to assure compliance with a curriculum consistent with measured aptitudes and interests. In many states, such rehabilitation programs as mobility training are administered under state auspices but contracted to private agencies for operational purposes.

In many countries of the world, the blind receive no financial or other support from their governments and are either cared for by their families or left to manage by themselves in any way they can.

REFERENCES

GENERAL

Baghdassarian SA, Tabbara KF: Childhood blindness in Lebanon. *Am J Ophthalmol* 1975;**79:**827.

Brand M: The care of the eye. In: *The Star.* National Hansen's Disease Center, 1980.

Choyce DP: Blindness in leprosy. *Trop Doct* (Jan) 1973;**3:**16.

Dawson CR, Jones BR, Tarizzo ML: *Guide to Trachoma Control in Programmes for the Prevention of Blindness.* World Health Organization, 1981.

Faye EE (editor): *Clinical Low Vision,* 2nd ed. Little, Brown, 1984.

Ffytche TJ: Role of iris changes as a cause of blindness in lepromatous leprosy. *Br J Ophthalmol* 1981;**65:**231.

Ghafour IM, Allan D, Foulds WS: Common causes of blindness and visual handicap in the west of Scotland. *Br J Ophthalmol* 1983;**67:**209.

Hobbs, HE, Choyce DP: The blinding lesions of leprosy. *Lepr Rev* 1971;**42:**131.

Jones BR: General obstacles to the prevention of blindness. *Trans Ophthalmol Soc UK* 1978;**98:**316.

Jones BR: The prevention of blindness from trachoma. *Trans Ophthalmol Soc UK* 1975;**95:**16.

Lariviere M et al: Double-blind study of ivermectin and diethylcarbamazine in African onchocerciasis patients with ocular involvement. *Lancet* 1985;**2:**174.

Law FW: World Health Day: 7 April 1976. *Br J Ophthalmol* 1976;**60:**231.

Lim ASM, Jones BR (editors): World's major blinding conditions. *Vision* 1982;**1:**1. [Entire issue.]

MacKay DM: The psychology of seeing. *Trans Ophthalmol Soc UK* 1973;**93:**391.

Marron JA, Bailey IL: Visual factors and orientation-mobility performance. *Am J Optom Physiol Opt* 1982;**59:**413.

Nizetić B: Prevention of "blindness": Potentialities of a systems analysis approach. *Acta Ophthalmol (Copenh)* 1974;**52:**134.

Onchocerciasis. (Editorial.) *Br J Ophthalmol* 1976;**60:**1.

Phillips CI et al: Blindness in schoolchildren: Importance of heredity, congenital cataract, and prematurity. *Br J Ophthalmol* 1987;**71:**578.

Pirie A: Vitamin A deficiency and child blindness in the developing world. *Proc Nutr Soc* 1983;**42:**53.

The Prevention of Blindness: Report of a WHO Study Group. World Health Organization Technical Report Series 518, 1973. [Entire issue.]

Roy FH: World blindness: Definition, incidence and major treatable causes. *Ann Ophthalmol* 1974;**6:**1049.

Sommer A: *Nutritional Blindness: Xerophthalmia and Keratomalacia.* Oxford Univ Press, 1982.

Sommer A et al: Xerophthalmia and anterior segment blindness among preschool-age children in El Salvador. *Am J Ophthalmol* 1976;**80:**1066.

Strategies for the Prevention of Blindness in National Programmes: A Primary Health Care Approach. World Health Organization, 1984.

Tabbara KF, Badr IA: Changing pattern of childhood blindness in Saudi Arabia. *Br J Ophthalmol* 1985;**69:**312.

Taylor HR et al: Treatment of onchocerciasis: The ocular effects of ivermectin and diethylcarbamazine. *Arch Ophthalmol* 1986;**104:**863.

ADDITIONAL REFERENCES & SOURCES

Division for the Blind and Physically Handicapped, Library of Congress.

Recording for the Blind, New York.

World Health Magazine (Jan) 1983.

Principles of Management of Common Ocular Disorders

25

Daniel Vaughan, MD

It is not necessary to refer every patient with an eye disease to an ophthalmologist for treatment. In general, sties, bacterial conjunctivitis, superficial trauma to the lids, cornea, and conjunctiva, and superficial corneal foreign bodies can be treated just as effectively by the internist or general physician as by the ophthalmologist. On the other hand, more serious eye diseases or symptoms such as the following should be referred as soon as possible for specialized care: iritis, glaucoma, retinal detachment, strabismus, eye pain or blurred vision of undetermined origin, double vision, and corneal trauma or infection.

In the management of acute ocular disorders, it is most important to establish a definitive diagnosis before prescribing treatment. ''All red eyes are not pinkeye,'' is a useful maxim, and the physician must be alert for the more serious iritis, keratitis, or glaucoma (see chart on inside front cover). The common practice of prescribing ''shotgun'' topical antibiotic combinations containing corticosteroids is to be discouraged, principally because of the inherent danger of incautious steroid treatment.

This chapter is an attempt to summarize the basic principles and techniques of diagnosis and management of common ocular problems. All of the disorders discussed here are dealt with in greater detail elsewhere in this book.

OFFICE EQUIPMENT & SUPPLIES

Basic Equipment

A great many specialized instruments have been devised for the investigation of eye disorders. However, most diseases of the eye can be diagnosed with the aid of a few relatively simple instruments:

(1) Hand flashlight.
(2) Binocular loupe.
(3) Ophthalmoscope.
(4) Visual acuity chart (Snellen).
(5) Tonometer. (Tonometry should be performed on all patients over 20 years of age having a physical examination.)

Basic Medications
A. Local Anesthetics:
1. Proparacaine 0.5%.
2. Tetracaine 0.5%.

B. Dyes: Sterile fluorescein papers, rose bengal solution.

C. Mydriatics: Phenylephrine 2.5% is a satisfactory mydriatic when the examiner wishes to obtain a clearer view of the lens, vitreous, or ocular fundus.

D. Miotics: Pilocarpine 1%.

E. Antibacterial Agents: Sulfisoxazole 4% ophthalmic solution or ointment; and gentamicin 0.3% solution or ointment.

HISTORY & PHYSICAL EXAMINATION

History

When taking a history from a patient who presents with an eye problem, a useful initial question is, ''How do your eyes bother you?'' After the patient has described the present difficulty, inquire specifically about glasses, blurred vision, pain, red eyes, double vision, trauma to the eyes or head, headaches, and ''eyestrain.'' Information concerning the patient's general health is also relevant, particularly with regard to diabetes mellitus and hypertension. Since many eye diseases have a genetic pattern, the family history should be obtained. The patient's age and occupation are important factors in many ocular difficulties. Patients with glasses should be asked how long it has been since their prescription was changed.

Physical Examination

An adequate gross physical examination of the eye can be performed easily and quickly with a minimum of equipment (see above). By far the most important single examination is visual acuity testing in each eye. This should be done on all patients and the results noted in the clinical record. Visual acuity is tested at a distance of 6 meters (20 feet) using the Snellen chart. It is usually noted with and without glasses. However, corrected visual acuity has greater significance, since it is presumably the best possible visual acuity.

Inspection is facilitated by adequate illumination and should include a mental note of the patient's age, body build, and the structure of the head, face, and eyelids (eg, a patient with Marfan's syndrome is tall and thin and has long fingers). Bell's palsy and acromegaly may also be noted. Observe the eyes grossly for evidence of exophthalmos or enophthalmos.

Using a hand flashlight, examine the lids, conjunctivas, and corneas to rule out inflammation. Observe for icteric scleras (eg, hepatitis), pale conjunctivas (anemia), tumors, and scars. The pupillary light response should also be noted at this time. Gross disorders of ocular movements can be observed by having the patient follow the light of a moving flashlight by moving the eyes to the right, left, up, down, and inward while holding the head in fixed position.

Pressure over the tear sac will produce a mucoid or purulent discharge if significant infection is present.

With the ophthalmoscope, one can judge the clarity of the aqueous, lens, and vitreous as well as the appearance of the optic nerve, macula, retina, retinal blood vessels, and choroid. The ophthalmoscopic examination is facilitated by dim illumination in the examining room and a strong, well-focused light in the ophthalmoscope. If the ocular fundi cannot be easily inspected through the normal pupil, the pupil should be dilated. *Caution:* Before instilling the mydriatic, examine the anterior chamber by oblique illumination with a hand light (see Fig 12–8). If the anterior chamber is shallow (iris and lens quite close to the cornea), dilation of the pupils should be performed only by an ophthalmologist, since in these cases dilation may precipitate an attack of acute glaucoma.

In any patient over 20 years of age, tonometry should be performed as a screening test for glaucoma. Determining the intraocular pressure by finger palpation of the eyes (tactile tension) is not a reliable procedure.

BACTERIOLOGIC & MICROSCOPIC EXAMINATION

In the management of all serious external eye infections, the first step is to obtain a stained smear of the exudate. In conjunctivitis, for example, the scraping is taken directly from the conjunctival surface, and in corneal ulcer the scraping is taken directly from the advancing border of the lesion. The equipment necessary for the study of stained smears is as follows: sterile spatula, glass slides, stains (methylene blue, Wright's, Gram's, and Giemsa's), microscope, light, and immersion oil. Pull down on the patient's lower lid to expose the conjunctiva, make 3–4 horizontal scrapings, and smear on a clean glass slide. Allow to dry in air, fix with methanol, and stain. Prior instillation of local anesthetic drops minimizes discomfort from the scraping.

Cultures and antibiotic sensitivity studies should be done in *all* cases of corneal ulcer and in severe cases of bacterial conjunctivitis.

Study of the stained smear is far more important than culturing in the average ocular infection, since by this means one can immediately determine whether the causative agent is bacterial, viral, fungal, or allergic and because in some instances the exact cause can be determined on the spot. This information serves as a guide to treatment. For example, if pneumococci are found, almost any type of antibiotic will be effective, whereas staphylococcal infection will require more specific measures. If there is considerable inflammation of the conjunctiva, if no bacteria are found, and if monocytes are present in increased numbers in the smear, a diagnosis of viral conjunctivitis can be made, and the physician knows that the condition will probably last 10–14 days with or without treatment. If many eosinophils are noted in the stained conjunctival smear, the conjunctivitis is probably due to allergy.

TREATMENT OF SPECIFIC EYE CONDITIONS

LIDS

Marginal Blepharitis

Marginal blepharitis is the most common disorder of the lids. The most important factor in its treatment is cleanliness, which is best maintained by rubbing the scales from the eyelid margins daily with a wet cotton applicator or clean washcloth or by scrubbing the lid margin and the base of the eyelashes with baby shampoo. Since this disorder is frequently associated with dandruff, vigorous efforts to keep the scalp clean are warranted. Specific antibiotic ointment should be applied to the lid margins once daily at bedtime when the condition is associated with microbial infection.

Internal Hordeolum

This common condition is essentially a meibomian gland abscess caused by infection with *Staphylococcus aureus*. The treatment is similar to that of a boil elsewhere on the body. Warm compresses should be applied for 15 minutes 3–4 times daily, followed by the instillation of sulfonamide or antibiotic ointment. Incision or expression is required when the hordeolum is pointing. If the hordeolum points toward the conjunctival surface, the incision should be a vertical one on the conjunctival side to avoid cutting across the meibomian glands. If the hordeolum is pointing on the lid side, a horizontal incision is made through the skin, since most of the lines of the skin in this region are horizontal.

External Hordeolum (Sty)

Infection of Zeis's or Moll's glands (sty) is smaller and more superficial than internal hordeolum (meibomian gland abscess). Pain and redness are the principal symptoms. Treatment is similar to that outlined for internal hordeolum.

Chalazion

A chalazion is a nontender lipogranulomatous inflammation of a meibomian gland. It should be excised by an ophthalmologist.

Dacryocystitis

A. In Adults: Acute dacryocystitis in adults usually implies that the nasolacrimal duct is completely blocked. Systemic administration of penicillin is effective treatment. Local treatment is generally ineffective. Operation is indicated if the infection does not respond to medical treatment. Dacryocystorhinostomy is the operation of choice for the prevention of recurrences of dacryocystitis.

B. In Infants: In infantile dacryocystitis, the tear sac should be massaged 3–4 times daily. Following the massage, instill sulfonamide or antibiotic drops into the conjunctival sac. If this is not successful, probing of the nasolacrimal duct by an ophthalmologist is indicated.

Tumors

Verrucae and papillomas are common and can usually be easily excised as well by the general physician as by the ophthalmologist as long as they are not near the lid margin. All lid tumors should be examined microscopically to rule out malignancy. Improper excision of tumors near the lid margin may result in lid abnormalities.

CONJUNCTIVA

Hyperemia of the conjunctival vessels is the most common cause of red eyes. Smog, smoke, and other irritants found in the environment may cause hyperemia of the conjunctival vessels. Local vasoconstrictors or cold compresses may be helpful in alleviating the symptoms and the redness.

Conjunctivitis caused by allergy can be helped by local vasoconstrictors and cold compresses. Topical corticosteroid drops may be used in severe cases under ophthalmologic supervision.

Conjunctivitis due to microbial agents—bacterial, viral, fungal, chlamydial, or parasitic—may be treated specifically after proper identification of the agent. Because treatment with ointments may cause blurring of vision for half an hour after instillation, eye drops are prescribed during the day; ointment can be used at bedtime to ensure prolonged effect during the sleeping hours. Patients are cautioned to wash their hands frequently and not to touch their eyes. This is to prevent spread of infection to the other eye as well as to other people. Individual washcloths and towels should be used. Systemic therapy may be indicated in certain forms of conjunctivitis (eg, chlamydial).

CORNEA

All corneal conditions except superficial foreign bodies should be treated by an ophthalmologist.

Corneal Foreign Bodies

Note the time and place of the accident and what the patient was doing when it occurred. Visual acuity testing—if possible, before treatment is instituted—is important for legal as well as medical reasons in all cases.

If the patient complains of a foreign body sensation and gives a consistent history, there usually is one even though it may not be readily visible on the initial examination. However, if oblique illumination is used with the hand flashlight, almost all foreign bodies can be detected. If no corneal foreign bodies are seen and the patient continues to have a foreign body sensation, instill a local anesthetic and turn the upper lid to exclude the possibility of an upper tarsal conjunctival foreign body. If there is no conjunctival foreign body, stain the cornea with fluorescein paper. When the corneal foreign body is found, remove it with a wet cotton applicator or spud under good illumination, using an ocular loupe if one is available. Instill gentamicin ointment to prevent contamination with a gram-negative or gram-positive organism. It is not necessary to patch the eye, but it is essential that the patient be observed on the following day to exclude the possibility of secondary infection of the crater. If no infection occurs, the corneal wound will heal by epithelial regeneration. If infection occurs, the wound area may take weeks or months to heal.

Untreated infection may cause severe corneal ulceration with consequent marked visual loss. Early infection is manifested by a white necrotic area around the foreign body crater and a slight gray exudate. *Note:* These patients should be referred immediately to an ophthalmologist.

Corneal Abrasions

The history should be taken and visual acuity tested before treatment. A patient with a corneal abrasion complains of severe pain, especially with movement of the lid over the cornea. The surface of the cornea may be examined with a light and loupe. If an abrasion is suspected but cannot be seen, stain the cornea with sterile 2% fluorescein solution. The area of corneal abrasion will have a deeper green stain than the surrounding cornea.

Instill gentamicin ophthalmic ointment. Apply a tight pressure bandage to prevent movement of the lid and resultant irritation of the abraded corneal area. Bed rest may be necessary. The patient should be observed on the following day to be certain that the cornea is healing. Corneal abrasions heal in 24–72 hours if a pressure bandage is properly applied. In contrast to corneal foreign body wounds, there is little chance of infection. The main dangers are delayed healing and recurrent corneal erosion due to imperfect healing. Do not use corticosteroids or topical anesthetics in any form of physical injury of the cornea. Systemic analgesics may be necessary in certain cases.

UVEAL TRACT

Any uveal tract disorder may lead to permanent visual impairment. Therefore, the treatment should be supervised by an ophthalmologist.

Acute Anterior Uveitis (Iritis)

This is the most common disorder of the uveal tract and can easily be confused with both conjunctivitis and acute glaucoma. Treatment with local cycloplegics and steroids is usually effective within 10 days. However, recurrences are common.

Posterior Uveitis

This disorder is more difficult to diagnose than anterior uveitis, and treatment is much less effective.

Neoplasms of the Uveal Tract

Melanoma is a primary tumor of the uveal tract. Its usual location is in the posterior choroid, where it can be seen with the ophthalmoscope. The method of treatment is determined by the size, location, and growth characteristics of the melanoma. If a melanoma is situated in the iris, iridectomy is usually successful in removing the growth.

VITREOUS

One of the most common of eye complaints is "spots before the eyes." These are usually due to vitreous opacities (visible upon ophthalmoscopic examination). In the absence of significant pathologic findings in the vitreous or retina, the patient may be reassured that they are not serious, only "little spots floating in the jellylike fluid [vitreous] inside the eye."

There is no treatment. With time, the opacities tend to fall inferiorly in the vitreous and thus out of the patient's line of sight. The examiner must bear in mind that vitreous floaters are occasionally the forerunners of retinal detachment.

RETINA

Retinal Detachment

This is an extremely important condition to keep in mind, since the diagnosis is fairly simple, and surgery is often effective if undertaken soon after onset. A complaint of sudden loss of vision, a shower of floaters, "soot," "lightning flashes," or "a curtain coming up [or down] in front of my eye," is an indication for examination with the ophthalmoscope through a dilated pupil for the presence of retinal detachment. This is particularly true if the patient is myopic, has undergone cataract surgery, or has sustained recent trauma.

A patient with retinal detachment should be hospitalized without delay and prepared for surgery. During transportation, a patient with retinal detachment should keep both eyes closed to avoid undue ocular movement. The area of the detachment should be in the dependent position. For example, the patient with a superior temporal retinal detachment of the right eye should be supine with the head turned to the right; if the right inferior nasal retina is detached, the patient should be transported sitting up with the head turned to the left.

Retinoblastoma

Retinoblastoma is the most common intraocular tumor in childhood. Any child with a suspected retinoblastoma should be referred to the ophthalmologist for prompt treatment.

LENS

Cataract

There is no medical treatment for cataract. The only treatment is lens extraction, which is indicated when visual acuity decreases to the point where the patient can no longer lead a normal life. Congenital cataracts should be removed as early as possible to prevent amblyopia.

Dislocated Lens

Lens dislocation may be genetically determined (eg, as one component of Marfan's syndrome) or may be caused by trauma. Visual impairment and secondary glaucoma are the principal indications for lens removal.

OPTIC NERVE

Optic Neuritis

Optic neuritis occurs as a manifestation of several neurologic diseases. It may be the first sign of multiple sclerosis. The presenting complaint is sudden loss of central vision with pain on moving the globe. On ophthalmoscopic examination, the optic disk may appear normal or may be slightly elevated, with increased vascularity. Systemic corticosteroid treatment has not been effective.

The vision ordinarily returns to normal in a matter of weeks.

Papilledema

Papilledema is most commonly caused by increased intracranial pressure, malignant hypertension, or thrombosis of the central retinal vein. It is manifested as an elevation of the optic disk and dilatation of the veins in the optic disk area. Parapapillary hemorrhages may occur. Papilledema can be observed easily with the ophthalmoscope through an undilated pupil. Intracranial tumors in the posterior fossa characteristically produce papilledema because of their blocking effect on the cerebrospinal fluid. Conversely, frontal lobe tumors usually do not produce papilledema. The rate of onset of papilledema after increased intracranial pressure produced by trauma (eg, subdural hematoma) is extremely variable and is of course related to the magnitude of the process. Moderate degrees of papilledema will not affect visual acuity, but the blind spots will be enlarged as shown by central visual field testing.

Optic Atrophy

In this condition, the disk is pale or white. Optic atrophy is usually an end-stage process for which no treatment is available. (See fuller discussion in Chapter 15.)

Visual Field Loss
in Intracranial Diseases

Some tumors of the central nervous system that produce gross visual defects in moderately advanced but still treatable stages can be suspected by the general physician on the basis of confrontation field tests. These include pituitary tumors, meningiomas, and posterior fossa tumors. These patients should be referred to a neurosurgeon for treatment.

STRABISMUS

There are 3 principal objectives in the treatment of strabismus: (1) to develop good visual acuity in each eye; (2) to straighten the eyes, for cosmetic purposes; and (3) to develop coordinate function of the 2 eyes (binocular vision). The best time to initiate nonsurgical treatment of a strabismus patient is by age 6 months. If treatment is delayed beyond this time, the child will favor the straight eye and suppress the image in the other eye; this results in failure of visual development (amblyopia) in the deviating eye. In such a case, patching of the good eye should be instituted without delay.

If the child is under 6 years of age and has an amblyopic eye, the amblyopia can be cured by patching the good eye. At 1 year of age, patching may be successful within 1 week; at 6 years, it may take a year to achieve the same result, ie, to equalize the visual acuity in the 2 eyes.

There is no firm rule about the proper time for surgery. Some surgeons operate as early as age 6 months; in some cases, there may be valid reasons for deferring strabismus surgery. If the visual acuity is equal and the eyes are made reasonably straight with surgery (or with glasses, as in the case of accommodative esotropia), eye exercises (orthoptics) may assist the patient in learning to use the eyes together. This is the seldom achieved ideal result in strabismus therapy. The prognosis is more favorable for strabismus with onset at age 2 or 3 than for strabismus present at birth; better for divergent (outward deviation of the eyes) than for convergent (inward deviation) strabismus; and better for intermittent than for constant strabismus.

GLAUCOMA

Ninety to 95% of glaucoma cases are of the chronic open-angle type. There are no symptoms in the early stages of open-angle glaucoma. The best means of detection is by routine tonometry and ophthalmoscopic inspection of the optic disk in all persons old enough to cooperate. Chronic glaucoma comes on insidiously and causes slowly progressive loss of peripheral vision by damaging the optic nerve. The response to antiglaucoma eye drops is usually good, and surgery is seldom necessary.

Acetazolamide and other carbonic anhydrase inhibitors (eg, dichlorphenamide) have been shown to be extremely effective in inhibiting the production of aqueous by the ciliary body. Consequently, they are helpful as preoperative adjuncts in the treatment of acute glaucoma and in the management of secondary glaucoma. Because of their side effects (particularly renal calculi), long-term therapy of open-angle glaucoma with such drugs is not advisable.

Epinephrine, 0.5–2%, when instilled as drops into the conjunctival sac, lowers the intraocular pressure.

Timolol is one of several beta-adrenergic agents effective in lowering the intraocular pressure by decreasing aqueous production. It is available as drops containing 0.25% and 0.5%.

Pilocarpine continues to be a commonly used antiglaucoma drop.

Laser trabeculoplasty is indicated if topical treatment is ineffective (see Chapter 12).

It is essential to diagnose glaucoma before significant visual loss has occurred, since visual field loss is not reversible. Tonometry, ophthalmoscopy, visual field tests, and gonioscopy are the most important procedures in evaluating and treating a glaucoma patient.

Approximately 5% of cases are angle-closure glaucoma, which produces pain, injection, and blurred vision. The patient seeks treatment immediately because of the pain. Acute glaucoma is treated by laser iridotomy. The laser treatment is preceded by intensive miotic therapy and carbonic anhydrase inhibitors over a period of hours. If miotics and carbonic anhydrase inhibitors do not lower the intraocular pressure sufficiently, glycerin or isosorbide by mouth or intravenous mannitol will nearly always do so within a few hours. Laser iridotomy is occasionally indicated as a preventive measure in patients with normal intraocular pressures who have extremely narrow anterior chamber angles, who are at risk for acute angle-closure glaucoma.

TRAUMA

Chemical Conjunctivitis & Keratitis

This is best treated with irrigation of the eyes with isotonic saline solution or water immediately after exposure. It is wise not to try to neutralize an acid or alkali by using its chemical counterpart, as the heat generated by the reaction may cause further damage. If the chemical irritant is an alkali, the irrigation should be continued for at least 1 hour; this is because alkalies are not precipitated by the proteins of the eye, as acids are, but tend to linger in the tissues, producing further damage for hours after exposure. A local anesthetic solution is instilled before the irrigation to relieve pain. The pupil should be dilated with 5% homatropine or 0.2% scopolamine solution. Collagenase inhibitors such as sodium edetate (EDTA) or acetylcysteine (Mucomyst) are now being used in the treatment of severe alkali burns. Acetylcysteine is available as 10% or 20% solution in a preparation suitable for ophthalmic use. Sodium edetate solution must be specially prepared for the purpose. The patient's own serum (full strength or diluted 2:1) may also be used for its lubricant and mild anticollagenase activity. The patient must be watched carefully for such complications as symblepharon, corneal scarring, closure of the puncta, and secondary infection. Soft contact lenses may sometimes be helpful in such patients.

Lids

Lacerations of the lids not involving the lid margins, no matter how deep, can be sutured just as any other skin laceration. If the lid margin is involved, whether the canaliculi are also involved or not, the patient should be referred for specialized care; permanent notching of the lid margin may occur if the edges are not properly sutured.

Conjunctiva

In minor lacerations of the conjunctiva, sutures are not necessary. To prevent infection, instill an antibiotic 2–3 times a day until the laceration is healed.

Cornea, Sclera; Intraocular Foreign Bodies

The best emergency treatment for a laceration of the cornea or sclera or an intraocular foreign body is to bandage the eye lightly and cover the bandage with a metal shield that rests on the orbital bones superiorly and inferiorly and is held in place with tape passing over the shield from the forehead to the cheek. Examination, manipulation, and eye movement should be kept to the absolute minimum, since any undue pressure on the eye may cause extrusion of the intraocular contents.

OCULAR EMERGENCIES

Ocular emergencies may be classified as true emergencies and urgent cases. A true emergency is defined as one in which a few hours' delay in treatment can lead to permanent ocular damage or extreme discomfort to the patient. An urgent case is one in which treatment should be started as soon as possible but in which a delay of a few days can be tolerated.

TRUE EMERGENCIES

Trauma

Corneal foreign bodies and corneal abrasions must be treated early in order to relieve the progressively more severe pain and irritation. Lacerations of the eyeball should be sutured as soon as possible in order to avoid extrusion of the internal contents of the eye. Intraocular foreign bodies should be removed without delay. It is sometimes possible to remove them through the point of entry with a magnet. Because the ocular media become cloudy if the foreign body is not removed, a foreign body that is visible with the ophthalmoscope shortly after the injury might not be visible several hours or a day later. These procedures are best undertaken by an ophthalmologist.

A foreign body beneath the upper lid is suggested by blepharospasm and a history of foreign body but no foreign body that is visible. Evert the lid by grasping the lashes gently and exerting pressure in the midportion of the outer surface of the upper lid with a cotton applicator. If a foreign body is present on the tarsal conjunctiva, it can be easily seen when the lid is everted and then removed with a wet cotton applicator.

Corneal Ulcer

Corneal tissue is a good culture medium for bacteria, particularly *Pseudomonas aeruginosa*. Specific treatment of any corneal wound or infection by an ophthalmologist should be instituted as soon as possible to avoid corneal perforation and possible loss of the eye.

Severe Conjunctivitis

Most cases of conjunctivitis are not urgent. One exception to this rule is gonococcal conjunctivitis, which has the serious complication of corneal ulceration; a delay in treatment of 1–2 days may result in corneal ulceration or perforation.

Orbital Cellulitis

Orbital cellulitis may be complicated by brain abscess. Immediate treatment with systemic antibiotics is indicated. The bacteriology of orbital cellulitis is similar to that of sinusitis. For example, pneumococci, staphylococci, and *Haemophilus* species are common invaders and require intensive systemic antibiotic therapy.

Chemical Burns

Chemical burns of the external ocular tissues must be treated immediately by copious irrigation with sterile water or saline, if available, or tap water, for at least 5 minutes. Do not use chemical antidotes, since the heat generated by the reaction may increase the degree of injury. After irrigation, instill sterile local anesthetics as necessary to relieve pain, and dilate the pupil. Local corticosteroid therapy may limit the degree of corneal damage. These patients should be referred to an ophthalmologist as soon as possible after injury.

Acute Iritis

Severe acute iritis causes extreme pain and photophobia. The pupil should be dilated as soon as possible to prevent the formation of posterior synechiae, which further increase the possibility of secondary cataract and glaucoma. Slit lamp examination is necessary to confirm the diagnosis.

Acute Glaucoma

If the intraocular pressure is unusually high (60–100 mm Hg), permanent optic nerve damage can occur within 24–48 hours. Therefore, these patients should be referred immediately for definitive care.

Occlusion of the Central Retinal Artery

This is a true emergency because the retina is completely without blood as long as the artery is occluded, and the visual receptors in the retina will degenerate within 30–60 minutes if the flow of blood is not restored. The diagnosis is based upon a history of sudden, complete, painless loss of vision in one eye in an older person and the following ophthalmoscopic findings: pallor of the optic disk, edema of the macula, cherry-red fovea, bloodless arterioles that may be difficult to detect, and "boxcar" segmentation of the blood in the veins.

The best treatment (of value only when the patient is seen within 30–60 minutes of onset) is to pass a sharp instrument such as a No. 11 Bard-Parker blade or No. 30 needle (see p 396) into the anterior chamber. The knife is inserted at the limbus and passed into the anterior chamber on a plane with the iris. The objective is to permit the extrusion of some of the anterior chamber fluid (aqueous) without striking the lens with the knife. This sudden decrease in the intraocular pressure may restore the flow of blood in the central retinal artery. No treatment is required for the wound. There are some favorable reports on the use of anticoagulants in cases of partial occlusion of the central retinal artery or its branches.

Retinal Detachment

Retinal detachment is a true emergency if the macula is threatened. If the macula is detached, permanent loss of central vision usually occurs even though the retina is eventually reattached successfully by surgical means.

URGENT CASES

Strabismus or Anisometropia in a Preschool Child With Amblyopia

The sense of sight develops from birth to about 6 years of age. If a child tends to favor one eye as a result of strabismus or anisometropia, vision may fail to develop in the other eye. These children should be treated without delay with glasses and alternate patching of the eyes. Surgery is performed if indicated after visual acuity has been equalized in the 2 eyes.

Chronic Glaucoma

Antiglaucoma therapy should be instituted without delay in order to decrease the intraocular pressure and preserve the remaining visual field.

Vitreous Hemorrhage

A patient with hemorrhage into the vitreous body should be referred, as the hemorrhage may later clear to reveal a retinal detachment.

Unilateral Exophthalmos of Recent Origin

Exophthalmos most commonly occurs in association with thyroid disease. In some cases of hyperthyroidism, it develops only after thyroidectomy. Unilateral exophthalmos may also be due to an orbital tumor, cavernous sinus thrombosis, or carotid cavernous fistula. These disorders are treatable.

Acute Dacryocystitis

Early treatment with warm compresses and systemic antibiotics is usually effective. If not, surgery is indicated.

Ocular Tumors

Many tumors of the ocular adnexa can be completely excised if they are diagnosed in an early stage. Malignant intraocular tumors (except those of the iris) may require enucleation.

Optic Nerve Disorders

Optic nerve disorders are quite serious and may indicate accompanying intracranial or systemic disease. The patient should be examined from a neurologic as well as an ophthalmologic standpoint.

Sympathetic Ophthalmia

With the availability of effective steroid treatment, sympathetic ophthalmia is now a condition that should be referred for immediate local and systemic corticosteroid or other immunosuppressive therapy. Sympathetic ophthalmia should be suspected if the patient has inflammation in both eyes and a history of penetrating injury to one eye.

PRINCIPLES OF ANTIBIOTIC & CHEMOTHERAPEUTIC TREATMENT OF OCULAR INFECTIONS

In the treatment of infectious eye disease, eg, conjunctivitis, one should always use the drug that is most effective, least likely to cause complications, least likely to be used systemically at a later date, and least expensive. Of the available antibacterial agents, the sulfonamides come closest to meeting these specifications. Two reliable sulfonamides are sulfisoxazole and sodium sulfacetamide. The sulfonamides have the added advantage of low allergenicity. They are available in ointment or solution form.

If sulfonamides are not effective, the antibiotics can be used. One of the most effective broad-spectrum antibiotics for ophthalmic use is gentamicin. It has some effect against gram-negative as well as gram-positive organisms. Other antibiotics frequently used are erythromycin, tetracycline, bacitracin, and polymyxin. Combined bacitracin-polymyxin ointment is often used prophylactically for the protection it affords against both gram-positive (bacitracin) and gram-negative (polymyxin) organisms.

The great majority of antibiotic and chemotherapeutic medications for eye infections are administered locally. Systemic administration is required for all intraocular infections, corneal ulcer, chlamydial conjunctivitis (trachoma and inclusion blennorrhea), orbital cellulitis, dacryocystitis, and any serious external infection that does not respond to local treatment.

Ointments have greater therapeutic effectiveness than solutions, since in this way contact can be maintained for at least 1 hour. However, they do have the disadvantage of causing blurred vision; where this must be avoided, solutions should be used.

Before one can determine the drug of choice, the causative organisms must be known. For example, a pneumococcal corneal ulcer will respond to treatment with a sulfonamide or any broad-spectrum antibiotic, but this is not true in the case of corneal ulcer due to *P aeruginosa,* which responds only to vigorous treatment with polymyxin, colistin, gentamicin, or tobramycin. Another example is staphylococcal dacryocystitis; staphylococci not sensitive to penicillin are most likely to be suceptible to erythromycin or methicillin.

Caution: It is well to keep in mind that the antibiotics, like the steroids, when used over a prolonged period of time in bacterial corneal ulcers, favor the development of secondary fungal infection of the cornea. This is another reason for using the sulfonamides whenever they are adequate for the purpose.

COMMON TECHNIQUES USED IN THE TREATMENT OF OCULAR DISORDERS

Liquid Medications
Place the patient in a sitting position with both eyes open and looking up. Pull down slightly on the lower lid and instill 1 drop in the lower cul-de-sac. The patient is then asked to look down while finger contact on the lower lid is maintained. Do not let the patient squeeze the eye shut.

Ointments
Ointments are instilled in the same way as liquids. While the patient is looking down, lift out the lower lid to trap the medication in the conjunctival sac. The lids should be kept closed for at least 1 minute to allow the ointment to melt.

Eye Bandages
Eye bandages should be applied firmly enough to hold the lid fairly securely against the cornea. A single patch consisting of gauze-covered cotton is usually sufficient. A wraparound head bandage is seldom necessary. Tape is passed from the cheek to the forehead. If more pressure is desired, use 2 or 3 patches.

Warm Compresses
Use a clean towel or washcloth soaked in hot tap water well below the temperature that will burn the thin skin covering the eyelids. Warm compresses are usually applied for 15 minutes 4 times a day. The therapeutic rationale is to increase blood flow to the affected area and decrease pain and inflammation.

Removal of Superficial Corneal Foreign Body
The main considerations are good illumination, magnification, anesthesia, position of the patient, and sterile technique. If possible, the patient's visual acuity is always recorded first.

The patient may be in the sitting or supine position. The examiner should use a loupe unless a slit lamp is available. An assistant should direct a strong flashlight into the eye with the rays of light striking the cornea at an oblique angle. The examiner may then see the corneal foreign body and remove it with a wet cotton applicator. If this is not successful, the foreign body may be removed with a metal spud while the lids are held apart with the other hand to prevent blinking. An antibacterial ointment is instilled after the foreign body has been removed. For more specific anti-infective measures, see Chapter 26.

Most patients are more comfortable without a patch on the eye after removal of a foreign body.

Note: It is essential to see the patient the next day to be certain that no infection has occurred and that healing is under way.

Home Medication

At home, the same techniques should be used as described above except that drops should be instilled with the patient in the supine position. Experienced patients (eg, those with glaucoma) are usually quite skillful in self-administration of eye drops.

COMMON PITFALLS TO BE AVOIDED IN THE MANAGEMENT OF OCULAR DISORDERS

Dangers in the Use of Local Anesthetics

Unsupervised self-administration of local anesthetics is dangerous because the patient may further injure an anesthetized eye without knowing it. Furthermore, most anesthetics delay healing. **Caution:** Do not give patients local anesthetics to take home with them. Eye pain should be controlled by systemic analgesics.

Errors in Diagnosis

Of these the most common is a diagnosis of conjunctivitis when the correct diagnosis is iritis (anterior uveitis), glaucoma, or corneal ulcer (especially herpes simplex). The differentiation between iritis and acute glaucoma may be difficult also.

Misuse of Atropine

Atropine must never be used in routine diagnosis or treatment. It causes cycloplegia (paralysis of the ciliary muscle) of about 14 days' duration and can precipitate an attack of glaucoma if the patient has a narrow anterior chamber angle.

Dangers of Local Corticosteroid Therapy

Local ophthalmologic corticosteroid preparations, eg, prednisolone, are often used for their anti-inflammatory effect on the conjunctiva, cornea, and iris. Although it is true that a patient with conjunctivitis, corneal inflammation, or iritis can be made more comfortable with local corticosteroids, it must be stressed that the corticosteroids are associated with 4 very serious complications when used in the eye over a long period of time: herpes simplex keratitis, open-angle glaucoma, cataract formation, and fungal infection. The most common complications are herpes simplex keratitis and glaucoma. Corticosteroids enhance the activity of the herpes simplex virus, apparently by increasing the destructive effect of collagenase on the collagen of the cornea. This is evidenced by the fact that perforation of the cornea occasionally occurs when the corticosteroids are used during the more active stage of a herpes simplex corneal infection. Corneal perforation was a very rare complication of dendritic keratitis before the corticosteroids came into general use. In the treatment of any corneal inflammation, particularly if the corneal epithelium is not intact, the prolonged use of corticosteroids is sometimes complicated by fungal infection (eg, *Candida albicans*), and this may lead to loss of the eye. Topical corticosteroids can cause or aggravate open-angle glaucoma and, less commonly, can produce cataracts.

For these reasons, although the corticosteroids are valuable in the treatment of ocular disease, any patient on whom they are being used should be watched carefully for the development of complications. The corticosteroids should not be used unless specifically indicated, eg, in iritis, certain types of keratitis, and acute allergic disorders.

Use of Contaminated Eye Medications

The external coats of the eye, including the sclera and the corneal epithelium, are resistant to infection. However, once the corneal epithelium or sclera is broken by trauma, the tissues become markedly susceptible to bacterial infection. For this reason, ophthalmic solutions that may be used in injured eyes must be prepared with the same degree of caution as fluids intended for intravenous administration.

Sterile, single-use disposable units of the common ophthalmic solutions should be used whenever liquid medication is instilled into an injured eye. For routine use in intact eyes, nearly all eye medications are now available in small plastic containers. It is perfectly safe to use these provided they are not kept a long time after opening and are not contaminated accidentally.

Overtreatment

Some patients with chronic conjunctivitis or keratitis may be made worse by overtreatment with topical medications. If a patient is not improving as expected, make certain the preservative in the local medication is not the cause.

REFERENCES

Claoué CMP, Ménage MJ, Easty DL: Severe herpetic keratitis: I. Prevalence of visual impairment in a clinic population. *Br J Ophthalmol* 1988;**72**:530.

Cogan DG: *Ophthalmic manifestations of Systemic Vascular Disease.* Saunders, 1974.

Deutsch TA, Feller DB: *Paton and Goldberg's Management of Ocular Injuries,* 2nd ed. Saunders, 1985.

Ellis PP, Smith DL: *Ocular Therapeutics and Pharmacology,* 7th ed. Mosby, 1985.

Ernest TJ (editor): *Year Book of Ophthalmology* 1987. Year Book, 1988.

Fraunfelder FT: *Drug-Induced Ocular Side Effects and Drug Interactions,* 2nd ed. Lea & Febiger, 1982.

Gardiner PA: *ABC of ophthalmology: Accidents and first*

aid. (ABC of Ophthalmology Series.) *Br Med J* 1978;**2:**1347.

Harrington DO: *The Visual Fields: A Textbook and Atlas of Clinical Perimetry,* 5th ed. Mosby, 1981.

Havener WH: *Ocular Pharmacology,* 5th ed. Mosby, 1983.

Henkind P et al (editorial consultants): *Physicians' Desk Reference (PDR) for Ophthalmology,* 16th ed. Medical Economics, 1988.

Keeney AH: *Ocular Examination: Basis and Techniques,* 2nd ed. Mosby, 1976.

Kennedy RH, Brubaker RF: Traumatic hyphema in a defined population. *Am J Ophthalmol* 1988;**106:**123.

Lariviere M et al: Double-blind study of invermectin and diethylcarbamazine in African onchocerciasis patients with ocuar involvement. *Lancet* 1985;**2:**174.

Macewen CJ: Sport-associated eye injury: A casualty department survey. *Br J Ophthalmol* 1987;**71:**701.

Kolker AE, Hetherington J: *Becker-Shaffer's Diagnosis and Therapy of the Glaucomas,* 5th ed. Mosby, 1983.

Miller NR (editor): *Walsh & Hoyt's Clinical Neuro-ophthalmology,* 4th ed. 3 vols. Williams & Wilkins, 1982, 1984, 1987.

Miller SJ: *Parson's Diseases of the Eye,* 17th ed. Churchill Livingstone, 1984.

Morgan SJ: Chemical burns of the eye: Causes and management. *Br J Ophthalmol* 1987;**71:**854.

Newell FW: *Ophthalmology: Principles and Concepts,* 6th ed. Mosby, 1986.

Owsley C, Sloane ME: Contrast sensitivity, acuity, and the perception of "real-world" targets. *Br J Ophthalmol* 1987;**71:**791.

Phillips CI et al: Blindness in schoolchildren: Importance of heredity, congenital cataract, and prematurity. *Br J Ophthalmol* 1987;**71:**578.

Rothova A et al: Clinical features of acute anterior uveitis. *Am J Ophthalmol* 1987;**103:**137.

Taylor HR et al: Treatment of onchocerciasis: The ocular effects of ivermectin and diethylcarbamazine. *Arch Ophthalmol* 1986;**104:**863.

Tuulonen A, Niva A-K, Alanko HI: A controlled five-year follow-up study of laser trabeculoplasty as primary therapy for open-angle glaucoma. *Am J Ophthalmol* 1987;**104:**334.

Commonly Used Eye Medications

26

Philip P. Ellis, MD

The following is intended to serve as a brief formulary of commonly used ophthalmic drugs. Standard pharmacology and physiology texts should be consulted for more detailed information.

TOPICAL ANESTHETICS

Topical anesthetics are useful for several diagnostic and therapeutic procedures, including tonometry, removal of foreign bodies or sutures, gonioscopy, conjunctival scraping, and minor surgical operations on the cornea and conjunctiva. One or 2 instillations are usually sufficient, but the dosage may be repeated during the procedure.

Tetracaine, proparacaine, and benoxinate are the most commonly used topical anesthetics. For practical purposes, they can be said to have equivalent anesthetic potency.

Other available topical anesthetic solutions include piperocaine (Metycaine) 2%, and cocaine 1–4%.

Note: Topical anesthetics should never be prescribed for home use, since prolonged application may cause corneal complications and mask serious ocular disease.

Tetracaine Hydrochloride (Pontocaine)
Preparations: Solution, 0.5.
Dosage: 1 drop and repeat as necessary.
Onset and duration of action: Anesthesia occurs within 1 minute and lasts for 15–20 minutes.
Comment: Stings considerably on instillation.

Proparacaine Hydrochloride (Ophthaine, others)
Preparation: Solution, 0.5%.
Dosage: 1 drop and repeat as necessary.
Onset and duration of action: Anesthesia begins within 20 seconds and lasts 10–15 minutes.
Comment: Least irritating of the topical anesthetics.

Benoxinate Hydrochloride
Preparation: Solution, 0.4%.
Dosage: 1 drop and repeat as necessary.
Onset and duration of action: Anesthesia begins within 1 or 2 minutes and lasts for 10–15 minutes.

Comment: Activity and duration of action are approximately equivalent to those of proparacaine. Benoxinate is the only anesthetic compatible with fluorescein. These 2 agents are available in a combined solution (Fluress) for use prior to applanation tonometry.

LOCAL ANESTHETICS FOR INJECTION

Lidocaine, procaine, and mepivacaine are commonly used local anesthetics for eye surgery. Longer-acting agents such as bupivacaine and etidocaine are often mixed with other local anesthetics to prolong the duration of effect. Local anesthetics are extremely safe when used with discretion, but the physician must be aware of the potential systemic toxic action when rapid absorption occurs from the site of the injection, with excessive dosage, or following inadvertent intravascular injection.

The addition of hyaluronidase encourages spreading of the anesthetic and shortens the onset to as little as 1 minute. For these reasons, hyaluronidase is commonly used in retrobulbar injections prior to cataract extraction. Up to 4 mL may be injected behind the globe with relative safety. Injectable anesthetics are used by ophthalmologists most commonly in older patients, who may be susceptible to cardiac arrhythmias; therefore, epinephrine should not be used in concentrations greater than 1:200,000.

Lidocaine Hydrochloride (Xylocaine)
Owing to its rapid onset and longer action (1–2 hours), lidocaine has become the most commonly used local anesthetic. It is approximately twice as potent as procaine. Thirty mL of 1% solution, without epinephrine, may be used safely. In cataract surgery, 20 mL is more than adequate. The maximum safe dose is 4.5 mg/kg without epinephrine and 7 mg/kg with epinephrine.

Procaine Hydrochloride (Novocaine)
Preparations: Solution, 1 and 2%.
Dosage: Approximately 50 mL of a 1% solution can be safely injected without systemic effects. The maximum safe dose is 10 mg/kg.
Duration of action: 45–60 minutes.

Mepivacaine Hydrochloride
(Carbocaine, others)
Preparations: Solution, 1 and 2%.
Dosage: Infiltration and nerve block, up to 20 mL of 1 or 2% solution.
Duration of action: Approximately 2 hours.
Comment: Carbocaine is similar to lidocaine in potency. It is usually used in patients who are allergic to lidocaine. The maximum safe dose is 7 mg/kg.

Bupivacaine Hydrochloride
(Marcaine, Sensorcaine)
Preparations: Solution, 0.25, 0.5, and 0.75%.
Dosage: The 0.75% solution has been used most frequently in ophthalmology. The maximum safe dose in an adult is 250 mg with epinephrine and 200 mg without epinephrine. Bupivacaine is frequently mixed with an equal amount of lidocaine.
Onset and duration of action: The onset of action is slower than that of lidocaine, but it persists much longer (up to 4–6 hours).

Etidocaine Hydrochloride
(Duranest)
Preparations: Solution, 1 and 1.5%.
Dosage: The maximum safe dose of etidocaine is 4 mg/kg without epinephrine and 5.5 mg/kg with epinephrine. This agent is frequently mixed with lidocaine for local anesthesia in ophthalmic surgery.
Onset and duration of action: The onset of action is slower than that of lidocaine but more rapid than that of bupivacaine. The duration of action is approximately twice as long as that of lidocaine.

MYDRIATICS & CYCLOPLEGICS

Mydriatics and cycloplegics both dilate the pupil. In addition, cycloplegics cause paralysis of accommodation (patient unable to see near objects, eg, printed words). They are commonly used drugs in ophthalmology, singly and in combination. Their prime uses are (1) for dilating the pupils to facilitate ophthalmoscopy; (2) for paralyzing the muscles of accommodation, particularly in young patients, as an aid in refraction; and (3) for dilating the pupil and paralyzing the muscles of accommodation in uveitis to prevent synechia formation and relieve pain and photophobia. Since mydriatics and cycloplegics both dilate the pupil, they should be used with extreme caution in eyes with narrow anterior chamber angles since either a mydriatic or a cycloplegic can cause angle-closure glaucoma in such eyes.

1. MYDRIATICS
(Sympathomimetics)

Phenylephrine is a mydriatic with no cycloplegic effect.

Phenylephrine Hydrochloride
(Neo-Synephrine, others)
Preparations: Solution, 2.5 and 10%.
Dosage: 1 drop and repeat in 5–10 minutes.
Onset and duration of action: The effect usually occurs within 30 minutes after instillation and lasts 2–3 hours.
Comment: Phenylephrine is used both singly and with cycloplegics to facilitate ophthalmoscopy, in treatment of uveitis, and to dilate the pupil prior to cataract surgery. It is used almost to the exclusion of all other mydriatics. If a patient is allergic to phenylephrine, hydroxyamphetamine hydrobromide (Paredrine) may be substituted. The 10% solution should not be used in newborn infants, in cardiac patients, or in patients receiving reserpine, guanethidine, or tricyclic antidepressants, because of increased susceptibility to the vasopressor effects.

2. CYCLOPLEGICS
(Parasympatholytics)

Atropine Sulfate
Preparations: Solution, 0.25–2%; ointment, 0.5 and 1%.
Dosage: For refraction in children, instill 1 drop of 0.25–0.5% solution or a ¼-inch ribbon of ointment in each eye twice a day for 1 or 2 days before the examination and then 1 hour before the examination.
Onset and duration of action: The onset of action is within 30–40 minutes. A maximum effect is reached in about 2 hours. The effect lasts for up to 2 weeks in a normal eye, but in the presence of acute inflammation the drug must be instilled 2–3 times daily to maintain its effect.
Toxicity: Atropine drops must be used with caution to avoid toxic reactions resulting from systemic absorption. Restlessness and excited behavior with dryness and flushing of the skin of the face, dry mouth, fever, inhibition of sweating, and tachycardia are prominent toxic symptoms, particularly in young children.
Comment: Atropine is an effective and long-acting cycloplegic. In addition to its use for cycloplegia in children, atropine is applied topically 2–3 times daily in the treatment of iritis. It is also used to maintain a dilated pupil after intraocular surgical procedures.

Scopolamine Hydrobromide
Preparation: Solution, 0.25%.
Dosage: 1 drop 2 or 3 times daily.
Onset and duration of action: Cycloplegia occurs in about 40 minutes and lasts for 3–5 days when scopolamine is used as an aid to refraction in normal eyes. The duration of action is much shorter in inflamed eyes.
Toxicity: Scopolamine occasionally causes diz-

ziness and disorientation, mainly in older people.
Comment: Scopolamine is an effective cycloplegic. It is used in the treatment of uveitis, in
refraction of children, and postoperatively.

Homatropine Hydrobromide
Preparations: Solution, 1, 2, and 5%.
Dosage: For refraction, 1 drop in each eye and
repeat 2 or 3 times at intervals of 10–15 minutes.
Onset and duration of action: Maximal cycloplegic effect lasts for about 3 hours, but complete
recovery time is about 36–48 hours. In certain
cases, the shorter action is an advantage over
scopolamine and atropine.
Toxicity: Sensitivity and side effects associated
with the topical instillation of homatropine are
rare.

Cyclopentolate Hydrochloride
(Cyclogyl, others)
Preparations: Solution, 0.5, 1, and 2%.
Dosage: For refraction, 1 drop in each eye and
repeat after 10 minutes.
Onset and duration of action: The onset of dilatation and cycloplegia is within 30–60 minutes.
The duration of action is less than 24 hours.
Comment: Cyclopentolate is more popular than
homatropine and scopolamine in refraction because of its shorter duration of action. Occasionally, neurotoxicity may occur, manifested by
incoherence, visual hallucinations, slurred
speech, and ataxia. These reactions are more
common in children.

Tropicamide
(Mydriacyl, others)
Preparations: Solution, 0.5 and 1%.
Dosage: 1 drop of 1% solution 2 or 3 times at 5-
minute intervals.
Onset and duration of action: The time required to reach the maximum cycloplegic effect
is usually 20–25 minutes, and the duration of this
effect is only 15–20 minutes; therefore, the timing of the examination after instilling tropicamide
is important. Complete recovery requires 5–6
hours.
Comment: Tropicamide is an effective mydriatic
with weak cycloplegic action and is therefore
most useful for ophthalmoscopy.

Cyclopentolate Hydrochloride-
Phenylephrine Hydrochloride
(Cyclomydril)
Preparation: Solution, 1.2% cyclopentolate hydrochloride and 1% phenylephrine hydrochloride.
Dosage: 1 drop every 5–10 minutes for 2 or 3
doses. Pressure should be applied over nasolacrimal sac after drop instillation to minimize systemic absorption.
Onset and duration of action: Mydriasis and

some cycloplegia occur within the first 3–6 minutes. The duration of action is usually less than
24 hours. This drug combination is of particular
value for pupillary dilation in examination of
premature and small infants.

DRUGS USED IN THE TREATMENT OF GLAUCOMA

The concentration used and the frequency of instillation should be individualized on the basis of to-
nometric measurements. Use the smallest dosage that
effectively controls the intraocular pressure and prevents optic nerve damage.

1. DIRECT-ACTING CHOLINERGIC (PARASYMPATHOMIMETIC) DRUGS

Pilocarpine Hydrochloride
Preparations: Solution, 0.5–6%; gel, 4%. Also
available in a sustained-release system (Ocusert).
Dosage: 1 drop up to 6 times a day; a ½-inch
strip of gel in lower conjunctival cul-de-sac at
bedtime.
Comment: Pilocarpine was introduced in 1976
and is still a commonly used antiglaucoma drug.

Carbachol
Preparations: Solution, 0.75–3%.
Dosage: 1 drop in each eye 3–4 times a day.
Comment: Carbachol is poorly absorbed through
the cornea and usually is used if pilocarpine is
ineffective. Its duration of action is 4–6 hours.
If benzalkonium chloride is used as the vehicle,
the penetration of carbachol is significantly increased.

2. INDIRECT-ACTING REVERSIBLE ANTICHOLINESTERASE DRUGS

Physostigmine Salicylate
(Eserine)
Preparations: Solution, 0.25–0.5%.
Dosage: 1 drop 3 or 4 times a day.
Comment: A high incidence of allergic reactions
has limited the use of this old but effective anti-
glaucoma drug. It can be combined in the same
solution with pilocarpine.

Neostigmine Bromide
(Prostigmin)
Preparations: Solution, 2.5–5%.
Dosage: 1 or 2 drops in each eye 2–6 times a
day.

3. INDIRECT-ACTING IRREVERSIBLE ANTICHOLINESTERASE DRUGS

These drugs are strong and long-lasting and are used
when other antiglaucoma medications fail to control

the intraocular pressure. The miosis produced is extreme. Local irritation is common, and phospholine iodide is believed to be cataractogenic in some patients. Pupillary block may occur. (See p 198.)

Isoflurophate (Floropryl)
Preparation: Ointment, 0.025%.
Dosage: A ¼-inch strip of ointment inside lower eyelid once or twice daily.

Echothiophate Iodide (Phospholine Iodide)
Preparations: Solution, 0.03–0.25%.
Dosage: 1 drop once or twice daily or less often, depending upon the response.
Comment: Echothiophate iodide is a long-acting drug similar to isoflurophate that has the advantages of being water-soluble and causing less local irritation. Systemic toxicity may occur in the form of cholinergic stimulation, including salivation, nausea, vomiting, and diarrhea.

Demecarium Bromide (Humorsol)
Preparations: Solution, 0.125 and 0.25%.
Dosage: 1 drop once or twice a day.
Comment: Systemic toxicity similar to that associated with echothiophate iodide may occur.

4. ADRENERGIC (SYMPATHOMIMETIC) DRUGS

In the treatment of glaucoma, epinephrine has the advantages of long duration of action (12–72 hours) and no miosis, which is especially important in patients with incipient cataracts (effect on vision not accentuated). At least 25% of patients develop local allergies; others complain of headache and heart palpitation (less common with dipivefrin).

Epinephrine acts by increasing outflow of aqueous humor.

Some of the preparations available for use in open-angle glaucoma are listed below. The dosage is the same for all, ie, 1 drop once or twice daily:

Epinephryl borate (Epinal, Eppy/N), 0.5 and 1%.
Epinephrine bitartrate (Epitrate, Murocoll), 1% and 2%.
Epinephrine hydrochloride (Epifrin, Glaucon), 0.25, 0.5, 1, and 2%.
Dipivefrin (Propine), 0.1%.

5. BETA-ADRENERGIC BLOCKING DRUGS

Timolol Maleate (Timoptic)
Preparations: Solution, 0.25 and 0.5%.
Dosage: 1 drop of 0.25% solution twice daily. Increase to 1 drop of 0.5% solution in each eye twice daily if needed.

Comment: Timolol maleate is a nonselective beta-adrenergic blocking agent applied topically for treatment of open-angle glaucoma, aphakic glaucoma, and some types of secondary glaucoma. A single application can lower the intraocular pressure for 12–24 hours. Timolol has been found to be effective in some patients with severe glaucoma inadequately controlled by maximum tolerated antiglaucoma therapy with other drugs. The drug does not affect pupillary size or visual acuity. Although timolol is usually well tolerated, it should be prescribed cautiously for patients with known contraindications to systemic use of beta-adrenergic blocking drugs (eg, asthma, heart failure). (See discussion of side effects, below.)

Betaxolol Hydrochloride (Betoptic)
Preparation: Solution, 0.5%.
Dosage: 1 drop twice daily.
Comment: Betaxolol has comparable efficacy to timolol in the treatment of glaucoma. Its relative beta-1 receptor selectivity reduces the risk of pulmonary side effects, particularly in patients with reactive airway disease.

Levobunolol Hydrochloride (Betagan)
Preparation: Solution, 0.5%.
Dosage: 1 drop twice daily.
Comment: Levobunolol is a nonselective beta-1 and beta-2 blocker. It has comparable effects to timolol in the treatment of glaucoma.

6. CARBONIC ANHYDRASE INHIBITORS

Inhibition of carbonic anhydrase in the ciliary body reduces the secretion of aqueous. The oral administration of carbonic anhydrase inhibitors is especially useful in reducing the intraocular pressure in selected cases of open-angle glaucoma and can be used with some effect in angle-closure glaucoma.

The carbonic anhydrase inhibitors in use are sulfonamide derivatives. Oral administration produces the maximum effect in approximately 2 hours; intravenous administration, in 20 minutes. The duration of maximal effect is 4–6 hours following oral administration.

The carbonic anhydrase inhibitors are used in patients whose intraocular pressure cannot be controlled with eye drops. They are valuable for this purpose but have many undesirable side effects, including potassium depletion, gastric distress, diarrhea, exfoliative dermatitis, renal stone formation, shortness of breath, fatigue, acidosis, and tingling of the extremities. Since the advent of timolol and laser therapy, carbonic anhydrase inhibitors are being used less frequently.

Acetazolamide
(Diamox)
Preparations and dosages:
Oral: Tablets, 125 and 250 mg; give 125–250 mg 2–4 times a day (dosage not to exceed 1 g in 24 hours). Sustained-release capsules, 500 mg; give 1 capsule once or twice a day.

Parenteral: May give 500-mg ampules intramuscularly or intravenously for short periods in patients who cannot tolerate the drug orally.

Dichlorphenamide
(Daranide)
Preparation: Tablets, 50 mg.

Dosage: Give a priming dose of 100–200 mg followed by 100 mg every 12 hours until the desired response is obtained. The usual maintenance dosage for glaucoma is 25–50 mg 3–4 times daily. The total daily dosage should not exceed 300 mg daily.

Ethoxzolamide
Preparation: Tablets, 125 mg.
Dosage: 125 mg 2–4 times daily.

Methazolamide (Neptazane)
Preparation: Tablets, 50 mg.
Dosage: 50–100 mg 2 or 3 times daily (total not to exceed 600 mg/d).

7. OSMOTIC AGENTS

Hyperosmotic agents such as urea, mannitol, and glycerin are used to reduce intraocular pressure by making the plasma hypertonic to aqueous humor. These agents are generally used in the management of acute (angle-closure) glaucoma and occasionally in pre- or postoperative surgery when reduction of intraocular pressure is indicated. The dosage for all is approximately 1.5 g/kg.

Urea
(Ureaphil)
Preparation: 30% solution of lyophilized urea in invert sugar.

Dosage: 1–1.5 g/kg intravenously.

Onset and duration of action: Maximum hypotensive effect occurs in about 1 hour and lasts 5–6 hours.

Toxicity: Accidental extravasation at the injection site may cause local reactions ranging from mild irritation to tissue necrosis.

Mannitol
(Osmitrol)
Preparation: 20% solution in water.
Dosage: 1.5–2 g/kg intravenously.
Onset and duration of action: Maximum hypotensive effect occurs in about 1 hour and lasts 5–6 hours.

Glycerin
(Glyrol, Osmoglyn)
Preparations and dosage: Glycerin is usually given orally as 50% solution with water, orange juice, or flavored normal saline solution over ice (1 mL of glycerin weighs 1.25 g). Dose is 1–1.5 g/kg.

Onset and duration of action: Maximum hypotensive effect occurs in 1 hour and lasts 4–5 hours.

Toxicity: Nausea, vomiting, and headache occasionally occur.

Comment: Oral administration and the absence of diuretic effect are significant advantages of glycerin over the other hyperosmotic agents.

TOPICAL CORTICOSTEROIDS

Indications

Topical corticosteroid therapy is indicated for inflammatory conditions of the anterior segment of the globe. Some examples are allergic conjunctivitis, uveitis, episcleritis, scleritis, phlyctenulosis, superficial punctate keratitis, interstitial keratitis, and vernal conjunctivitis.

Administration & Dosage

The corticosteroids and certain derivatives vary in their anti-inflammatory activity. The relative potency of prednisolone to hydrocortisone is 4 times; of dexamethasone and betamethasone, 25 times. The side effects are not decreased with the higher-potency drugs even though the therapeutic dosage is lower.

The duration of treatment will vary with the type of lesion and may extend from a few days to several months.

Initial therapy for a severely inflamed eye consists of instilling drops every 1 or 2 hours during waking hours. When a favorable response is observed, gradually reduce the dosage and discontinue as soon as possible.

Caution: The steroids enhance the activity of the herpes simplex virus, as shown by the fact that perforation of the cornea occasionally occurs when they are used in the eye for treatment of herpes simplex keratitis. Corneal perforation was an extremely rare complication of herpes simplex keratitis before the steroids came into general use. Other side effects of local steroid therapy are fungal overgrowth, cataract formation (unusual), and open-angle glaucoma (common). These effects are produced to a lesser degree with systemic steroid therapy. Any patient receiving local ocular corticosteroid therapy or long-term systemic corticosteroid therapy should be under the care of an ophthalmologist.

A partial list of the available topical corticosteroids for ophthalmologic use is as follows:

Hydrocortisone acetate suspension, 2.5%; ointment, 0.5%.

Prednisolone acetate suspension, 0.125% and 1%.
Prednisolone sodium phosphate solution, 0.125% and 1%.
Dexamethasone sodium phosphate suspension, 0.1%; ointment, 0.05%.
Medrysone suspension, 1%.
Fluorometholone suspension, 0.1% and 0.25%.

MIXTURES OF CORTICOSTEROIDS & ANTI-INFECTIVE AGENTS

There are numerous commercial products containing fixed-dose combinations of corticosteroids and one or more anti-infective agents. They are used by ophthalmologists chiefly to treat conditions in which both agents may be required, eg, marginal keratitis due to a combined staphylococcal infection and allergic reaction, blepharoconjunctivitis, and phlyctenular keratoconjunctivitis. They are also used postoperatively.

These mixtures should not be used to treat conjunctivitis or blepharitis due to unknown causes. They should not be used as substitutes solely for anti-infective agents but only when a clear indication for corticosteroids exists as well. Mixtures of steroids and anti-infective agents may cause all of the same complications that occur with the topical steroid preparations alone.

NONSTEROIDAL ANTI-INFLAMMATORY AGENTS

Occasionally, nonsteroidal anti-inflammatory agents are used to treat ocular inflammatory disorders. Topical preparations of antiprostaglandins have been approved for use only in reducing miosis occurring during intraocular surgery and presumed to be secondary to release of prostaglandins.

Preparation: Flurbiprofen sodium (Ocufen), 0.03%.

OTHER DRUGS USED IN THE TREATMENT OF ALLERGIC CONJUNCTIVITIS

Cromolyn Sodium (Opticrom)
Preparation: Solution, 4%.
Dosage: 1 drop 4–6 times a day.
Comment: Cromolyn is useful in the treatment of many types of allergic conjunctivitis. Response to therapy usually occurs within a few days but sometimes not until treatment is continued for several weeks. Cromolyn acts by inhibiting the release of histamine and SRS-A (slow-reacting substance of anaphylaxis) from mast cells. It is not useful in the treatment of acute symptoms. Soft contact lenses should not be worn during treatment with cromolyn.

ANTI-INFECTIVE OPHTHALMIC DRUGS

1. TOPICAL ANTIBIOTIC SOLUTIONS & OINTMENTS

Antibiotics are commonly used in the treatment of external ocular infection, including bacterial conjunctivitis, styes, marginal blepharitis, and bacterial corneal ulcers. The frequency of use is related to the severity of the condition. Antibiotic treatment of intraocular infection is discussed in Table 26–1.

Table 26–1. Doses of selected antimicrobials in endophthalmitis.[1,2]

	Topical Concentration	Subconjunctival Dose	Usual Adult Intravenous		Intravitreal Dose
			Dose	Frequency	
Amphotericin B (Fungizone)	0.15–0.5%		Varies[3]	Varies[3]	0.005–0.01 mg
Cefamandole (Mandol)	50 mg/mL	75 mg	1 g	6–8 h[4]	1–2 mg
Cefazolin (Ancef, Kefzol)	50 mg/mL	100 mg	1 g	6–8 h	2 mg
Clindamycin (Cleocin)	20 mg/mL	30 mg	0.5–1 g	8 h	0.25 mg
Gentamicin (Garamycin)	8–15 mg/mL	20 mg	70–100 mg	8 h[4]	0.1–0.2 mg
Methicillin (Staphcillin)	1%	100 mg	1 g	6 h	2 mg
Miconazole (Monistat)	10 mg/mL	5 mg	200–600 mg	8 h	0.025 mg
Tobramycin (Nebcin)	8–15 mg/mL	20 mg	70–100 mg	8 h[4]	0.5 mg

[1] Modified and reproduced, with permission, from Parke DW, Brinton GS: Endophthalmitis. In: *Infections of the Eye.* Tabbara KF, Hyndiuk RA (editors). Little, Brown, 1986.
[2] Higher doses have been recommended in some cases by some authors. These doses are considered appropriate by the authors based on drug toxicity studies.
[3] Dose and frequency determined on case-by-case basis.
[4] Nephrotoxic; dose adjusted based on creatinine clearance and weight.

Bacitracin, neomycin, polymyxin, erythromycin, tetracycline, gentamicin, and tobramycin are the most commonly used topical antibiotics. They are used separately and in combination as solutions and as ointments.

Bacitracin

Preparation: Ointment, 500 units/g. Commercially available in combinations with bacitracin and polymyxin B.

Comment: Most gram-positive organisms are sensitive to bacitracin. It is not used systemically because of nephrotoxicity.

Erythromycin

Erythromycin ointment, 0.5% is an effective agent, particularly in staphylococcal conjunctivitis. May be used instead of silver nitrate in prophylaxis of ophthalmia neonatorum.

Neomycin

Preparations: Solution, 2.5–5 mg/mL; ointment, 3.5–5 mg/g. Commercially available in combinations with bacitracin and polymyxin B.

Dosage: Apply ointment or drops 3 or 4 times daily. Solutions containing 50–100 mg/mL have been used for corneal ulcers.

Comment: Effective against gram-negative and gram-positive organisms. Neomycin is usually combined with some other drug to widen its spectrum of activity. It is best known in ophthalmologic practice as Neosporin, both in ointment and solution form, in which it is combined with polymyxin and bacitracin. Contact skin sensivity develops in 5% of patients if the drug is continued for longer than a week.

2. TOPICAL PREPARATIONS OF SYSTEMIC ANTIBIOTICS

Topical use of the antibiotics commonly used systemically should be avoided if possible, because sensitization of the patient may interfere with future systemic use. However, in certain instances clinical judgment overrides this principle if the drug is particularly effective locally and the disorder is serious. A prime example of this is tetracycline in the treatment of trachoma, the commonest eye infection in the world.

Tetracyclines

Preparations: Solution, 10 mg/mL; ointment, 10 mg/g.

Comment: Tetracycline, oxytetracycline, and chlortetracycline have limited uses in ophthalmology because their effectiveness is so often impaired by the development of resistant strains. Solutions of these compounds are unstable with the exception of Achromycin in sesame oil, which is widely used in the treatment of tra-

choma. Ointment may be used for prophylaxis of ophthalmia neonatorum.

Gentamicin (Garamycin, Genoptic, Gentacidin)

Preparations: Solution, 3 mg/mL; ointment, 3 mg/g.

Comment: Gentamicin is widely accepted for use in serious ocular infections, especially corneal ulcers caused by gram-negative organisms. It is also effective against many gram-positive staphylococci but is not effective against streptococci.

Tobramycin (Tobrex)

Preparations: Solution, 3 mg/mL; ointment, 3 mg/g.

Comment: Similar antimicrobial activity to gentamicin but more effective against streptococci. Best reserved for treatment of *Pseudomonas* keratitis, for which it is more effective.

Chloramphenicol

Preparations: Solution, 5–10 mg/mL; ointment, 10 mg/g.

Comment: Chloramphenicol is effective against a wide variety of gram-positive and gram-negative organisms. It rarely causes local sensitization, but cases of aplastic anemia have occurred with long-term therapy.

3. COMBINATION ANTIBIOTIC AGENTS

Several ophthalmic preparations are available that contain a mixture of antibiotics.

Drug	Trade Name
Bacitracin and polymyxin B	Polysporin, Ocumycin
Bacitracin (gramicidin), neomycin, and polymyxin B	Mycirtracin, Neosporin Ocutricin, AK-Spore
Oxytetracycline and polymyxin B	Terramycin-Polymyxin B
Neomycin and polymyxin B	Statrol

4. SULFONAMIDES

The sulfonamides are the most commonly used drugs in the treatment of bacterial conjunctivitis. Their advantages include (1) activity against both gram-positive and gram-negative organisms, (2) relatively low cost, (3) low allergenicity, and (4) the fact that their use is not complicated by secondary fungal infections, as sometimes occurs following prolonged use of antibiotics.

The commonest sulfonamides employed are sulfisoxazole and sulfacetamide sodium.

Sulfacetamide Sodium (Sulamyd)

Preparations: Ophthalmic solution, 10 and 30%; ointment, 10%.

Dosage: Instill 1 drop frequently, depending upon the severity of the conjunctivitis.

Sulfisoxazole
(Gantrisin)
Preparations: Ophthalmic solution, 4%; ointment, 4%.
Dosage: As for sulfacetamide sodium (above).

5. TOPICAL ANTIFUNGAL AGENTS

Natamycin
(Natacyn)
Preparation: 5% suspension.
Dosage: Instill 1 drop every 1–2 hours.
Comment: Effective against filamentary and yeast forms. Initial drug of choice for most mycotic corneal ulcers.

Nystatin
(Mycostatin)
Not available in ophthalmic ointment form, but the dermatologic preparation (100,000 units/g) is not irritating to ocular tissues and can be used in the treatment of fungal infection of the eye.

Amphotericin B
(Fungizone)
More effective than nystatin but not available in ophthalmic ointment form. The dermatologic preparation is highly irritating. A solution (0.5–1.5 mg/mL of distilled water in 5% dextrose) must be made up in the pharmacy from the powdered drug. Many patients have extreme ocular discomfort following application of this drug.

Miconazole
(Monistat)
A 1% solution is available in the form of an intravenous preparation that may be applied directly into the eye. The drug is not available in an ophthalmologic form.

6. ANTIVIRAL AGENTS

Idoxuridine
(Dendrid, Herplex, Stoxil)
Preparations: Ophthalmic solution, 0.1%; ointment, 0.5%.
Dosage: 1 drop every hour during the day and every 2 hours at night. With improvement (as determined by fluorescein staining), the frequency of instillation is gradually reduced. The ointment may be used 4–6 times daily, or the solution may be used during the day and the ointment at bedtime.
Comment: Used in the treatment of herpes simplex keratitis. Epithelial infection usually improves within a few days. Therapy should be continued for 3 or 4 days after apparent healing.

Many ophthalmologists still prefer to denude the affected corneal epithelium and not use idoxuridine.

Vidarabine
(Adenine Arabinoside, Vira-A)
Preparation: Ophthalmic ointment, 3%.
Dosage: In herpetic epithelial keratitis, apply 4 times daily for 7–10 days.
Comment: Vidarabine is effective against herpes simplex virus but not other RNA or DNA viruses. It is effective in some patients unresponsive to idoxuridine. Vidarabine interferes with viral DNA synthesis. The principal metabolite is arabinosylhypoxanthine (Ara-Hx). The drug is effective against herpetic corneal epithelial disease and has limited efficacy in stromal keratitis or uveitis. It may cause cellular toxicity and delay corneal regeneration. The cellular toxicity is less than that of idoxuridine.

Trifluridine
(Viroptic)
Preparation: 1% solution.
Dosage: One drop every 2 hours (maximum total, 9 drops daily).
Comment: Acts by interfering with viral DNA synthesis. More soluble than either idoxuridine or vidarabine and probably more effective in stromal disease.

Acyclovir
(Zovirax)
Acyclovir (acycloguanosine) is a new antiviral agent, which shows great promise in the treatment of herpes simplex and herpes zoster infections. It is phosphorylated initially by virus-specified thymidine kinase to acyclovir monophosphate and then by cellular kinases to acyclovir triphosphate, which inhibits viral DNA polymerase. Thus, there is a marked selectivity for virus-infected cells. Acyclovir has low toxicity except for crystal deposition in renal tubules when used at high doses or when urine output is poor. No commercial ophthalmic preparation is currently available in the USA; a topical product available for treatment of genital herpes should not be used in the eye. An oral preparation is available that may be used for treatment of selected herpes zoster ocular infections.

DIAGNOSTIC DYE SOLUTIONS

Sodium Fluorescein
Preparations: Solution, 2%, in single-use disposable units; as sterile paper strips; as 10% sterile solution for intravenous use in fluorescein angiography.
Dosage: 1 drop.

Comment: Used as a diagnostic agent for detection of corneal epithelial defects, in applanation tonometry, and in fitting contact lenses.

Rose Bengal
Preparation: Solution, 1%.
Dosage: 1 drop.
Comment: Used in diagnosis of keratoconjunctivitis sicca; the mucous shreds and devitalized corneal epithelium stain with rose bengal.

TEAR REPLACEMENT & LUBRICATING AGENTS

Methylcellulose and related chemicals, polyvinyl alcohol and related chemicals, and gelatin are used in the formulation of artificial tears, ophthalmic lubricants, contact lens solutions, and gonioscopic lens solutions. These agents are particularly useful in the treatment of keratoconjunctivitis sicca. (See Chapter 4.)

To increase viscosity and prolong corneal contact time, methylcellulose is sometimes added to eye solutions (eg, pilocarpine).

VASOCONSTRICTORS & DECONGESTANTS

There are many commercially available OTC (over-the-counter) ophthalmic vasoconstrictive agents. The active ingredients in these agents usually are either ephedrine 0.123%, naphazoline 0.012–0.1%, phenylephrine 0.12%, or tetrahydrozoline 0.05–0.15%.

These agents constrict the superficial vessels of the conjunctiva and relieve redness. They also relieve minor surface irritation and itching of the conjunctiva, which can represent a response to noxious or irritating agents such as smog, swimming pool chlorine, etc. Products also are available that contain an antihistamine, antazoline phosphate 0.25–0.5%, or pheniramine maleate 0.3%.

CORNEAL DEHYDRATING AGENTS

Dehydrating solutions and ointments applied topically to the eye reduce corneal edema by creating an osmotic gradient in which the tear film is made hypertonic to the corneal tissues. Temporary clearing of corneal edema results.
Preparations: Anhydrous glycerin (Ophthalgan), hypertonic sodium chloride 2% and 5% (Absorbonac, Hypersal, Muro-128)
Dosage: 1 drop to clear cornea. May be repeated every 3–4 hours.

OCULAR & SYSTEMIC SIDE EFFECTS OF DRUGS

F.T. Fraunfelder, MD, & S. Martha Meyer, BS

Both systemically and topically administered drugs can produce adverse ocular effects, and topical ophthalmic preparations occasionally lead to systemic effects if too much active ingredient is absorbed. Preservatives in drugs may also be associated with side effects.

Tables 26–2 to 26–4 list possible ocular and systemic side effects of some ocular and systemic medications. This is not in any way a complete listing of all drugs and their side effects. The information has been compiled from various sources. Physicians are advised to consult product labels, the references at the end of this chapter, and other appropriate sources for further information.

SYSTEMIC SIDE EFFECTS OF TIMOLOL

One example of an ocular drug with which serious side effects may occur is timolol. Timolol by topical administration is the most commonly used antiglaucoma medication in the world and has been associated with severe, even fatal, reactions. Plasma drug concentrations sufficient to cause systemic beta-adrenoceptor blocking effects can occasionally result from ocular administration. When topical ocular timolol is administered in infants, blood levels are often more than 6 times what minimum therapeutic levels would be if the drug were given orally for some other condition; these high blood levels may be present for many hours after administration. If the lacrimal system is not closed during administration, an estimated 80% of a timolol eye drop is absorbed from the nasal mucosa and passes almost directly into the vascular system. Because the drug can reach target organs before it is detoxified in the liver, the blood level following topical ophthalmic administration is proportionately higher than when the drug is given orally, as in hypertension. A genetic fault in the oxidative metabolism of beta blockers has been detected in some patients, and significantly higher levels of plasma concentrations develop in poor metabolizers.

Cardiopulmonary histories should be taken for candidates for beta-blocker glaucoma therapy. Pulmonary function studies should be considered in patients with bronchoconstrictive disease, and electrocardiograms should be ordered on selected patients with cardiac disease. Specifically, the precautions set forth in the package insert should be heeded carefully. Patients with known bronchial asthma, chronic respiratory or cardiovascular disease, or sinus bradycardia should avoid using timolol. The drug should be used with

Table 26–2. Possible adverse ocular effects of systemic drugs.

Drug	Adverse Effects	Drug	Adverse Effects
Allopurinol	Cataract	Ketamine	Nystagmus
Amiodarone	Corneal opacity	Methyldopa	Conjunctivitis
Amphetamines	Elevation of intraocular pressure	Monoamine oxidase inhibitors	Optic atrophy
Antibiotics	Conjunctivitis, keratitis		
Anticholinergics	Elevation of intraocular pressure	Morphine	Optic neuritis
Anticoagulants	Retinal hemorrhage	Nalidixic acid	Papilledema
Barbiturates	Conjunctivitis, Stevens-Johnson syndrome, ptosis, optic atrophy	Naproxen	Corneal opacity
		Oral contraceptives	Retinal occlusion, retinal hemorrhage, retinal edema, retinal vasospasm, corneal edema, nystagmus, papilledema
Busulfan	Cataract		
Cardiac glycosides	Retinal degeneration		
Chloral hydrate	Conjunctivitis		
Chlorambucil	Papilledema	Penicillamine	Extraocular muscle paralysis, ptosis, optic neuritis
Chloramphenicol	Optic atrophy, optic neurits		
Chloroquine	Corneal opacity, retinal degeneration	Phenothiazines	Conjunctival deposits, corneal opacity, oculogyric crisis, pigmentation of lens, retinal degeneration
Chlorpropamide	Stevens-Johnson syndrome, corneal opacity, extraocular muscle paralysis		
		Phenylbutazone	Conjunctivitis, keratitis, retinal hemorrhage
Clofazimine	Conjunctival deposits, corneal opacity		
Corticosteroids	Elevation of intraocular pressure, cataract	Phenytoin	Nystagmus, extraocular muscle paralysis
Diazepam	Nystagmus	Quinacrine	Conjunctival deposits
Disulfiram	Optic neuritis	Quinine	Retinal edema, retinal vasodilation followed by vasoconstriction
Ethambutol	Optic neuritis		
Gold salts	Conjunctival deposits, corneal opacity, nystagmus, pigmentation of lens	Rifampin	Optic neurtis
		Salicylates	Nystagmus, retinal hemorrhage
		Streptomycin	Optic neuritis
Guanethidine	Ptosis	Sulfonamides	Conjunctivitis, Stevens-Johnson syndrome, retinal hemorrhage
Haloperidol	Contaract		
Hexamethonium	Retinal vasodilation	Tetracycline	Papilledema
Indomethacin	Corneal opacity	Tricyclic antidepressants	Elevation of intraocular pressure
Iodoquinol	Optic atrophy	Vitamin A	Conjunctival deposits, papilledema
Isoniazid	Optic neuritis	Vitamin D	Conjunctival deposits, corneal opacity
Isotretinoin	Conjunctivits, corneal opacity, papilledema		

caution in patients receiving other systemic beta-blocking agents.

WAYS TO DIMINISH SYSTEMIC SIDE EFFECTS

One important principle in avoiding systemic side effects from topical ophthalmic medications is to prevent overdosing. The physician should prescribe the lowest concentration of medication that will be therapeutically effective. Only 1 drop of medication is needed at each dosage, since the volume the eye can hold is less than 1 drop.

The proper method of topical administration of ophthalmic medications is as follows:

Position the patient with head tilted back toward the ceiling. Grasp the lower eyelid below the lashes and gently pull the lid away from the eye (Fig 26–1). Instill 1 drop of medication into the inferior cul-de-sac nearest the involved area, being careful not to touch the lashes or eyelids and thus avoid contamination (Fig 26–2). The lower eyelid should then be gently lifted to make contact with the upper lid (Fig 26–3). Patients should position their heads so that gravity will keep the drug where medically indicated. The eyelids should be kept closed for 3 minutes or more to prevent blinking, which pumps the drug into

the nose and increases systemic absorption. The patient should be shown how to obstruct the lacrimal drainage system with firm pressure over the inner corner of the closed eyelids (Fig 26–4). Excess medication in the medial canthus should be blotted away before pressure is released or the eyelids opened. The patient receiving multiple topical medications should wait 10 minutes between doses, so that the first drug will not be washed out of the eye by the second.

NATIONAL REGISTRY OF DRUG-INDUCED OCULAR SIDE EFFECTS

The National Registry of Drug-Induced Ocular Side Effects is a clearinghouse of drug information on ocular toxicology. The principle underlying its establishment is the assumption that the suspicions of practicing clinicians regarding possible ocular toxicity of drugs can be pooled to increase the data base and decrease the lag time in recognizing adverse responses. Physicians who wish to report suspected adverse drug reactions or would like to receive references pertaining to the data in Tables 26–2 to 26–4 should call or write the Department of Ophthalmology, Oregon Health Sciences University, 3181 S.W. Sam Jackson Park Road, Portland, OR 97201, (503) 279–8456.

Table 26–3. Possible adverse systemic effects of topical ocular medications.

Medication	Adverse Effects
Anesthetics, topical local	
Benoxinate	Allergic reactions, anaphylactic reactions, convulsions, faintness, hypotension, syncope
Proparacaine	Same as benoxinate
Tetracaine	Same as benoxinate
Antibiotics	
Chloramphenicol	Allergic reactions; bone marrow depression, including aplastic anemia; gastrointestinal symptoms
Chlortetracycline	Photosensitivity, skin discoloration
Sulfacetamide	Photosensitivity, Stevens-Johnson syndrome
Sulfamethizole	Same as sulfacetamide
Sulfisoxazole	Same as sulfacetamide
Tetracycline	Same as chlortetracycline
Anticholinergics	
Atropine	Confusion, dermatitis, dry mouth, excitement, fever, flushed skin, hallucinations, psychosis, tachycardia, thirst
Cyclopentolate	Amnesia, ataxia, convulsions, disorientation, dysarthria, fever, hallucinations, psychosis
Homatropine	Same as atropine
Scopolamine	Same as atropine
Tropicamide	Same as cyclopentolate
Anticholinesterases, long-acting	
Demecarium	Abdominal cramps, diarrhea, fatigue, nausea, rhinorrhea, weight loss
Echothiophate	Same as demecarium
Isoflurophate	Same as demecarium
Anticholinesterases, short-acting	
Neostigmine	Abdominal cramps, depigmentation, diarrhea, nausea, vomiting
Physostigmine	Same as neostigmine
Beta-adrenoceptor blocking agent	
Timolol	Asthma, bradycardia, cardiac arrhythmia, confusion, depression, dizziness, dyspnea, hallucinations, impotence, myasthenia, psychosis
Parasympathomimetics	
Carbachol	Abdominal cramps, diarrhea, hypotension, increased salivation, muscle tremors, nausea, respiratory distress, rhinorrhea, slurred speech, sweating, vomiting, weakness
Pilocarpine	Same as carbachol
Sympathomimetics	
Ephedrine	Cardiac arrhythmia, hypertension, palpitations, subarachnoid hemorrhage, tachycardia
Epinephrine	Same as ephedrine
Hydroxyamphetamine	Same as ephedrine
Phenylephrine	Same as ephedrine

Table 26–4. Possible adverse ocular effects of topical ocular medications.

Medication	Adverse Effects
Anesthetics, local	
Butacaine	Allergic reactions, corneal opacity, decreased corneal wound healing, iritis
Proparacaine	Same as butacaine
Tetracaine	Same as butacaine
Antibiotics	
Chlortetracycline	Allergic reactions, corneal, corneal discoloration
Neomycin	Allergic reactions, follicular conjunctivitis, keratitis
Tetracycline	Same as chlortetracycline
Anticholinergics	
Cyclopentolate	Angle-closure glaucoma, blurred vision, photophobia
Tropicamide	Same as cyclopentolate
Anticholinesterases, long-acting	
Demecarium	Accommodative spasm, cataract, depigmentation of lids, iris cysts, lacrimal outflow obstruction
Echothiophate	Same as demecarium
Isoflurophate	Same as demecarium
Anti-inflammatory agents	
Corticosteroids	Cataracts, corneal thinning, decreased corneal wound healing, glaucoma, infection
Antivirals	
Idoxuridine	Cicatricial pseudopemphigoid, keratitis, lacrimal outflow obstruction
Trifluridine	Same as idoxuridine
Vidarabine	Same as idoxuridine
Beta-adrenoceptor blocking agent	
Timolol	Blepharoconjunctivitis, corneal anesthesia, diplopia, dry eyes, keratitis, ptosis
Parasympathomimetic	
Pilocarpine	Accommodative spasm, cicatricial pseudopemphigoid, corneal haze (gel), myopia, retinal detachment
Preservatives	
Benzalkonium chloride	Allergic reactions, corneal opacity, keratitis
Phenylmercuric nitrate	Same as benzalkonium chloride
Thimerosal	Same as benzalkonium chloride
Sympathomimetics	
Dipivefrin	Allergic reactions, angle-closure glaucoma, follicular conjunctivitis
Epinephrine	Cicatricial pseudopemphigoid; cystoid macular edema; discoloration of cornea, conjunctiva, and soft contact lens; lacrimal outflow obstruction

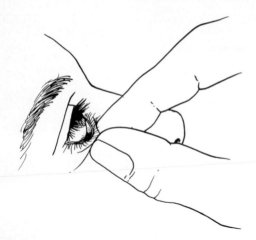

Figure 26–1. With the patient's head tilted back toward the ceiling, grasp the lower eyelid below the lashes and gently pull the lid away from the eye.

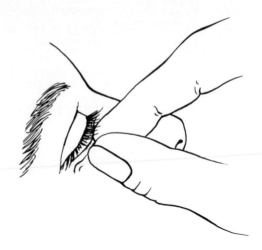

Figure 26–3. While the patient is looking downward, gently lift the lower eyelid to make contact with the upper lid.

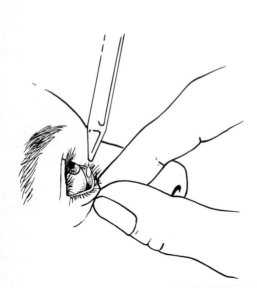

Figure 26–2. One drop of solution or a "match head" amount of ointment should be placed in the inferior cul-de-sac, without touching the bottle to the lashes or eyelids (to prevent contamination).

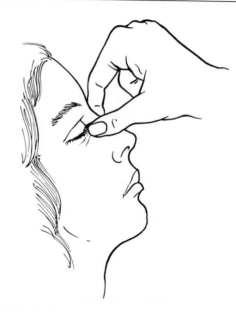

Figure 26–4. For 3 minutes or more, firm pressure is maintained with the forefinger or thumb over the inner corner of the closed eyelids. Any excess medication should be blotted away before pressure is released or the eye is opened.

REFERENCES

American Medical Association: *Drug Evaluations,* 6th ed. Saunders, 1987.

Baum J: Therapy for ocular bacterial infection. *Trans Ophthalmol Soc UK* 1986;**105:**69.

Davidson SI, Rennie IG: Ocular toxicity from systemic drug therapy: An overview of clinically important adverse reactions. *Med Toxicol* 1986;**1:**217.

Dukes MN, Beeley L (editors): *Side Effects of Drugs,* 11th ed. Elsevier, 1987.

Ellis PP: *Ocular Therapeutics and Pharmacology,* 7th ed. Mosby, 1985.

Foster CS: Evaluation of topical cromolyn sodium in the treatment of vernal keratoconjunctivitis: From the

Cromolyn Sodium Collaborative Study Group. *Ophthalmology* 1988;**95**:194.

Fraunfelder FT: *Drug-Induced Ocular Side Effects and Drug Interactions,* 3rd ed. Lea & Febiger, 1989.

Fraunfelder FT, Roy FH (editors): *Current Ocular Therapy,* 2nd ed. Saunders, 1984.

Grant WM: *Toxicology of the Eye,* 3rd ed. Thomas, 1986.

Havener WH: *Ocular Pharmacology,* 5th ed. Mosby, 1983.

Kahán A: Developmental implications of ocular pharmacology. *Pharmacol Ther* 1985;**28**:163.

Koneru PB et al: Oculotoxicities of systemically administered drugs. *J Ocular Pharmacol* 1986;**2**:385.

Lamberts DW, Potter DE (editors): *Clinical Ocular Pharmacology.* Little, Brown, 1987.

Lee VH, Robinson JR: Topical ocular drug delivery: Recent developments and future challenges. *J Ocular Pharmacol* 1986;**2**:67.

Leopold IH: Recent developments in chemotherapy of ocular disease. *J Ocular Pharmacol* 1986;**2**:185.

McCloskey RV: Topical antimicrobial agents and antibiotics for the eye. *Med Clin North Am* 1988;**72**:717.

Palmer EA: How safe are ocular drugs in pediatrics? *Ophthalmology* 1986;**93**:1038.

Penna EP, Tabbara KF: Oxybuprocaine keratopathy: A preventable disease. *Br J Ophthalmol* 1986;**70**:202.

Sears ML (editor): *Pharmacology of the Eye.* Springer-Verlag, 1984.

Sears ML, Tarkkanen A (editors): *Surgical Pharmacology of the Eye.* Raven Press, 1985.

Shuster JN: Side effects of commonly used glaucoma medications. *Geriatr Ophthalmol* 1986;**2**:30.

Zun LS et al: Formulary of commonly used ophthalmologic medications. *Emerg Med Clin North Am* 1988;**6**:121.

27

Lasers in Ophthalmology

James B. Wise, MD

Ophthalmology was the first surgical specialty to utilize laser energy in patient treatment, and it still accounts for more laser operations than any other specialty. Unlike other body tissues, the optical media of the eye are transparent, allowing laser light to be focused upon the intraocular structures without the need for endoscopy. By use of laser therapy, treatment of a number of serious ocular diseases has become much safer and more effective.

OCULAR LASER SYSTEMS

The word "laser" is an acronym for *l*ight *a*mplification by *s*timulated *e*mission of *r*adiation. A laser consists of a transparent crystal rod (solid-state laser) or a gas- or liquid-filled cavity (gas or fluid laser) constructed with a fully reflective mirror at one end and a partially reflective mirror at the other. Surrounding the rod or cavity is an optical or electrical source of energy that will raise the energy level of the atoms within the rod or cavity to a high and unstable level—called a population inversion—from which the excited atoms will spontaneously decay back to a lower energy level, releasing their excess energy in the form of light. This light can be emitted in any direction. In the laser cavity, however, light emitted in the long axis of the cavity can bounce back and forth between the mirrors, setting up a standing wave that stimulates the remaining excited atoms to release their energy into the standing wave, producing an intense beam of light that exits the cavity through the partially reflective mirror. The light beam thus produced is all of the same wavelength (monochromatic), with all of the light waves in phase with each other (coherent). The light waves follow closely parallel courses, with almost no tendency to spread out with distance.

These unique properties of laser light allow the beam to be focused down to extremely small spots, resulting in very high energy densities that are the basis of the tissue-altering effects. In some lasers, such as the Q-switched Nd:YAG laser, all the light energy is released in a few nanoseconds to produce temperatures in excess of 10,000 °C at the point of focus.

MECHANISMS OF LASER EFFECTS

Photocoagulation

The principal lasers used in ophthalmic therapy are the thermal lasers, which depend upon absorption of the laser light by tissue pigments. The absorbed light is converted into heat, thus raising the temperature of the target tissue high enough to coagulate and denature the cellular components. These lasers can be used to destroy intraocular neovascularization, as in diabetic retinopathy; to shrink collagen, increasing tension in the trabecular meshwork or iris for treatment of retinal holes; and, at higher energy levels, to evaporate tissue and thus produce perforations, as in laser iridotomy. Although the original—now obsolete—ruby laser photocoagulator produced a pulse duration of about 1 ms, the laser photocoagulators now in use operate in continuous mode or very rapidly pulsed (thermal) mode. The blue-green argon laser is the workhorse of this class. Because laser light is monochromatic, selective absorption into specific tissues is possible with some wavelengths, sparing other tissues. Examples are the argon laser in green-only mode, the red krypton laser, the yellow and orange wavelengths of the tunable dye laser, and the infrared beam of the neodymium:YAG laser in thermal mode.

Photodisruption

Photodisruptor lasers are the other major class of ophthalmic lasers. They release a giant pulse of energy with a pulse duration of a few nanoseconds. When this pulse is focused to a 15–25 μm spot, so that the nearly instantaneous light pulse exceeds a critical level of energy density, "optical breakdown" occurs in which the temperature rises so high (about 10,000 °C) that electrons are stripped from atoms, resulting in a physical state known as a plasma. This plasma expands with momentary pressures as high as 10 kilobars (150,000 psi), exerting a cutting effect upon the ocular tissues. Because the initial plasma size is so small, it has little total energy and produces little effect away from the point of focus. Though a significant shock wave is produced, studies on polyethylene membranes indicate that direct contact with the plasma is required for cutting tissue.

Photodisruptors are used principally for perforating

cloudy posterior capsules after cataract extraction and for performing laser iridotomy. The only commercial ophthalmic laser of this class is the Q-switched neodymium:YAG laser. Mode-locked neodymium:YAG lasers are still in use but are no longer being manufactured.

Photoevaporation

Photoevaporator lasers are represented by the carbon dioxide laser, which produces a long-wavelength infrared heat beam. The beam is absorbed by water and therefore will not enter the interior of the eye. This laser can evaporate away surface lesions such as lid tumors and can be used for bloodless incisions in skin or sclera, but it causes too much scarring to be useful for ocular plastic surgery. The carbon dioxide laser beam can also be delivered through probes for contact photoincision and photocoagulation within the eye.

Photodecomposition

Photodecomposition lasers produce very short wavelength ultraviolet light that interacts with the chemical bonds of biologic materials, breaking the bonds and converting biologic polymers into small molecules that diffuse away. These lasers collectively are called **excimer** (''excited dimer'') lasers because the cavity contains 2 gases, such as argon and fluorine, that react into unstable molecules which then emit the laser light. At present experimental with no approved human uses, they offer the possibility of altering the focusing strength of the eye by ultraprecise corneal incisions or by precise recontouring of the corneal surface via computer-controlled ablation of the thin layers of the cornea.

THERAPEUTIC APPLICATIONS

Retinal Photocoagulation

Retinal photocoagulation was the first application of ophthalmic lasers and evolved from use of the xenon arc photocoagulator for this purpose.

Diabetic Retinopathy

Many patients with long-term diabetes mellitus will gradually develop diffuse obliteration of the retinal microcirculation—especially of the capillaries—resulting in generalized retinal ischemia. This ischemia state leads to retinal neovascularization, which is at least partly mediated by diffusible vasoproliferative factors released from the ischemic retina into the ocular fluids. The first sign of diabetic retinopathy is the appearance of tiny intraretinal microaneurysms, typically just temporal to the macula and along the arcades. This is followed by flat neovascularization with blot hemorrhages and round neovascular clumps, then by feathery neovascular tufts that can grow on the retina (retinal rubeosis) or spread from the disk. The proliferative stage is entered when these tufts leave

the plane of the retina and begin to grow up into the vitreous either from the retinal surface or from the disk. Proliferating scar tissue sheets now appear, spreading on the retinal surface and extending up into the vitreous; and as these sheets exert traction upon the abnormal vessels, vitreous hemorrhage occurs and accelerates the fibrotic process. The progressive vitreous traction then leads to retinal detachment and blindness. Vision can also be impaired by macular edema and exudates from leaking paramacular microaneurysms.

Laser treatment is performed in 2 ways. Focal photocoagulation of the abnormal vessels with argon blue-green or argon green laser light can be used to stop hemorrhage, destroy threatening neovascular areas, and thrombose leaking aneurysms. However, focal treatment alone is not sufficient because the neovascularization tends to recur and because elevated neovascularization off the disk or elsewhere cannot be treated. The second method of treatment, called panretinal photocoagulation or retinal ablation, consists of peppering the entire retina, except for the area within the arcades, with 500-μm laser burns placed one or 2 burn widths apart (Fig 27–1). This treatment uses 1000–2000 burns, usually delivered over 2–4 sessions of treatment, with the sessions given about 2 weeks apart. While the exact mechanism of action is unproved, panretinal photocoagulation causes the neovascular areas to wither away so that the retinopathy becomes inactive and new vessels cease to appear. Direct treatment of neovascularization is not necessary with this method, as ablation with the krypton red laser is quite effective even though this wavelength is poorly absorbed by hemoglobin. The treatment must be given in sessions of 500–600 burns each because excessive treatment at one time can cause uveitis, macular edema, exudative retinal detachment, and even shallowing of the anterior chamber with angle closure. Panretinal photocoagulation properly used is highly effective in producing regression of neovascularization, but established fibrosis will remain and can continue to produce retinal traction. Vitreous hemorrhage can prevent treatment of the retina with the laser. Therefore, panretinal photocoagulation should be used as soon as high-risk characters are noted, before irreversible changes have occurred. These high-risk characters include rapid increase in neovascularization associated with signs of ischemia (cotton-wool spots, occluded or very narrow vessels), macular edema, retinal rubeosis, and early proliferations from disk or retina. Laser therapy should be given before significant visual decrease has occurred—and certainly before advanced changes such as vitreous hemorrhage and fibrosis occur. Because timely laser therapy is so effective in preventing blindness in diabetes, any diabetic with retinopathy greater than scattered microaneurysms should be seen on a regular basis by a laser-qualified ophthalmologist.

Central Retinal Vein Thrombosis

Central retinal vein thrombosis produces the classic

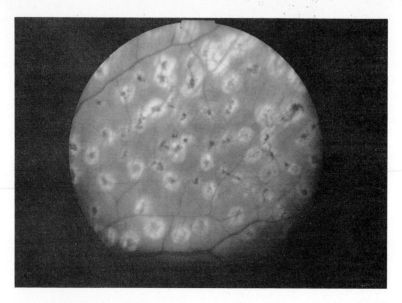

Figure 27–1. Argon laser photocoagulation scars in the retina.

fundus appearance of papilledema, marked venous dilatation, and almost confluent retinal hemorrhages. While these changes can progress to retinal neovascularization, vitreous hemorrhage, and fibrosis, a more common complication is the development of neovascular glaucoma. If severe retinal ischemia is present on fluorescein angiography, there is a 60% chance of this complication. In neovascular glaucoma, substances produced by the ischemic retina diffuse forward and stimulate formation of a fibrovascular membrane that grows across the iris surface and covers the trabecular meshwork, resulting in glaucoma characterized by very high pressures, pain, and marked resistance to medical and surgical therapy, so that enucleation of the blind painful eye may be required. Panretinal photocoagulation, preferably with the krypton red laser to avoid preretinal fibrosis caused by heat absorption in the hemorrhages, can greatly reduce the incidence of neovascular glaucoma in ischemic central retinal vein thrombosis. Once neovascular glaucoma is present, adequate panretinal photocoagulation will usually cause regression of anterior segment neovascularization, allowing glaucoma to be controlled medically or by filtering surgery. Unfortunately, established neovascular glaucoma is often associated with corneal edema, miosis, or hyphema, all of which rule out laser therapy, so that only cyclodestructive procedures or enucleation can be used. Because established neovascular glaucoma is so resistant to treatment, prophylactic krypton red laser photocoagulation is advised in all cases of ischemic central retinal vein thrombosis. Visual acuity 20/200 or less, when combined with the classic blood-and-thunder fundus, is nearly always evidence of ischemia severe enough to warrant prophylactic panretinal photocoagulation.

Branch Retinal Vein Thrombosis

This condition varies from tiny localized areas of venous congestion and hemorrhage to hemiretinal involvement from thrombosis of the superior or inferior division of the central retinal vein. Typically, the occlusion occurs at an arteriovenous crossing, where an artery is compressing the vein. Neovascular glaucoma is rare in branch vein thrombosis, and the principal complications are chronic macular edema and development of neovascularization followed by vitreous hemorrhage. Prophylactic krypton red scatter photocoagulation in the area of ischemia reduces the chance of these complications, and focal argon laser photocoagulation can destroy established neovascular areas.

Retinal Tears

When a peripheral retinal tear occurs, usually due to senile vitreous degeneration causing vitreous traction, the patient often notices the sudden appearance of floaters. The tear can cause retinal detachment, but if promptly detected it can be walled off by applying a ring of laser burns around it to create adhesion of the adjacent attached retina to the pigment epithelium. If detachment has occurred, so that the retina is no longer apposed to the pigment epithelium, surgery will be required for treatment. Prompt examination is therefore indicated in any eye with sudden onset of floaters.

Macular Degeneration & Related Diseases

The principal layers of the sensory lining of the eye are the sensory retina, the pigment epithelium, Bruch's membrane, and the choroid. Bruch's membrane forms a barrier layer between the pigment epithelium and the choriocapillaris, which is the capillary layer of the choroid. If Bruch's membrane deteriorates or is damaged, capillary nets can grow through the break beneath the pigment epithelium, at first causing exudative pigment epithelial detachment with distortion and edema of the overlying retina and then later causing hemorrhage and fibrosis with destruction of the retinal function in that area.

The macular retina is especially likely to develop Bruch's membrane breaks and neovascularization, though these changes can occur anywhere in the fundus. The most frequent cause is age-related macular degeneration, which begins as asymptomatic yellowish deposits (drusen) in the macular area. As the years advance, pigment epithelial atrophy and clumping are seen, and finally Bruch's membrane breaks appear, leading to fluid leaks, neovascularization, fibrosis, and loss of central vision.

This condition is the leading cause of legal blindness in the older population. Bruch's membrane breaks and neovascular nets can occur at sites of old chorioretinitis from childhood histoplasmosis, toxoplasmosis, and various other inflammatory disorders. They can develop from traumatic choroidal ruptures even in children and can occur in a host of hereditary diseases involving the retina. If sub-pigment epithelial neovascular nets are located away from the central foveal area, they can be destroyed by careful laser photocoagulation.

The yellow macular pigment (xanthophyll) strongly absorbs blue light, weakly absorbs green light, and does not absorb yellow, orange, or red light. Hemoglobin strongly absorbs blue, green, yellow, and orange light, but very weakly absorbs red light. Melanin absorbs all visible wavelengths. Selective absorption of laser energy is therefore possible. If the neovascular net has melanin pigment in it or is bleeding, krypton red laser light allows deep penetration to the choriocapillaris, without hemoglobin or xanthophyll absorption. If the net does not have much melanin and has not bled, argon green or dye laser yellow or orange will be absorbed by hemoglobin to coagulate the net, but the scattered light will not be absorbed by xanthophyll.

The whole neovascular net must be heavily treated for control. Unfortunately, in many cases the net is already under the fovea at the time of diagnosis, or bleeding is already so extensive that laser treatment is not possible. Early diagnosis is therefore of utmost importance in this group of diseases, and patients at risk must diligently look for and report the small blurs and distortions of vision that are the first signs of neovascular growth. Fluorescein angiography can then be used to demonstrate the retinal circulation, including areas of neovascularization and abnormal vascular permeability.

Glaucoma

Treatment of both open-angle and angle-closure (closed-angle) glaucoma has been radically altered by availability of effective laser techniques.

A. Angle–Closure Glaucoma: In primary angle closure, aqueous flow though the pupil is blocked by contact of the lens with the posterior surface of the iris. The resulting pressure in the posterior chamber forces the peripheral iris forward into contact with the trabecular meshwork, blocking outflow and increasing intraocular pressure. While the classic, dramatic acute glaucoma attack is usually considered the prototype of angle closure, acute attacks are actually rare. Creeping or subacute angle closure is much more common, especially in darkly pigmented eyes, and can occur with a normal central anterior chamber depth. Angle closure can be determined only by examining the angle, which is usually done by slit lamp gonioscopy through a contact lens containing a mirror. Because angle closure causes approximately three-fourths of all the glaucoma in the Asian countries, worldwide it is probably the most common type of glaucoma. Secondary pupillary block can be caused by a pseudophakos, by vitreous, or by fibrotic tissue.

Surgical iridectomy was the standard treatment for angle closure for decades but carried the risks of hemorrhage, infection, anesthetic accidents, and even sympathetic ophthalmia. Studies of ruby laser iridotomy began in animals in 1964, but not until 1975 was an effective argon laser technique developed for human eyes. Laser iridotomy was made more effective by the Abraham contact lens, whose 66-diopter focusing button increased iris energy density by a factor of 2.67. The recently introduced Wise iridotomy-sphincterotomy lens has a 103-diopter button that gives the highest energy density possible with a practical contact lens—7.79 times the energy density through a plano contact lens and 2.92 times that through the Abraham lens. With these high energy densities, laser iridotomy is nearly 100% successful with either the argon laser or the Q-switched Nd:YAG laser, failing only when the cornea is so cloudy that the laser cannot be focused upon the iris. With the argon laser, the beam is focused through the Wise lens upon the far peripheral iris fibers, which are cut in a line parallel to the limbus by multiple shots at 0.01 s or 0.02 s of exposure and energy levels of about 1 watt (Fig 27–2). With the Nd:YAG laser, iridotomy can be done through the Wise lens by a high-power single-point method using about 8 mJ per shot in a single shot or a 2- or 3-shot burst—or it can be done by cutting the far peripheral iris fibers in a line parallel to the limbus with multiple shots at 1–1.5 mJ.

The argon laser is preferable for dark-brown thick irises, which tend to bleed with the Nd:YAG laser, while light blue irises do not absorb argon laser energy well and are more easily perforated with the Nd:YAG laser. Because of its safety, laser iridotomy can be done not only for established angle closure but whenever progressive pupillary block is occurring, before irreversible damage from angle closure has occurred.

B. Primary Open–Angle Glaucoma: This is the most common type of glaucoma in Western societies and is characterized by painless, gradual reduction in trabecular meshwork function with decreasing outflow, increasing intraocular pressure, progressive cupping of the optic nerve, and insidious loss of visual field leading ultimately to blindness. In the past, treat-

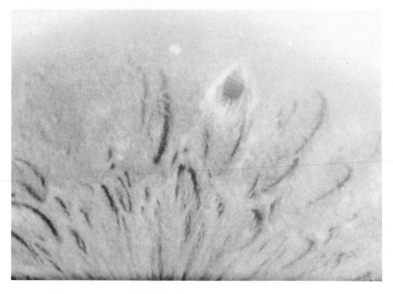

Figure 27–2. Laser iridotomy.

ment has consisted of medical therapy, followed by fistulizing surgery if the medical therapy was not effective. Because surgery is associated with a significant incidence of cataract formation, flat chambers, hemorrhage, and other complications, patients were subjected to the expense and side effects of very heavy medical therapy and often developed severe glaucoma field loss before the risks of surgery were accepted. In the first attempts to treat open-angle glaucoma, laser perforations of the meshwork were created with the Q-switched ruby laser by Krasnov and with the argon laser by Hager, by Worthen, and by Teichmann and others. Though temporary pressure reductions did occur, the perforations quickly closed with recurrent elevation of pressure.

By 1976, laser trabeculopuncture or trabeculotomy had been discontinued by all of these investigators. In 1976, Wise originated a new concept of laser glaucoma therapy, initially called laser trabecular tightening and now known as laser trabeculoplasty. This consists of spacing 100 or more nonperforating argon laser burns 360 degrees around the trabecular meshwork, using 0.1 s burn duration, 50-μm spot size, and enough energy to produce a small bubble or blanch. The heat of the laser burns shrinks the collagen in the tissues of the trabecular ring, reducing the circumference and therefore the diameter of the trabecular ring, pulling the trabecular layers apart, and reopening the intertrabecular spaces and Schlemm's canal. Growth of new trabecular cells may also occur.

Trabeculoplasty increases outflow but has no influence upon aqueous secretion. Though in some eyes the abnormal meshwork can continue to deteriorate, with late failure requiring filtration surgery, control of glaucoma for 10 years and for 12 years (Wise, unpublished data) has been observed. Most of the eyes continue to require medical therapy, and the value of trabeculoplasty lies in avoiding or greatly postponing the risk of filtration surgery. The only significant side effects are a rise in pressure for 1–4 hours in about one-third of eyes (preventable by oral glycerol or by apraclonidine drops) and a rise in pressure for 1–3 weeks in about 4% of treated eyes. To reduce the severity of these pressure rises, many laser surgeons do trabeculoplasty in 180 degrees of the trabecular meshwork, treating the other 180 degrees about 4 weeks later.

Laser Photomydriasis & Laser Sphincterotomy

For a variety of reasons—but most frequently because of long-term miotic therapy—the pupil can become fixed at a very small size, reducing vision and interfering with pupillary dilation for retinal examination or treatment. Multiple laser burns 200 μm in diameter placed in a ring outside the pupil will produce temporary enlargement, but marked uveitis and intraocular pressure rises can occur and the dilating effect disappears over time. A better method is argon laser sphincterotomy, in which one or more linear cuts across the iris sphincter are made by focusing the argon laser through the Wise iridotomy-sphincterotomy lens and using numerous shots at 0.01 s of exposure and about 1 watt of energy. This produces permanent enlargement of the pupil with less irritation. Energy levels must be kept low to avoid lens burns. The Nd:YAG laser at very low energy levels can be used to cut persistent nonpigmented bridging strands.

Posterior Capsulotomy After Cataract Surgery

Cataract surgery consists of removing the natural lens of the eye when it has become clouded due to age or disease. If lens removal alone is done, the eye has lost an important focusing element and the uncorrected vision is quite blurred. The strong cataract glasses required to correct this aphakic state produce considerable visual distortion and field limitation. Lens replacement with an artificial intraocular implant lens is therefore an attractive concept, promising full-time vision and normal visual field. However, an intraocular lens implant is a foreign body placed within a very delicate organ, and this foreign body must be tolerated for the remainder of the patient's life. To be tolerated, the intraocular lens must be supported in such a way that it does not migrate and does not chronically rub against or irritate the vascular or nervous structures in the anterior segment. The only supporting structure that meets these requirements is the capsule of the lens. In extracapsular cataract surgery, the anterior capsule and all of the contents of the cataractous lens are removed, leaving the peripheral and posterior portions of the capsule in place, supported by the zonule. The intraocular lens optic bears supporting fibers, usually arcs of polypropylene or polymethylmethacrylate. By compressing the supports, the entire lens assembly can be inserted into the cavity of the lens capsule, where mild fibrosis will firmly fix the supporting fibers so that the IOL cannot move and does not touch blood vessels or nerves.

However, an intact posterior capsule will frequently opacify. In the past, primary capsulotomy at surgery was often performed to avoid the need for a second operation to perform surgical capsulotomy. An intact posterior capsule for at least the first few weeks postoperatively is desirable, because the intact capsule significantly reduces the incidence of complications. If this intact capsule later opacifies, Q-switched Nd:YAG laser pulses can be focused just posterior to the capsule to produce a central capsulotomy without surgically invading the eye. Careful focus through a condensing contact lens is necessary to avoid damage to the IOL. By allowing posterior capsules to be left intact at surgery routinely, laser capsulotomy has significantly improved the overall results of cataract surgery.

Cutting Vitreous Bands & Opacities

After incision or laceration of the cornea, vitreous strands can come through the pupil and become attached to the cornea, causing pupillary distortion, chronic uveitis, and sometimes cystoid macular edema. These bands can be cut with the Q-switched Nd:YAG laser, either directly through the cornea, by focusing on the band through a condensing contact lens such as the Wise lens; or in the angle, by focusing through the mirror of a condensing goniolens such as the Trokel lens or the Lasag CGA lens. Multiple shots at minimal optical breakdown levels should be used to minimize concussion to cornea and iris. Eyes with chronic cystoid macular edema have improved after cutting of vitreocorneal bands.

Localized opacities and bands in the anterior vit-

reous can be cut with the Nd:YAG laser to clear the visual axis or reduce traction upon the retina. Most of the time, however, the vitreous abnormalities are widespread, and surgical vitrectomy is required.

Vaporization of Lid Tumors

The carbon dioxide laser has been used to bloodlessly remove both benign and malignant lid tumors. However, because of scarring, lack of a histologic specimen, and inability to assess margins, laser treatment appears inferior to other methods in most cases.

INVESTIGATIONAL USES OF OPHTHALMIC LASERS

Cyclophotocoagulation

Glaucoma refractory to the usual operative procedures can sometimes be controlled by direct destruction of the ciliary processes, usually by cryosurgery. The ciliary processes can be photocoagulated directly through the pupil in aniridia or traumatic mydriasis, but only the anterior tips can be treated. When delivered through a fiberoptic probe passed through the pars plana during vitrectomy, extensive argon laser cyclocoagulation has given good results in one series. Transconjunctival cyclocoagulation has been done by Beckman, using a high-energy ruby laser, and by Frankhauser, using a thermal-mode Nd:YAG laser. Good results have been reported, but multiple treatments are usually required, and the equipment is specialized and very expensive.

Laser Sclerostomy

To avoid the surgical and anesthetic hazards of filtering surgery for glaucoma, numerous investigators have attempted to achieve scleral perforation by laser light energy. In 1969, L'Esperance injected colloidal carbon (India ink) into the peripheral cornea and then perforated that area by directing the argon laser across the anterior chamber with a mirrored goniolens. Similar attempts have been made by March by absorbing thermal Nd:YAG into intracorneal silver oxide (argyrol). This method was abandoned because argyrol is not formulated or approved as safe for injection. March has also studied argon laser energy absorbed by fluorescein and krypton red laser absorbed by methylene blue. L'Esperance and Beckman have used the carbon dioxide laser to bloodlessly perforate sclera and iris during filtering surgery for neovascular glaucoma. Gaasterland, among others, has perforated the sclera in animals with excimer, visible, and infrared laser energy by contact intraocular delivery through optical fibers passed across the anterior chamber or by contact extraocular delivery by passing the fibers beneath the conjunctiva.

With all these methods, surgical or laser iridectomy must also be done to prevent iris from occluding the sclerostomy. None have been shown to be as effective as or safer than standard surgical methods. The principal cause of failure in glaucoma surgery is not fistula closure but episcleral scarring. During surgery, this can be anticipated by excision and undermining of Tenon's capsule, which is not possible with laser sclerostomy.

Argon or Nd:YAG laser treatment has been successfully used to remove membranes occluding surgical sclerostomies.

Refractive Surgery

The excimer lasers, particularly the 193-nm-wavelength argon fluoride laser, can evaporate tissue very cleanly with almost no damage to cells adjacent to the cut. Precise corneal incisions can therefore be

made for radial keratotomy for myopia and for trephining the recipient and donor corneas in penetrating keratoplasty. The argon fluoride laser can also be used with multiple pulses and progressively changing spot size to evaporate successive thin layers of the cornea, offering the possibility of computer-controlled recontouring of the cornea to precisely correct even large refractive errors. Patterned area ablation of rabbit and of moneky corneas has been successful, and initial difficulties with surface scarring have been overcome.

Human trials are now beginning on blind eyes. While much study remains to be done, safe and permanent correction of refractive errors may prove to be possible.

REFERENCES

Abraham RK, Miller GL: Outpatient argon laser iridectomy for angle closure glaucoma: A two-year study. *Trans Am Acad Ophthalmol Otolaryngol* 1975;**79**:529.

Abraham RK, Munnerlyn CR: Laster iridotomy: Improved methodology with a new iridotomy lens. *Ophthalmology* 1979;**86(Suppl)**:126.

Beckman H, Waeltermann J: Transscleral ruby laser cyclocoagulation. *Am J Ophthalmol* 1984;**98**:788.

Branch Vein Occlusion Study Group: Argon laser scatter photocoagulation for prevention of neovascularization and vitreous hemorrhage in branch vein occlusion: A randomized clinical trial. *Arch Ophthalmol* 1986;**104**:34.

Gaasterland DE et al: Ab interno and ab externo filtering operations by laser contact surgery. *Ophthalmic Surg* 1987;**18**:254.

Goldberg MF, Jampol LM: Knowledge of diabetic retinopathy before and 18 years after the Airlie House symposium on treatment of diabetic retinopathy. *Ophthalmology* 1987;**94**:741.

Hanna KD et al: Excimer laser keratectomy for myopia with a rotating-slit delivery system. *Arch Ophthalmol* 1988;**106**:245.

Klapper RM et al: Transscleral neodymium:YAG thermal cyclophotocoagulation in refractory glaucoma: A preliminary report. *Ophthalmology* 1988;**95**:719.

Krasnov MM: Laser puncture of anterior chamber angle in glaucoma. *Am J Ophthalmol* 1973;**75**:674.

L'Esperance FA Jr: Laser trabeculosclerostomy. In: *Ophthalmic Lasers: Photocoagulation, Photoradiation, and Surgery,* 2nd ed. Mosby, 1982.

Macular Photocoagulation Study Group: Argon laser photocoagulation for neovascular maculopathy: Three-year results for randomized clinical trials. *Arch Ophthalmol* 1986;**104**:694.

Magargal LE et al: Neovascular glaucoma following central retinal vein obstruction. *Ophthalmology* 1981;**88**:1095.

Patel A et al: Endolaser treatment of the ciliary body for uncontrolled glaucoma. *Ophthalmology* 1986;**93**:825.

Vogel A et al: Cavitation bubble dynamics and acoustic transient generation in ocular surgery with pulsed neodymium:YAG lasers. *Ophthalmology* 1986;**93**:1259.

Wise JB: Iris sphincterotomy, iridotomy, and synechiotomy by linear incision with the argon laser. *Ophthalmology* 1985;**92**:641.

Wise JB: Low-energy linear-incision neodymium:YAG laser iridotomy versus linear-incision argon laser iridotomy: A prospective clinical investigation. *Ophthalmology* 1987; **94**:1531.

Wise JB: Management of the glaucomas with argon laser (laser trabeculoplasty). *Highlights Ophthalmol* 1985; **1**:456.

Wise JB: Ten year results of laser trabeculoplasty: Does the laser avoid glaucoma surgery or merely defer it? *Eye* 1987;**1**:45.

Wise JB, Munnerlyn CR, Erickson PJ: A high-efficiency laser iridotomy-sphincterotomy lens. *Am J Ophthalmol* 1986;**101**:546.

Wise JB, Witter SL: Argon laser therapy for open-angle glaucoma: A pilot study. *Arch Ophthalmol* 1979;**97**:319.

Appendix I:
Visual Standards

INDUSTRIAL VISUAL EVALUATION[*]

The following mathematical calculation of loss of visual efficiency is used for legal and industrial cases, particularly in determination of compensation for injury.[†]

Calculation of total visual efficiency is based on 3 factors of equal importance: percentage loss of visual acuity, percentage loss of visual field, and percentage loss of coordinated ocular movements. Percentage loss of visual acuity in one eye does not represent the individual's total disability; even a total loss of one eye would not represent a 50% disability if the remaining eye were normal. Many people lead normal lives with one eye.

For evaluation of industrial visual efficiency, therefore, 3 visual functions are measured and mathematically coordinated: (1) visual acuity, (2) visual field, and (3) ocular motility (diplopia field, binocular field).

Visual Acuity

Distance and near vision are weighted evenly.

For purposes of calculating total visual acuity loss, near visual acuity is equally as important as distance acuity.

Example: If the distance acuity is 20/80 and the subject can read Jaeger 6—

$$\frac{40 + 50}{2} = \text{45\% visual acuity loss, or 55\% visual acuity efficiency}$$

Visual Field

A white test object is used in 8 meridians as diagrammed on p 420. This can be done with a 3-mm object at 0.33 m, using a perimeter. A full field rep-

---

[*]Modified and reproduced, with permission, from *Arch Ind Health* 1955;**12**:439. For further explanation of the reasons behind the statistics and a legal discussion, see Spaeth EB: *Trans Am Acad Ophthalmol Otolaryngol* 1957;**61**:592.

[†]The method described here may differ from government standards for defining reduced vision in assessing eligibility for compensation, which vary from state to state. The State Department of Industrial Relations (or its equivalent) can be contacted for data.

AMA Method of Estimation of Percentage Visual Loss (Using Best Correcting Spectacle Lens)

Distance	
Distance Visual Acuity	**% Loss**
20/20	0
20/25	5
20/40	15
20/50	25
20/80	40
20/100	50
20/160	70
20/200	80
20/400	90

Near	
Jaeger Test Type	**% Loss**
1	0
2	0
3	10
6	50
7	60
11	85
14	95

resents 100% function. (Illumination should be at least 120 lux.)

Ocular Motility

The extent of diplopia in the various directions of gaze is best determined using a tangent screen at 1 meter. A small test light is used and diplopia plotted along the 3 meridians above the horizontal 10, 20, and 30 degrees from fixation. Diplopia fields are also plotted on the horizontal meridians and the 3 meridians below, 10, 20, 30, and 40 degrees from the straight-ahead position. Diplopia within the central 20 degrees represents 100% loss of motility efficiency of one eye, since this condition usually requires patching one eye. If diplopia is not present in the central 20 degrees, loss of ocular motility is calculated from a field diagram showing percentage loss. This value is then subtracted from 100 and expressed as "80% motility efficiency," etc.

The inferior fields are weighted heavily, since this is the position of the eyes in reading. Diplopia away from fixations in other quadrants is considered much less important.

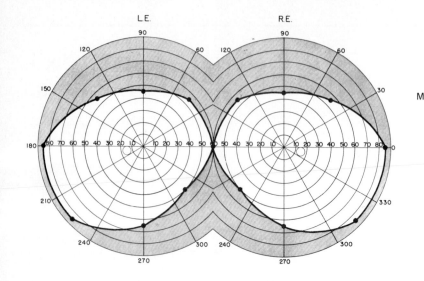

Minimum Legal Visual Field

Minimal Normal Field:
Temporally	85°
Down and temporally	85°
Down	65°
Down and nasally	50°
Nasally	60°
Up and nasally	55°
Up	45°
Up and temporally	55°
Full field	= 500°

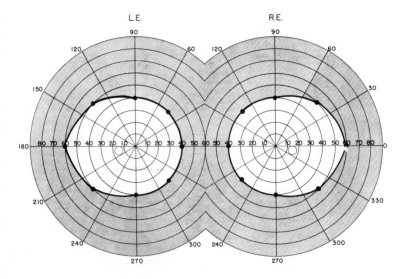

Twenty-eight Percent Loss

Moderate Loss of Field:
Temporally	60°
Down and temporally	50°
Down	40°
Down and nasally	40°
Nasally	40°
Up and nasally	40°
Up	40°
Up and temporally	50°
	360°

$$\frac{360 \times 100}{500} = \text{72\% field remaining, or 28\% field loss}$$

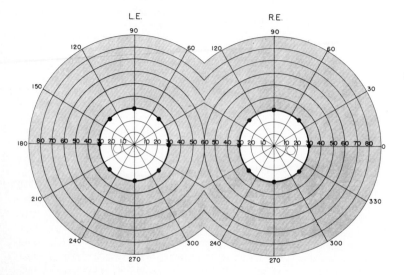

Fifty-two Percent Loss

Severe Loss of Field:
Temporally	30°
Down and temporally	30°
Down	30°
Down and nasally	30°
Nasally	30°
Up and nasally	30°
Up	30°
Up and temporally	30°
	240°

$$\frac{240 \times 100}{500} = \text{48\% field remaining, or 52\% field loss}$$

Visual Efficiency (VE) of One Eye

The percentages of efficiency for the 3 measurements are multiplied to give the total visual efficiency.

Example: **Visual acuity = 73%**
Visual field = 57%
Motility = 90%

Visual Efficiency (VE) of 2 Eyes

The 2 eyes are calculated separately; the better eye is weighted 3 times and the poorer eye once. Thus, one blind eye and one normal eye give 75% visual efficiency.

$$\frac{3 \times (\% \text{ VE better eye}) + \% \text{ VE in worse eye}}{4}$$

$$= \text{binocular VE } (\%)$$

Example: RE = 90%; LE = 30%.

$$\frac{3 \times 90 + 30}{4} = 75\% \text{ binocular VE}$$

VISUAL STANDARDS FOR THE ARMED FORCES[*]

The visual acuity requirements outlined below apply for all branches of the services. For aircraft pilots, service academy candidates, and some other officer assignments, the requirements are much more rigid.

Standards for Disqualification

Any strabismus of 40 prism diopters or more uncorrectable by lenses to less than 40 diopters is disqualifying, as is the presence of diplopia. Any active or progressive disease of the eyes is disqualifying even though the minimal visual standards can be met.

Minimal Standards

Distance visual acuity must correct to one of the following: (1) 20/40 in one eye and 20/70 in the other; (2) 20/30 in one eye and 20/100 in the other; (3) 20/20 in one eye and 20/400 in the other.

Near visual acuity must correct to at least J-6 in the better eye.

VISUAL STANDARDS FOR DRIVERS' LICENSES IN THE USA

States have varying visual standards for persons applying for drivers' licenses. Failure to meet certain minimum standards may result in suspension of driving privileges or denial of license unless a certificate is obtained from an ophthalmologist or optometrist.

[*]Subject to change. Medical Officers for Recruitment at military hospitals or induction centers are supplied with the latest data.

In recent years there has been a trend toward higher standards and more periodic visual testing, especially in persons over age 70.

EDUCATIONAL VISUAL STANDARDS IN THE USA

Twelve percent of the pupils in elementary schools have significant eye difficulty, but no more than one in 1000 requires special educational facilities because of severe visual deficiencies. Although a medical examination is mandatory for school children in all states because of assessments required by Public Law 94-142, ophthalmologic examinations are seldom included. It has therefore been found necessary to devise procedures by which it will be possible, without a highly specialized staff, to give preliminary screening tests.

The Snellen test is the single most important test. Visual acuity tests may be given by nurses, parents, or trained volunteer teachers. Visual acuity testing of preschool children is far more important than visual acuity testing of school-age children. Testing should be performed as early as possible, preferably no later than $3\frac{1}{2}$–4 years of age.

Even if a child has a significant visual handicap, it is best to try regular school. If the student cannot keep up with regular schoolwork, special "sight-saving" classes are necessary.

Education of Visually Handicapped Children

Education must be provided for partially seeing pupils at all school levels. (For educational purposes, a partially seeing child is one who has a corrected visual acuity of 20/70 or less in the better eye.) Experience indicates that it is best to establish the first class on an elementary school level, since the earlier help is given the better will be the prospect of success. In communities in which the school population is too small to warrant the establishment of more than one class, it may be advisable to give the advantages of the special class to children above the second grade, since much less close eye work is required in the first and second grades and a great deal of material in large, clear print is available for younger children. In general, well-motivated partially sighted children have good learning potential.

Education of Blind Children

Children with poor visual acuity who are unable to take advantage of ordinary visual educational methods are entered either in special schools for the blind, where emphasis is placed upon learning by touch (Braille), or (preferably) in integrated schools where facilities are available for special training but where the child is not deprived of all contact with normal persons in the same age group.

Appendix II:
Practical Factors in Illumination

The physical aspects of illumination discussed below are of practical interest to the physician who may be called upon to evaluate the adequacy of light sources in factories, shops, schoolrooms, and homes. Of principal interest is light **intensity,** conventionally measured in lux. One lux is equal to 1 lumen per square meter. Lux can be measured directly with special light meters.

Proper illumination minimizes eyestrain and increases the speed and efficiency of reading. Poor lighting does not cause eye disease but increases eye fatigue. The most common error students make in adjusting their lighting arrangement is to place a desk lamp opposite them on the desk. From this position the light is reflected into the reader's eyes, causing glare. For reading, the best light source is an incandescent or fluorescent lamp coming from above that produces a diffuse light with a minimum of glare and shadows. For writing, the light source should be so adjusted that the shadow of the arm and hand on the page is eliminated.

The most common sources of light are daylight, incandescent light, and fluorescent light. Daylight is an excellent light source but quite variable, and it is difficult to control its intensity. Incandescent lamps simulate daylight and provide a steady, diffuse flow of light. Ordinary fluorescent tubes operate on an alternating current that causes flickering, but it is possible to link 2 fluorescent tubes in a couple so adjusted that when one is on the up-phase the other is on the down-phase, thus eliminating the flicker.

Illumination Factors Affecting Visibility

A. Intensity: The amount of illumination is directly related to reading efficiency. A reader employing 80 lux reads much more slowly and less efficiently than if a 500-lux source were utilized. The following minimum intensities are recommended (assuming that all undue reflections resulting in glare have been eliminated): reading black print on white paper, 500–650 lux; schoolrooms, 500–650 lux at the desk and 650–800 lux at the blackboard; passageways, halls, and closets, 80 lux; eye charts, 1350–1700 lux; operating room illumination at the point of surgery, 5000 lux.

There is a close relationship between a person's age and the magnification and illumination required. Because they have great powers of accommodation, children can read small print in semidarkness by holding the page close to their eyes. (This does not hurt the child's eyes although it may bother the parents.) On the other hand, a 48-year-old, slightly farsighted presbyope cannot read under ordinary illumination without magnifying glasses because the power of accommodation has been lost. Using a stronger light bulb or taking the printed material into sunlight makes reading possible in such cases. The presbyope also can improve visual performance by holding printed matter farther away. ("I need longer arms.")

The basic requirement in illumination is to have enough light to see by. Once this is accomplished, the intensity of illumination and the magnification (eyeglasses) can be adjusted to increase the efficiency of visual performance.

The intensity of light on an object is inversely proportionate to the square of the distance from the light source. Therefore, if a reading lamp 0.6 m (2 feet) from the page is moved to a distance of 1.2 m (4 feet), there will be 4 times less light on the page.

B. Contrast: It is much easier to read black letters on a white page than black letters on a blue page. Eye fatigue is minimized when the surroundings are about 30–40% darker than the object being observed. Thus, in watching a television screen it is best not to have a completely darkened room.

C. Diffuseness: Shadows and spotlight phenomena should be avoided. However, diffuseness is overdone by manufacturers of indirect lighting fixtures. Indirect "reading lamps" are usually inadequate because of the vastly decreased amount of illumination on the printed page. This can be demonstrated by observing the unwarranted amount of light cast on the ceiling by the average indirect reading lamp.

D. Age of Subject: Illumination requirements and age are closely related, as evidenced by the increased illumination required by the 45-year-old presbyope compared with a teenage daughter. Although it is not recommended, children in the 7–16 age group can read adequately in semidarkness, whereas the same person 30 years later may be able to read the telephone book only by "taking it to the window." Conversely, many people in the 50- to 65-year range who require full correction for their presbyopia can still read fine print without glasses in sunlight.

In general, illumination should be sufficient to perform the task at hand efficiently and comfortably.

Appendix III:
Rehabilitation of the Visually Handicapped & Special Services Available to the Blind

Although no completely reliable statistics are available, the most widely used estimates place the legally blind population of the USA at 2.24 per thousand (ie, approximately 500,000). Approximately 50,000 become legally blind annually, and 'many others have enough visual loss to constitute a serious employment problem.

Blindness does not necessarily imply helplessness. Individual adjustment to marked visual impairment or total blindness varies with age at onset, temperament, education, economic resources, and many other factors. The older patient, for example, may accept blindness quite stoically, whereas for the younger patient the vocational or social impact of blindness is often catastrophic. Blindness is accepted more easily by persons who are born blind and by persons of any age who lose their vision gradually rather than suddenly.

The responsibility of the physician clearly does not end with the diagnosis, prevention, and treatment of ocular disorders that might result in blindness. The physician caring for the patient who is suddenly faced with actual or imminent blindness is in a position to be of great assistance. When blindness is a possibility but is not inevitable (eg, during acute ocular inflammation), optimism and reassurance are warranted. However, it is unwise to offer false hopes or to delay "breaking the news" when blindness is inevitable. If it is certain that blindness will occur, it is important to extend to the distraught patient as well as to the patient's family the warmth, understanding, encouragement, and assistance so desperately needed. The physician should be alert to the severe depressive reactions that may occur.

It is especially important to assist the patient in making the adjustment to blindness while some vision is still present. Early referral to rehabilitation agencies is essential for recently blinded adults and those with irreversible progressive visual loss. Training programs or reeducation for the many changes involved in daily living and employment are greatly simplified if the patient has the partial support provided by even limited vision.

It may be valuable to have the patient talk with a blind person who has made a satisfactory adjustment to blindness.

Many special services are available for blind persons. The aim of the rehabilitation program is to enable the patient to lead as nearly normal a life as possible. Approximately 5000 blind persons in the USA are rehabilitated and obtain paid employment each year. An additional larger number of blind homemakers are able to perform their household duties without assistance or are able to live independently of others.

The physician should work actively with both the patient and the family and with other professional people concerned with rendering services to the blind.

Rehabilitation must be individualized. Guide dogs, for example, may be extremely valuable for certain persons but totally unsatisfactory for others. The methods of sightless reading and writing must be adapted to the capabilities, needs, and preferences of each patient. Mobility training is most important; several universities[*] have undergraduate and postgraduate programs in mobility training for the blind.

State Services

The physician should be familiar with the many special services available to the blind. Services vary from state to state but may be illustrated by the diversified programs for the blind conducted by the State of California.[†]

A. Educational Services for the Blind:

1. California School for the Blind–A residential school for general education from kindergarten through the secondary grades; also provides field service, guidance, and assistance to preschool children and students in advanced courses.

2. California State Library–A repository for magazines and books in raised type (Moon and Braille), talking books and machines for use with the

---

[*]Undergraduate level programs are at Cleveland State University in Ohio, Florida State University in Florida, and Stephen F. Austin University in Texas. Graduate programs are at Boston University, California State University (Los Angeles), Northern Colorado University, San Francisco State University, University of Arkansas, University of Wisconsin, and Western Michigan State University.

[†]The services referred to are those provided by public-sponsored agencies for the blind and do not include the many religious organizations, private or voluntary health and welfare agencies, sheltered workshops, and community and recreational facilities.

books, casettes and tapes, games adapted for use by the blind, and writing appliances. These materials may be secured directly from the library or by mail (postage-free).

3. Office of Special Education–Coordinates the establishment and operation of special public school programs for visually handicapped children throughout the state. This program enables blind and partially seeing students to live at home and attend school with normal children.

4. Clearinghouse Depository for Handicapped Students–Instructional aids for visually handicapped students in public or nonprofit private schools that comply with the Civil Rights Act. Also serves as a referral service on educational materials for visually handicapped students.

B. Reader Services for Blind Students: Provides reader services for blind students in high schools, junior colleges, vocational training schools, colleges, and universities.

C. Rehabilitation Services for the Blind:

1. Field rehabilitation services–Counselor-teachers provide services to the blind within their homes or in hospitals and other institutions so that individuals may learn the skills necessary to meet the demands of daily living. Counseling in adjustment to blindness is given to the visually disabled person and the family.

2. Orientation Center for the Blind (State of California Department of Rehabilitation)–Provides intensive orientation and prevocational training, including training in techniques of daily living and travel, physical conditioning, sensory training, instruction in Braille, typing, and business methods, and training in hand and machine work, homemaking, and other vocationally useful skills. Limited residence facilities are available.

3. Vocational Rehabilitation Service–Provides, for the adult blind, vocational counseling to help work out suitable employment objectives, supervised vocational training, and job placement. The following services may also be provided if needed for employment and if the applicant is unable to pay for them: medical and surgical treatment, including hospitalization; prosthetic appliances and glasses; maintenance and transportation while undergoing treatment or training; and tools or equipment needed in training, job placement, or self-employment.

4. Business enterprise program–Assists blind persons to establish and operate vending stands, snack bars, and cafeteria or other businesses they may be qualified to operate.

D. Social Welfare Programs for the Blind:

1. Supplemental Security Income (SSI)–Financial assistance paid by state and federal governments to blind persons who, because of loss or impairment of sight, are unable to provide themselves with the necessities of life.

2. Aid to Potentially Self-Supporting Blind–Financial assistance by the county and state to the adult blind who, because of loss or impairment of

sight, are unable fully to provide themselves with the necessities of life but who are working on a plan for self-support.

3. Prevention of Blindness–A program designed to prevent blindness or restore vision by providing necessary medical or surgical treatment through MediCal (Medicaid in other states) and other federal, state, and local funds.

4. Counseling and support programs–County Social Service Departments provide help to visually handicapped persons through locating needed services and, when necessary, paying for in-home chore workers.

E. Provisions for Prevention of Blindness, Preventive Medicine Services Branch (California State Department of Health):

1. Prevention of blindness in newborn infants–Enforces legal requirement of (1) silver nitrate or antibiotic prophylaxis for the eyes as a preventive measure against ophthalmia neonatorum; (2) prenatal serologic test of parents for syphilis; and (3) control of excessive use of oxygen in the care of premature infants as a preventive measure against retinopathy of prematurity.

2. Control of communicable diseases apt to cause loss of vision–Requires reporting, isolation, treatment, and control of ophthalmia neonatorum, trachoma, and syphilis.

3. Aid to Physically Handicapped Children (California Children's Service)–Provides for the necessary medical care of children suffering from eye conditions leading to loss of vision if the parents or legal guardians are unable to meet these costs in whole or in part.

F. Guide Dogs for the Blind: The State Board of Guide Dogs for the Blind (California State Department of Consumer Affairs) was established for the purpose of ensuring that guide dogs are trained and that their owners also are trained to use the dogs as guides. Minimum requirements, licensing, and supervision of guide dog schools are functions of the Board.

National Services

The following organizations will provide information and send literature and catalogs upon request:

(1) American Foundation for the Blind, 15 West 16th Street, New York 10011. Provides information on almost all phases of problems of the blind; sells special watches, home appliances, etc, for the blind.

(2) American Printing House for the Blind, 1839 Frankfort Avenue, PO Box 6085, Louisville, Kentucky 40206-0085. Prints and sells Braille publications.

(3) Guide Dogs for the Blind, Inc., PO Box 1200, San Rafael, California 94915. Training of guide dogs and training of blind persons to use dogs as guides.

(4) The Hadley School for the Blind, Inc., 700 Elm Street, Winnetka, Illinois 60093. Provides free home-study courses from elementary level into college, vocational and avocational training, Braille and other

useful skills. Accredited by National Home Study Council, National Accreditation Council, and North Central Association of Colleges and Schools. Affiliate member of National University Extension Association.

(5) Howe Press of Perkins School for the Blind, 175 North Beacon Street, Watertown, Massachusetts 02172. Manufactures and distributes internationally the Perkins Brailler (portable Braille typewriter) and Braille paper. Also children's stories in a special Braille edition, games, mathematical aids, Braille maps, music, and Braille writing appliances.

(6) Library of Congress. Extensive collection of books and magazines in Braille, on disk, and on cassette available free to visually impaired US citizens. Materials and playback equipment are distributed through a system of network libraries in each state. (Consult local library for specific addresses.) Music materials only are circulated directly from the Library (Division for the Blind and Physically Handicapped, 1291 Taylor Street, NW, Washington, DC 20542).

(7) Rehabilitation Services Administration, Division for the Blind and Visually Handicapped, US Department of Health and Human Services, 330 C Street, SW, Room 3229, Washington, DC 20201. Conducts a nationwide program for the vocational rehabilitation of the blind; provides pamphlets and other information regarding rehabilitation services available to the blind.

(8) *Readers Digest*. Publishes *Readers Digest* in Braille and on records for the Talking Book; may be secured from the American Printing House for the Blind.

(9) Recording for the Blind, Inc., 545 Fifth Avenue, Suite 204, New York 10017. Records textbooks and educational materials free of charge for blind persons for educational, vocational, or professional use.

(10) The Seeing Eye, Inc., PO Box 375, Morristown, New Jersey 07960. First organization in USA to provide guide dogs for qualified blind persons (1929).

(11) Central Blind Rehabilitation Center (124), Veterans Administration Hospital, Hines, Illinois 60141. Provides rehabilitation program lasting up to 18 weeks for veterans. VA Blind Rehabilitation Centers also located at Veterans Administration Hospitals in West Haven, Connecticut, and Palo Alto, California. Round trip transportation of veteran generally paid by Veterans Administration.

(12) Xavier Society for the Blind, 154 East 23rd Street, New York 10010, provides free periodical and library service in Braille, large print, and cassette or open reel tape recordings to any interested blind or partially sighted reader. Catalogs available on request.

American Foundation for the Blind. 1987–88 Catalog of Publications.

Carroll TJ: *Blindness*. Little, Brown, 1961.

Cholden L: *Psychiatric Aspects of Informing the Patient of Blindness*. American Academy of Ophthalmology and Otolaryngology, Instruction Section, Course No. 221, 1953.

Cholden L: *Some Psychiatric Problems in the Rehabilitation of the Blind*. Bulletin of the Menninger Clinic, Vol. 18, No. 3, May 1954.

Faye EE (editor): *Clinical Low Vision*, 2nd ed. Little, Brown, 1984.

Gloor B, Brückner R: *Rehabilitation of the Visually Disabled and the Blind at Different Ages*. University Park Press, 1980.

Hoehne CW, Cull JG, Hardy RE: *Ophthalmological Considerations in the Rehabilitation of the Blind*. Thomas, 1980.

If Blindness Occurs. The Seeing Eye, Inc.

Mallinson GG (editor): *Blindness 1977–78*. American Association of Workers for the Blind, Inc., 1978.

Sekuler R, Kline D, Dimukes K: *Aging and Human Visual Function*. Alan R. Liss, 1982.

Stetten D Jr: Coping with blindness. *N Engl J Med* 1981; **305:**458.

US Department of Health, Education and Welfare: *Support for Vision Research: Interim Report of the National Advisory Eye Council, 1976*. National Institutes of Health, DHEW Publication No. (NIH) 76-1098.

Glossary of Terms Relating to the Eye[*]

Accommodation: The adjustment of the eye for seeing at different distances, accomplished by changing the shape of the lens through action of the ciliary muscle, thus focusing a clear image on the retina.

Agnosia: Inability to recognize common objects despite an intact visual apparatus.

Albinism: A hereditary deficiency of pigment in the retinal pigment epithelium, iris, and choroid.

Amaurosis fugax: Transient recurrent unilateral loss of vision.

Amblyopia: Reduced visual acuity (uncorrectable with lenses) in the absence of detectable anatomic defect in the eye or visual pathways.

Ametropia: See Refractive error.

Amsler grid: A chart with vertical and horizontal lines used for testing the central visual field for scotomas.

Angiography: A diagnostic test in which a substance is injected so that the vascular system can be examined.

Aniridia: Congenital absence of the iris.

Anisocoria: Unequal pupillary size.

Aniseikonia: A condition in which the image seen by one eye differs in size or shape from that seen by the other.

Anisometropia: Difference in refractive error of the eyes.

Anophthalmos: Absence of a true eyeball.

Anterior chamber: Space filled with aqueous bounded anteriorly by the cornea and posteriorly by the iris.

Aphakia: Absence of the crystalline lens.

Aqueous: Clear, watery fluid that fills the anterior and posterior chambers.

Asthenopia: Eye fatigue from muscular, environmental, or psychologic causes.

Astigmatism: Refractive error that prevents the light rays from coming to a point focus on the retina because of different degrees of refraction in the various meridians of the cornea or crystalline lens.

Axis: The meridian specifying the orientation of a cylindric lens.

Binocular vision: Ability of the eyes to focus on one object and to fuse the 2 images into one.

Bitot's spots: Keratinization of the bulbar conjunctiva near the limbus, resulting in a raised spot—a feature of vitamin A deficiency.

Blepharitis: Inflammation of the eyelids.

Blepharoptosis: Drooping of the eyelid.

Blepharospasm: Involuntary spasm of the lids.

Blind spot: "Blank" area in the visual field, corresponding to the light rays that come to a focus on the optic nerve.

Blindness: In the USA, the usual definition of blindness is corrected visual acuity of 20/200 or less in the better eye, or a visual field of no more than 20 degrees in the better eye.

Buphthalmos: Large eyeball in infantile glaucoma.

Canal of Schlemm: A circular modified venous structure in the anterior chamber angle.

Canaliculus: Small tear drainage tube in inner aspect of upper and lower lids leading from the puncta to the common canaliculus and then to the tear sac.

Canthotomy: Usually implies lateral canthotomy—cutting of the lateral canthal tendon for the purpose of widening the palpebral fissure.

Canthus: The angle at either end of the eyelid aperture; specified as outer and inner.

Cataract: An opacity of the crystalline lens.

Cataract extraction: Removal of a cataract, either by removal of the lens complete with its capsule (intracapsular cataract extraction), or by removal of the lens contents after opening the capsule (extracapsular cataract extraction).

Chalazion: Granulomatous inflammation of a meibomian gland.

Chemosis: Conjunctival edema.

Choroid: The vascular middle coat between the retina and sclera.

Ciliary body: Portion of the uveal tract between the iris and the choroid. It consists of ciliary processes and the ciliary muscle.

Coloboma: Congenital cleft due to the failure of some portion of the eye or ocular adenexa to complete growth.

Color blindness: Diminished ability to perceive differences in color.

Concave lens: Lens having the power to diverge rays of light; also known as diverging, reducing, negative, or minus lens, denoted by the sign $(-)$.

Cones and rods: Two kinds of retinal receptor cells. Cones are concerned with visual acuity and color discrimination; rods, with peripheral vision under decreased illumination.

Conjunctiva: Mucous membrane that lines the posterior aspect of the eyelids and the anterior sclera.

Convergence: The process of directing the visual axes of the eyes to a near point.

Convex lens: Lens having power to converge rays of light and to bring them to a focus; also known as converging, magnifying, or plus lens, denoted by the sign $(+)$.

---

[*]See also Definitions of Strabismus, Chapter 13, and Glossary of Genetic Terms, Chapter 19.

Cornea: Transparent portion of the outer coat of the eyeball forming the anterior wall of the anterior chamber.

Corneal contact lenses: Thin lenses that fit directly on the cornea under the eyelids.

Corneal graft (keratoplasty): Operation to restore vision by replacing a section of opaque cornea with transparent cornea, either involving the full thickness of the cornea (penetrating keratoplasty) or only a superficial layer (lamellar keratoplasty).

Cornea: May be from the same human (autograft), another human (homograft), or another species (heterograft).

Cover test: A method of determining the presence and degree of phoria or tropia by covering one eye with an opaque object, thus eliminating fusion.

Cross cylinder: A specialized spherocylindric lens used to measure astigmatism.

Crystalline lens: A transparent biconvex structure suspended in the eyeball between the aqueous and the vitreous. Its function is to bring rays of light to a focus on the retina. Accommodation is produced by variations in the magnitude of this effect. (Now usually called simply the lens.)

Cycloplegic: A drug that temporarily puts the ciliary muscle at rest, paralyzing accommodation.

Cylindric lens: A segment of a cylinder the refractive power of which varies in different meridians.

Dacryocystitis: Infection of the lacrimal sac.

Dacryocystorhinostomy: A procedure by which a communication is made between the nasolacrimal duct and the nasal cavity to relieve an obstruction in the nasolacrimal duct, or sac.

Dark adaptation: The ability to adjust to decreased illumination.

Diopter: Unit of measurement of refractive power of lenses.

Diplopia: Seeing one object as two.

"E" test: A system of testing visual acuity in illiterates, particularly preschool children.

Ectropion: Turning out of the eyelid.

Emmetropia: Absence of refractive error.

Endophthalmitis: Extensive intraocular infection.

Enophthalmos: Abnormal retrodisplacement of the eyeball.

Entropion: A turning inward of the eyelid.

Enucleation: Complete surgical removal of the eyeball.

Epicanthus: Congenital skin fold that overlies the inner canthus.

Eiphora: Tearing.

Esophoria: A tendency of the eyes to turn inward.

Esotropia: A manifest inward deviation of the eyes.

Evisceration: Removal of the contents of the eyeball.

Exenteration: Removal of the entire contents of the orbit, including the eyeball and lids.

Exophoria: A tendency of the eyes to turn outward.

Exophthalmos: Abnormal protrusion of the eyeball.

Exotropia: A manifest outward deviation of the eyes.

Far Point: The point at which the eye is focused when accommodation is completely relaxed.

Farsightedness: See Hyperopia.

Field of vision: The entire area that can be seen without shifting the gaze.

Floaters: Small dark particles in the vitreous.

Focus: A point to which rays of light are brought together to form an image; focal distance is the distance between a lens and its focal point.

Folliculosis: Chronic conjunctivitis characterized by multiple lymphatic nodules.

Fornix: The junction of the palpebral and bulbar conjunctiva.

Fovea: Depression in the macula adapted for most acute vision.

Fundus: The posterior portion of the eye visible through an ophthalmoscope.

Fusion: Coordinating the images received by the 2 eyes into one image.

Glaucoma: Disease characterized by abnormally increased intraocular pressure, optic atrophy, and loss of visual field.

Gonioscopy: A technique of examining the anterior chamber angle, utilizing a corneal contact lens, magnifying device, and light source.

Hemianopia: Blindness of one-half the field of vision of one or both eyes.

Heterophoria (phoria): A tendency of the eyes to deviate.

Heterotropia: See Strabismus.

Hippus: Exaggerated spontaneous rhythmic movements of the iris.

Hordeolum, external (sty): Infection of the glands of Moll or Zeis.

Hordeolum, internal: Meibomian gland infection.

Hyperopia, hypermetropia (farsightedness): A refractive error in which the focus of light rays from a distant object is behind the retina.

Hyperphoria: A tendency of the eyes to deviate upward.

Hypertropia: A manifest deviation of one eye in relation to the other.

Hyphema: Blood in the anterior chamber.

Hypopyon: Pus in the anterior chamber.

Hypotony: Abnormally soft eye from any cause.

Injection: Congestion of blood vessels.

Iris: Colored, circular membrane, suspended behind the cornea and immediately in front of the lens.

Ishihara color plates: A test for color vision based on the ability to trace patterns in a series of multicolored charts.

Isopter: An object for testing visual fields. Isopters can be of different colors and sizes and are used to differentiate relative visual field defects from absolute defects.

Jaeger test: A test for near vision using lines of various sizes of type.

Keratitis: Inflammation of the cornea.

Keratoconus: Cone-shaped deformity of the cornea.

Keratomalacia: Corneal softening, usually associated with avitaminosis A.

Keratometer: An instrument for measuring the curvature of the cornea, used in fitting contact lenses.

Keratopathy, bullous: Swelling of the cornea with painful blisters in the epithelium due to corneal hydration.

Keratoplasty: See Corneal graft.

Keratoprosthesis: Plastic implant surgically placed in an opaque cornea to achieve an area of optical clarity.

Keratotomy: An incision in the cornea. Radial keratotomy is a procedure in which radial incisions are made in the cornea to correct myopia.

Koeppe nodule: Accumulation of epithelioid cells on the posterior cornea in uveitis.

Lacrimal sac: The dilated area at the junction of the nasolacrimal duct and the canaliculi.

Lens: A refractive medium having one or both surfaces curved. (See also Crystalline lens.)

Leukoma: Dense corneal opacity due to any cause.

Limbus: Junction of the cornea and sclera.

Macula: Moderately dense corneal opacity due to any cause.

Macula lutea: The small avascular area of the retina surrounding the fovea, often having yellow pigment.

Maddox rod: A red lens composed of parallel series of strong cylinders through which a point of light is viewed as a red line—used to measure phorias.

Magnification: The ratio of the size of an image to the size of its object.

Megalocornea: Abnormally large cornea (> 13 mm in diameter).

Metamorphopsia: Wavy distortion of vision.

Microphthalmos: Abnormal smallness of the eyeball.

Miotic: A drug causing pupillary constriction.

Mydriatic: A drug causing pupillary dilatation.

Myopia (nearsightedness): A refractive error in which the focus for light rays from a distant object is anterior to the retina.

Near point: The point at which the eye is focused when accommodation is fully active.

Nearsightedness: See Myopia.

Nebula: Slight corneal opacity due to any cause.

Nystagmus: An involuntary, rapid movement of the eyeball that may be horizontal, vertical, rotatory, or mixed.

Oculist or ophthalmologist: Terms used interchangeably; a physician who is a specialist in diseases of the eye.

Ophthalmia neonatorum: Conjunctivitis in the newborn.

Ophthalmoscope: An instrument with a special illumination system for viewing the inner eye, particularly the retina and associated structures.

Optic atrophy: Optic nerve degeneration.

Optic disk: Ophthalmoscopically visible portion of the optic nerve.

Optic nerve: The nerve that carries visual impulses from the retina to the brain.

Optician: One who makes or deals in eyeglasses or other optical instruments and who fills prescriptions for glasses and contact lenses.

Optometrist: A nonmedical person trained in the measurement of refraction of the eye.

Orbital cellulitis: Inflammation of the tissues surrounding the eye.

Orthoptist: One who measures ocular muscle imbalances and gives corrective exercises.

Oscillopsia: The subjective illusion of movement of objects that occurs with some types of nystagmus.

Palpebral: Pertaining to the eyelid.

Pannus: Infiltration of the cornea with blood vessels.

Panophthalmitis: Inflammation of the entire eyeball.

Papilledema: Swelling of the optic disk.

Papillitis: Optic nerve head ischemia or inflammation that is ophthalmoscopically visible when acute.

Partially seeing child: For educational purposes, a partially seeing child is one who has a corrected visual acuity of 20/70 or less in the better eye.

Perimeter: An instrument for measuring the field of vision.

Peripheral vision: Ability to perceive the presence, motion, or color of objects outside of the direct line of vision.

Phakomatoses: A group of hereditary diseases characterized by the presence of spots, cysts, and tumors in various parts of the body—eg, Recklinghausen's disease, Von Hippel-Lindau disease, tuberous sclerosis.

Phlyctenule: Localized lymphocytic infiltration of the conjunctiva.

Phoria: See Heterophoria.

Photocoagulation: A method of using light energy to cause inflammation of the retina and choroid for treatment of certain types of retinal disorders, particularly retinal vascular diseases.

Photophobia: Abnormal sensitivity to light.

Photopsia: Appearance of sparks or flashes within the eye due to retinal irritation.

Phthisis bulbi: Atrophy of the eyeball with blindness and decreased intraocular pressure, due to end-stage intraocular disease.

Placido's disk: A disk with concentric rings used to determine the regularity of the cornea by observing the ring's reflection on the corneal surface.

Poliosis: Absence of pigment in the hair, resulting in white eyelashes.

Posterior chamber: Space filled with aqueous anterior to the lens and posterior to the iris.

Presbyopia ("old sight"): Physiologically blurred near vision, commonly evident soon after age 40, due to reduction in the power of accommodation.

Prism: A wedge of transparent material that deviates light rays without changing their focus.

Prism diopter: The unit of prism power in deviating light rays.

Pseudoisochromatic charts: Charts with colored dots of various hues and shades forming numbers, letters, or patterns, used for testing color discrimination.

Pseudophakia: Presence of an artificial intraocular lens implant following cataract extraction.

Pterygium: A triangular growth of tissue that extends from the conjunctiva over the cornea.

Ptosis: Drooping of the eyelid.

Puncta: External orifices of the upper and lower canaliculi.

Pupil: The round hole in the center of the iris that corresponds to the lens aperture in a camera.

Refraction: (1) Deviation in the course of rays of light in passing from one transparent medium into another of different density. (2) Determination of refractive errors of the eye and correction by glasses.

Refractive error (ametropia): An optical defect that prevents light rays from being brought to a single focus on the retina.

Refractive keratoplasty: Surgery of the cornea to correct optical defects.

Refractive index: The ratio of the speed of light in a vacuum to the speed of light in a given material.

Refractive media: The transparent parts of the eye having refractive power.

Retina: Innermost coat of the eye, consisting of the sensory retina, which is composed of light-sensitive neural elements connecting to other neural cells, and the pigment epithelium.

Retinal detachment: A separation of the neurosensory retina from the pigment epithelium and choroid.

Retinitis pigmentosa: A hereditary degeneration and atrophy of the retina.

Retinoscope: An instrument specially designed for refracting an eye objectively.

Rods: See Cones and rods.

Schlemm's canal: A narrow channel in the anterior chamber angle that drains aqueous to the aqueous veins.

Sclera: The white part of the eye—a tough covering that, with the cornea, forms the external protective coat of the eye.

Scleral spur: The protrusion of sclera into the anterior chamber angle.

Scotoma: A blind or partially blind area in the visual field.

Slit lamp: A combination light and microscope for examination of the eye, principally the anterior segment.

Snellen chart: Used for testing central visual acuity. It consists of lines of letters or numbers, in graded sizes drawn to Snellen measurements.

Sphincterotomy: A surgical incision of the iris sphincter muscle.

Staphyloma: A thinned part of the coat of the eye, causing protrusion.

Strabismus (heterotropia, tropia): A manifest deviation of the eyes.

Sty: See Hordeolum, external.

Symblepharon: Adhesions between the bulbar and palpebral conjunctiva.

Sympathetic ophthalmia: Inflammation in one eye following traumatic inflammation in the fellow eye.

Synechia: Adhesion of the iris to cornea (anterior synechia) or lens (posterior synechia).

Syneresis: Degenerative process within a gel, involving a drawing together of particles of the dispersed medium, separation of the medium, and shrinkage of the gel.

Tarsorrhaphy: A surgical procedure by which the upper and lower lid margins are united.

Tonometer: An instrument for measuring intraocular pressure.

Trabeculectomy: Surgical removal of a portion of the trabeculum.

Trachoma: A serious form of infectious keratoconjunctivitis.

Trichiasis: Inversion and rubbing of the eyelashes against the globe.

Tropia: See Strabismus.

Uvea (uveal tract): The iris, ciliary body, and choroid.

Uveitis: Inflammation of one or all portions of the uveal tract.

Vergence: The amount of coming together—or speading apart—of a bundle of light rays, measured in diopters.

Visual acuity: Measure of the acuteness of vision; the finest of detail that the eye can distinguish.

Visual axis: An imaginary line that connects a point in space (point of fixation) with fovea centralis.

Vitiligo: Localized patchy decrease or absence of pigment on the skin.

Vitreous: Transparent, colorless mass of soft, gelatinous material filling the eyeball behind the crystalline lens.

Xerosis: Drying of tissues lining the anterior surface of the eye.

Zonule: The numerous fine tissue strands that stretch from the ciliary processes to the crystalline lens equator (360 degrees) and hold the lens in place.

Zonulolysis: Lysis of the zonule, as with chymotrypsin, to facilitate removal of the lens in intracapsular cataract surgery.

SUBJECT INDEX

NOTE: Page numbers in bold face type indicate a major discussion. A *t* following a page number indicates tabular material and an *i* following a page number indicates an illustration. Drugs are listed under their generic names. When a drug trade name is listed, the reader is referred to the generic drug name.

A scan ultrasonography, 52–53, 52*i*
"A" and "V" syndromes, **223–224**
A-pattern, in dry eye syndrome, 71
Abducens nerve, 14*i*, 232
   extraocular muscles supplied by,
     11, 207
   palsy (paralysis of), **221–222**, 268
   peripheral and intermediate con-
     nections of nuclei of, 267
Abduction, definition of, 207
Aberrations, visual, 20
Abetalipoproteinemia, retinitis pig-
     mentosa caused by, 173
Abiotrophic disease, definition of,
     341
Abrasions
   corneal, **344–345**
     management of, 391–392
   of lids, **343–344**
Abscess. *See specific type or struc-*
     ture involved
AC/A ratio, high, accommodative
     esotropia caused by, 221
Acanthamoeba, keratitis caused by,
     114
Accommodation, 364
   amplitude of, 364
   definition of, 426
   manipulation of in heterophoria,
     227
   range of, 364
Acetazolamide in glaucoma, 393,
     403
   acute angle-closure, 199–200
   open-angle, 197
Acetylcysteine, in chemical conjunc-
     tivitis and keratitis, 394
Acid
   burns caused by, 347
     conjunctivitis and, 95
     scleral injury caused by, 129
     scleritis caused by, 128*t*
   conjunctivitis caused by, 94–95
Acidosis, in methanol poisoning, 254
Acne rosacea, **314**
   ocular rosacea and, 95
   scleritis and, 128*t*
Acquired, definition of, 341
Acquired immunodeficiency syn-
     drome, **304–306**
   clinical findings in, 305–306
   posterior uveitis in, 141
   prevention of, 304–305
   transmission of, 304–305

Acrobrachycephaly, 333
Acrocephaly, 333
Acropachy, thyroid, 294
Actinomyces israelii canaliculitis, 65,
     65*i*
   conjunctivitis secondary to, 98
Acuity, visual. *See* Visual acuity
Acyclovir, 406
   in herpes simplex keratitis, 112
Adduction, definition of, 207
Adenine arabinoside. *See* Vidarabine
Adenoviruses
   epidemic keratoconjunctivitis
     caused by, 84–85
   keratitis caused by, 113
   pharyngoconjunctival fever caused
     by, 84
   uveitis caused by, 135*t*
Adie's syndrome, 262
Adnexa, anatomy of, **1–4**
Afferent pupillary defect, **262**, 263*i*
After-cataract, **150**
After-image test, 216
Age, illumination requirements af-
     fected by, 422
Age-related cataract, **145–146**
Age-related macular degeneration,
     180–182
   exudative, 181–182
   nonexudative, 180–181
Agnosia, definition of, 426
AIDS. *See* Acquired immunodefi-
     ciency syndrome
Aids, low vision. *See* Low vision
     aids
Alacrima, 64
   dry eye syndrome and, 68*t*
   in Riley-Day syndrome, 64
Albinism, **312**, 332
   definition of, 426
Albumin, in tear fluid, 67
Alcohol, amblyopia caused by, 252–
     254
Alignment, testing of, 24
Alkali
   burns caused by, 347
   conjunctivitis caused by, 94–95
   scleral injury caused by, 129
   scleritis caused by, 128*t*
Alleles, 336
   definition of, 341
   dominant, 336
   recessive, 336

Allergic conjunctivitis. *See* Immuno-
     logic conjunctivitis
Allergic rhinitis, conjunctivitis and,
     90–91
Allopurinol, adverse ocular effects
     of, 408*i*
Alpers' disease, optic atrophy in,
     255
Alternate cover test, 213
Amaurosis fugax, 272–273
   causes of, 282
   definition of, 426
   retinal emboli causing, 281–282
Amaurotic pupil, 262, 264*i*
Amblyopia
   alcohol causing, 252–254
   in children, 334
   definition of, 426
   drug toxicity causing, 254
   early diagnosis of, 371
   methanol poisoning causing, 254
   neurogenic ptosis and, 59
   prevention of, **370–371**
   in strabismus, 211
   tobacco causing, 252–254
   toxic-nutritional, **252–254**
   treatment of, 217
   as urgent case, 395
Ametropia, 21
   definition of, 426, 428
Amikacin, in keratitis, 109*t*
Amiodarone
   adverse ocular effects of, 408*i*
   ocular complications of systemic
     use of, 315
Amoxicillin, with clavulanic acid, in
     orbital cellulitis, 234
Amphetamines, adverse ocular ef-
     fects of, 408*i*
Amphotericin B, 404*t*, 406
   in candidal conjunctivitis, 88
   in choroiditis caused by histoplas-
     mosis, 140
   in keratitis, 109*t*
   in mucormycosis of orbit, 235
Ampicillin
   in keratitis, 109*t*
   in orbital cellulitis, 234
Amsler grid, **39–40**, 42*i*
   definition of, 426
   in low vision testing, 376–377
Amyloidosis
   diffuse uveitis and, 141*t*
   dry eye syndrome and, 68*t*